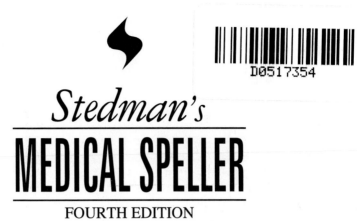

Stedman's
MEDICAL SPELLER
FOURTH EDITION

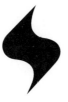

Stedman's

MEDICAL SPELLER

FOURTH EDITION

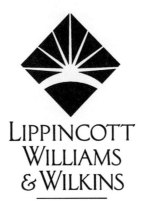

LIPPINCOTT
WILLIAMS
& WILKINS

Publisher: Julie K. Stegman
Senior Product Manager: Eric Branger
Associate Managing Editor: Amy Millholen
Production Coordinator: Jason Delaney
Typesetter: Peirce Graphic Services, LLC.
Printer & Binder: Malloy Litho, Inc.

Library of Congress Cataloging-in-Publication Data

Stedman's medical speller.— 4th ed.
    p. ; cm. — (Stedman's word book series)
  Includes bibliographical references.
  ISBN 0-7817-5448-8
 1. Medicine—Terminology. 2. English language—Orthography and spelling.
I. Lippincott Williams & Wilkins. II. Title: Medical speller. III. Series: Stedman's
word books.
  [DNLM: 1. Medicine—Terminology—English. W 15 S812 2005]
R123.S7 2005
610'.1'4—dc22

2004006940
04
1 2 3 4 5 6 7 8 9 10

Contents

Acknowledgments

An important part of our editorial process is the involvement of medical transcriptionists — as advisors, reviewers, and/or editors.

We extend special thanks to Jeanne Bock, CSR, MT, who edited the manuscript and updated appendix material; and to Helen Littrell, CMT, who edited the format to make it consistent with that of our other Word Books. As always, Barb Ferretti played an integral role in the process by assisting with the content for this reference and by providing a final quality check.

As with all our *Stedman's* word references, this resource incorporates the suggestions and expertise of our many contacts in the medical transcriptionist community. Thanks to all of our advisory board participants, reviewers, and editors; AAMT meeting attendees; and others who have written us with requests and comments — keep talking, and we'll keep listening.

Publisher's Preface

Stedman's Medical Speller, Fourth Edition, offers an authoritative assurance of quality and exactness to the wordsmiths of the healthcare professions—medical transcriptionists, medical editors, writers, and copyeditors, health information management personnel, court reporters, and the many other users and producers of medical documentation.

This new edition, with more than 96,000 entries, includes the *Stedman's Word Book Series* trademarks: cross-indexing by first and last word, A-Z format with main entries and subentries, and appendix material for additional comprehension and application of the terminology.

Perfect as a solid reference for the beginning and professional medical transcriptionist, medical writer and editor, and the court reporter, *Stedman's Medical Speller, Fourth Edition,* is the first place to start when looking for comprehensive, up-to-date medical spelling information. Incorporating information from references like *Stedman's Electronic Medical Dictionary* and *Stedman's Concise Medical Dictionary for the Health Professions, Stedman's Medical Speller, Fourth Edition,* is better than ever. This new edition's valuable appendix section has also been updated and includes Common Prefixes, Suffixes, and Combining Forms; Ligaments; Muscles; Common Professional Titles and Degrees; and Common Medical Abbreviations and Acronyms. Finally, as always, we have done a thorough review of the content to ensure all information is accurate and relevant for the medical language professional.

We at Lippincott Williams & Wilkins strive to provide you with the most up-to-date and accurate word references available. Your use of this Word Book will prompt new editions, which we will publish as often as updates and revisions justify. We welcome your suggestions for improvements, changes, corrections, and additions—whatever will make this *Stedman's* product more useful to you. Please complete the postage-paid card in this book for future suggestions and recommendations, or visit us online at www.stedmans.com.

Explanatory Notes

Medical transcription is an art as well as a science. Both approaches are needed to correctly interpret the dictation of a physician, whose language is a product of education, training, and experience. This variety in medical language means that there are several acceptable ways to express certain terms, including jargon. *Stedman's Medical Speller, Fourth Edition,* provides variant spellings and phrasings for many terms. These elements, in addition to complete cross-indexing, make *Stedman's Medical Speller, Fourth Edition,* a valuable resource for determining the validity of terms as they are encountered.

Alphabetical Organization

Alphabetization of main entries is letter by letter as spelled, ignoring punctuation, spaces, prefixed numbers, or other characters. Greek letters are spelled out and placed in alphabetical order. For example:

Eglis gland	**alpha-blocker**
1E globulin	**alphadione**
ego	**alpha-fetoprotein (AFP)**
ego-alien	**alpha-ketoglutarate**

In subentry alphabetization, the abbreviated singular form or the spelled-out plural form of the noun main entry word is ignored.

Format and Style

All main entries are in **boldface** to expedite locating a sought-after term, to enhance distinction between main entries and subentries, and to relieve the textual density of the pages.

Irregular plurals and variant spellings are shown on the same line as the singular or preferred form of the word. For example:

hallex, pl. hallices
facet, facette

Hyphenation

As a rule of style, multiple eponyms (e.g., Mears-Rubash approach) are hyphenated. Also, hyphens have been added between a manufacturer and one or more eponyms (e.g., Vital-Metzenbaum dissecting scissors). Please note that in many cases, hyphenation is a question of style, not of accuracy, and thus is a matter of choice.

Possessives

Possessive forms have been dropped in this reference for the sake of consistency and conformance with the guidelines of the American Association for Medical Transcription (AAMT) and other groups. Please note, however, that in many cases, retaining the possessive, like hyphenating, is a question of style, not of accuracy, and thus is a matter of choice. To form the possessive of a word, simply add the apostrophe or apostrophe "s" to the end of the word.

Cross-indexing

The word list is in an index-like main entry-subentry format that contains two combined alphabetical listings:

(1) A *noun* main entry-subentry organization, which is typical of the A-Z section of medical dictionaries like *Stedman's:*

family	**period**
cancer f.	absolute refractory p.
extended f.	amblyogenic p.
gene f.	uritical p.

(2) An *adjective* main entry-subentry organization, which lists words and phrases as you hear them. The main entries are the adjectives or modifiers in a multiword term. The subentries are the nouns around which the terms are constructed and to which the adjectives or modifiers pertain:

decidual

  d. cast

  d. cell

  d. endometritis

superficial

  s. brachial artery

  s. branch

  s. dorsal vein

This format provides the user with more than one way to locate and identify a multiword term. For example:

debt

  oxygen d.

oxygen

  o. debt

pessary

  cube p.

  Mayer p.

Mayer

  M. hemalum stain

  M. pessary

This format also allows the user to see together all terms that contain a particular descriptor, as well as all types, kinds, or variations of a noun entity. For example:

deprivation

  d. amblyopia

  androgen d.

  d. dwarfism

  emotional d.

  sensory d.

gonad

  g. dose

  female g.

  indifferent g.

  male g.

  g. nucleus

Wherever possible, abbreviations are separately defined and cross-referenced. For example:

MAT

  multifocal atrial tachycardia

multifocal
   m. atrial tachycardia (MAT)

tachycardia
   multifocal atrial t. (MAT)

α (*var. of* alpha)
A
    A band
    A bile
    A cell
    A chain
    A disc
    A fiber
    A wave
2A
    multiple endocrine neoplasia, type 2A (MEN2A)
AA
    amino acid
aa3
    cytochrome aa3
AAA
    abdominal aortic aneurysm
Aagenaes syndrome
A-aO2 difference
AAR
    antigen-antibody reaction
Aaron sign
Aarskog-Scott syndrome
A1, A2 segment
AASH
    adrenal androgen-stimulating hormone
AAV
    adeno-associated virus
Ab
    antibody
abacterial thrombotic endocarditis
Abadie sign
abampere
abapical pole
abarognosis
abarticular gout
abasia
    atactic a.
    ataxic a.
    choreic a.
    paralytic a.
    spastic a.
    trembling a.
    a. trepidans
abasia-astasia
abasic
abatement
abatic
abaxial
abaxile
Abbe flap
Abbott
    A. artery
    A. method
    A. stain
    A. tube
abciximab
ABC leads
abcoulomb
abdomen
    acute a.
    carinate a.
    doughy a.
    navicular a.
    a. obstipum
    protuberant a.
    scaphoid a.
    surgical a.
abdominal
    a. angina
    a. aorta
    a. aortic aneurysm (AAA)
    a. aortic plexus
    a. apoplexy
    a. aura
    a. ballottement
    a. canal
    a. cavity
    a. dropsy
    a. external oblique muscle
    a. fibromatosis
    a. fissure
    a. fistula
    a. gestation
    a. guarding
    a. hernia
    a. hysterectomy
    a. hysteropexy
    a. hysterotomy
    a. incision
    a. internal oblique muscle
    a. lymph node
    a. migraine
    a. muscle deficiency syndrome
    a. myomectomy
    a. nephrectomy
    a. nephrotomy
    a. ostium
    a. ovariotomy
    a. pad
    a. pool
    a. pregnancy
    a. pressure
    a. pulse
    a. reflex
    a. region
    a. respiration
    a. retractor
    a. ring

abdominal *(continued)*
    a. sac
    a. salpingectomy
    a. salpingotomy
    a. section
    a. splenectomy
    a. testis
    a. tuberculosis
    a. typhoid
    a. zone
abdominalis
    anulus a.
abdominis
    angina a.
    cavum a.
abdominocardiac reflex
abdominocentesis
abdominocyesis
abdominocystic
abdominogenital
abdominohysterectomy
abdominohysterotomy
abdominojugular reflux
abdominopelvic
    a. cavity
    a. splanchnic nerve
abdominoperineal resection (APR)
abdominoplasty
abdominoscopy
abdominoscrotal
abdominothoracic
    a. arch
    a. incision
abdominovaginal hysterectomy
abdominovesical
abduce
abducens
    a. eminence
    a. nerve
    a. nucleus
    a. oculi
abducent nerve
abduct
abduction
abductor
    a. digiti minimi
    a. digiti minimi muscle
    a. hallucis muscle
    a. pollicis brevis muscle
    a. pollicis longus muscle
    a. spasmodic dysphonia
Abegg rule
Abell-Kendall method
Abelson murine leukemia virus
abembryonic
abenteric
Abernethy
    A. fascia
    A. operation

aberrant
    a. bile duct
    a. bundle
    a. complex
    a. ductule
    a. ganglion
    a. goiter
    a. hemoglobin
    a. obturator artery
    a. regeneration
    a. ureter
    a. ventricular conduction
aberrantes
    ductus a.
aberrantia
    Ferrein vasa a.
aberration
    chromatic a.
    chromosome a.
    color a.
    coma a.
    curvature a.
    dioptric a.
    distortion a.
    heterosomal a.
    intrachromosomal a.
    lateral a.
    longitudinal a.
    mental a.
    meridional a.
    monochromatic a.
    optical a.
    spherical a.
aberrometer
abetalipoproteinemia
abeyance
abfarad
ABG
    arterial blood gas
abhenry
abiotic
abiotrophy
abirritation
ablastemic
ablastin
ablate
ablation
    electrode catheter a.
    endometrial a.
    laparoscopic uterosacral nerve a.
ablepharia
abluent
ablution
abnerval
abneural
abnormal
    a. occlusion
    a. psychology
    a. ST segment

abnormality
    figure-of-8 a.
    no significant a.
ABO
    ABO antigen
    ABO blood group
    ABO factor
    ABO hemolytic disease
abohm
aborad
aboral
abort
aborted
    a. ectopic pregnancy
    a. systole
aborticide
abortient
abortifacient
abortigenic
abortion
    ampullar a.
    complete a.
    criminal a.
    elective a.
    habitual a.
    illegal a.
    imminent a.
    incomplete a.
    induced a.
    inevitable a.
    infected a.
    menstrual extraction a.
    missed a.
    natural a.
    a. rate
    recurrent a.
    septic a.
    spontaneous a.
    therapeutic a.
    threatened a.
    tubal a.
abortionist
abortive
    a. neurofibromatosis
    a. transduction
abortus
    a. bacillus
    Brucella a.
aboulia
above
    a. elbow (A-E)
    a. knee (A-K)

ABP
    androgen binding protein
ABPA
    allergic bronchopulmonary aspergillosis
ABR
    auditory brainstem response
    ABR audiometry
abrachia
abrachiocephalia
abrachiocephaly
abrade
abraded wound
Abrahams sign
Abrams heart reflex
abrasion
    air a.
    brush burn a.
    corneal a.
    gingival a.
abrasiveness
abrasive strip
abreact
abreaction
abrupt exacerbation
abruption
abruptio placentae
abscess
    acute a.
    alveolar a.
    amebic a.
    apical periodontal a.
    appendiceal a.
    axillary a.
    Bartholin a.
    Bezold a.
    bicameral a.
    blind a.
    bone a.
    Brodie a.
    buccal space a.
    bursal a.
    caseous a.
    cheesy a.
    cholangitic a.
    chronic a.
    cold a.
    collar-button a.
    crypt a.
    dental a.
    dentoalveolar a.
    diffuse a.
    Douglas a.

NOTES

abscess *(continued)*
    dry a.
    Dubois a.
    embolic a.
    encapsulated a.
    encysted a.
    fecal a.
    follicular a.
    gas a.
    gingival a.
    glandular a.
    gravitation a.
    gummatous a.
    helminthic a.
    hematogenous a.
    hemorrhagic a.
    hot a.
    hypostatic a.
    idiopathic a.
    ischiorectal a.
    lateral alveolar a.
    lateral periodontal a.
    marginal a.
    mastoid a.
    mediastinal a.
    metastatic a.
    migrating a.
    miliary a.
    mural a.
    myocardial a.
    otitic a.
    parapharyngeal a.
    perforating a.
    periappendiceal a.
    periarticular a.
    peritoneal a.
    peritonsillar a.
    phlegmonous a.
    Pott a.
    primary a.
    psoas a.
    pulmonary a.
    pyemic a.
    recrudescent a.
    residual a.
    ring a.
    satellite a.
    secondary a.
    septicemic a.
    serous a.
    shirt-stud a.
    stellate a.
    stercoraceous a.
    stercoral a.
    stitch a.
    strumous a.
    subaponeurotic a.
    subpectoral a.
    subscapular a.

    subungual a.
    sudoriferous a.
    sudoriparous a.
    suture a.
    Tornwaldt a.
    tropical a.
    tuberculous a.
    tuboovarian a.
    tympanitic a.
    verminous a.
    wandering a.
abscise
abscissa
abscission
absconsio
abscopal effect
absence
    congenital ossicular a.
    myoclonic a.
    protein induced by vitamin K a.
    pure a.
    a. seizure
    simple a.
absent state
absinthe
absinthin
absinthium
absinthol
absolute
    a. agraphia
    a. alcohol
    atmosphere a.
    a. cell increase
    a. dehydration
    a. glaucoma
    a. hemianopia
    a. humidity
    a. hydration
    a. hyperopia
    a. intensity threshold acuity
    a. latency
    a. leukocytosis
    a. pressure
    a. refractory period
    a. scale
    a. scotoma
    a. sterility
    a. temperature
    a. terminal innervation ratio
    a. threshold
    a. unit
    a. viscosity
    a. zero
absorb
absorbable
    a. dressing
    a. gelatin film
    a. gelatin sponge
    a. surgical suture

absorbance
absorbancy index
absorbed dose
absorbefacient
absorbency
absorbent
   a. cotton
   a. point
   a. system
   a. vessel
absorber head
absorption
   a. band
   a. cell
   a. chromatography
   a. coefficient
   a. collapse
   cutaneous a.
   disjunctive a.
   electron resonance a.
   external a.
   a. fever
   fluorescent treponemal antibody a. (FTA-ABS)
   interstitial a.
   a. line
   a. spectrum
absorptive cell
absorptivity
   molar a.
abstergent
abstinence
   a. symptom
   a. syndrome
abstract
   a. intelligence
   structured a.
   a. thinking
abstraction
abstriction
abterminal
abulia
abulic
abundance
abuse
   chemical a.
   child a.
   drug a.
   elder a.
   ethanol a.
   inhalant a.
   laxative a.

   mixed drug a.
   polydrug a.
   polypharmacy a.
   polysubstance a.
   psychoactive substance a.
   sexual a.
   spousal a.
   spouse a.
   substance a.
   tobacco a.
abutment
   auxiliary a.
   ball-and-socket a.
   dovetail stress-broken a.
   intermediate a.
   isolated a.
ABVD
   Adriamycin, bleomycin, vinblastine, and dacarbazine
abvolt
abzyme
ACA
   adenocarcinoma
AC/A
   accommodative convergence-accommodation
acalculia
acampsia
acantha
acanthamebiasis
Acanthamoeba medium
acanthamoebiasis
acanthella
acanthesthesia
Acanthia lectularia
acanthion
acanthocephaliasis
acanthocyte
acanthocytosis with chorea
acanthoid
acantholysis
acanthoma
   clear cell a.
acanthomatous ameloblastoma
acanthomeatal line
acanthopelvis
acanthopodia
acanthor
acanthorrhexis
acanthosis
   glycogenic a.
   a. nigricans

NOTES

acanthotic
acanthrocyte
acanthrocytosis
acapnia
acapnial alkalosis
acarbose
acardia
acardiac
acardius
    a. acephalus
    a. amorphus
    a. anceps
acariasis
acaricide
acarid
Acaridae
acaridan
acaridiasis
Acarina
acarine
acarinosis
acarodermatitis
acaroid
acarology
acarophobia
Acarus
    A. balatus
    A. folliculorum
    A. gallinae
    A. hordei
acaryote
acatalasemia
acatalasia
acathectic
acathexia
acathexis
acathisia
acaudal
acaudate
ACC
    anodal closure contraction
accelerans
accelerant
accelerated
    a. conduction
    a. eruption
    a. hypertension
    a. reaction
    a. rejection
acceleration
    angular a.
    linear a.
acceleration-deceleration injury
accelerator
    a. factor
    a. fiber
    a. globulin
    linear a. (LINAC)
    a. nerve

    proserum prothrombin conversion a.
    prothrombin a.
    serum prothrombin conversion a.
accelerin
accelerometer
accentuator
acceptor
    alcohol dehydrogenase a.
    hydrogen a.
    a. RNA
    a. splicing site
access
    arteriovenous a.
    a. opening
    venovenous a.
accessoria
    mamma a.
accessorius
    lien a.
accessory
    a. adrenal
    a. atrium
    a. auricle
    a. breast
    a. canal
    a. cell
    a. cephalic vein
    a. chromosome
    a. cuneate nucleus
    a. flexor muscle
    a. flocculus
    a. hemiazygos vein
    a. lacrimal gland
    a. meningeal artery
    a. meningeal branch
    a. molecule
    a. nasal cartilage
    a. nerve lymph node
    a. nerve trunk
    a. nipple
    a. obturator artery
    a. olivary nucleus
    a. organ
    a. pancreas
    a. pancreatic duct
    a. parotid gland
    a. phrenic nerve
    a. placenta
    a. plantar ligament
    a. process
    a. quadrate cartilage
    a. root
    a. saphenous vein
    a. sign
    a. spleen
    a. suprarenal gland
    a. symptom
    a. thyroid gland
    a. tragus

a. tubercle
a. vertebral vein
a. visual apparatus
a. visual structure
a. volar ligament
accident
cardiac a.
cardiovascular a.
car versus pedestrian a.
cerebrovascular a. (CVA)
motor vehicle a. (MVA)
a. neurosis
accidental
a. host
a. hypothermia
a. image
a. murmur
a. myiasis
a. parasite
a. symptom
accident-prone
acclimating fever
acclimation
acclimatization
accommodating resistance
accommodation
amplitude of a.
histologic a.
negative a.
positive a.
pupils equal, react to light and a.
 (PERLA)
pupils equal, round, react to light
 and a. (PERRLA)
range of a.
a. reflex
relative a.
accommodative
a. asthenopia
a. convergence
a. convergence-accommodation
 (AC/A)
a. convergence-accommodation ratio
a. insufficiency
a. palsy
a. spasm
a. strabismus
accompanying vein
accordion graft
accouchement forcé
accoucheur hand
accrementition

accreta
placenta a.
accretio cordis
accretionary growth
accretion line
accrochage
accumulation
a. analysis
a. disease
ACDF
anterior cervical discectomy and fusion
ACE
angiotensin-converting enzyme
acebutolol
aceclidine
acedapsone
acedia
acefylline piperazine
ACEI
angiotensin-converting enzyme inhibitor
acellular
acelom
acelomate
acelomatous
acenesthesia
acenocoumarin
acenocoumarol
acentric
a. chromosome
a. fragment
a. occlusion
acephalgic migraine
acephalia
acephaline
acephalism
acephalobrachia
acephalocardia
acephalocheiria
acephalochiria
acephalocyst
acephalogasteria
acephalopodia
acephalorrhachia
acephalostomia
acephalothoracia
acephalous
acephalus
acardius a.
a. acormus
a. dibrachius
a. dipus
a. monobrachius

NOTES

7

acephalus *(continued)*
a. monopus
a. sympus
acephaly
acerbity
acerola
acervuline
acervulus
acestoma
acesulfame
acetabula (*pl. of* acetabulum)
acetabular
a. artery
a. branch
a. cup
a. fossa
a. labrum
a. lip
a. margin
a. notch
acetabulectomy
acetabuli
incisura a.
acetabuloplasty
acetabulum, pl. **acetabula**
acetaldehyde
activated a.
acetal phosphatide
acetamide
acetamidobenzoate
deanol a.
acetaminophen poisoning
acetaminosalol
acetanilid poisoning
acetarsol
acetarsone
acetate
active a.
aluminum a.
amphetamine a.
cortisol a.
cupric a.
deoxycorticosterone a.
dequalinium a.
desmopressin a.
flecainide a.
fludrocortisone a.
guanabenz a.
a. kinase
lead a.
leuprolide a.
medroxyprogesterone a.
megestrol a.
melengestrol a.
a. replacement factor
a. thiokinase
acetate-CoA ligase
acetazolamide
acetenyl

acetic
a. acid
a. aldehyde
a. amide
a. fermentation
a. solution
aceticoceptor
acetify
acetimeter
acetoacetate
acetoacetic acid
acetoacetyl-CoA
acetoacetyl-coenzyme A
acetoacetyl-CoA thiolase
acetoacetyl-coenzyme A (acetoacetyl-CoA)
acetoin
acetokinase
acetolysis
acetometer
acetone
a. body
a. compound
a. fixative
a. test
acetone-insoluble antigen
acetonemia
acetonemic
acetonide
fluocinolone a.
acetonitrile
acetonuria
aceto-orcein stain
acetophenide
algestone a.
alphasone a.
acetosoluble
acetous fermentation
acetowhitening
acetum
aceturate
acetyl
a. chloride
a. phosphate
a. value
acetyl-activating enzyme
acetylase
acetylation
acetylcarbromal
acetylcholine chloride
acetylcholinesterase (AChE)
acetyl-CoA
acetyl-coenzyme A
acetyl-CoA acetyltransferase
acetyl-CoA ligase
acetyl-CoA synthetase
acetyl-CoA thiolase
acetyl-coenzyme A (acetyl-CoA)
acetyldigitoxin
acetyldigoxin

acetylmethadol
acetylornithine deacetylase
acetylsalicylate
    antipyrine a.
acetylsalicylic acid (ASA)
acetyltransferase
    acetyl-CoA a.
    carnitine a.
    choline a.
    lipoate a.
ACF
    acute care facility
achalasia
    cricopharyngeal a.
    esophageal a.
Achard syndrome
Achard-Thiers syndrome
AChE
    acetylcholinesterase
ache
    bone a.
    stomach a.
acheilia
acheilous
acheiria
acheiropody
acheirous
Achenbach syndrome
achievable
    as low as reasonably a. (ALARA)
achievement
    a. age
    a. motive
    a. quotient
    a. test
Achilles
    A. bursa
    A. tendon
    A. tendon reflex
achillobursitis
achillodynia
achillorrhaphy
achillotenotomy
achillotomy
achilous
achiral
achiropody
achirous
achlorhydria
achlorhydric anemia
achlorophyllous

Acholeplasma
    A. axanthum
    A. laidlawii
acholia
acholic
acholuria
acholuric jaundice
achondrogenesis type IA, IB, II
achondroplasia
    homozygous a.
achondroplastic dwarfism
achordal
achordate
achoresis
achrestic anemia
achroacyte
achrodextrin
achromacyte
achromasia
achromat
achromatic
    a. apparatus
    a. figure
    a. lens
    a. objective
    a. threshold
    a. vision
achromatin
achromatinic
achromatism
achromatocyte
achromatolysis
achromatophil
achromatophilia
achromatopia
achromatopsia, achromatopsy
    atypical a.
    complete a.
    incomplete a.
achromatosis
achromatous
achromaturia
achromia parasitica
achromic
achromocyte
achromophil
achromophilic, achromophilous
achromotrichia
achroodextrin
achylia
    a. gastrica
    a. pancreatica

NOTES

achylous
acicular
acid
    acetic a.
    acetoacetic a.
    acetylsalicylic a. (ASA)
    acidic amino a.
    activated amino a.
    activated carboxylic a.
    activated fatty a.
    adenylic a.
    agaric a.
    a. agglutination
    a. alcohol
    aliphatic a.
    alpha-amino a.
    alpha-aminosuccinic a.
    alpha-ketoglutaric a.
    alpha-lipoic a. (ALA)
    amino a. (AA)
    arabic a.
    argininosuccinic a.
    arsenic a.
    ascorbic a.
    aspartic a.
    aspergillic a.
    basic amino a.
    benzoic a.
    bile a.
    boric a.
    Brønsted a.
    butyric a.
    caprylic a.
    carbamic a.
    carbolic a.
    carbonic a.
    a. carboxypeptidase
    catechinic a.
    a. cell
    choleic a.
    cholic a.
    cis-aconitic a.
    citric a.
    complementary ribonucleic a.
     (cRNA)
    conjugate a.
    cyanuric a.
    cysteic a.
    cytidylic a.
    dehydroacetic a.
    dehydrocholic a.
    deoxyadenylic a. (dAMP)
    deoxycholic a.
    deoxycytidylic a.
    deoxyguanylic a.
    a. deoxyribonuclease
    deoxyribonucleic a. (DNA)
    deoxythymidylic a.
    a. dextran

    a. dextrin
    d-galacturonic a.
    diacetic a.
    diacetyltannic a.
    dibasic amino a.
    diethenoid fatty a.
    difenoxylic a.
    dihydroascorbic a.
    dihydropteroic a.
    diluted acetic a.
    diluted hydrochloric a.
    dilute phosphoric a.
    dimethyl iminodiacetic a. (HIDA)
    djenkolic a.
    a. dyspepsia
    edetic a.
    elaidic a.
    eleostearic a.
    erucic a.
    essential amino a.
    essential fatty a.
    a. etch cemented splint
    ethacrynic a.
    ethanoic a.
    eugenic a.
    fatty a.
    fibric a.
    flavianic a.
    flufenamic a.
    folic a.
    folinic a.
    formic a.
    formiminoglutamic a.
    frangulic a.
    free fatty a. (FFA)
    a. fuchsin
    fumaric a.
    fuming nitric a.
    fuming sulfuric a.
    fusidic a.
    G a.
    gadoleic a.
    gallic a.
    gentisic a.
    gibberellic a.
    glacial acetic a.
    glacial phosphoric a.
    a. gland
    glucoascorbic a.
    gluconic a.
    glucuronic a.
    glutaconic a.
    glutamic a.
    glutaric a.
    glyceric a.
    glycerophosphoric a.
    glycocholic a.
    glycolic a.
    glyconic a.

glycuronic a.
glyoxylic a.
guanylic a.
heparinic a.
hexacosanoic a.
hexadecanoic a.
hexonic a.
hexuronic a.
hippuric a.
homogentisic a.
homoprotocatechuic a.
homovanillic a.
hyalobiuronic a.
hyaluronic a.
hydrobromic a.
hydrochloric a.
hydroxamic a.
hydroxy a.
hydroxyacetic a.
hydroxyfatty a.
hydroxynervonic a.
hydroxytoluic a.
hygric a.
hypobromous a.
hypochlorous a.
hypophosphorous a.
ibotenic a.
iduronic a.
imino a.
a. indigestion
indolic a.
infectious nucleic a.
inorganic a.
inosinic a.
a. intoxication
iobenzamic a.
iocetamic a.
iodic a.
iodogorgoic a.
iodopanoic a.
ioglycamic a.
iopanoic a.
iophenoic a.
iophenoxic a.
iothalamic a.
isethionic a.
isobutyric a.
isocitric a.
isocyanic a.
isonicotinic a.
isosuccinic a.
isovaleric a.

itaconic a.
kainic a.
keto a.
ketopantoic a.
ketosuccinic a.
kinic a.
kojic a.
kynurenic a.
lactic a.
lactobacillic a.
lauric a.
levulic a.
levulinic a.
Lewis a.
lignoceric a.
linoleic a.
linolenic a.
linolic a.
lipoic a.
lithic a.
lithocholic a.
lysergic a.
lysophosphatidic a.
maleic a.
malic a.
malonic a.
a. maltase
mandelic a.
mannuronic a.
meconic a.
mefenamic a.
melissic a.
mercaptoacetic a.
mercapturic a.
metaperiodic a.
metaphosphoric a.
methacrylic a.
methylmalonic a.
mevalonic a.
molybdic a.
nalidixic a.
n-capric a.
n-caproic a.
N-carbamoylaspartic a.
nervonic a.
neuraminic a.
nicotinic a.
nitric a.
nitrous a.
nonessential amino a.
nucleic a.
organic a.

NOTES

acid *(continued)*
    orotic a.
    orthophosphoric a.
    osmic a.
    oxalic a.
    oxaloacetic a.
    oxalosuccinic a.
    a. oxide
    palmitoleic a.
    pantothenic a.
    a. perfusion test
    phenaceturic a.
    phenylacetic a.
    phenylaceturic a.
    phenyllactic a.
    phenylpyruvic a.
    a. phosphatase
    phosphoenolpyruvic a.
    phosphoric a.
    phosphotungstic a.
    pimelic a.
    polyenoic a.
    propionic a.
    prostanoic a.
    pyruvic a.
    a. radical
    a. reaction
    a. red 87, 91
    a. reflux test
    retinoic a.
    ribonucleic a. (RNA)
    ribothymidylic a.
    a. rigor
    salicylic a.
    a. salt
    saturated fatty a. (SFA)
    a. seromucoid
    sialic a.
    a. stain
    stearic a.
    a. sulfate
    sulfonic a.
    sulfuric a.
    tannic a.
    a. tartrate
    taurocholic a.
    teichoic a.
    thiosulfuric a.
    a. tide
    triacetic a.
    trichloroacetic a.
    unsaturated fatty a.
    ureidosuccinic a.
    uric a.
    uridylic a.
    urocanic a.
    vanillylmandelic a.
    vitamin A1 a.
    a. wave

acid-ash diet
acid-base
    a.-b. balance
    a.-b. equilibrium
acid-citrate-dextrose
acidemia
    fumaric a.
    hyperpipecolic a.
    isovaleric a.
    lactic a.
acid-etched restoration
acid-fast
    a.-f. bacillus (AFB)
    a.-f. smear (AFS)
acidic
    a. amino acid
    a. dye
acidified serum test
acidify
acidity
acidophil
    a. adenoma
    a. cell
    a. granule
acidophile
acidophilic leukocyte
acidophilus
    Lactobacillus a.
    a. milk
acidosis
    carbon dioxide a.
    compensated respiratory a.
    diabetic a.
    hypercapnic a.
    hyperchloremic a.
    lactic a.
    metabolic a.
    renal tubular a.
    respiratory a.
    starvation a.
    uremic a.
acidotic
acidulous
aciduria
    d-glyceric a.
    glycolic a.
    mevalonic a.
aciduric
acinar
    a. carcinoma
    a. cell
    a. cell tumor
Acinetobacter calcoaceticus
acini *(pl. of acinus)*
acinic
    a. cell adenocarcinoma
    a. cell carcinoma
aciniform
acinitis

acinose
acinotubular gland
acinous
  a. cell
  a. gland
a-c interval
acinus, pl. acini
  liver a.
  pulmonary a.
ackee poisoning
aclasia
aclasis
ACLF
  adult congregate living facility
ACLS
  advanced cardiac life support
acme
acmesthesia
acne
  adolescent a.
  a. artificialis
  bromide a.
  a. cachecticorum
  chlorine a.
  a. ciliaris
  colloid a.
  common a.
  a. conglobata
  a. cosmetica
  cystic a.
  a. erythematosa
  a. fulminans
  a. generalis
  halogen a.
  a. hypertrophica
  a. indurata
  iodide a.
  a. keloid
  a. keratosa
  a. medicamentosa
  a. necrotica miliaris
  a. neonatorum
  occupational a.
  a. papulosa
  pomade a.
  a. punctata
  a. pustulosa
  a. rosacea
  steroid a.
  summer a.
  tropical a.
  a. varioliformis

  a. venenata
  a. vulgaris
acneiform, acneform
acnemia
acnes
  Corynebacterium a.
acokanthera
acolous
aconitase
aconitate hydratase
aconite
aconitine
acorea
acormus
  acephalus a.
acorn-tipped catheter
Acosta disease
acoustic
  a. agraphia
  a. aphasia
  a. area
  a. capsule
  a. cell
  a. crest
  a. enhancement
  a. ganglion
  a. hypoesthesia
  a. immittance
  a. impedance
  a. labyrinth
  a. lemniscus
  a. lens
  a. meatus
  a. nerve
  a. neurilemoma
  a. neurinoma
  a. neuroma
  a. papilla
  a. pressure
  a. radiation
  a. reference level
  a. reflex
  a. reflex threshold
  a. schwannoma
  a. shadow
  a. spot
  a. stimulation test
  a. stria
  a. tetanus
  a. tolerance
  a. tooth
  a. trauma

NOTES

acoustic *(continued)*
    a. trauma hearing loss
    a. tubercle
    a. tumor
    a. vesicle
acoustical surround
acousticofacial ganglion
acousticopalpebral reflex
acousticophobia
acoustics
acquired
    a. agammaglobulinemia
    a. albinism
    a. centric
    a. centric relation
    a. character
    a. drive
    a. eccentric relation
    a. enamel cuticle
    a. epileptic aphasia
    a. hemolytic anemia
    a. hemolytic icterus
    a. hernia
    a. hyperlipoproteinemia
    a. hypogammaglobulinemia
    a. ichthyosis
    a. immunity
    a. immunodeficiency syndrome (AIDS)
    a. leukoderma
    a. leukopathia
    a. megacolon
    a. methemoglobinemia
    a. nevus
    a. pellicle
    a. reflex
    a. sensitivity
    a. toxoplasmosis
    a. tufted angioma
acquisition
    gradient-recalled a.
acral lentiginous melanoma
acrania
acranial
acranius
Acrel ganglion
acribometer
acridine
    a. dye
    a. orange
    a. yellow
acrid poison
acriflavine
acrimonia
acrimony
acrinol
acrisorcin
acritical
acroagnosis

acroanesthesia
acroarthritis
acroasphyxia
acroataxia
acroblast
acrobrachycephaly
acrocentric chromosome
acrocephalia
acrocephalic
acrocephalopolysyndactyly
acrocephalosyndactyly
acrocephalous
acrocephaly
acrochordon
acrocinesia, acrokinesia
acrocinesis
acrocontracture
acrocyanosis
acrocyanotic
acrodermatitis
    a. chronica atrophicans
    a. continua
    a. enteropathica
    a. perstans
acrodermatosis
acrodont
acrodynia
acrodynic erythema
acrodysesthesia
acrodysostosis
acroesthesia
acrofacial
    a. dysostosis
    a. syndrome
acrogenous
acrogeria
acrognosis
acrohyperhidrosis
acrohyperkeratosis
    focal a.
acrokeratoelastoidosis
acrokeratosis
acrokinesia *(var. of* acrocinesia)
acromegalia
acromegalic gigantism
acromegalogigantism
acromegaloidism
acromegaly
acromelalgia
acromelia
acromelic dwarfism
acromesomelia
acromesomelic dwarfism
acrometagenesis
acromial
    a. anastomosis
    a. angle
    a. arterial network
    a. artery

a. articular surface
a. branch
a. end
a. extremity
a. facet
a. part
a. plexus
a. process
a. reflex
acromicria
acromioclavicular
a. disc
a. joint
a. ligament
acromiocoracoid
acromiohumeral
acromion
a. presentation
a. process
acromioplasty
acromioscapular
acromiothoracic artery
acromphalus
acromyotonia
acromyotonus
acroosteolysis
acropachy
acropachyderma
acroparesthesia syndrome
acropetal
acrophobia
acropigmentation
acropleurogenous
acropustulosis
infantile a.
acroscleroderma
acrosclerosis
acrosin
acrosomal
a. cap
a. granule
a. vesicle
acrosome
acrosomin
acrospiroma
eccrine a.
acroteric
acrotic
acrotism
acrotrophodynia
acrotrophoneurosis
acrylate

acrylic
a. resin
a. resin base
a. resin tooth
a. resin tray
ACT
activated clotting time
act
compulsive a.
impulsive a.
Individuals with Disabilities
Education A.
ACTH
adrenocorticotropic hormone
little ACTH
ACTH stimulation test
ACTH-producing adenoma
actin filament
acting out
actinic
a. cheilitis
a. conjunctivitis
a. dermatitis
a. granuloma
a. keratitis
a. keratosis
a. porokeratosis
a. prurigo
a. ray
a. reticuloid
actinide element
actinides
actinium emanation
actinobacillosis
Actinobacillus
A. *actinomycetemcomitans*
A. *lignieresii*
actinodermatitis
actinohematin
Actinomadura
A. *africana*
A. *latina*
A. *madurae*
A. *pelliertieri*
actinomycelial
Actinomyces
A. *bovis*
A. *israelii*
A. *naeslundii*
A. *odontolyticus*
A. *viscosus*

NOTES

actinomyces
  Weigert stain for a.
actinomycetemcomitans
  Actinobacillus a.
  Haemophilus a.
actinomycetes
actinomycetoma
actinomycin A, C, D, F1
actinomycoma
actinomycosis
actinomycotic appendicitis
actinophage
actinophytosis
actinosin
actinotherapy
action
  ball valve a.
  calorigenic a.
  cumulative a.
  a. current
  a. potential
  quit tam a.
  sparing a.
  specific a.
  specific dynamic a.
  a. tremor
activated
  a. acetaldehyde
  a. amino acid
  a. atom
  a. carbon dioxide
  a. carboxylic acid
  a. charcoal
  a. choline
  a. clotting time (ACT)
  a. fatty acid
  a. glucose
  a. glycol aldehyde
  a. hydrogen
  a. macrophage
  a. partial thromboplastin time
    (aPTT)
  a. resin
  a. sludge
  a. sludge method
  a. state
activation
  a. analysis
  EEG a.
  energy of a.
  feedback a.
  feed-forward a.
  gene a.
  Gibbs energy of a.
activator
  catabolite gene a.
  plasminogen a.
  tissue plasminogen a. (TPA, t-PA,
    tPA)

active
  a. acetate
  a. aldehyde
  a. anaphylaxis
  a. carbon dioxide
  a. caries
  a. center
  a. chronic hepatitis
  a. congestion
  a. cool-down
  a. electrode
  a. formaldehyde
  a. formate
  a. formyl
  a. glycoaldehyde
  a. hyperemia
  a. immunity
  a. immunization
  a. inflammation
  a. labor
  a. length-tension curve
  a. medium
  a. methionine
  a. methyl
  a. movement
  a. mutant
  a. placebo
  a. principle
  a. prophylaxis
  a. psychoanalysis
  a. pyruvate
  a. recovery
  a. repressor
  a. site
  a. splint
  a. succinate
  a. sulfate
  a. transport
  a. treatment
  a. vasoconstriction
  a. vasodilation
activity
  a. adaptation
  asynchronous a.
  background a.
  blocking a.
  a. coefficient
  a.'s of daily living (ADL)
  a.'s of daily living scale
  discrete a.
  functional a.
  a. grading
  a. group
  insulinlike a. (ILA)
  intrinsic sympathomimetic a. (ISA)
  involuntary a.
  nonsuppressible insulinlike a.
  optic a.
  optical a.

a. pattern analysis
physical a.
plasma renin a.
pulseless electrical a.
specific a.
a. synthesis
triggered a.
actomyosin
actual cautery
acuity
absolute intensity threshold a.
aculeate
acumentin
acuminate
acuminatum
condyloma a.
acuology
acupressure
acupuncture anesthesia
acusis
acustica
area a.
acuta
myositis epidemica a.
acute
a. abdomen
a. abdominal series
a. abscess
a. adrenocortical insufficiency
a. African sleeping sickness
a. alcoholism
a. angle
a. anterior poliomyelitis
a. appendicitis
a. ascending paralysis
a. ataxia
a. bacterial endocarditis
a. brachial radiculitis
a. bulbar poliomyelitis
a. cardiovascular disease (ACVD)
a. care facility (ACF)
a. care hospital
a. cellular rejection
a. chalazion
a. cholecystitis
a. chorea
a. compression triad
a. contagious conjunctivitis
a. crescentic glomerulonephritis
a. cutaneous leishmaniasis
a. decubitus ulcer
a. delirium

a. disseminated encephalomyelitis
a. epidemic conjunctivitis
a. epidemic leukoencephalitis
a. febrile neutrophilic dermatosis
a. febrile polyneuritis
a. fibrinous pericarditis
a. fulminating meningococcal septicemia
a. fulminating meningococcemia
a. glaucoma
a. goiter
a. hallucinatory paranoia
a. hemorrhagic conjunctivitis
a. hemorrhagic encephalitis
a. hemorrhagic glomerulonephritis
a. hemorrhagic pancreatitis
a. histoplasmosis
a. hypokalemic nephropathy
a. idiopathic polyneuritis
a. inclusion body encephalitis
a. infectious nonbacterial gastroenteritis
a. inflammation
a. inflammatory demyelinating polyradiculoneuropathy
a. inflammatory polyneuropathy
a. intermittent porphyria
a. interstitial nephritis
a. interstitial pneumonia
a. interstitial pneumonitis
a. invasive aspergillosis
a. isolated myocarditis
a. lobar nephrosis
a. lymphocytic leukemia (ALL)
a. malaria
a. mania
a. massive liver necrosis
a. multifocal placoid pigment epitheliopathy
a. myocardial infarction (AMI)
a. necrotizing encephalitis
a. necrotizing hemorrhagic encephalomyelitis
a. necrotizing hemorrhagic leukoencephalitis
a. necrotizing hemorrhagic leukoencephalopathy
a. necrotizing myelitis
a. necrotizing ulcerative gingivitis (ANUG)
a. on chronic symptoms
a. organic brain syndrome

NOTES

17

acute *(continued)*
  a. parenchymatous hepatitis
  a. phase protein
  a. phase reactant
  a. phase reaction
  a. phase response
  a. poststreptococcal
    glomerulonephritis
  a. primary hemorrhagic
    meningoencephalitis
  a. promyelocytic leukemia
  a. pulmonary alveolitis
  a. pyelonephritis
  a. radiation syndrome
  a. recurrent rhabdomyolysis
  a. reflex bone atrophy
  a. renal failure (ARF)
  a. respiratory disease (ARD)
  a. respiratory distress (ARD)
  a. respiratory distress syndrome
    (ARDS)
  a. respiratory failure (ARF)
  a. retinal necrosis (ARN)
  a. rheumatic arthritis
  a. rhinitis
  a. rickets
  a. salivary adenitis
  a. scalp cellulitis
  a. schizophrenia
  a. schizophrenic episode
  a. sensory motor axonal neuropathy
  a. sensory-motor axonal neuropathy
  a. situational reaction
  a. splenic tumor
  a. stress reaction
  a. transverse myelitis
  a. trypanosomiasis
  a. tuberculosis
  a. urticaria
  a. viral conjunctivitis
  a. yellow atrophy
ACVD
  acute cardiovascular disease
  arteriosclerotic cardiovascular disease
acyanotic
acyclic compound
acycloguanosine
acyclovir
acyl-ACP dehydrogenase
acyl-activating enzyme
acyladenylate
acylamidase
  aryl a.
acylation
acylcarnitine
acyl carrier protein
acyl-CoA
  acyl-coenzyme A

acyl-CoA dehydrogenase
acyl-CoA synthetase
acyl-coenzyme A (acyl-CoA)
acylmercaptan bond
acyltransferase
  glycine a.
  lecithin a.
  lecithin-cholesterol a. (LCAT)
  lysolecithin-lecithin a.
  lysophosphatidic acid a.
acyltransferases
acystia
AD
  admitting diagnosis
  advance directive
adacrya
adactylous
adactyly
adamantine membrane
adamantinoma
  pituitary a.
Adamkiewicz
  artery of A.
Adam's apple
adamsite
Adams position
Adams-Stokes
  A.-S. disease
  A.-S. syncope
  A.-S. syndrome
adansonian classification
adaptation
  activity a.
  dark a.
  a. disease
  light a.
  photopic a.
  retinal a.
  scotopic a.
  a. syndrome of Selye
adapter
adaptive
  a. behavior
  a. behavior scale
  a. enzyme
  a. hypertrophy
adaptometer
adaptor hypothesis
adaxial
ADC
  AIDS dementia complex
addict
addiction
  alcohol a.
addictive drug
Addis
  A. count
  A. test

Addison
    A. anemia
    A. clinical plane
    A. disease
Addison-Biermer disease
addisonian
    a. anemia
    a. crisis
    a. syndrome
addition
    a. compound
    a. mutation
addition-deletion mutation
additive
    a. effect
    a. model
additivity
    causal a.
    interlocal a.
    intralocal a.
addressin ligand
adducent
adducin
adduct
adducta
    coxa a.
adduction
adductor
    a. brevis muscle
    a. canal
    a. compartment
    a. hallucis muscle
    a. hiatus
    a. longus muscle
    a. magnus muscle
    a. minimus muscle
    a. pollicis muscle
    a. reflex
    a. spasmodic dysphonia
    a. tubercle
adductovarus
    metatarsus a.
adductus
    metatarsus a.
adelomorphous
adenalgia
adendric
adendritic
adenectomy
adenectopia
adenemphraxis
Aden fever

adeniform
adenine
    a. arabinoside
    a. deaminase
    a. deoxyribonucleotide
    a. nucleotide
    a. phosphoribosyltransferase
adenitis
    acute salivary a.
    cervical a.
    mesenteric a.
    phlegmonous a.
adenization
adenoacanthoma
adenoameloblastoma
adeno-associated virus (AAV)
adenoblast
adenocarcinoma (ACA)
    acinic cell a.
    alveolar a.
    a. in Barrett esophagus
    bronchiolar a.
    bronchioloalveolar a.
    clear cell a.
    mammary a.
    mesonephric a.
    papillary a.
    polypoid a.
    a. in situ
adenocellulitis
adenochondroma
adenocystoma
adenocyte
adenodiastasis
adenodynia
adenofibroma
adenofibromyoma
adenofibrosis
adenogenous
adenohypophysial
adenohypophysis
adenohypophysitis
    lymphocytic a.
adenoid
    a. cancer
    a. cystic carcinoma
    a. facies
    a. hypertrophy
    a. squamous cell carcinoma
    a. tissue
    a. tumor
adenoidal-pharyngeal-conjunctival virus

NOTES

adenoidectomy
adenoiditis
adenolike
    gallus a. (GAL)
adenolipoma
adenolipomatosis
adenolymphocele
adenolymphoma
adenoma
    acidophil a.
    ACTH-producing a.
    adnexal a.
    adrenocortical a.
    apocrine a.
    basal cell a.
    basophil a.
    bronchial mucous gland a.
    canalicular a.
    chromophil a.
    chromophobe a.
    chromophobic a.
    colloid a.
    embryonal a.
    eosinophil a.
    fibroid a.
    a. fibrosum
    follicular a.
    Fuchs a.
    gonadotropin-producing a.
    growth hormone-producing a.
    hepatic a.
    hepatocellular a.
    Hürthle cell a.
    invasive pituitary a.
    lactating a.
    macrofollicular a.
    mammosomatotroph cell a.
    microfollicular a.
    oncocytic a.
    papillary cystic a.
    prolactin-producing a.
    sebaceous a.
    a. sebaceum
    villous a.
adenomatoid odontogenic tumor
adenomatosis
    erosive a.
    familial multiple endocrine a.
    fibrosing a.
    pulmonary a.
adenomatous
    a. goiter
    a. hyperplasia
    a. polyp
    a. polyposis coli
adenomegaly
adenomere
adenomyoma
adenomyosis uteri

adenoneural
adenopathy
adenophlegmon
adenosalpingitis
adenosarcoma
adenosatellite virus
adenose
adenosine
    a. cyclic phosphate
    a. deaminase
    a. diphosphate
    a. 5′-diphosphate (ADP)
    a. kinase
    a. monophosphate (AMP)
    a. monophosphate deaminase
    a. nucleosidase
    a. tetraphosphate
    a. triphosphatase
    a. triphosphate
adenosis
    blunt duct a.
    fibrosing a.
    microglandular a.
    sclerosing a.
adenosquamous carcinoma
adenosyl
adenosylcobalamin
adenotomy
adenotonsillectomy
adenous
adenovirus
adenylate
    aminoacyl a.
    a. cyclase
    a. kinase
adenyl cyclase
adenylic acid
adeps, pl. adipes
    a. lanae
    a. renis
adequal cleavage
adequate stimulus
adermia
adermogenesis
ADH
    antidiuretic hormone
adherence
    immune a.
    a. syndrome
adherens
    fascia a.
    macula a.
adherent
    a. cell
    a. leukoma
    a. pericardium
    a. placenta
adhering junction
adhesin

A

adhesio interthalamica
adhesiolysis
adhesion
    amnionic a.
    a. dyspepsia
    fibrinous a.
    fibrous a.
    interthalamic a.
    membranous a.
    a. molecule
    a. phenomenon
    primary a.
    secondary a.
    a. test
adhesiotomy
adhesive
    a. absorbent dressing
    a. arachnoiditis
    a. atelectasis
    a. bandage
    a. capsulitis
    a. inflammation
    a. otitis
    a. pericarditis
    a. peritonitis
    a. phlebitis
    a. pleurisy
    a. tape
    a. tenosynovitis
    a. vaginitis
adiabatic
adiadochocinesia
adiadochocinesis
adiadochokinesis
adiaphoresis
adiaphoretic
adiaphoria
adiaspiromycosis
adiaspore
adiastole
adiathermancy
Adie
    A. pupil
    A. syndrome
adiemorrhysis
adipes (*pl. of* adeps)
adipis
adipocellular
adipoceratous
adipocere
adipocyte
adipofibroma

adipogenesis
adipogenic
adipogenous
adipoid
adipokinetic hormone
adipokinin
adipometer
adiponecrosis
adiposa
    blepharoptosis a.
adiposalgia
adipose
    a. capsule
    a. cell
    a. degeneration
    a. fold
    a. fossa
    a. infiltration
    a. sarcoma
    a. tissue
    a. tumor
adiposis
    a. cardiaca
    a. cerebralis
    a. dolorosa
    a. orchica
    a. tuberosa simplex
    a. universalis
adiposity
adiposogenital
    a. degeneration
    a. dystrophy
    a. syndrome
adiposogenitalis
    dystrophia a.
adiposum
    cor a.
    corpus a.
adiposuria
adiposus
    arcus a.
adipsy, adipsia
aditus
    laryngeal a.
adjacent angle
adjustable
    a. articulator
    a. axis face-bow
    a. occlusal pivot
adjustment disorder
adjuvant
    a. chemotherapy

NOTES

adjuvant *(continued)*
    double-emulsion a.
    Freund complete a.
    Freund incomplete a.
    oil emulsion a.
    a. therapy
    a. vaccine
ADL
    activities of daily living
adlerian
    a. psychoanalysis
    a. psychology
Adler test
admaxillary gland
admedial
admedian
admission
    prior to a.
admittance
admitting
    a. diagnosis (AD)
    a. physician
admixture
    venous a.
adnata
    alopecia a.
adnatum
    filiform a.
adnerval
adneural
adnexa
    a. oculi
    a. uteri
adnexal
    a. adenoma
    a. carcinoma
adnexectomy
adnexitis
adnexopexy
adnexum
adolescence
    avoidant disorder of a.
adolescent
    a. acne
    a. albuminuria
    a. cataract
    a. crisis
    a. medicine
    a. round back
adoptive
    a. immunity
    a. immunotherapy
ADP
    adenosine 5′-diphosphate
    ADP ribosylation
ADR
    adverse drug reaction
adrenal
    accessory a.

    a. androgen
    a. androgen-stimulating hormone (AASH)
    a. apoplexy
    a. body
    a. capsule
    a. cortex
    a. cortex injection
    a. cortical carcinoma
    a. cortical syndrome
    a. crisis
    a. gland
    a. hermaphroditism
    a. hypertension
    a. hypoplasia
    a. leukodystrophy
    Marchand a.
    a. neoplasm
    a. rest
    a. virilism
    a. virilizing syndrome
    a. weight factor
adrenalectomy
adrenaline
    a. oxidase
    a. reversal
adrenalism
adrenalitis
adrenalone
adrenalopathy
adrenarche
adrenergic   Glaucoma
    a. agonist
    a. amine
    a. blockade
    a. bronchodilator
    a. fiber
    a. neuronal blocking agent
    a. neurotransmitter
    a. receptor
adrenic
adrenoceptive
adrenoceptor
adrenocortical
    a. adenoma
    a. hormone
    a. insufficiency
adrenocorticohyperplasia
adrenocorticoid
adrenocorticomimetic
adrenocorticotropic, adrenocorticotrophic
    a. hormone (ACTH)
    a. peptide
    a. releasing factor
adrenocorticotropin
adrenogenic
adrenogenital syndrome
adrenogenous
adrenoleukodystrophy

adrenolytic
adrenomedullary hormone
adrenomegaly
adrenomimetic amine
adrenomyeloneuropathy
adrenopathy
adrenopause
adrenoprival
adrenoreactive
adrenoreceptor
adrenotoxin
adrenotropic, adrenotrophic
    a. hormone
adrenotropin
Adriamycin, bleomycin, vinblastine, and
  dacarbazine (ABVD)
Adson
    A. forceps
    A. maneuver
    A. test
adsorb
adsorbate
adsorbent
adsorption
    a. chromatography
    immune a.
    a. theory
    a. theory of narcosis
adsternal
adterminal
adult
    a. congregate living facility
    (ACLF)
    a. foveomacular retinal dystrophy
    a. hypophosphatasia
    a. lactase deficiency
    a. medulloepithelioma
    a. pseudohypertrophic muscular
    dystrophy
    a. respiratory distress syndrome
    (ARDS)
    a. rickets
    a. T-cell leukemia
    a. T-cell lymphoma
    a. teratoma
    a. tuberculosis
adulterant
adulteration
adultomorphism
adult-onset diabetes
adultorum
    scleredema a.

advance
    a. beneficiary notice
    a. directive (AD)
advanced
    a. cardiac life support (ACLS)
    a. multiple-beam equalization
    radiography (AMBER)
advancement
    capsular a.
    a. flap
    maxillary a.
adventitia
    membrana a.
adventitial
    a. cell
    a. dermis
    a. neuritis
adventitious
    a. albuminuria
    a. breath sounds
    a. bursa
    a. cyst
    a. lung sounds
adverse
    a. drug event
    a. drug reaction (ADR)
    a. effect
adversive movement
advice
    against medical a. (AMA)
advocate
    patient a.
adynamia episodica hereditaria
adynamic ileus
A-E
  above elbow
    A-E amputation
Aeby plane
Aedes
    A. *aegypti*
    A. *albopictus*
    A. *atlanticus*
    A. *caballus*
    A. *dorsalis*
    A. *leucocelaenus*
    A. *melanimon*
    A. *mitchellae*
    A. *nigromaculis*
    A. *polynesiensis*
    A. *sollicitans*
    A. *taeniorhynchus*
    A. *triseriatus*

NOTES

Aedes (continued)
    A. *trivittatus*
    A. *variegatus*
    A. *vexans*
aegypti
    Aedes a.
aegyptius
    Haemophilus a.
aequorin
aerate
aeration
aerendocardia
aerial
    a. mycelium
    a. sickness
aerobe
    obligate a.
aerobic
    a. capacity
    a. dehydrogenase
    a. power
    a. respiration
    a. system
aerobics
aerobiology
aerobioscope
aerobiosis
aerobiotic
aerocele
aerocolpos
aerodermectasia
aerodontalgia
aerodontia
aerodynamic
    a. size
    a. theory
aerodynamics
aeroembolism
aerofaciens
    Eubacterium a.
aerogastria
    blocked a.
aerogen
aerogenes
    Enterobacter a.
    Pasteurella a.
aerogenesis
aerogenic tuberculosis
aerogenous
aeromedicine
aeromonad
Aeromonas hydrophila
aero-odontalgia
aero-odontodynia
aeropause
aerophagia
aerophagy
aerophil
aerophile

aerophilic
aerophilous
aerophobia
aeropiesotherapy
aeroplankton
aerosialophagy
aerosinusitis
aerosis
aerosol
    a. generator
    mainstream a.
    sidestream a.
    a. therapy
aerosolization
aerospace medicine
aerotaxis
aerotherapeutics
aerotherapy
aerotitis media
aerotolerant
aerotonometer
aerotropism
aesculapian
Aesculapius
    staff of A.
aesculin
aesthesiometer
aestival
aestivoautumnal fever
AFB
    acid-fast bacillus
afebrile
afetal
affect
    apathetic a.
    blunt a.
    blunted a.
    congruent a.
    a. displacement
    a. display
    euphoric a.
    flat a.
    a. hunger
    impaired a.
    inappropriate a.
    labile a.
    a. memory
    restricted a.
    a. spasm
affection
affective
    a. disorder
    a. personality
    a. psychosis
    a. tone
affectivity
affectomotor
afferent
    a. fiber

a. glomerular arteriole
a. loop
a. loop syndrome
a. lymphatic
a. nerve
a. vessel
affinity
a. antibody
a. chromatography
a. column
affinous
affirmation
affusion
AFH
anterior facial height
afibrillar cementum
afibrinogenemia
congenital a.
aflatoxicosis
aflatoxin
AFORMED
alternating, failure of response,
mechanical, to electrical depolarization
AFORMED phenomenon
AFP
alpha-fetoprotein
African
A. endomyocardial fibrosis
A. furuncular myiasis
A. hemorrhagic fever
A. histoplasmosis
A. sleeping sickness
A. tick-bite fever
A. tick fever
A. trypanosomiasis
africana
Actinomadura a.
AFS
acid-fast smear
afterbirth
aftercare
afterchroming
aftercontraction, after-contraction
aftercurrent, after-current
afterdischarge, after-discharge
aftereffect, after-effect
aftergilding
afterimage
afterimpression
afterload
a. matching

a. reduction
ventricular a.
afterloading
a. radiation
a. screw
aftermath
aftermovement, after-movement
after-nystagmus
afterpains, after-pains
afterperception
afterpotential, after-potential
diastolic a.
aftersensation
aftersound, after-sound
aftertaste, after-taste
aftertouch
afunctional occlusion
afzelii
Borrelia a.
A/G
albumin-globulin
A/G ratio
against medical advice (AMA)
agalactia
agalactorrhea
agalactosis
agalactous
agamete
agamic
agammaglobulinemia
acquired a.
Bruton a.
agamocytogeny
agamogenesis
agamogenetic
agamogony
agamous
aganglionic
aganglionosis
agapism
agar
bile salt a.
birdseed a.
blood a.
Bordet-Gengou potato blood a.
brain-heart infusion a.
chocolate a.
cornmeal a.
Czapek solution a.
Endo a.
eosin-methylene blue a.
MacConkey a.

NOTES

agar *(continued)*
    Novy and MacNeal blood a.
    Sabouraud dextrose a.
    Thayer-Martin a.
agaric
    a. acid
    deadly a.
    fly a.
Agaricus
agaropectin
agarose
Ag-AS stain
agastric
agastroneuria
age
    achievement a.
    anatomical a.
    basal a.
    Binet a.
    bone a.
    childbearing a.
    chronologic a.
    developmental a.
    emotional a.
    fertilization a.
    gestational a.
    menstrual a.
    mental a.
    ovulational a.
    skeletal a.
agene process
agenesis
    anorectal a.
    gonadal a.
    ovarian a.
    renal a.
    vaginal a.
agenetic fracture
agenitalism
agenosomia
agent
    adrenergic neuronal blocking a.
    alkylating a.
    alpha-adrenergic blocking a.
    antianxiety a.
    antidyskinetic a.
    antifoaming a.
    antipsychotic a.
    atypical antipsychotic a.
    bacteriostatic a.
    beta-adrenergic blocking a.
    Bittner a.
    blister a.
    blocking a.
    calcium channel-blocking a.
    cardioprotective a.
    chemotherapeutic a.
    chimpanzee coryza a.
    cholinergic a.
    contrast a.
    cycle-specific a.
    cytoprotective a.
    delta a.
    disclosing a.
    Eaton a.
    embedding a.
    enterokinetic a.
    F a.
    fertility a.
    foamy a.
    ganglionic blocking a.
    high osmolar contrast a. (HOCA)
    initiating a.
    inotropic a.
    low osmolar contrast a. (LOCA)
    luting a.
    mood stabilizing a.
    myoneural blocking a.
    neuroleptic a.
    nonionic contrast a.
    A. Orange
    physical a.
    Pittsburgh pneumonia a.
    promoting a.
    slow channel-blocking a.
agerasia
age-related macular degeneration
age-specific rate
ageusia
    central a.
    peripheral a.
ageustia
agger
    a. nasi
    a. perpendicularis
    a. valvae venae
agglomeration
agglutinant
agglutinate
agglutinating antibody
agglutination
    acid a.
    bacteriogenic a.
    cold a.
    cross a.
    false a.
    group a.
    immune a.
    indirect a.
    a. test
agglutinative thrombus
agglutinin
    blood group a.
    chief a.
    cold a.
    cross-reacting a.
    flagellar a.
    group a.

H a.
immune a.
incomplete a.
major a.
minor a.
O a.
partial a.
saline a.
serum a.
agglutinogen
blood group a.
agglutinogenic
agglutinophilic
agglutogen
agglutogenic
aggrecan
aggregate
a. anaphylaxis
a. gland
proteoglycan a.
aggregated
a. lymphatic follicle
a. lymphatic nodule
a. lymphoid nodule
aggregation
familial a.
aggregometer
aggressin
aggression
aggressive
a. angiomyxoma
a. infantile fibromatosis
a. instinct
a. manner
a. treatment
aging
amyloidosis of a.
clonal a.
agitated
a. depression
a. melancholia
agitolalia
agitophasia
aglomerular
aglossia
aglossia-adactylia syndrome
aglossostomia
aglutition
aglycon
aglycone
aglycosuria
aglycosuric

agminated gland
agminate gland
agnathia
agnathous
agnea
Agnew-Verhoeff incision
agnogenic myeloid metaplasia
agnosia
auditory a.
color a.
finger a.
gustatory a.
localization a.
olfactory a.
spatial a.
tactile a.
time a.
visual a.
agomphiasis
agomphious
agomphosis
agonadal
agonal
a. clot
a. infection
a. leukocytosis
a. rhythm
a. thrombosis
a. thrombus
agonist
adrenergic a.
cholinergic a.
muscarinic a.
narcotic a.
prostaglandin a.
agonist-antagonist
narcotic a.-a.
agony
agoraphobia
agoraphobic
agraffe
agrammatica
agrammatism
agrammatologia
agranular
a. cortex
a. endoplasmic reticulum
a. leukocyte
agranulocyte
agranulocytic angina
agranulocytosis
agranuloplastic

NOTES

agraphia
    absolute a.
    acoustic a.
    amnemonic a.
    atactic a.
    constructional a.
    literal a.
agraphic
agretope
agrypnotic
ague
    brass founder's a.
AGUS
    atypical glandular cell of undetermined
     significance
agyiophobia
agyria
AH
    AH conduction time
    AH interval
ahaustral
Ahumada-del Castillo syndrome
ahylognosia
AIc
    hemoglobin AIc
Aicardi syndrome
aichmophobia
aid
    behind-the-ear hearing a.
    digital hearing a.
    ergogenic a.
    first a.
    hearing a.
    in-the-canal hearing a.
    in-the-ear hearing a.
AIDS
    acquired immunodeficiency syndrome
    AIDS dementia
    AIDS dementia complex (ADC)
AIDS-related
    AIDS-r. complex (ARC)
    AIDS-r. virus
ailurophobia
ainhum
air
    a. abrasion
    alveolar a.
    ambient a.
    a. bladder
    a. block glaucoma
    a. boot
    a. bronchogram
    a. cell
    complemental a.
    complementary a.
    a. conduction
    a. contrast barium enema
    a. cushion sign
    a. dose

    a. embolism
    functional residual a.
    a. hunger
    liquid a.
    a. medical transport
    minimal a.
    a. pollution
    reserve a.
    residual a.
    a. sac
    a. sickness
    a. splint
    supplemental a.
    a. syringe
    a. thermometer
    tidal a.
    a. tube
    a. vesicle
air-bone gap
airborne infection
airbrasive technique
air-conditioner lung
air-fluidized bed
air-gap
    a.-g. radiography
    a.-g. technique
airplane splint
airport malaria
airsickness
air-slaked lime
airspace
airspace-filling pattern
airtrapping
airway
    anatomic a.
    anatomical a.
    a. anatomy
    conducting a.
    esophageal obturator a.
    Guedel a.
    lower a.
    a. management
    nasopharyngeal a.
    a. obstruction
    oropharyngeal a.
    a. pattern
    a. pressure release ventilation
    a. resistance
    upper a.
Airy disc
ajacis
    Delphinium a.
A-K
    above knee
    A-K amputation
akamushi
    a. disease
    Leptotrombidium a.
akanthion

akaryocyte
akaryote
akathisia
akeratosis
Akerlund deformity
akinesia
    a. algera
    a. amnestica
    spinal a.
akinesic
akinesis
akinesthesia
akinetic
    a. mutism
    a. seizure
aknemia
ALA
   alpha-lipoic acid
ala, pl. **alae**
    a. auris
    a. nasi
alactic oxygen debt
Alagille syndrome
alalia
alalic
Aland Island albinism
alanine
    a. aminotransferase (ALT)
    a. racemase
    a. transaminase
alanine-glucose cycle
alanine-glyoxylate aminotransferase
alanine-oxomalonate aminotransferase
alanosine
Alanson amputation
alantin
alantol
alant starch
alanyl
alar
    a. artery
    a. chest
    a. fold
    a. incision
    a. lamina
    a. ligament
    a. plate
    a. process
    a. spine
ALARA
   as low as reasonably achievable
alarm reaction

alaryngeal speech
alastrim
alata
    scapula a.
alba
    linea a.
    lochia a.
    materia a.
    miliaria a.
    pityriasis a.
Albarran
    A. gland
    A. test
Albers-Schönberg disease
Albert
    A. diphtheria stain
    A. position
    A. suture
albicans
    Candida a.
    corpus a.
albiduria
albidus
Albini nodule
albinism
    acquired a.
    Aland Island a.
    cutaneous a.
    Forsius-Eriksson a.
    Nettleshop-Falls a.
    ocular a.
    red a.
    rufous a.
albinotic
albinuria
Albinus muscle
albocinereous
albopictus
    Aedes a.
    Dermacentor a.
Albrecht bone
Albright
    A. disease
    A. hereditary osteodystrophy
    A. syndrome
albuginea
    tunica a.
albugineotomy
albugineous
albumin
    a. A, B
    Bence Jones a.

NOTES

29

albumin *(continued)*
    blood a.
    bovine serum a. (BSA)
    dried human a.
    egg a.
    iodinated 131I human serum a.
    iodinated 125I serum a.
    macroaggregated a.
    normal human serum a.
    serum a.
albuminate
    iron a.
albuminaturia
albumin-globulin (A/G)
    a.-g. ratio
albuminiferous
albuminiparous
albuminized iron
albuminocytologic dissociation
albuminogenous
albuminoid
albuminolysis
albuminoptysis
albuminoreaction
albuminorrhea
albuminous
    a. cell
    a. gland
    a. swelling
albuminuria
    adolescent a.
    adventitious a.
    Bamberger a.
    benign a.
    cardiac a.
    colliquative a.
    dietetic a.
    essential a.
    false a.
    febrile a.
    functional a.
    intermittent a.
    lordotic a.
    nephrogenous a.
albuminuric retinitis
albuterol
alcapton
alcaptonuria, alkaptonuria
alcaptonuric, alkaptonuric
Alcian blue
alclofenac
alclometasone
Alcock canal
alcogel
alcohol
    absolute a.
    acid a.
    a. addiction
    allyl a.

a. amnestic syndrome
amyl a.
anhydrous a.
a. automatism
benzyl a.
bile a.
butyl a.
dehydrated a.
a. dehydrogenase
a. dehydrogenase acceptor
a. dehydrogenase NADP+
denatured a.
dihydric a.
dilute a.
a. diuresis
ethyl a.
farnesene a.
fatty a.
furfuryl a.
glyceryl a.
grain a.
isopropyl a.
ketone a.
methyl a.
monohydric a.
primary a.
propyl a.
secondary a.
tertiary a.
trihydric a.
a. withdrawal delirium
alcoholate
alcohol-glycerin fixative
alcoholic
    a. cardiomyopathy
    a. cirrhosis
    a. dementia
    a. deterioration
    a. extract
    a. fermentation
    a. hyalin
    a. hyaline body
    a. myocardiopathy
    a. paranoia
    a. pneumonia
    a. polyneuropathy
    a. psychosis
    a. tincture
    a. withdrawal tremor
alcoholism
    acute a.
    chronic a.
alcoholization
alcoholophobia
alcoholysis
aldehyde
    acetic a.
    activated glycol a.
    active a.

angular a.
benzoic a.
betaine a.
formic a.
glyceric a.
mcthyl a.

Alder
A. anomaly
A. body

aldimine
alditol
aldocortin
aldohexose
aldoketomutase
aldolase
deoxyribosephosphate a.

aldol condensation
aldopentose
aldose
aldosterone antagonist
aldosteronism
idiopathic a.
primary a.
secondary a.

aldosteronogenesis
aldosteronopenia
aldotetrose
aldotriose
aldoxime
Aldrich syndrome
aldrin
alecithal ovum
alemmal
Aleppo boil
aleukemia
aleukemic
a. leukemia
a. myelosis

aleukemoid
aleukia
aleukocytic
aleukocytosis
aleurioconidium
aleuriospore
aleuron
aleuronate
aleuronoid
Alexander
A. disease
A. hearing impairment
A. law

alexia
incomplete a.

alexic
alexin unit
alexithymia
alfa
epoetin a.

alfacalcidol
algae
blue-green a.

algal
algefacient
algera
akinesia a.
analgesia a.
dyskinesia a.

algesia
algesic
algesichronometer
algesimeter
algesiogenic
algesiometer
algesthesia
algesthesis
algestone acetophenide
algetic
algicide
algid
a. malaria
a. pernicious fever
a. stage

algin
alginate
calcium a.

alginolyticus
Vibrio a.

algiomotor
algiomuscular
algiovascular
algodystrophy
algogenesia
algogenesis
algogenic
algoid cell
algolagnia
algology
algometer
algometry
algophilia
algophobia
algorithm
algoscopy

NOTES

algospasm
algovascular
alible
Alice in Wonderland syndrome
alicyclic compound
alienation
alienia
aliform
alignment
    a. curve
    a. mark
    postural a.
aliment
alimentary
    a. apparatus
    a. canal
    a. diabetes
    a. glycosuria
    a. hyperinsulinism
    a. lipemia
    a. osteopathy
    a. pentosuria
    a. system
    a. therapy
    a. tract
    a. tract smear
alimentation
    forced a.
alinasal
alinement
alinjection
aliphatic
    a. acid
    a. compound
alipoid
alipotropic
aliquant
aliquot
alisphenoid cartilage
alizarin
    a. cyanin
    a. indicator
    a. purpurin
    a. red S
alkadiene
alkalemia
alkalescent
alkali
    caustic a.
    a. denaturation test
    a. earth metal
    fixed a.
    a. reserve
    a. therapy
alkalimetry
alkaline
    a. earth element
    a. earths
    a. milk drip

    a. phosphatase
    a. reaction
    a. reflux gastritis
    a. RNase
    a. tide
    a. water
    a. wave
alkaline-ash diet
alkaline toluidine blue O
alkalinity
alkalinization
alkalinuria
alkalitherapy
alkalization
alkalizer
alkaloid
    ergot a.
    fixed a.
    imidazole a.
alkalosis
    acapnial a.
    altitude a.
    compensated metabolic a.
    compensated respiratory a.
    hypokalemic a.
    metabolic a.
    respiratory a.
    uncompensated a.
alkalotic
alkaluria
alkane
alkapton
alkaptonuria (*var. of* alcaptonuria)
alkaptonuric (*var. of* alcaptonuric)
alkatriene
alkavervir
alkene
alkenyl
alkide
alkyl
    arylated a.
alkylamine
alkylating agent
alkylation
ALL
    acute lymphocytic leukemia
allachesthesia
allantoate deiminase
allantochorion
allantoenteric diverticulum
allantogenesis
allantoic
    a. bladder
    a. cyst
    a. diverticulum
    a. fluid
    a. sac
    a. stalk
    a. vesicle

A

allantoid membrane
allantoidoangiopagous twin
allantoidoangiopagus
allantoin
allantoinase
allantoinuria
allantois
Allarton operation
allaxis
allele
    codominant a.
allelic
    a. exclusion
    a. gene
allelism
allelocatalysis
allelocatalytic
allelochemicals
allelomorph
allelomorphic
allelomorphism
allelotaxis
allelotaxy
Allen
    A. cognitive level scale
    A. test
Allen-Doisy
    A.-D. test
    A.-D. unit
Allen-Masters syndrome
allergen
allergenic extract
allergic
    a. bronchopulmonary aspergillosis
    (ABPA)
    a. conjunctivitis
    a. contact dermatitis
    a. coryza
    a. cystitis
    a. eczema
    a. extract
    a. granulomatosis
    a. granulomatous angiitis
    a. inflammation
    a. purpura
    a. reaction
    a. rhinitis
    a. salute
    a. stomatitis
    a. urticaria
allergies (pl. of allergy)
allergist

allergization
allergized
allergology
allergosis
allergy, pl. allergies
    atopic a.
    bacterial a.
    cold a.
    contact a.
    delayed a.
    drug a.
    immediate a.
    latent a.
    no known allergies (NKA)
    no known drug allergies (NKDA)
    physical a.
    polyvalent a.
allesthesia
allethrin
allethrolone
Allgrove syndrome
allied health professional
alligator
    a. forceps
    a. skin
Allingham ulcer
Allis forceps
alliteration
all or none law
alloalbuminemia
alloantibody
alloantigen
allobarbital
allocentric
allochiria, allocheiria
allocholesterol
allochroic
allochroism
allocortex
allodiploid
allodynia
alloerotic
alloerotism
alloesthesia
allogamy
allogeneic
    a. antigen
    a. graft
    a. inhibition
allogenic
allogotrophia

NOTES

allograft
    living related a.
    living unrelated a.
    a. rejection
allogroup
allohexaploid
allohydroxylysine
alloimmune
alloisoleucine
alloisomer
allokeratoplasty
allokinesis
allolactose
allolalia
allomeric function
allomerism
allometron
allomone
allomorphism
allongement
allopath
allopathic keratoplasty
allopathist
allopathy
allopentaploid
allophasis
allophenic
allophore
allophthalmia
alloplasia
alloplast
alloplasty
alloploid
alloploidy
allopolyploid
allopolyploidy
allopregnane
allopsychic
allopurinol
allorhythmia
allorhythmic
allose
allosensitization
allosome
allosteric
    a. enzyme
    a. site
allosterism
allostery
allotetraploid
allotherm
allothreonine
allotope
allotopia
allotransplantation
allotriodontia
allotriosmia
allotriploid
allotrope

allotrophic
allotropic
allotropism
allotropy
allotype
    Gm a.
    Km a.
allotypic
    a. determinant
    a. marker
allowance
    recommended daily a.
alloxan diabetes
alloxantin
alloxuremia
alloxuria
alloy
    eutectic a.
    gold a.
allspice oil
all-trans-retinal
allyl alcohol
Almeida disease
almond oil
aloe
aloetin
alogia
aloin
alopecia
    a. adnata
    androgenic a.
    a. areata
    a. capitis totalis
    cicatricial a.
    a. circumscripta
    congenital a.
    a. congenitalis
    congenital sutural a.
    female pattern a.
    a. hereditaria
    hereditary a.
    a. leprotica
    a. liminaris frontalis
    lipedematous a.
    male pattern a.
    a. marginalis
    a. medicamentosa
    a. mucinosa
    patterned a.
    a. pityrodes
    a. prematura
    a. presenilis
    pressure a.
    scarring a.
    a. senilis
    a. symptomatica
    a. syphilitica
    a. totalis
    a. toxica

traction a.
a. triangularis
a. triangularis congenitalis
a. universalis
x-ray a.
alopecic
Alpers disease
alpha, α
a. amylase
a. angle
a. blocking
a. cell
a. error
a. fiber
a. granule
interferon a.
a. methyl dopa
a. particle
a. radiation
a. ray
a. rhythm
a. substance
A. test
a. unit
a. wave
alpha-adrenergic
a.-a. blocking agent
a.-a. receptor
alpha-adrenoceptor antagonist
alpha-amino acid
alpha-aminosuccinic acid
alpha-blocker
alphadione
alpha-fetoprotein (AFP)
alpha-ketoglutarate
alpha-ketoglutaric acid
alpha-lipoic acid (ALA)
alpha-oxidation
alphaprodine
alphasone acetophenide
Alphavirus
alpidem
Alpine scurvy
Alport syndrome
alprazolam
alprostadil
ALS
amyotrophic lateral sclerosis
Alström syndrome
ALT
alanine aminotransferase

alta
patella a.
ALT:AST ratio
Altemeier operation
alteplase
alteration
modal a.
alterative inflammation
altercursive intubation
alteregoism
alternans
auditory a.
auscultatory a.
concordant a.
cycle length a.
discordant a.
electrical a.
pulsus a.
alternate
a. binaural loudness balance test
a. cover test
a. day strabismus
a. hemianesthesia
alternating
a. calculus
a. current
a., failure of response, mechanical,
to electrical depolarization
(AFORMED)
a. hemiplegia
a. light test
a. mydriasis
a. pulse
a. strabismus
a. suture
a. tremor
alternation
cardiac a.
concordant a.
discordant a.
electrical a.
alternative
a. hypothesis
a. inheritance
a. medicine
a. splicing
a. tremor
alternator
alternocular
altitude
a. alkalosis
a. chamber

NOTES

altitude (*continued*)
    a. disease
    a. erythremia
    a. sickness
altitudinal hemianopia
Altmann
    A. anilin-acid fuchsin stain
    A. fixative
    A. granule
    A. theory
Altmann-Gersh method
alum
    burnt a.
    cake a.
    chrome a.
    dried a.
    exsiccated a.
    ferric a.
    iron a.
    a. whey
alum-hematoxylin
alumina
    hydrated a.
aluminate
    bismuth a.
aluminated
aluminon
aluminosis
aluminum
    a. acetate
    a. aspirin
    a. group
    a. hydrate
    a. hydroxide
    a. hydroxide gel
    a. penicillin
    a. phosphate
    a. phosphate gel
    a. subacetate
Alu sequence
alveoalgia, alveolalgia
alveolar
    a. abscess
    a. adenocarcinoma
    a. air
    a. air equation
    a. angle
    a. arch
    a. atrophy
    a. body
    a. bone
    a. border
    a. bronchiole
    a. canal
    a. cell
    a. cell carcinoma
    a. crest
    a. dead space

    a. duct
    a. duct emphysema
    a. edema
    a. foramen
    a. gas
    a. gas equation
    a. gingiva
    a. gland
    a. hydatid cyst
    a. index
    a. macrophage
    a. mucosa
    a. osteitis
    a. pattern
    a. periosteum
    a. point
    a. pore
    a. process
    a. ridge
    a. sac
    a. septum
    a. soft part sarcoma
    a. supporting bone
    a. ventilation
    a. yoke
alveolar-arterial oxygen tension difference
alveolar-capillary membrane
alveolate
alveolectomy
alveoli (*pl. of* alveolus)
alveolingual
alveolitis
    acute pulmonary a.
    chronic fibrosing a.
    cryptogenic fibrosing a.
    extrinsic allergic a.
    fibrosing a.
alveolobuccal
    a. groove
    a. sulcus
alveolocapillary
    a. block
    a. membrane
alveoloclasia
alveolodental
    a. canal
    a. ligament
    a. membrane
alveololabial
    a. groove
    a. sulcus
alveololabialis
alveololingual
    a. groove
    a. sulcus
alveolonasal line
alveolopalatal

alveoloplasty
    interradicular a.
    intraseptal a.
alveoloschisis
alveolotomy
alveolus, pl. alveoli
    a. dentalis
    pulmonary a.
    alveoli pulmonis
alveoplasty
alveus
alymphia
alymphocytosis
alymphoplasia
    thymic a.
Alzheimer
    A. dementia
    A. disease
    A. fibril
    A. sclerosis
    A. stain
    A. type I, II astrocyte
alzyme
AMA
    against medical advice
amacrine cell
Amadori rearrangement
amalgam
    a. carrier
    marginal integrity of a.
    a. matrix
    a. strip
    a. tattoo
amalgamate
amalgamation
amalgamator
amalonatica
    Citrobacter a.
Amanita
    A. muscaria
    A. phalloides
Am antigen
amaranth solution
amaranthum
amarine
amaroid
amaroidal
amarum
amastia
amastigote
amathophobia
amatoxin

amaurosis
    diabetic a.
    a. fugax
amaurotic
    a. cat eye
    a. mydriasis
    a. nystagmus
    a. pupil
amaxophobia
amazia
amazon thorax
ambageusia
ambenonium chloride
AMBER
    advanced multiple-beam equalization
    radiography
amber
    a. codon
    a. mutant
    a. mutation
    a. suppressor
Amberg lateral sinus line
ambidexterity
ambidextrism
ambidextrous
ambient
    a. air
    a. cistern
ambiguity
    genital a.
ambiguous
    a. atrioventricular connection
    a. external genitalia
ambilateral
ambilevous
ambisexual
ambisinister
ambisinistrous
ambivalence
ambivalent
ambivert
amblyaphia
amblygeustia
amblyogenic period
Amblyomma
    A. americanum
    A. cajennense
    A. hebraeum
    A. maculatum
    A. variegatum
amblyopia
    anisometropic a.

NOTES

amblyopia *(continued)*
    crossed a.
    deprivation a.
    a. ex anopsia
    hysterical a.
    meridional a.
    nocturnal a.
    pattern distortion a.
    suppression a.
    tobacco-alcohol a.
amblyopic
amblyoscope
    major a.
    Worth a.
amboceptor unit
ambomalleal
ambrosin
Ambu bag
ambucetamide
ambulance service
ambulant
    a. edema
    a. erysipelas
    a. plague
ambulation
ambulatory
    a. anesthesia
    a. automatism
    a. care
    a. patient group
    a. plague
    a. schizophrenia
    a. surgery
    a. typhoid
ambuphylline
amcinonide
ameba, pl. **amebae, amebas**
amebacide
amebiasis
    canine a.
    a. cutis
    hepatic a.
amebic
    a. abscess
    a. colitis
    a. dysentery
    a. granuloma
    a. vaginitis
amebicidal
amebicide
amebiform
amebiosis
amebism
amebocyte
ameboid
    a. cell
    a. movement
ameboididity

ameboidism
ameboma
amebula
amebule
ameburia
amelanotic melanoma
amelia
    brachial a.
    complete a.
    unilateral a.
amelioration
ameloblast
ameloblastic
    a. adenomatoid tumor
    a. fibroma
    a. fibrosarcoma
    a. layer
    a. odontoma
    a. sarcoma
ameloblastoma
    acanthomatous a.
    follicular a.
    multicystic a.
    plexiform a.
ameloblastomatous craniopharyngioma
amelodental junction
amelodentinal junction
amelogenesis
amelogenin
amenia
amenorrhea
    dietary a.
    emotional a.
    exercise-induced a.
    hyperprolactinemic a.
    hypophysial a.
    hypothalamic a.
    lactation a.
    physiologic a.
    pituitary a.
    primary a.
    secondary a.
    traumatic a.
amenorrhea-galactorrhea syndrome
amenorrheal
amenorrheic
amentia
    Stearns alcoholic a.
amential
American
    A. leishmaniasis
    A. tarantula
    A. trypanosomiasis
americanum
    Amblyomma a.
americium
amerism
ameristic

Ames
    A. assay
    A. test
amethopterin
ametria
ametropia
    axial a.
    index a.
ametropic
AMI
    acute myocardial infarction
amiantaceous
amianthoid
Amici
    A. line
    A. stria
amicrobic
amicroscopic
amidase
amide
    acetic a.
    angiotensin III a.
amidine
amidinotransferase
    glycine a.
amidohydrolase
amimia
aminase
    fumaric a.
    guanine a.
aminate
amination
amine
    adrenergic a.
    adrenomimetic a.
    biogenic a.
    a. oxidase
    a. precursor uptake, decarboxylase
     (APUD)
    pressor a.
    primary a.
    secondary a.
    sympathetic a.
    sympathomimetic a.
    tertiary a.
    vasoactive a.
aminergic
amino
    a. acid (AA)
    a. acid dehydrogenase
    a. acid oxidase
    a. sugar

aminoacidemia
aminoacid-tRNA ligase
aminoaciduria
    hyperbasic a.
aminoacyl adenylate
amlnoacylase
aminobenzene
aminobenzoate
    butyl a.
aminoglycoside antibiotic
aminolysis
aminopeptidase
aminopherase
aminorex
amino-terminal
aminotransferase
    alanine a. (ALT)
    alanine-glyoxylate a.
    alanine-oxomalonate a.
    aspartate a. (AST)
aminotriazole
aminotripeptidase
aminoxide
    eserine a.
aminuria
amithiozone
amitosis
amitotic
amitrole
amlodipine
ammeter
Ammon
    A. fissure
    A. horn
    A. prominence
ammonemia
ammonia
    a. assimilation
    a. detoxication
    a. fixation
ammoniac
ammoniacal urine
ammonia-lyase
ammoniated
    a. mercuric chloride
    a. mercury
    a. tincture
ammoniemia
ammonium
    a. benzoate
    a. carbonate
    a. chloride

NOTES

ammoniuria
ammonolysis
ammonotelia
ammonotelic
ammonotelism
amnemonic agraphia
amnesia
    anterograde a.
    auditory a.
    elective a.
    emotional a.
    lacunar a.
    localized a.
    olfactory a.
    posttraumatic a.
    retrograde a.
    transient global a.
    traumatic a.
amnesiac
amnesic, amnestic
    a. aphasia
    a. syndrome
amnestica
    akinesia a.
amnii
    liquor a.
amniocardiac vesicle
amniocele
amniocentesis
amniochorial
amniochorionic
amnioembryonic junction
amniogenesis
amniogenic cell
amniography
amnio-hook
amnioinfusion
amnioma
amnion
    a. nodosum
    a. ring
amnionic
    a. adhesion
    a. amputation
    a. band
    a. band syndrome
    a. cavity
    a. corpuscle
    a. duct
    a. ectoderm
    a. fluid
    a. fluid embolism
    a. fluid index
    a. fluid syndrome
    a. fold
    a. raphe
    a. sac
amnionitis
amniorrhea

amniorrhexis
amnioscope
amnioscopy
Amniota
amniotic
    a. band
    a. fluid
    a. hernia
amniotome
amniotomy
amobarbital
A-mode
amoebapore
amoebocyte
amoeboid
amok, amuck
amorph
amorpha
    pars a.
amorphagnosia
amorphia
amorphism
amorphosynthesis
amorphous
    a. hydroxyapatite
    a. insulin zinc suspension
    a. phosphorus
    a. selenium plate
    a. silicon
amorphus
    acardius a.
amoxapine
amoxicillin
AMP
    adenosine monophosphate
    cyclic AMP
    AMP deaminase
amperage
ampere
Ampère postulate
amperometry
ampheclexis
amphetamine
    a. acetate
    a. phosphate
amphiarthrodial
amphiarthrosis
amphiaster
amphibolic fistula
amphibolous fistula
amphicelous
amphicentric
amphichroic
amphichromatic
amphicyte
amphid
amphidiploid
amphikaryon
amphileukemic

amphimicrobe
amphimictic
amphimixis
amphinucleolus
amphion
amphipathic
amphiphilic
amphiphobic
amphiprotic solvent
amphistome
amphitrichate
amphitrichous
amphitypy
amphixenosis
amphochromatophil, amphochromatophile
amphochromophil, amphochromophile
amphocyte
ampholyte
amphomycin
amphophil, amphophile
   a. granule
amphophilic, amphophilous
amphoric
   a. rale
   a. resonance
   a. respiration
   a. voice
   a. voice sound
amphoriloquy
amphorophony
amphoteric
   a. electrolyte
   a. element
   a. reaction
amphotericin B
amphoterism
amphotropic virus
ampicillin
amplexus
amplification
   genetic a.
   linear a.
amplifier
   a. host
   image a.
amplitude
   a. of accommodation
   a. of convergence
   a. image
   a. of pulse
ampoule
amprotropine phosphate

ampule, ampul
ampulla
   biliaropancreatic a.
   bony a.
   duodenal a.
   Henle a.
   hepatopancreatic a.
   lactiferous a.
   membranous a.
   rectal a.
   Thoma a.
   a. of Vater
ampullar
   a. abortion
   a. pregnancy
ampullary
   a. aneurysm
   a. crest
   a. crus
   a. cupula
   a. fold
   a. groove
   a. membranous limb
   a. sulcus
ampullitis
ampullula
amputation
   A-E a.
   A-K a.
   Alanson a.
   amnionic a.
   aperiosteal a.
   B-E a.
   Bier a.
   birth a.
   B-K a.
   bloodless a.
   Callander a.
   Carden a.
   central a.
   cervical a.
   Chopart a.
   cinematic a.
   cineplastic a.
   circular a.
   congenital a.
   consecutive a.
   a. in continuity
   double flap a.
   dry a.
   Dupuytren a.
   eccentric a.

NOTES

amputation *(continued)*
    elliptical a.
    excentric a.
    Farabeuf a.
    flap a.
    flapless a.
    forequarter a.
    Gritti-Stokes a.
    guillotine a.
    Guyon a.
    Hancock a.
    Hey a.
    hindquarter a.
    immediate a.
    intermediate a.
    interpelviabdominal a.
    interscapulothoracic a.
    intrauterine a.
    Jaboulay a.
    kineplastic a.
    Kirk a.
    knee disarticulation a.
    a. knife
    Krukenberg a.
    Larrey a.
    Le Fort a.
    linear a.
    Lisfranc a.
    Mackenzie a.
    major a.
    Malgaigne a.
    mediotarsal a.
    Mikulicz-Vladimiroff a.
    minor a.
    a. neuroma
    oblique a.
    oval a.
    periosteoplastic a.
    Pirogoff a.
    pulp a.
    racket a.
    root a.
    spontaneous a.
    Stokes a.
    subperiosteal a.
    Syme a.
    Teale a.
    transverse a.
    traumatic a.
    Tripier a.
amputee
amrinone lactate
Amsel criteria
Amsler
    A. chart
    A. grid
    A. test
Amsterdam syndrome
amuck *(var. of* amok)

amusia
    instrumental a.
Amussat
    A. valve
    A. valvula
amychophobia
amycolatum
    Corynebacterium a.
amyelencephalia
amyelencephalic
amyelencephalous
amyelia
amyelic
amyelinated
amyelination
amyelinic
amyeloic
amyelonic
amyelous
amygdala, pl. **amygdalae**
    a. cerebelli
amygdalase
amygdalin
amygdaline
amygdaloclaustral area
amygdaloid
    a. body
    a. complex
    a. fossa
    a. nucleus
    a. tubercle
amygdalopiriform transition area
amygdalose
amygdaloside
amyl
    a. alcohol
    a. hydrate
    a. nitrite
    a. valerate
amylaceous corpuscle
amylaceum
    corpus a.
amylase
    alpha a.
amylase-creatinine clearance ratio
amylasuria
amylemia
amylene
    a. chloral
    a. hydrate
amylic fermentation
amylin
amylodextrin
amylogenesis
amylogenic body
amyloglucosidase
amyloid
    a. angiopathy
    a. corpuscle

a. degeneration
a. kidney
a. nephrosis
a. protein
a. tongue
a. tumor
amyloidoma
amyloidosis
a. of aging
chronic a.
a. cutis
familial a.
focal a.
hereditary a.
lichen a.
lichenoid a.
light chain-related a.
macular a.
a. of multiple myeloma
nodular a.
primary a.
renal a.
secondary a.
senile a.
amylolysis
amylolytic
amylomaltase
amylopectin
amylopectinosis
amylophagia
amyloplast
amylopsin
amylorrhea
amylose
amylosuria
amylum
amyluria
amyoesthesia
amyoesthesis
amyoplasia congenita
amyostasia
amyostatic
amyosthenia
amyosthenic
amyotaxy
amyotonia congenita
amyotrophic
a. cachexia
a. lateral sclerosis (ALS)
amyotrophy, amyotrophia
diabetic a.

hemiplegic a.
neuralgic a.
amyous
amyxorrhea
ANA
antinuclear antibody
anabiosis
anabiotic cell
anabolic steroid
anabolism
anabolite
anacamptometer
anacatadidymus
anacatesthesia
anacidity
anaclasis
anaclitic
a. depression
a. psychotherapy
anacrotic
a. limb
a. notch
a. pulse
anacrotism
anacusis, anakusis
anadenia ventriculi
anadicrotic pulse
anadicrotism
anadidymus
anadipsia
anadrenalism
anadromous
anaerobe
facultative a.
obligate a.
anaerobic
a. cellulitis
a. dehydrogenase
a. pneumonia
a. power
a. respiration
anaerobiosis
anaerobiotic
anaerogenic
anaerophyte
anaeroplasty
anagen effluvium
anagenesis
anagenetic
anagogy
anakatadidymus
anakmesis

NOTES

anakusis (*var. of* anacusis)
anal
    a. atresia
    a. canal
    a. cleft
    a. column
    a. crypt
    a. cushion
    a. duct
    a. erotism
    a. fascia
    a. fissure
    a. fistula
    a. gland
    a. membrane
    a. orifice
    a. pecten
    a. phase
    a. pit
    a. plate
    a. reflex
    a. region
    a. sinus
    a. skin tag
    a. speculum
    a. sphincter
    a. transitional zone
    a. triangle
    a. valve
    a. verge
analbuminemia
analeptic enema
analgesia
    a. algera
    conduction a.
    a. dolorosa
    inhalation a.
    patient-controlled a. (PCA)
    spinal a.
analgesic
    a. cuirass
    a. nephritis
    a. nephropathy
analgesimeter
analgetic
analis
    pecten a.
anality
anallergic
analog, analogue
    enzyme a.
analogous
analphalipoproteinemia
analysand
analysis, pl. **analyses**
    accumulation a.
    activation a.
    activity pattern a.

    bioelectrical impedance a.
    biomechanical a.
    bite a.
    blood gas a.
    bradykinetic a.
    breath a.
    cephalometric a.
    character a.
    cluster a.
    content a.
    decision a.
    didactic a.
    discriminant a.
    displacement a.
    distributive a.
    Downs a.
    ego a.
    Fourier a.
    gastric a.
    intention-to-treat a.
    interaction process a.
    Kaplan-Meier a.
    linkage a.
    Northern blot a.
    occlusal a.
    pedigree a.
    qualitative a.
    quantitative a.
    regression a.
    segregation a.
    Southern blot a.
    transactional a.
    a. of variance (ANOVA)
    volumetric a.
    Western blot a.
    zoo blot a.
analyst
analyte
analytic
    a. chemistry
    a. psychiatry
    a. study
    a. therapy
analytical
    a. psychology
    a. sensitivity
    a. specificity
analyzer
    batch a.
    centrifugal fast a.
    CO_2 a.
    continuous flow a.
    discrete a.
    kinetic a.
    pulse height a.
analyzing rod
analyzor
anamnesis

anamnestic
    a. reaction
    a. response
anamnionic, anamniotic
anamorph
anamorphosis
ananastasia
anancasm
anancastia
anancastic
anandria
anangioplasia
anangioplastic
ANAP
    anionic neutrophil-activating peptide
anaphase lag
anaphia
anaphoresis
anaphoretic
anaphrodisiac
anaphylactic
    a. antibody
    a. intoxication
    a. reaction
    a. shock
anaphylactica
    enteritis a.
anaphylactogen
anaphylactogenesis
anaphylactogenic
anaphylactoid
    a. crisis
    a. purpura
    a. shock
anaphylatoxin inactivator
anaphylaxis
    active a.
    aggregate a.
    antiserum a.
    chronic a.
    generalized a.
    inverse a.
    local a.
    passive a.
    systemic a.
anaphylotoxin
anaplasia
anaplastic
    a. astrocytoma
    a. carcinoma
    a. cell
    a. large cell lymphoma

    a. malignant teratoma
    a. oligodendroglioma
anaplastology
anaplerosis
anaplerotic reaction
anapophysis
anaptic
anarithmia
anarthria
anarthritic rheumatoid disease
anasarca
    fetoplacental a.
anasarcous
anastigmat
anastigmatic
anastole
anastomose
anastomosing
    a. fiber
    a. vessel
anastomosis, pl. anastomoses
    acromial a.
    aneurysm by a.
    antiperistaltic a.
    arteriolovenular a.
    a. arteriolovenularis
    a. arteriovenosa
    arteriovenous a.
    Béclard a.
    bevelled a.
    Billroth I, II a.
    Brackin a.
    Braun a.
    calcaneal a.
    cavopulmonary a.
    Clado a.
    a. clamp
    Coffey a.
    conjoined a.
    crucial a.
    cruciate a.
    cubital a.
    Damus-Stancel-Kaye a.
    elliptical a.
    end-to-end a.
    Furniss a.
    Galen a.
    genicular a.
    Haight a.
    Hofmeister-Pólya a.
    Hoyer a.
    Hyrtl a.

NOTES

anastomosis (*continued*)
    intermesenteric arterial a.
    intestinal a.
    isoperistaltic a.
    Jacobson a.
    Martin-Gruber a.
    microvascular a.
    peristaltic a.
    postcostal a.
    precostal a.
    Riolan a.
    Roux-en-Y a.
    Schmidel a.
    sequential a.
    side-to-end a.
    side-to-side a.
    sutureless a.
    terminoterminal a.
    ureteroileal a.
anastomotic
    a. branch
    a. fiber
    a. stricture
    a. ulcer
    a. vein
    a. vessel
anastral
anatomic
    a. airway
    a. conjugate
    a. crown
    a. dead space
    a. pathology
    a. position
    a. snuffbox
    a. sphincter
    a. tooth
    a. tubercle
    a. wart
anatomical
    a. age
    a. airway
    a. conjugate
    a. crown
    a. element
    a. position
    a. root
    a. wart
anatomicomedical
anatomicopathologic
anatomicosurgical
anatomist
anatomy
    airway a.
    artificial a.
    artistic a.
    clastic a.
    clinical a.
    comparative a.

    dental a.
    descriptive a.
    developmental a.
    functional a.
    general a.
    gross a.
    living a.
    macroscopic a.
    medical a.
    microscopic a.
    pathological a.
    radiological a.
    regional a.
    special a.
    surface a.
    surgical a.
    topographic a.
    ultrastructural a.
anatopism
anatoxic
anatoxin
anatricrotic
anatricrotism
anatripsis
anatriptic
anatrophic nephrotomy
anaxon
anaxone
anazoturia
ANCA
    antineutrophil cytoplasmic antibody
AnCC
    anodal closure contraction
anceps
    acardius a.
ancestor
    leading a.
anchorage
    cervical a.
    a. dependence
    extraoral a.
    intermaxillary a.
    intramaxillary a.
    intraoral a.
anchorin
anchoring
    a. fibril
    a. villus
anchor splint
anchusin
ancillary
    a. port
    a. services
ancipital
ancipitate
ancipitous
ancon
anconad
anconal fossa

anconeal
anconeus muscle
anconoid
ancrod
Ancylostoma
    A. braziliense
    A. caninum
    A. duodenale
    A. tubaeforme
ancylostomatic
ancylostomiasis
    cutaneous a.
ancyroid
Andernach ossicle
Andersch
    A. ganglion
    A. nerve
Anders disease
Andersen disease
Anderson
    A. and Goldberger test
    A. splint
Anderson-Collip test
andersoni
    Dermacentor a.
Andes virus
andira
Andral decubitus
andrenosterone
andriatrics
andriatry
androblastoma
androgen
    adrenal a.
    a. binding protein (ABP)
    a. deprivation
    a. insensitivity syndrome
    a. resistance syndrome
    a. unit
androgenesis
androgenic
    a. alopecia
    a. hormone
    a. steroid
    a. zone
androgenous
androgynism
androgynoid
androgynous
androgyny

android
    a. obesity
    a. pelvis
andrology
andromedotoxin
andromorphous
andropathy
andropause
androphobia
androstane
androstanediol
androstanedione
androstene
androstenediol
androstenedione
androstenol
androstenolone
androsterone
anecdotal
anechoic chamber
anelectrotonic
anelectrotonus
Anel method
anemia
    achlorhydric a.
    achrestic a.
    acquired hemolytic a.
    Addison a.
    addisonian a.
    angiopathic hemolytic a.
    aplastic a.
    asiderotic a.
    autoimmune hemolytic a.
    Bartonella a.
    Belgian Congo a.
    Biermer a.
    brickmaker's a.
    chlorotic a.
    congenital aplastic a.
    congenital dyserythropoietic a.
    congenital Heinz body hemolytic a.
    congenital hypoplastic a.
    congenital nonregenerative a.
    Cooley a.
    cow milk a.
    crescent cell a.
    deficiency a.
    Diamond-Blackfan a.
    dilution a.
    dimorphic a.
    diphyllobothrium a.
    drepanocytic a.

NOTES

anemia *(continued)*
    dyshemopoietic a.
    Ehrlich a.
    elliptocytary a.
    elliptocytotic a.
    equine infectious a.
    erythroblastic a.
    erythronormoblastic a.
    essential a.
    exercise-induced a.
    Faber a.
    false a.
    familial hypoplastic a.
    familial microcytic a.
    familial pyridoxine-responsive a.
    Fanconi a.
    feline infectious a.
    fish tapeworm a.
    folic acid deficiency a.
    goat's milk a.
    a. gravis
    ground itch a.
    Heinz body a.
    hemolytic a.
    hemorrhagic a.
    hookworm a.
    hyperchromatic a.
    hyperchromic a.
    hypochromic microcytic a.
    hypoferric a.
    hypoplastic a.
    infectious a.
    iron deficiency a.
    isochromic a.
    lead a.
    leukoerythroblastic a.
    local a.
    macrocytic achylic a.
    malignant a.
    Marchiafava-Micheli a.
    megaloblastic a.
    megalocytic a.
    metaplastic a.
    microangiopathic hemolytic a.
    microcytic a.
    microdrepanocytic a.
    milk a.
    myelopathic a.
    myelophthisic a.
    neonatal a.
    a. neonatorum
    normochromic a.
    normocytic a.
    pernicious a.
    profound a.
    refractory a.
    sickle cell a.
    sideroachrestic a.
    sideroblastic a.
    spherocytic a.
    sports a.
    spur cell a.
    traumatic a.
    tropical a.
    tunnel a.

anemic
    a. anoxia
    a. halo
    a. hypoxia
    a. infarct
    a. murmur
    a. polyneuritis
    a. urine

anemometer
anemonol
anemophobia
anemotrophy
anencephalia
anencephalic
anencephalous
anencephaly
anenterous
anenzymia
anephric
anepiploic
anergasia
anergastic
anergia
anergic leishmaniasis
anergy
    cutaneous a.
    negative a.
    positive a.

aneroid manometer
anerythroplasia
anerythroplastic
anerythroregenerative
anesthecinesia
anesthekinesia
anesthesia
    acupuncture a.
    ambulatory a.
    axillary a.
    balanced a.
    basal a.
    block a.
    brachial a.
    caudal a.
    cervical a.
    circle absorption a.
    closed a.
    compression a.
    conduction a.
    continuous epidural a.
    continuous spinal a.
    crossed a.
    dental a.
    diagnostic a.

differential spinal a.
dissociated a.
dissociative a.
a. dolorosa
electric a.
cndotrachcal a.
epidural a.
extradural a.
facial a.
field block a.
fractional epidural a.
fractional spinal a.
general a.
girdle a.
glove a.
gustatory a.
high spinal a.
hyperbaric spinal a.
hypobaric spinal a.
hypotensive a.
hypothermic a.
hysterical a.
infiltration a.
inhalation a.
insufflation a.
intercostal a.
intramedullary a.
intranasal a.
intraoral a.
intraosseous a.
intraspinal a.
intratracheal a.
intravenous a.
intravenous regional a.
isobaric spinal a.
local a.
low spinal a.
a. machine
nerve block a.
nonrebreathing a.
open drop a.
patient-controlled a. (PCA)
peridural a.
perineural a.
rebreathing a.
a. record
rectal a.
refrigeration a.
regional a.
retrobulbar a.
saddle block a.
segmental a.

semiclosed a.
semiopen a.
spinal a.
splanchnic a.
stocking a.
surgical a.
tactile a.
thermal a.
thermic a.
topical a.
traumatic a.
unilateral a.
visceral a.
anesthesiologist
anesthesiology
anesthetic
    a. circuit
    a. depth
    a. ether
    flammable a.
    a. gas
    general a.
    a. index
    inhalation a.
    intravenous a.
    a. leprosy
    local a.
    primary a.
    secondary a.
    a. shock
    a. vapor
anesthetist
    certified registered nurse a.
anesthetization
anesthetize
anestrous ovulation
anestrum
anestrus
anethopath
anetoderma
    Jadassohn-Pellizzari a.
aneuploid
aneuploidy
aneurine pyrophosphate
aneurolemmic
aneurysm
    abdominal aortic a. (AAA)
    ampullary a.
    a. by anastomosis
    aortic sinus a.
    arteriosclerotic a.
    arteriovenous a.

NOTES

aneurysm *(continued)*
  atherosclerotic a.
  axial a.
  benign bone a.
  Bérard a.
  berry a.
  cardiac a.
  Charcot-Bouchard a.
  cirsoid a.
  compound a.
  congenital cerebral a.
  consecutive a.
  coronary artery a.
  cylindroid a.
  diffuse a.
  dissecting a.
  ductal a.
  ectatic a.
  embolic a.
  embolomycotic a.
  endogenous a.
  erosive a.
  exogenous a.
  false a.
  fusiform a.
  hernial a.
  infraclinoid a.
  intracavernous a.
  intracranial a.
  miliary a.
  mycotic a.
  a. needle
  Park a.
  phantom a.
  Pott a.
  racemose a.
  Rasmussen a.
  saccular a.
  sacculated a.
  subclinoid a.
  supraclinoid a.
  syphilitic a.
  varicose a.
aneurysmal
  a. bone cyst
  a. bruit
  a. cough
  a. murmur
  a. phthisis
  a. sac
  a. thrill
  a. varix
aneurysmatic
aneurysmectomy
aneurysmograph
aneurysmoplasty
aneurysmorrhaphy
aneurysmotomy

ANF
  antinuclear factor
  atrial natriuretic factor
angelica root
Angelman syndrome
Angelucci syndrome
angel wing
Anger camera
angiectasia
  congenital dysplastic a.
angiectasis
angiectatic
angiectopia
angiitis
  allergic granulomatous a.
  consecutive a.
  frosted branch a.
  hypersensitivity a.
angina
  abdominal a.
  a. abdominis
  agranulocytic a.
  crescendo a.
  a. cruris
  a. decubitus
  a. of effort
  false a.
  Heberden a.
  hypercyanotic a.
  intestinal a.
  a. inversa
  Ludwig a.
  lymphatic a.
  a. lymphomatosa
  a. pectoris
  preinfarction a.
  Prinzmetal a.
  unstable a.
  variant a.
  Vincent a.
  walk-through a.
anginal
anginiform
anginoid
anginophobia
anginosa
  scarlatina a.
anginose scarlatina
anginous
angioarchitecture
angioblast
angioblastic
  a. cell
  a. cyst
angioblastoma of Nakagawa
angiocardiocinetic
angiocardiography
  exercise radionuclide a.

gated radionuclide a.
radionuclide a.
angiocardiokinetic
angiocardiopathy
angiocholitis
angiocyst
angioderm
angiodysgenetic myelomalacia
angiodysplasia
angiodystrophy, angiodystrophia
angioedema
hereditary a.
angioelephantiasis
angioendothelioma
angioendotheliomatosis
angiofibrolipoma
angiofibroma
juvenile a.
angiofibrosis
angiofollicular mediastinal lymph node hyperplasia
angiogenesis factor
angiogenic
angioglioma
angiogliomatosis
angiogliosis
angiogram
projection a.
angiographic
angiography
aortic arch a.
biplane a.
a. catheter
cerebral a.
coronary a.
digital subtraction a. (DSA)
emission a.
fluorescein a.
indocyanine green a.
interventional a.
magnetic resonance a. (MRA)
magnification a.
peripheral a.
pulmonary a.
radionuclide a.
subtraction a.
angiohyalinosis
angiohypertonia
angiohypotonia
angioid streak
angioimmunoblastic
a. lymphadenopathy

a. lymphadenopathy with dysproteinemia
angioinvasive
angiokeratoma
diffuse a.
Fordyce a.
Mibelli a.
angiokeratosis
angiokinesis
angiokinetic
angioleiomyoma
angiolipofibroma
angiolipoma
angiolith
angiolithic
a. degeneration
a. sarcoma
angiologia
angiology
angiolupoid
angiolymphoid hyperplasia
angiolysis
angioma
acquired tufted a.
capillary a.
cavernous a.
cherry a.
a. serpiginosum
spider a.
telangiectatic a.
venous a.
angiomatoid
angiomatosis
bacillary a.
cephalotrigeminal a.
cerebroretinal a.
congenital dysplastic a.
cutaneomeningospinal a.
encephalotrigeminal a.
angiomatous
angiomegaly
angiomyocardiac
angiomyofibroma
angiomyolipoma
angiomyoma
angiomyopathy
angiomyosarcoma
angiomyxoma
aggressive a.
angioneurectomy
angioneuropathy

NOTES

angioneurotic
    a. anuria
    a. dermatosis
    a. edema
angioneurotomy
angioosteohypertrophy syndrome
angioparalysis
angioparalytic neurasthenia
angioparesis
angiopathic
    a. hemolytic anemia
    a. neurasthenia
angiopathy
    amyloid a.
    cerebral amyloid a.
    congophilic a.
    giant cell hyaline a.
angiophacomatosis, angiophakomatosis
angioplany
angioplasty
    a. balloon
    percutaneous transluminal a. (PTA)
    percutaneous transluminal
      coronary a. (PTCA)
angiopoiesis
angiopoietic
angiorrhaphy
angiosarcoma
angiosclerotica
    dysbasia a.
    myasthenia a.
angioscope
angioscopy
angioscotoma
angioscotometry
angiosis
angiosome
angiospasm
angiospastic
angiospastica
    dysbasia a.
angiostenosis
angiostrongylosis
angiotelectasia
angiotelectasis
angiotensin
    a. III amide
    a. I, II, III
    a. precursor
    a. receptor
    a. receptor blocker
angiotensinase
angiotensin-converting
    a.-c. enzyme (ACE)
    a.-c. enzyme inhibitor (ACEI)
angiotensinogen
angiotensinogenase
angiotomy
angiotonia

angiotribe
angiotrophic
angitis
angle
    acromial a.
    acute a.
    adjacent a.
    alpha a.
    alveolar a.
    anorectal a.
    apical a.
    axial a.
    basilar a.
    Bennett a.
    beta a.
    biorbital a.
    Broca basilar a.
    Broca facial a.
    buccal a.
    buccoocclusal a.
    cardiodiaphragmatic a.
    cardiohepatic a.
    cardiophrenic a.
    carrying a.
    cavity line a.
    cavosurface a.
    cephalic a.
    cephalomedullary a.
    cerebellopontine a.
    A. classification
    A. classification of malocclusion
    a. of convergence
    costal a.
    costophrenic a.
    costovertebral a. (CVA)
    costoxiphoid a.
    craniofacial a.
    critical a.
    cusp a.
    Daubenton a.
    a. of deviation
    disparity a.
    distal a.
    duodenojejunal a.
    a. of eccentricity
    epigastric a.
    ethmoid a.
    facial a.
    filtration a.
    flip a.
    Frankfort-mandibular incisor a.
    frontal a.
    a. of Fuchs
    gamma a.
    hypsiloid a.
    impedance a.
    incident a.
    incisal guide a.
    infrasternal a.

iridocorneal a.
Jacquart facial a.
kappa a.
limiting a.
line a.
Louis a.
Lovibond a.
Ludwig a.
lumbosacral a.
mastoid a.
maxillary a.
medial a.
mesial a.
metafacial a.
meter a.
pelvivertebral a.
point a.
pubic a.
a. recession
sternal a.
sternoclavicular a.
subpubic a.
a. suture
ureterovesical a. (UVA)
urethrovesical a.
venous a.
visual a.
angle-closure glaucoma
angor
a. nocturnus
a. ocularis
a. pectoris
Ångström
Ångström law
Ångström scale
Ångström unit
angstrom
angular
a. acceleration
a. aldehyde
a. aperture
a. artery
a. cheilitis
a. conjunctivitis
a. convolution
a. curvature
a. gyrus
a. incision
a. incisure
a. methyl
a. notch
a. sphincter

a. spine
a. stomatitis
a. vein
angularis
dens a.
incisura a.
angulation
apex anterior a.
apex posterior a.
angulus
anhaphia
anhedonia
anhepatic jaundice
anhepatogenous jaundice
anhidrosis
anhidrotic ectodermal dysplasia
anhistic
anhistous
anhydrase
carbonic a.
anhydration
anhydride
carbonic a.
coumaric a.
anhydroleucovorin
anhydrosugar
anhydrous
a. alcohol
a. chloral
a. lanolin
ani (*pl. of* anus)
aniacinamidosis
aniacinosis
anicteric
a. leptospirosis
a. viral hepatitis
a. virus hepatitis
anidean
anideus
embryonic a.
anidous
anileridine
anilide
anilinction
anilinctus
aniline
a. blue
a. fuchsin
a. gentian violet
a. red
anilingus
anilinism

NOTES

anilinophil
anilinophile
anilinophilous
anilism
animal
    a. black
    a. charcoal
    control a.
    conventional a.
    a. dextran
    a. force
    a. graft
    Houssay a.
    a. magnetism
    a. model
    a. pole
    a. protein factor
    a. psychology
    a. soap
    a. starch
    a. toxin
    a. wax
animalcule
anima mundi
animation
    suspended a.
animatism
animism
animus
AN interval
anion
    a. exchange
    a. exchanger
    a. gap
anion-exchange resin
anionic neutrophil-activating peptide
  (ANAP)
anionotropy
aniridia
anisakiasis
anisakid
anisate
anise
aniseikonia
anisic
anisindione
anisoaccommodation
anisochromasia
anisochromatic
anisocoria
    essential a.
anisocytosis
anisodactylous
anisodactyly
anisogamy
anisognathous
anisokaryosis
anisole
anisomastia

anisomelia
anisometropia
anisometropic amblyopia
anisopiesis
anisorrhythmia
anisosphygmia
anisosthenic
anisotonic
anisotropic
    a. disc
    a. lipid
anitrata
    Lingelsheimia a.
Anitschkow
    A. cell
    A. myocyte
ankle
    a. bone
    a. clonus
    a. jerk
    a. joint
    a. reflex
    a. region
ankle-foot orthosis
ankyloblepharon
ankylodactyly, ankylodactylia
ankyloglossia superior syndrome
ankylomele
ankylopoietic
ankylosed tooth
ankylosing
    a. hyperostosis
    a. spondylitis
ankylosis
    artificial a.
    bony a.
    capsular a.
    dental a.
    extracapsular a.
    false a.
    fibrous a.
    intracapsular a.
    ligamentous a.
    partial a.
    spurious a.
    true a.
ankylostomiasis
ankylotic
ankyrin
ankyroid
anlage
anneal
annealing
    a. lamp
    a. tray
annectent gyrus
annelid
annellide
annelloconidium

annexa
annexal
annihilation radiation
annular (*var. of* anular)
annularis
    lichen planus a.
    lipoatrophia a.
annuloaortic ectasia
annuloplasty ring
annulorrhaphy
annulospiral
    a. ending
    a. organ
annulus (*var. of* anulus)
AnOC
    anodal opening contraction
anochromasia
anococcygeal
    a. body
    a. ligament
    a. nerve
anocutaneous line
anodal
    a. closure contraction (ACC, AnCC)
    a. current
    a. opening contraction (AnOC, AOC)
anode
    a. ray
    rotating a.
anoderm
anodic
anodontia
anodontism
anodyne
anoetic
anogenital
    a. band
    a. raphe
anomalad
anomalies (*pl. of* anomaly)
anomaloscope
anomalous
    a. atrioventricular excitation
    a. complex
    a. conduction
    a. mitral arcade
    a. pulmonary venous connection
    a. retinal correspondence
    a. trichromatism

    a. uterus
    a. viscosity
anomalus
    Hoplopsyllus a.
anomaly, pl. anomalies
    Alder a.
    Aristotle a.
    asplenia with cardiovascular anomalies
    Chédiak-Steinbrinck-Higashi a.
    developmental a.
    Ebstein a.
    eugnathic a.
    Freund a.
    Hegglin a.
    May-Hegglin a.
    Rieger a.
    Shone a.
    urogenital sinus a.
anomer
anomeric carbon
anomia
anomic aphasia
anomie
anonychia
anonychosis
anonyma
anonymous vein
Anopheles
anophelicide
anophelifuge
anopheline
anophelism
anophthalmia
anophthalmos
anoplasty
anopsia
    amblyopia ex a.
anorchia
anorchism
anorectal
    a. agenesis
    a. angle
    a. dressing
    a. flexure
    a. junction
    a. lymph node
    a. spasm
    a. syndrome
anorectic, anoretic
anorectoperineal muscle
anorexia nervosa

NOTES

anorexiant
anorexic
anorexigenic
anorgasmia
anorgasmy
anorthography
anoscope
    Bacon a.
anosigmoidoscopy
anosmia
    hypogonadism with a.
anosmic
anosodiaphoria
anosognosia
anosognosic
    a. epilepsy
    a. seizure
anospinal center
anosteoplasia
anostosis
anotia
ANOVA
    analysis of variance
anovesical
anovular
    a. menstruation
    a. ovarian follicle
anovulation
anovulational menstruation
anovulatory cycle
anoxemia test
anoxia
    anemic a.
    anoxic a.
    diffusion a.
    gastric a.
    histotoxic a.
    a. neonatorum
    stagnant a.
anoxic anoxia
ANP
    atrial natriuretic peptide
    ANP clearance receptor
Anrep
    A. effect
    A. phenomenon
ansa
    a. cervicalis
    Haller a.
    Henle a.
    lenticular a.
ansae nervorum spinalium
ansate
Ansbacher unit
anserina
    cutis a.
anserine
    a. bursa
    a. bursitis

anserinus
    pes a.
ansiform lobule
Anson-McVay operation
ansoparamedian fissure
ansotomy
ant
    black imported fire a.
    fire a.
    harvester a.
    red imported fire a.
antacid
antagonism
    bacterial a.
antagonist
    aldosterone a.
    alpha-adrenoceptor a.
    associated a.
    calcium a.
    competitive a.
    enzyme a.
    folic acid a.
    insulin a.
    leukotriene receptor a.
    opioid a.
antagonistic
    a. muscle
    a. reflex
antalgesia
antalgic gait
antalkaline
antaphrodisiac
antaphroditic
antarthritic
antasthenic
antasthmatic
antatrophic
antebrachial fascia
antebrachium
antecardium
antecedent
    plasma thromboplastin a.
    a. sign
antecubital space
antefebrile
anteflex
anteflexion
antegonial notch
antegrade
    a. block
    a. cardioplegia
    a. conduction
    a. cystography
    a. pyelography
    a. urography
antemortem
    a. clot
    a. thrombus
antenatal diagnosis

antepartum
anteposition
antepyretic
anterior
    a. acoustic stria
    a. ampullary nerve
    a. amygdaloid area
    a. antebrachial nerve
    a. antebrachial region
    a. aphasia
    a. apprehension test
    a. articular surface
    a. asynclitism
    a. atlantooccipital membrane
    a. auricular branch
    a. auricular groove
    a. auricular muscle
    a. auricular nerve
    a. auricular vein
    a. axillary fold
    a. axillary line
    a. axillary lymph node
    a. basal branch
    a. basal segment
    a. basal segmental artery
    a. basal vein
    a. border
    a. brachial region
    a. cardiac vein
    a. cardinal vein
    a. carpal region
    a. cecal artery
    a. central convolution
    a. central gyrus
    a. centriole
    a. cerebellar notch
    a. cerebral artery
    a. cerebral vein
    a. cervical discectomy and fusion (ACDF)
    a. cervical intertransversarii muscle
    a. cervical intertransverse muscle
    a. cervical region
    a. chamber
    a. chamber cleavage syndrome
    a. chamber trabecula
    a. choroidal artery
    a. choroiditis
    a. ciliary artery
    a. ciliary vein
    a. circumflex humeral artery
    a. circumflex humeral vein
    a. clear space
    a. clinoid process
    a. column
    a. communicating artery
    a. condyloid foramen
    a. conjunctival artery
    a. corneal dystrophy
    a. coronary periarterial plexus
    a. corticospinal tract
    a. costotransverse ligament
    a. cranial base
    a. cranial fossa
    a. cruciate ligament
    a. crural nerve
    a. crural region
    a. cubital region
    a. curvature
    a. cusp
    a. cutaneous branch
    a. deep cervical lymph node
    a. elastic lamina
    a. elastic layer
    a. embryotoxon
    a. ethmoidal air cell
    a. ethmoidal artery
    a. ethmoidal nerve
    a. external arcuate fiber
    a. facial height (AFH)
    a. facial vein
    a. fascicle
    a. fasciculus proprius
    a. femoral cutaneous nerve
    a. focal point
    a. fontanelle
    forceps a.
    a. fovea
    a. funiculus
    funiculus a.
    a. gray column
    a. gray commissure
    a. ground bundle
    a. guide
    a. horn
    a. horn cell
    a. humeral circumflex artery
    a. hypothalamic area
    a. hypothalamic nucleus
    a. hypothalamic region
    a. inferior cerebellar artery
    a. inferior iliac spine
    a. inferior renal segment
    a. intercostal artery

NOTES

anterior *(continued)*
- a. intercostal branch
- a. intercostal vein
- a. intermediate groove
- a. intermediate sulcus
- a. interosseous artery
- a. interosseous nerve
- a. interpositus nucleus
- a. interventricular artery
- a. interventricular branch
- a. interventricular groove
- a. interventricular sulcus
- a. intestinal portal
- a. intraoccipital joint
- a. intraoccipital synchondrosis
- a. jugular lymph node
- a. jugular vein
- a. junction line
- a. knee region
- a. labial artery
- a. labial branch
- a. labial commissure
- a. labial nerve
- a. labial vein
- a. lacrimal crest
- a. lateral malleolar artery
- a. lateral nasal branch
- a. limiting lamina
- a. limiting layer
- a. limiting ring
- a. lingual gland
- a. lip
- a. lobe
- a. longitudinal ligament
- a. lunate lobule
- a. medial malleolar artery
- a. median fissure
- a. median line
- a. mediastinal artery
- a. mediastinal lymph node
- a. mediastinoscopy
- a. mediastinotomy
- a. mediastinum
- a. medullary velum
- a. megalophthalmos
- a. meningeal artery
- a. meningeal branch
- a. meniscofemoral ligament
- musculus tibiofascialis a.
- a. myocardial infarction
- a. naris
- a. nasal spine
- a. neuropore
- a. occlusion
- a. ocular segment
- a. olfactory nucleus
- a. palatine arch
- a. palatine foramen
- a. palatine suture

- a. palpebral margin
- a. paracentral gyrus
- a. parietal artery
- a. parolfactory sulcus
- a. pectoral cutaneous branch
- a. pelvic exenteration
- a. perforated substance
- a. perforating artery
- a. perineum
- a. periventricular nucleus
- a. peroneal artery
- a. pharyngotomy
- a. pillar
- a. piriform gyrus
- a. pituitary gonadotropin
- a. pituitary-like hormone
- a. pole
- a. pontomesencephalic vein
- a. pyramid
- a. quadrigeminal body
- a. ramus
- a. raphespinal tract
- a. rectus muscle
- a. rhinoscopy
- a. rhizotomy
- a. sacrococcygeal ligament
- a. sacroiliac ligament
- a. sacrosciatic ligament
- a. scalene muscle
- a. scleritis
- a. sclerotomy
- a. scrotal nerve
- a. scrotal vein
- a. segmental artery
- a. semicircular canal
- a. septal branch
- a. serratus muscle
- a. sinus
- a. spinal artery
- a. spinocerebellar tract
- a. spinothalamic tract
- a. staphyloma
- a. sternoclavicular ligament
- a. superficial cervical lymph node
- a. superior alveolar artery
- a. superior alveolar nerve
- a. superior dental artery
- a. superior iliac spine
- a. superior pancreaticoduodenal artery
- a. superior renal segment
- a. superior segmental artery
- a. supraclavicular nerve
- a. talofibular ligament
- a. talotibial ligament
- a. tarsal tendinous sheath
- a. tegmental decussation
- a. temporal artery
- a. temporal branch

a. thalamic radiation
a. thalamic tubercle
a. thoracotomy
a. tibial bursa
a. tibial compartment syndrome
a. tibial lymph node
a. tibial muscle
a. tibial nerve
a. tibial recurrent artery
a. tibial vein
a. tibiofascial muscle
a. tibiofibular ligament
a. tibiotalar ligament
a. tooth
a. transverse temporal gyrus
a. trigeminothalamic tract
a. tympanic artery
a. urethra
a. urethral valve
a. urethritis
a. uveitis
a. vertebral vein
a. vestibular artery
a. vitrectomy
a. white commissure
anterius
    mediastinum a.
anterofacial dysplasia
anterograde
a. amnesia
a. block
a. conduction
a. memory
anteroinferior
a. myocardial infarction
a. surface
anterointernal
anterolateral
a. central artery
a. column
a. cordotomy
a. fontanelle
a. groove
a. myocardial infarction
a. striate artery
a. sulcus
a. surface
a. system
a. thalamostriate artery
a. tract
a. tractotomy
anterolisthesis

anteromedial
a. central artery
a. central branch
a. frontal branch
a. intermuscular septum
a. nucleus
a. thalamostriate artery
anteromedian groove
anteroposterior (AP)
a. diameter
a. dysplasia
a. facial dysplasia
a. projection
anteroseptal myocardial infarction
anterosuperior surface
anteroventral nucleus
antesystole
anteversion
anteverted
anthelix (*var. of* antihelix)
anthelmintic, anthelminthic
anthelone E, U
antheridium
anthiolimine
anthocyanin
anthracemia
anthracene
anthracic
anthracin
anthracis
    Bacillus a.
anthracoid
anthracosilicosis
anthracosis
anthracotic tuberculosis
anthracycline
anthralin
anthramucin
anthrapurpurin
anthrax
    cerebral a.
    cutaneous a.
    intestinal a.
a. septicemia
a. toxin
anthrone
anthropobiology
anthropocentric
anthropogenesis
anthropogenic, anthropogenetic
anthropogeny
anthropogony

NOTES

anthropography
anthropoid pelvis
anthropology
    criminal a.
    cultural a.
    dental a.
anthropometer
anthropometric
anthropometry
anthropomorphism
anthroponomy
anthroponotic cutaneous leishmaniasis
anthropopathy
anthropophilic
anthropophobia
anthroposcopy
anthroposomatology
anthropozoonosis
antiadrenergic
antiagglutinin
antialexin
antiallergic
antialopecia factor
antianaphylaxis
antiandrogen
antianemic
    a. factor
    a. principle
antiangiogenesis factor
antiantibody
antiantitoxin
antianxiety agent
antiarachnolysin
antiarrhythmic
antiarthritic
antiasthmatic
antiautolysin
antibacterial
antibasement
    a. membrane antibody
    a. membrane glomerulonephritis
    a. membrane nephritis
antibechic
antiberiberi
    a. factor
    a. vitamin
antibiont
antibiosis
antibiotic
    aminoglycoside a.
    bactericidal a.
    bacteriostatic a.
    beta-lactam a.
    broad-spectrum a.
    carbapenem a.
    cephalosporin a.
    a. enterocolitis
    fluoroquinolone a.
    glycopeptide a.

    lincosamide a.
    macrolide a.
    oral a.
    peptide a.
    polyene a.
    a. sensitivity
    a. sensitivity test
    sulfonamide a.
    tetracycline a.
    topical a.
antibiotic-resistant
antibiotin
anti–black-tongue factor
antiblennorrhagic
antibody (Ab)
    affinity a.
    agglutinating a.
    anaphylactic a.
    antibasement membrane a.
    anticardiolipin a.
    antiidiotype a.
    anti-MAG a.
    antineutrophil cytoplasmic a.
      (ANCA)
    antinuclear a. (ANA)
    antiphospholipid a.
    antithyroglobulin a.
    avidity a.
    bivalent a.
    blocking a.
    blood group a.
    catalytic a.
    cell-bound a.
    chimeric a.
    cold a.
    cold-reactive a.
    complement-fixing a.
    complete a.
    cross-reacting a.
    cytophilic a.
    cytotropic a.
    a. deficiency disease
    a. deficiency syndrome
    Donath-Landsteiner a.
    a. excess
    fluorescent a.
    fluorescent antinuclear a. (FANA)
    Forssman a.
    a. to the hepatitis B core antigen
      (HBcAb)
    a. to the hepatitis B e antigen
      (HBeAb)
    a. to the hepatitis B surface
      antigen (HBsAb)
    heterocytotropic a.
    heterogenetic a.
    heterophil a.
    homocytotropic a.
    human antimouse a.

idiotypic a.
immobilizing a.
incomplete a.
inhibiting a.
lymphocytotoxic a.
monoclonal a. (MAB, MoAb)
natural a.
neutralizing a.
normal a.
reaginic a.
univalent a.
antibody-combining site
antibody-dependent cell-mediated
cytotoxicity
antibrachial
antibrachium
antibromic
anticalculous
anticardiolipin antibody
anticarious
anticathexis
anticephalalgic
anticholagogue
anticholinergic
1-antichymotrypsin
anticipate
anticipation
anticlinal
anticnemion
anticoagulant
lupus a.
a. therapy
anticoding strand
anticodon
anticomplement
anticomplementary
a. factor
a. serum
anticontagious
anticonvulsant
anticonvulsive
anticurare
anticus
musculus tibiofascialis a.
anticytotoxin
antidepressant
antidermatitis factor
antidiabetic
antidiarrheal
antidiarrhetic
anti-D immunoglobulin

antidiuresis
antidiuretic hormone (ADH)
antidotal
antidote
chemical a.
mechanical a.
physiologic a.
antidromic
antidysenteric
antidyskinetic agent
antidysrhythmic
antidysuric
antiemetic
antienergic
antienzyme
antiepileptic
antiepithelial serum
antiestrogen
antiestrogenic
antifebrile
antifibrillatory
antifibrinolysin
antifibrinolytic
antifoaming agent
antifolic
antifungal
antigen
ABO a.
acetone-insoluble a.
allogeneic a.
Am a.
antibody to the hepatitis B core a.
(HBcAb)
antibody to the hepatitis B e a.
(HBeAb)
antibody to the hepatitis B
surface a. (HBsAb)
Au a.
Aus a.
Australia a.
autologous a.
bacterial a.
Bea a.
Becker a.
bi a.
Bile a.
blood group a.
By a.
CA-125 a.
CA-15-3 a.
CA-19-9 a.
capsular a.

NOTES

antigen *(continued)*
  carcinoembryonic a. (CEA)
  Casoni a.
  C carbohydrate a.
  cholesterinized a.
  Chra a.
  class I, II, III a.
  cluster of differentiation a.
  common a.
  complete a.
  conjugated a.
  D a.
  delta a.
  Dharmendra a.
  Di a.
  Duffy a.
  epithelial membrane a. (EMA)
  a. excess
  flagellar a.
  Forssman a.
  Fy a.
  G a.
  Ge a.
  Gerbich a.
  Gm a.
  Good a.
  Gr a.
  group a.
  H a.
  H-2 a.
  He a.
  heart a.
  hepatitis-associated a. (HAA)
  hepatitis B core a. (HBcAg)
  hepatitis B e a. (HBe, HBeAg)
  hepatitis B surface a. (HBsAg)
  heterogeneic a.
  heterogenetic a.
  heterogenic enterobacterial a.
  heterophil a.
  hexon a.
  Hikojima a.
  histocompatibility a.
  Ho a.
  homologous a.
  Hu a.
  human leukocyte a. (HLA)
  H-Y a.
  I a.
  incomplete a.
  a. interferon
  Jk a.
  Jobbins a.
  Js a.
  K a.
  Kell a.
  Kidd a.
  Km a.
  Kunin a.
  Kveim a.
  Kveim-Siltzbach a.
  Lan a.
  Le a.
  leukocyte common a.
  Levay a.
  Lu a.
  lymphocyte function associated a.
  lymphogranuloma venereum a.
  Lyt a.
  M a.
  Mc a.
  Mg a.
  Mitsuda a.
  M1, M2 a.
  MNSs a.
  mumps skin test a.
  O a.
  oncofetal a.
  organ-specific a.
  partial a.
  a. peptide
  proliferating cell nuclear a.
  prostate-specific a.
  sensitized a.
  somatic a.
  species-specific a.
  T a.
  tissue-specific a.
  tumor a.
  tumor-specific transplantation a.
  a. unit
antigen-antibody
  a.-a. complex
  a.-a. reaction (AAR)
antigen-binding site
antigenemia
antigenic
  a. competition
  a. complex
  a. determinant
  a. drift
  a. shift
  a. variation
antigenicity
antigenome
antigen-presenting cell
antigen-responsive cell
antigen-sensitive cell
antiglobulin test
antigonorrheic
antigravity muscle
anti-G suit
anti-HBc
anti-HBe
anti-HBs
antihelix, anthelix
  leg of a.
antihelminthic

antihemagglutinin
antihemolysin
antihemolytic
antihemophilic
    a. factor A, B
    a. globulin
    a. globulin A, B
    a. plasma
antihemorrhagic
    a. factor
    a. vitamin
antihistamine
antihistaminic
antihormone
antihuman
    a. globulin
    a. globulin test
antihydropic
antihypertensive
antihypnotic
antihypotensive
anti-icteric
antiidiotype
    a. antibody
    a. autoantibody
antiinflammatory
anti-insulin
antiketogenesis
antiketogenic
antikidney serum nephritis
anti-Lepore
    hemoglobin a.-L.
antileukocidin
antileukotoxin
antileukotriene
anti-Lewisite
    British a.-L.
antilipotropic
antilithic
antilobium
antiluteogenic
antilymphocyte
    a. globulin
    a. serum
antilysin
anti-MAG antibody
antimalarial
antimere
antimesenteric
antimetabolite
antimetropia
antimicrobial spectrum

antimitotic
antimongoloid
antimonid
antimonous oxide
anti-Monson curve
antimony
    a. chloride
    a. oxide
antimonyl
anti-müllerian hormone
antimuscarinic
antimutagen
antimutagenic
antimyasthenic
antimycotic
antinauseant
antineoplastic
antineoplastons
antineuritic
    a. factor
    a. vitamin
antineurotoxin
antineutrophil cytoplasmic antibody
  (ANCA)
antiniad
antinial
antinion
antinomy
antinuclear
    a. antibody (ANA)
    a. factor (ANF)
antiodontalgic
antioncogene
antioxidant
antipain
antiparallel strand
antiparasitic
antipedicular
antipediculotic
antipellagra factor
antiperiodic
antiperistalsis
antiperistaltic anastomosis
antipernicious anemia factor
antiperspirant
antiphagocytic
antiphlogistic
antiphobic
antiphospholipid
    a. antibody
    a. antibody syndrome
antiplasmin

NOTES

antiplatelet
antipneumococcic
antipodal cone
antipode
antiport
antiporter
anti-Pr cold autoagglutinin
antiprecipitin
antiprogestin
antiprothrombin
antipruritic
antipsychotic agent
antipurine
antipyogenic
antipyresis
antipyretic
antipyrimidine
antipyrine acetylsalicylate
antipyrotic
antirabies serum
antirachitic vitamin
antireflection coating
antireticular cytotoxic serum
antirheumatic
antiricin
antiruminant
antiscorbutic vitamin
antiseborrheic
antisecretory
antisense
    a. DNA
    a. drug
    a. RNA
    a. strand
    a. therapy
antisepsis
antiseptic dressing
antiserum
    a. anaphylaxis
    blood group a.
    heterologous a.
    homologous a.
antishock garment
antisialagogue
antisideric
antisocial
    a. personality
    a. personality disorder
antispasmodic
antistaphylococcic
antistaphylolysin
antisteapsin
antisterility
    a. factor
    a. vitamin
antistreptococcic
antistreptokinase
antistreptolysin
antitac

antitermination protein
antitetanic
antithenar
antithrombin
    a. III
    a. test
antithyroglobulin antibody
antithyroid
antitonic
antitoxic
    a. serum
    a. unit
antitoxigen
antitoxin
    bivalent gas gangrene a.
    bothropic a.
    Bothrops a.
    botulinum a.
    botulism a.
    bovine a.
    Crotalus a.
    despeciated a.
    diphtheria a.
    dysentery a.
    gas gangrene a.
    normal a.
    a. rash
    a. unit
antitoxinogen
antitragicus muscle
antitragohelicine fissure
antitragus
antitreponemal
antitrismus
antitrope
antitropic
antitrypsic
1-antitrypsin deficiency
antitrypsin deficiency
antitryptic index
antitumor
    a. enzyme
    a. protein
antitumorigenesis
antitussive
antityphoid
antivenene unit
antivenereal
antivenin
antiviral
    a. immunity
    a. protein
antivitamin
antivivisection
antixerophthalmic
antixerotic
Antoni type A, B neurilemoma
Anton syndrome
antra (*pl. of* antrum)

antral
    a. follicle
    a. lavage
    a. pouch
    a. sphincter
antrectomy
antroduodenectomy
antronasal
antrophose
antropyloric
antroscope
antroscopy
antrostomy
    intranasal a.
    intraoral a.
antrotomy
antrotonia
antrotympanic
antrum, pl. **antra**
    cardiac a.
    ethmoid a.
    antra ethmoidalia
    follicular a.
    mastoid a.
    maxillary a.
    pyloric a.
    tympanic a.
Antyllus method
ANUG
    acute necrotizing ulcerative gingivitis
anular, annular
    a. band
    a. cartilage
    a. cataract
    a. lesion
    a. ligament
    a. lipid
    a. pancreas
    a. placenta
    a. plexus
    a. pulley
    a. scleritis
    a. scotoma
    a. sphincter
    a. staphyloma
    a. stricture
    a. synechia
anulare
    erythema a.
anuloplasty
anulus, annulus
    a. abdominalis

    a. ciliaris
    a. conjunctivae
    a. femoralis
    a. fibrosus
    Haller a.
    a. hemorrhoidalis
    a. inguinalis profundus
    a. inguinalis superficialis
    mitral a.
    a. ovalis
    a. tympanicus
    a. umbilicalis
    a. urethralis
    a. of Zinn
anum
    per a.
anuria
    angioneurotic a.
    calculous a.
    obstructive a.
    renal a.
    suppressive a.
anuric
anus, pl. **ani**
    atresia ani
    Bartholin a.
    a. cerebri
    imperforate a.
    pruritus ani
    a. vesicalis
anvil sound
anxiety
    a. attack
    castration a.
    a. disorder
    a. dream
    existential a.
    free-floating a.
    a. hysteria
    a. neurosis
    neurotic a.
    a. reaction
    separation a.
    a. syndrome
    a. tension state
anxiolytic
anxious delirium
AOC
    anodal opening contraction
Aonchotheca
aorta, pl. **aortae**
    abdominal a.

NOTES

aorta *(continued)*
    ascending a.
    bifurcation of a.
    buckled a.
    descending thoracic a.
    double a.
    dynamic a.
    kinked a.
    overriding a.
    thoracic a.
aortal
aortalgia
aortarctia
aortartia
aortectasia
aortectasis
aortectomy
aortic
    a. arch
    a. arch angiography
    a. arch syndrome
    a. area
    a. atresia
    a. bifurcation
    a. body
    a. body tumor
    a. bulb
    a. coarctation
    a. curtain
    a. dissection
    a. dwarfism
    a. facies
    a. foramen
    a. glomera
    a. hiatus
    a. impression
    a. incompetence
    a. insufficiency
    a. isthmus
    a. knob
    a. knuckle
    a. lymphatic plexus
    a. murmur
    a. nerve
    a. nipple
    a. notch
    a. opening
    a. orifice
    a. ostium
    a. prosthesis
    a. reflex
    a. regurgitation
    a. root
    a. sac
    a. septal defect
    a. sinus
    a. sinus aneurysm
    a. spindle
    a. stenosis

    a. sulcus
    a. thrill
    a. valve
    a. vestibule
    a. window
aortica
    glomera a.
aorticopulmonary
    a. septal defect
    a. window
aorticorenal ganglion
aortic-pulmonic window
aortitis
    giant cell a.
aortoannular ectasia
aortocoronary bypass
aortogram
aortography
aortoiliac
    a. bypass
    a. occlusive disease
aortopathy
aortopexy
aortoplasty
aortoptosia
aortoptosis
aortopulmonary
    a. septum
    a. shunt
    a. window
aortorenal bypass
aortorrhaphy
aortosclerosis
aortostenosis
aortotomy incision
AP
    anteroposterior
    AP projection
A&P
    auscultation and percussion
apallesthesia
apallic
    a. state
    a. syndrome
apancreatic
aparalytic
aparathyreosis
aparathyroidism
apareunia
apathetic
    a. affect
    a. hyperthyroidism
    a. thyrotoxicosis
apathism
apathy
apatite calculus
A-pattern
    A-p. esotropia

A-p. exotropia
A-p. strabismus
A-P-C virus
ape
    a. fissure
    a. hand
apellous
apenteric
apepsinia
aperiodic biopolymer
aperiosteal amputation
aperistalsis
aperitive
apertognathia
apertometer
Apert syndrome
apertura
aperture
    angular a.
    a. diaphragm
    external acoustic a.
    frontal sinus a.
    inferior pelvic a.
    inferior thoracic a.
    laryngeal a.
    lateral a.
    median a.
    superior pelvic a.
apex, pl. **apices**
    a. anterior angulation
    a. auriculae
    a. beat
    a. pneumonia
    a. posterior angulation
    a. prostatae
    a. pulmonis
    a. radicis dentis
    a. satyri
    a. vesicae
apexcardiogram
apexcardiography
apexification
apexigraph
Apgar score
aphagia
aphakia
aphakic
    a. eye
    a. glaucoma
aphalangia
aphasia
    acoustic a.

    acquired epileptic a.
    amnesic a.
    anomic a.
    anterior a.
    associative a.
    ataxic a.
    auditory a.
    Broca a.
    conduction a.
    crossed a.
    expressive a.
    fluent a.
    functional a.
    global a.
    graphic a.
    graphomotor a.
    impressive a.
    jargon a.
    mixed a.
    motor a.
    nominal a.
    nonfluent a.
    posterior a.
    primary progressive a.
    receptive a.
    sensory a.
    total a.
    transcortical a.
    visual a.
    Wernicke a.
aphasiac
aphasic
aphasiologist
aphasiology
aphasmid
apheliotropism
apheresis
aphilopony
aphonia
    hysterical a.
    a. paralytica
    spastic a.
aphonic pectoriloquy
aphonous
aphotesthesia
aphrasia
aphrodisia
aphrodisiac
aphrodisiomania
aphrophilus
    Haemophilus a.
aphtha, pl. **apthae**

NOTES

aphtha *(continued)*
    Bednar aphthae
    herpetiform aphthae
    aphthae major
    Mikulicz aphthae
    aphthae minor
aphthoid
aphthosis
aphthous stomatitis
Aphthovirus
aphylactic
aphylaxis
apical
    a. angle
    a. area
    a. axillary lymph node
    a. bronchopulmonary segment
    a. cap
    a. complex
    a. dendrite
    a. dental foramen
    a. ectodermal ridge
    a. gland
    a. granuloma
    a. impulse
    a. infarction
    a. infection
    a. ligament
    a. lordotic projection
    a. periodontal abscess
    a. periodontal cyst
    a. periodontitis
    a. pneumonia
    a. pole
    a. process
    a. pulse
    a. segmental artery
    a. space
    a. vein
apical-aortic conduit
apicalis
apicectomy
apiceotomy
apices (*pl. of* apex)
apicitis
apicoectomy
apicolocator
apicolysis
apicoposterior
    a. artery
    a. bronchopulmonary segment
    a. vein
apicostome
apicostomy
apicotomy
apiculate
apiculus
apicurettage
apinealism

apiphobia
apituitarism
aplacental
aplanatic lens
aplanatism
aplasia
    congenital a.
    a. cutis congenita
    germinal a.
    gonadal a.
    nuclear a.
    retinal a.
    thymic a.
aplastic
    a. anemia
    a. lymph
apleuria
apnea
    a. attack
    central a.
    deglutition a.
    induced a.
    obstructive sleep a.
    peripheral a.
    sleep a.
apnea-hypopnea index
apneic
    a. oxygenation
    a. pause
apneumia
apneusis
apneustic breathing
apobiosis
apochromatic
    a. lens
    a. objective
apocrine
    a. adenoma
    a. carcinoma
    a. chromhidrosis
    a. hidrocystoma
    a. metaplasia
    a. miliaria
    a. sweat gland
apocrustic
apodal
apodia
apodous
apody
apoenzyme
apoferritin
apogamia
apogamy
apogee
apoinducer
apolar
    a. bond
    a. cell
    a. interaction

apolipoprotein
    a. A-I, -II, -IV
    a. B-100
    a. B-48
    a. B, D, E
    a. C-I, II, III
apomixia
aponeurectomy
aponeurogenic ptosis
aponeurorrhaphy
aponeurosis, pl. **aponeuroses**
    bicipital a.
    a. bicipitalis
    Denonvilliers a.
    epicranial a.
    a. epicranialis
    extensor a.
    lingual a.
aponeurositis
aponeurotic
    a. fibroma
    a. reflex
aponeurotica
    falx a.
aponeurotome
aponeurotomy
apophylaxis
apophysary point
apophysial, apophyseal
    a. fracture
    a. point
apophysis, pl. **apophyses**
    basilar a.
    lenticular a.
apophysitis
    calcaneal a.
apoplasmia
apoplectic
    a. cyst
    a. retinitis
apoplectiform
apoplexy
    abdominal a.
    adrenal a.
    bulbar a.
    cerebellar a.
    fulminating a.
    functional a.
    heat a.
    labyrinthine a.
    pontile a.
    splenic a.

apoprotein
apoptosis
aporepressor
aposome
apostaxis
aposthia
apostilb
apothanasia
apothecaries weight
apothecary
apothem, apotheme
apoxesis
apozem, apozema
apparatus
    accessory visual a.
    achromatic a.
    alimentary a.
    attachment a.
    Barcroft-Warburg a.
    Beckmann a.
    Benedict-Roth a.
    branchial a.
    central a.
    chromatic a.
    chromidial a.
    dental a.
    digestive a.
    genitourinary a.
    Golgi a.
    Haldane a.
    hyoid a.
    juxtaglomerular a.
    Kirschner a.
    Kjeldahl a.
    lacrimal a.
    masticatory a.
    mental a.
    Warburg a.
apparent viscosity
appearance
    cluster-of-grapes a.
    cushingoid a.
    eggshell a.
    finger-in-glove a.
    ground-glass a.
    pigtail a.
    shocklike a.
    stuck-on a.
    toxic a.
appendage
    atrial a.
    auricular a.

NOTES

appendage *(continued)*
    drumstick a.
    epiploic a.
    left auricular a.
    vesicular a.
appendalgia
appendectomy
    auricular a.
appendiceal abscess
appendicectasis
appendicectomy
appendices (*pl. of* appendix)
appendicis
appendicism
appendicitis
    actinomycotic a.
    acute a.
    bilharzial a.
    chronic a.
    focal a.
    foreign body a.
    fulminating a.
    gangrenous a.
    left-sided a.
    lumbar a.
    nonobstructive a.
    perforating a.
    subperitoneal a.
    suppurative a.
    verminous a.
appendicocele
appendicolith
appendicolithiasis
appendicolysis
appendicostomy
appendicovesicostomy
appendicular
    a. artery
    a. ataxia
    a. colic
    a. lymph node
    a. muscle
    a. skeleton
    a. vein
appendix, pl. appendices
    auricular a.
    ensiform a.
    epiploic a.
    a. epiploica
    fatty a.
    fibrous a.
    functional a.
    omental a.
    vermiform a.
    a. vermiformis
apperception
apperceptive mass
appersonation
appersonification

appestat
appetite juice
appetitive behavior
applanation tonometer
applanometry
apple
    Adam's a.
    bitter a.
    a. jelly nodule
    May a.
    a. oil
appliance
    craniofacial a.
    edgewise a.
    extraoral fracture a.
    Hawley a.
    intraoral fracture a.
    labiolingual a.
    light wire a.
    Roger Anderson pin fixation a.
applicator
appliqué form
Appolito operation
apposition
    bayonet a.
    a. suture
appositional growth
appraisal
    critical a.
    health risk a.
approach
    facial recess a.
    idiographic a.
    infratemporal a.
    middle fossa a.
    posterior fossa a.
    retrosigmoid a.
    transcochlear a.
    translabyrinthine a.
    transnasal a.
    transseptal a.
approach-approach conflict
approach-avoidance conflict
approximal surface
approximate
approximation suture
approximator
    rib a.
APR
    abdominoperineal resection
apractagnosia
apractic
apragmatism
apraxia
    articulatory a.
    childhood a.
    constructional a.
    cortical a.
    developmental a.

gait a.
ideokinetic a.
ideomotor a.
innervation a.
limb-kinetic a.
oral motor a.
verbal a.
apraxic
aproctia
aprofen, aprofene, aprophen
aprosody
aprosopia
aprotinin
apthae (*pl. of* aphtha)
aptitude test
aPTT
activated partial thromboplastin time
Apt test
APUD
amine precursor uptake, decarboxylase
APUD cell
apyknomorphous
apyrase
apyretic typhoid
apyrexia
apyrexial
aquagenic
a. pruritus
a. urticaria
aquaphobia
aquapuncture
aquatic
aquatile
Flavobacterium a.
aqueduct
cerebral a.
cochlear a.
Cotunnius a.
fallopian a.
a. veil
aqueductal intubation
aqueous
a. chamber
a. flare
a. humor
a. influx phenomenon
a. outflow
a. phase
a. solution
a. vaccine
a. vein
aquiparous

aquocobalamin
aquosity
aquosus
humor a.
arabic
a. acid
gum a.
arabin
arabinoside
adenine a.
cytosine a.
arachidic bronchitis
arachidonic acid cascade
arachis oil
arachnase
arachnephobia
arachnidism
necrotic a.
arachnodactyly
arachnoid
a. cyst
a. foramen
a. granulation
a. mater
a. membrane
a. villus
arachnoidal granulation
arachnoidea
a. mater
a. mater encephali
arachnoideae
granulationes a.
arachnoiditis
adhesive a.
basal a.
arachnolysin
arachnophobia
Aran-Duchenne disease
araneism
Arantius
A. ligament
A. nodule
A. ventricle
araphia
arbor
arborescent
arborization block
arborize
arboroid
arbovirus
ARC
AIDS-related complex

NOTES

arc
  auricular a.
  binauricular a.
  bregmatolambdoid a.
  crater a.
  flame a.
  interauricular a.
  longitudinal a.
  mercury a.
  a. perimeter
  reflex a.
arcade
  anomalous mitral a.
  arterial a.
  Flint a.
  intestinal arterial a.
  lower dental a.
  mandibular dental a.
  marginal a.
  maxillary dental a.
arcate
arc-flash conjunctivitis
arch
  abdominothoracic a.
  alveolar a.
  anterior palatine a.
  aortic a.
  arterial a.
  axillary a.
  a. bar
  a. bar fixation
  branchial a.
  carpal a.
  coracoacromial a.
  Corti a.
  cortical a.
  costal a.
  crural a.
  deep crural a.
  deep palmar arterial a.
  deep palmar venous a.
  deep plantar arterial a.
  dental a.
  dorsal carpal arterial a.
  dorsal venous a.
  double aortic a.
  expansion a.
  fallen a.
  fallopian a.
  femoral a.
  a. form
  glossopalatine a.
  Gothic a.
  Haller a.
  hemal a.
  hyoid a.
  iliopectineal a.
  inferior dental a.
  inferior palpebral arterial a.

  jugular venous a.
  labial a.
  Langer a.
  lateral longitudinal a.
  a. length
  a. length deficiency
  lingual a.
  longitudinal a.
  malar a.
  mandibular a.
  medial longitudinal a.
  medial lumbocostal a.
  neural a.
  palatoglossal a.
  palatopharyngeal a.
  palmar a.
  pharyngeal a.
  plantar a.
  posterior a.
  pubic a.
  superciliary a.
  superior dental a.
  tendinous a.
  vertebral a.
  a. wire
  zygomatic a.
archaic-paralogical thinking
arched crest
archenteric canal
archenteron
archeocerebellum
archeokinetic
archetype
archeus
archicerebellum
archicortex
archil
archin
archipallium
architectonics
architectural barrier
architecture
  bone a.
arch-loop-whorl system
archwire
arciform
  a. artery
  a. vein
arcon articulator
arctation
arcual
arcuata
  zona a.
arcuate
  a. artery
  a. crest
  a. eminence
  a. fasciculus
  a. fiber

A

a. incision
a. line
a. nucleus
a. popliteal ligament
a. pubic ligament
a. scotoma
a. uterus
a. vein
a. zone
arcuation
arcus
a. adiposus
a. cornealis
a. dentalis inferior
a. dentalis mandibularis
a. dentalis maxillaris
a. dentalis superior
a. ductus thoracici
a. palatoglossus
a. palatopharyngeus
a. palmaris
a. palmaris profundus
a. palmaris superficialis
a. palpebralis inferior
a. palpebralis superior
a. pedis
a. pedis longitudinalis
a. senilis
a. tendineus
a. zygomaticus
ARD
acute respiratory disease
acute respiratory distress
ardent
a. fever
a. spirit
ARDS
acute respiratory distress syndrome
adult respiratory distress syndrome
area
acoustic a.
a. acustica
amygdaloclaustral a.
amygdalopiriform transition a.
anterior amygdaloid a.
anterior hypothalamic a.
aortic a.
apical a.
association a.
auditory a.
bare a.
basal seat a.

body surface a. (BSA)
Broca parolfactory a.
Brodmann a.
catchment a.
cochlear a.
Cohnheim a.
contact a.
cribriform a.
denture-bearing a.
denture foundation a.
denture-supporting a.
dermatomic a.
dorsal hypothalamic a.
embryonal a.
embryonic a.
entorhinal a.
excitable a.
facial nerve a.
Flechsig a.
frontal a.
frontoorbital a.
fusion a.
gastric a.
genital a.
germinal a.
a. germinativa
Head a.
impression a.
inferior vestibular a.
insular a.
intermediate hypothalamic a.
Kiesselbach a.
Laimer-Haeckerman a.
lateral hypothalamic a.
lateral inferior hepatic a.
lateral superior hepatic a.
Little a.
macular a.
Martegiani a.
mitral a.
motor a.
Panum a.
performance a.
postcentral a.
precentral a.
prefrontal a.
Rolando a.
sensorimotor a.
silent a.
total body surface a.
triangular a.

NOTES

area *(continued)*
    trigger a.
    visual a.
areata
    alopecia a.
areflexia
    detrusor a.
arenacea
    corpora a.
arenaceous
areola, pl. **areolae**
    a. papillaris
    a. umbilici
    a. umbilicus
areolar
    a. choroiditis
    a. choroidopathy
    a. gland
    a. incision
    a. tissue
    a. tubercle
    a. venous plexus
areometer
ARF
    acute renal failure
    acute respiratory failure
argasid
Argas reflexus
argentaffin
    a. cell
    a. granule
argentaffine
argentaffinoma
argentation
argentic
Argentinean hemorrhagic fever
Argentine hemorrhagic fever virus
argentophil, argentophile
argentous
argentum
arginase
arginine
    a. deiminase
    a. glutamate
    a. vasopressin
argininosuccinic acid
argininosuccinicaciduria
argon laser
Argyll
    A. Robertson
    A. Robertson pupil
argyria
argyric
argyrism
argyrol
argyrophil, argyrophile
argyrophilic
    a. cell
    a. fiber

arhinia
Arias-Stella
    A.-S. effect
    A.-S. phenomenon
    A.-S. reaction
ariboflavinosis
aristotelian method
Aristotle anomaly
arithmetic mean
arithmomania
Arlt
    A. operation
    A. sinus
arm
    bar clasp a.
    brawny a.
    circumferential clasp a.
    clasp a.
    dynein a.
    nuchal a.
    a. phenomenon
armamentarium
Armanni-Ebstein
    A.-E. change
    A.-E. kidney
armarium
armed
    a. macrophage
    a. rostellum
arm-extension position
armillatus
    Armillifer a.
Armillifer armillatus
Armitage-Doll model
armor
    character a.
    a. heart
armored heart
armpit
Army
    A. alpha test
    A. beta test
ARN
    acute retinal necrosis
Arndt law
Arneth
    A. classification
    A. count
    A. formula
    A. index
    A. stage
Arnold
    A. body
    A. bundle
    A. canal
    foramen of A.
    A. ganglion
    A. nerve
    A. tract

Arnold-Chiari
    A.-C. deformity
    A.-C. malformation
    A.-C. syndrome
aromatase inhibitor
aromatic
    a. ammonia spirit
    a. bitter
    a. castor oil
    a. compound
    a. d-amino acid decarboxylase
    a. series
    a. water
aromatize
arotinoid
arousal
    a. function
    a. reaction
arrector pili muscle
arrest
    a. of active phase
    cardiac a.
    cardioplegic a.
    cardiopulmonary a.
    circulatory a.
    deep hypothermic a.
    a. of descent
    epiphysial a.
    heart a.
    a. of labor
    maturation a.
    a. signal
    sinus a.
arrested
    a. dental caries
    a. tuberculosis
Arrhenius
    A. equation
    A. law
Arrhenius-Madsen theory
arrhenoblastoma
arrhinencephaly, arrhinencephalia
arrhinia
arrhythmia
    cardiac a.
    continuous a.
    juvenile a.
    sinus a.
arrhythmic
arrhythmogenic

arrival
    dead on a. (DOA)
    prior to a.
arrow
    a. point tracing
    a. poison
arrowroot
Arruga forceps
arsacetin
arsenamide
arsenate
arseniasis
arsenic
    a. acid
    a. pigmentation
    a. trihydride
    a. trioxide
arsenical
    a. keratosis
    a. paralysis
    a. polyneuropathy
arsenicalism
arsenic-fast
arsenide, arseniuret
arsenious
arsenite
    copper a.
    cupric a.
arsenium
arseniuret (*var. of* arsenide)
arseniureted hydrogen
arsenotherapy
arsenoxide
arsonium
artefact
arteria, pl. **arteriae**
    arteriae atriales
    a. celiaca
    a. lusoria
    a. mediana
    a. pulmonalis
    a. quadrigeminalis
arterial
    a. arcade
    a. arch
    a. blood
    a. blood gas (ABG)
    a. bulb
    a. canal
    a. capillary
    a. catheter
    a. circle

NOTES

arterial *(continued)*
    a. cone
    a. duct
    a. flap
    a. forceps
    a. groove
    a. hyperemia
    a. hypotension
    a. ligament
    a. line
    a. murmur
    a. nephrosclerosis
    a. plexus
    a. sclerosis
    a. segment
    a. spasm
    a. spider
    a. switch operation
    a. tension
    a. thoracic outlet syndrome
    a. thrombosis
    a. vein
    a. wave
arterialization
arteriectasis, arteriectasia
arteriectomy
arterioatony
arteriocapillary sclerosis
arteriococcygeal gland
arteriogram
arteriographic
arteriography
    bronchial a.
    cerebral a.
arteriohepatic dysplasia
arteriolar
    a. nephrosclerosis
    a. network
    a. sclerosis
arteriole
    afferent glomerular a.
    capillary a.
    efferent glomerular a.
    inferior macular a.
    inferior temporal retinal a.
    medial a.
    middle macular a.
    postglomerular a.
    preglomerular a.
    superior macular a.
    superior nasal retinal a.
    superior temporal retinal a.
arteriolith
arteriolitis
    necrotizing a.
arteriolonecrosis
arteriolonephrosclerosis
arteriolosclerosis
arteriolosclerotic kidney

arteriolovenous
arteriolovenular
    a. anastomosis
    a. bridge
arteriolovenularis
    anastomosis a.
arteriomalacia
arteriometer
arteriomotor
arteriomyomatosis
arterionephrosclerosis
arteriopalmus
arteriopathy
    hypertensive a.
arterioplania
arterioplasty
arteriopressor
arteriorrhaphy
arteriorrhexis
arteriosclerosis
    coronary a.
    hyperplastic a.
    hypertensive a.
    medial a.
    Mönckeberg a.
    nodular a.
    a. obliterans
    peripheral a.
    senile a.
arteriosclerotic
    a. aneurysm
    a. cardiovascular disease (ACVD)
    a. gangrene
    a. kidney
    a. retinopathy
    a. vertigo
arteriospasm
arteriostenosis
arteriosus
    conus a.
    ductus a.
    major circulus a.
    persistent truncus a.
arteriotomy incision
arteriovenosa
    anastomosis a.
arteriovenous (AV, A-V)
    a. access
    a. anastomosis
    a. aneurysm
    a. carbon dioxide difference
    a. fistula
    a. nicking
    a. oxygen difference
    a. shunt
arteritis
    brachiocephalic a.
    coronary a.
    cranial a.

extracranial a.
giant cell a.
granulomatous a.
Heubner a.
Horton a.
intracranial granulomatous a.
a. nodosa
a. obliterans
obliterating a.
rheumatic a.
Takayasu a.
temporal a.
artery
Abbott a.
aberrant obturator a.
accessory meningeal a.
accessory obturator a.
acetabular a.
acromial a.
acromiothoracic a.
a. of Adamkiewicz
alar a.
angular a.
anterior basal segmental a.
anterior cecal a.
anterior cerebral a.
anterior choroidal a.
anterior ciliary a.
anterior circumflex humeral a.
anterior communicating a.
anterior conjunctival a.
anterior ethmoidal a.
anterior humeral circumflex a.
anterior inferior cerebellar a.
anterior intercostal a.
anterior interosseous a.
anterior interventricular a.
anterior labial a.
anterior lateral malleolar a.
anterior medial malleolar a.
anterior mediastinal a.
anterior meningeal a.
anterior parietal a.
anterior perforating a.
anterior peroneal a.
anterior segmental a.
anterior spinal a.
anterior superior alveolar a.
anterior superior dental a.
anterior superior
  pancreaticoduodenal a.
anterior superior segmental a.

anterior temporal a.
anterior tibial recurrent a.
anterior tympanic a.
anterior vestibular a.
anterolateral central a.
anterolateral striate a.
anterolateral thalamostriate a.
anteromedial central a.
anteromedial thalamostriate a.
apical segmental a.
apicoposterior a.
appendicular a.
arciform a.
arcuate a.
ascending cervical a.
ascending palatine a.
ascending pharyngeal a.
atrial a.
axillary a.
azygos a.
basilar a.
brachial a.
bronchial a.
buccal a.
buccinator a.
buckled innominate a.
calcaneal a.
calcarine a.
callosomarginal a.
caroticotympanic a.
carotid a.
carpal a.
caudal pancreatic a.
cavernous a.
cecal a.
celiac a.
central retinal a.
central sulcal a.
cerebellar a.
cerebral a.
cervicovaginal a.
Charcot a.
circumflex femoral a.
circumflex fibular a.
circumflex humeral a.
circumflex iliac a.
circumflex scapular a.
coiled a.
colic a.
collateral digital a.
collicular a.
comitant a.

NOTES

artery *(continued)*

common carotid a.
common cochlear a.
common hepatic a.
common iliac a.
common interosseous a.
common palmar digital a.
common plantar digital a.
communicating a.
conjunctival a.
coronary a.
cortical radiate a.
costocervical a.
cremasteric a.
cricothyroid a.
cystic a.
deep auricular a.
deep brachial a.
deep cervical a.
deep circumflex iliac a.
deep epigastric a.
deep lingual a.
deep plantar a.
deep temporal a.
deferential a.
descending genicular a.
descending palatine a.
descending scapular a.
digital collateral a.
distal medial striate a.
distributing a.
dolichoectatic a.
dorsal digital a.
dorsal interosseous a.
dorsalis pedis a.
dorsal metacarpal a.
dorsal metatarsal a.
dorsal nasal a.
dorsal pancreatic a.
dorsal scapular a.
dorsal thoracic a.
elastic a.
end a.
episcleral a.
esophageal a.
external carotid a.
external iliac a.
external mammary a.
external maxillary a.
external nasal a.
external pudendal a.
external spermatic a.
facial a.
femoral nutrient a.
fibular nutrient a.
frontal a.
frontopolar a.
gastric a.
gastroduodenal a.

gastroepiploic a.
gastroomental a.
genicular a.
glaserian a.
great anastomotic a.
greater palatine a.
greater pancreatic a.
great radicular a.
great segmental medullary a.
great superior pancreatic a.
helicine a.
hepatic a.
Heubner a.
highest intercostal a.
highest thoracic a.
humeral nutrient a.
hyaloid a.
hypogastric a.
ileal a.
ileocolic a.
iliac a.
iliolumbar a.
inferior alveolar a.
inferior dental a.
inferior epigastric a.
inferior gluteal a.
inferior hemorrhoidal a.
inferior hypophysial a.
inferior internal parietal a.
inferior labial a.
inferior laryngeal a.
inferior lateral genicular a.
inferior lingular a.
inferior lobar a.
inferior medial genicular a.
inferior mesenteric a.
inferior pancreatic a.
inferior pancreaticoduodenal a.
inferior phrenic a.
inferior rectal a.
inferior segmental a.
inferior suprarenal a.
inferior thyroid a.
inferior tympanic a.
inferior ulnar collateral a.
inferior vesical a.
infraorbital a.
infrascapular a.
innominate a.
insular a.
intercostal a.
interlobar a.
interlobular a.
intermediate temporal a.
internal auditory a.
internal carotid a.
internal iliac a.
internal mammary a.
internal maxillary a.

internal pudendal a.
internal spermatic a.
internal thoracic a.
intestinal a.
intrarenal a.
jejunal a.
juxtacolic a.
Kugel anastomotic a.
labyrinthine a.
lacrimal a.
lateral basal segmental a.
lateral circumflex femoral a.
lateral frontobasal a.
lateral inferior genicular a.
lateral malleolar a.
lateral nasal a.
lateral occipital a.
lateral orbitofrontal a.
lateral plantar a.
lateral sacral a.
lateral segmental a.
lateral splanchnic a.
lateral striate a.
lateral superior genicular a.
lateral tarsal a.
lateral thoracic a.
left anterior descending a.
left carotid a. (LCA)
left circumflex coronary a.
left colic a.
left coronary a.
left gastric a.
left gastroepiploic a.
left gastroomental a.
left hepatic a.
left marginal a.
left pulmonary a.
lenticulostriate a.
lesser palatine a.
lienal a.
lingual a.
lingular a.
long central a.
long posterior ciliary a.
long thoracic a.
lowest lumbar a.
lowest thyroid a.
lumbar a.
macular a.
mammillary a.
marginal a.
masseteric a.

mastoid a.
maxillary a.
medial basal segmental a.
medial circumflex femoral a.
medial collateral a.
medial commisural a.
medial femoral circumflex a.
medial frontobasal a.
medial inferior genicular a.
medial malleolar a.
medial occipital a.
medial orbitofrontal a.
medial plantar a.
medial segmental a.
medial striate a.
medial superior genicular a.
medial tarsal a.
median a.
median callosal a.
median commissural a.
median sacral a.
mediastinal a.
medium a.
medullary spinal a.
mental a.
metatarsal a.
middle cerebral a.
middle colic a.
middle collateral a.
middle genicular a.
middle hemorrhoidal a.
middle lobar a.
middle meningeal a.
middle rectal a.
middle sacral a.
middle suprarenal a.
middle temporal a.
musculophrenic a.
a. needle
nutrient a.
obturator a.
occipital a.
ophthalmic a.
ovarian a.
palpebral a.
perforating a.
pericardiacophrenic a.
perineal a.
peroneal a.
plantar metatarsal a.
polar temporal a.
popliteal a.

NOTES

artery *(continued)*
  prepancreatic a.
  princeps pollicis a.
  profunda brachii a.
  profunda femoris a.
  pterygomeningeal a.
  pulmonary a.
  radial collateral a.
  radialis indicis a.
  radial recurrent a.
  recurrent ulnar a.
  renal a.
  right descending pulmonary a.
  right gastric a.
  right pulmonary a.
  segmental a.
  short gastric a.
  sigmoid a.
  sphenopalatine a.
  splenic a.
  stylomastoid a.
  subclavian a.
  subcostal a.
  sublingual a.
  submental a.
  subscapular a.
  superficial brachial a.
  superior cerebellar a.
  supraorbital a.
  suprascapular a.
  supratrochlear a.
  sural a.
  terminal a.
  testicular a.
  thoracoacromial a.
  thoracodorsal a.
  transverse cervical a.
  transverse facial a.
  transverse scapular a.
  ulnar a.
  umbilical a.
  urethral a.
  uterine a.
  vaginal a.
  ventricular a.
  vertebral a.
  Wilkie a.
  zygomaticoorbital a.
arthralgia
  intermittent a.
  a. saturnina
arthralgic
arthrectomy
arthresthesia
arthritic
  a. atrophy
  a. calculus
  a. general pseudoparalysis

arthriticum
  tuberculum a.
arthritis, pl. **arthritides**
  acute rheumatic a.
  bacterial a.
  chronic absorptive a.
  chylous a.
  colitic a.
  a. deformans
  degenerative a.
  enteropathic a.
  erosive a.
  exudative a.
  filarial a.
  gonococcal a.
  gonorrheal a.
  gouty a.
  hemophilic a.
  hypertrophic a.
  Jaccoud a.
  juvenile chronic a.
  juvenile rheumatoid a.
  Lyme a.
  a. mutilans
  navicular a.
  neurogenic a.
  a. nodosa
  a. psoriasis
  psoriatic a.
  rheumatoid a.
  suppurative a.
arthrocele
arthrocentesis
arthrochondritis
arthroclasia
arthroconidium
arthrodesis
arthrodia
arthrodial
  a. articulation
  a. cartilage
  a. joint
arthrodynia
arthrodynic
arthrodysplasia
arthroendoscopy
arthroereisis
arthrogenous
arthrogram
arthrography
arthrogryposis multiplex congenita
arthrokatadysis
arthrokinematics
arthrolith
arthrolithiasis
arthrology, arthrologia
arthrolysis
arthrometer
arthrometry

A

arthroophthalmopathy
   hereditary progressive a.
arthropathia psoriatica
arthropathology
arthropathy
   diabetic a.
   Jaccoud a.
   long-leg a.
   neuropathic a.
   tabetic a.
arthroplasty
   Charnley hip a.
   gap a.
   interposition a.
   intracapsular temporomandibular
    joint a.
   total hip a.
   total joint a.
   total knee a.
arthropneumoradiography
arthropod
arthropodiasis
arthropodic
arthropodous
arthropyosis
arthrorisis
arthrosclerosis
arthroscope
arthroscopy
arthrosia
   exanthesis a.
arthrosis
arthrospore
arthrostomy
arthrosynovitis
arthrotome
arthrotomy
arthrotropic
arthrotyphoid
arthroxesis
Arthus
   A. phenomenon
   A. reaction
articular
   a. branch
   a. capsule
   a. cartilage
   a. cavity
   a. chondrocalcinosis
   a. circumference
   a. corpuscle
   a. crepitus

   a. crescent
   a. crest
   a. disc
   a. eminence
   a. facet
   a. fracture
   a. gout
   a. labrum
   a. lamella
   a. lip
   a. margin
   a. meniscus
   a. muscle
   a. nerve
   a. process
   a. rheumatism
   a. sensibility
   a. surface
   a. vascular circle
   a. vascular network
   a. vascular plexus
articularis
   a. cubiti muscle
   a. genus muscle
   meniscus a.
articulate
articulated skeleton
articulating paper
articulation
   arthrodial a.
   atlantooccipital a.
   balanced a.
   bicondylar a.
   cartilaginous a.
   compound a.
   condylar a.
   confluent a.
   cricoarytenoid a.
   cricothyroid a.
   cuneonavicular a.
   dental a.
   a. disorder
   distal radioulnar a.
   glenohumeral a.
   humeral a.
   humeroradial a.
   incudomalleolar a.
   incudostapedial a.
   interchondral a.
   intermetatarsal a.
   interphalangeal a.
   intertarsal a.

NOTES

articulation *(continued)*
    metacarpophalangeal a.
    metatarsophalangeal a.
    talonavicular a.
articulator
    adjustable a.
    arcon a.
articulatory apraxia
artifact
    chemical shift a.
    radiographic a.
    thermal a.
artifactitious
artifactual
artificial
    a. active immunity
    a. anatomy
    a. ankylosis
    a. Carlsbad salt
    a. crown
    a. dentition
    a. eye
    a. fever
    a. heart
    a. insemination
    a. intelligence
    a. kidney
    a. Kissingen salt
    a. labor
    a. larynx
    a. melanin
    a. membrane rupture
    a. nose
    a. pacemaker
    a. passive immunity
    a. pneumothorax
    a. pupil
    a. radioactivity
    a. respiration
    a. selection
    a. sphincter
    a. stone
    a. tears
    a. ventilation
artificialis
    acne a.
artistic anatomy
arycorniculate synchondrosis
aryepiglottic
    a. fold
    a. muscle
aryl acylamidase
arylamidase
arylated alkyl
arylsulfatase A, B deficiency
arytenoepiglottidean fold
arytenoid
    a. cartilage
    a. dislocation

    a. gland
    a. subluxation
    a. swelling
arytenoidectomy
arytenoiditis
arytenoidopexy
ASA
    acetylsalicylic acid
asbestoid
asbestos
    a. body
    a. cancer
    a. pneumoconiosis
    a. wart
asbestosis
ascariasis
ascaricide
ascarid
Ascaris lumbricoides
ascending
    a. aorta
    a. branch
    a. cervical artery
    a. cholangitis
    a. colon
    a. current
    a. degeneration
    a. frontal convolution
    a. frontal gyrus
    a. lumbar vein
    a. mesocolon
    a. myelitis
    a. neuritis
    a. palatine artery
    a. paralysis
    a. parietal convolution
    a. parietal gyrus
    a. pharyngeal artery
    a. pharyngeal plexus
    a. process
    a. pyelonephritis
ascertainment
    a. bias
    complete a.
    incomplete a.
Ascher
    A. aqueous influx phenomenon
    A. syndrome
Aschner
    A. phenomenon
    A. reflex
Aschner-Dagnini reflex
Aschoff
    A. body
    A. cell
    A. nodule
asci (*pl. of* ascus)
ascites
    chyliform a.

a. chylosus
chylous a.
fatty a.
gelatinous a.
hemorrhagic a.
milky a.
nephrogenic a.
ascitic
ascitogenous
ascocarp
ascogenous
ascogonium
Ascoli
A. reaction
A. test
ascomycetous
ascorbate-cyanide test
ascorbate oxidase
ascorbic acid
ascorbyl palmitate
ascospore
ASCUS
atypical squamous cell of undetermined
significance
ascus, pl. **asci**
asecretory
Aselli
A. gland
A. pancreas
asemasia
asepsis
aseptate
aseptic
a. fever
a. necrosis
a. surgery
asepticism
asequence
asexual
a. dwarfism
a. generation
a. reproduction
ash
bone a.
Ashby method
ashen
a. tuber
a. tubercle
a. wing
Asherman syndrome
ash-leaf macule
Ashman phenomenon

ashy
a. dermatitis
a. dermatosis
asialism
asialoglycoprotein receptor
Asian influenza
Asiatic
A. cholera
A. schistosomiasis
asiderotic anemia
asitia
Askanazy cell
Ask-Upmark kidney
**as low as reasonably achievable
(ALARA)**
asocial
aspartate aminotransferase (AST)
aspartic acid
aspect
facial a.
frontal a.
lateral a.
Asperger disorder
aspergillic acid
aspergillin
aspergilloma
aspergillosis
acute invasive a.
allergic bronchopulmonary a.
(ABPA)
chronic necrotizing a.
disseminated a.
Aspergillus
A. *clavatus*
endonuclease S1 A.
A. *flavus*
A. *fumigatus*
A. *nidulans*
A. *niger*
A. *terreus*
aspermatogenic sterility
aspermia
aspersion
aspheric lens
asphygmia
asphyxia
autoerotic a.
cyanotic a.
a. livida
local a.
a. neonatorum

NOTES

asphyxia *(continued)*
    sexual a.
    traumatic a.
asphyxial
asphyxiant
asphyxiate
asphyxiating
    a. thoracic chondrodystrophy
    a. thoracic dysplasia
    a. thoracic dystrophy
asphyxiation
aspidin
aspidinol
aspidium
aspidosamine
aspidospermine
aspirate
aspirating needle
aspiration
    a. biopsy
    fine-needle a. (FNA)
    level of a.
    meconium a.
    a. pneumonia
    silent a.
aspirator
aspirin
    aluminum a.
asplenia
    functional a.
    a. syndrome
    a. with cardiovascular anomalies
asplenic
asporogenous
asporous
asporulate
Assam fever
assassin bug
assault
    felonious a.
assay
    Ames a.
    biologic a.
    clonogenic a.
    competitive binding a.
    complement binding a.
    double antibody sandwich a.
    EAC rosette a.
    enzyme-linked immunosorbent a.
     (ELISA)
    Grunstein-Hogness a.
    hemizona a.
    hemolytic plaque a.
    immunochemical a.
    immunoradiometric a.
    indirect a.
    Jerne plaque a.
    Lowry-Folin a.
    Lowry protein a.

    radioimmunoprecipitation a.
    Raji cell a.
assertive
    a. conditioning
    a. training
assessment
    focused medical a.
    focused trauma a.
    health risk a.
    initial a.
    ongoing a.
    rapid medical a.
    rapid trauma a.
Assézat triangle
assident
    a. sign
    a. symptom
assignment
    sex a.
assimilable
assimilation
    ammonia a.
    a. pelvis
    a. sacrum
assistant
    dental a.
    medical a.
assist-control ventilation
assisted
    a. cephalic delivery
    a. circulation
    a. reproductive technology
    a. respiration
    a. ventilation
assistive
    a. listening device
    a. movement
Assmann tuberculous infiltrate
associate
    microbial a.
associated
    a. antagonist
    a. movement
association
    a. area
    clang a.
    a. constant
    a. cortex
    dream a.'s
    a. fiber
    free a.
    genetic a.
    independent practice a.
    law of a.
    loose a.'s
    loosening of a.'s
    a. mechanism
    a. system
    a. test

a. time
a. tract
associationism
associative
a. aphasia
a. reaction
a. strength
assortative mating
assortment
independent a.
assumption
a. of care
a. of risk
assurance
quality a.
AST
aspartate aminotransferase
astasia
astasia-abasia
astatic seizure
astatine
asteatosis cutis
astemizole
aster
astereognosis
asterion
asteriosaponin
asteriotoxin
asterixis
asternal
asternia
asteroid
a. body
a. hyalosis
asteroides
Nocardia a.
asthenia
asthenic
a. personality
a. personality disorder
asthenopia
accommodative a.
muscular a.
asthenopic
asthenospermia
asthenozoospermia
asthma
atopic a.
bronchial a.
bronchitic a.
cardiac a.
catarrhal a.

cotton-dust a.
a. crystal
dust a.
Elsner a.
exercise-induced a.
extrinsic a.
food a.
hay a.
Heberden a.
intrinsic a.
miller a.
miner's a.
Rostan a.
asthmatic bronchitis
asthmaticus
status a.
asthmatoid wheeze
asthma-weed
asthmogenic
astigmatic
a. dial
a. lens
astigmatism
a. against the rule
compound hyperopic a.
compound myopic a.
corneal a.
hyperopic a.
irregular a.
lenticular a.
mixed a.
myopic a.
regular a.
retinal a.
simple a.
a. with the rule
astigmatometry
astigmia
astigmometry
Astler-Coller classification
astomatous
astomia
astomous
A-strabismus
astragalar
astragalectomy
astragalocalcanean
astragalofibular
astragaloscaphoid
astragalotibial
astral fiber
astrapophobia

NOTES

astriction
astringent
astroblast
astroblastoma
astrocele
astrocyte
Alzheimer type I, II a.
fibrillary a.
fibrous a.
gemistocytic a.
protoplasmic a.
astrocytoma
anaplastic a.
cerebellar a.
desmoplastic cerebral a.
fibrillary a.
gemistocytic a.
grade I–IV a.
juvenile cerebellar a.
low grade a.
pilocytic a.
astrocytosis cerebri
astroependymoma
astroglia cell
astroid
astrokinetic
astrosphere
Astwood test
asverin
asyllabia
asylum
asymbolia
asymmetric
a. chondrodystrophy
a. disulfide
a. fetal growth restriction
a. motor neuropathy
asymmetrus
janiceps a.
asymmetry
asymptomatic
a. neurosyphilis
a. pyelonephritis
asymptotic
asynchronous
a. activity
a. pulse generator
asynclitism
anterior a.
posterior a.
asyndesis
asynechia
asynergic
asynergy
asynesia, asynesis
asystematic
asystole, asystolia
asystolic

atactic
a. abasia
a. agraphia
atactilia
ataractic
ataraxia
ataraxic
atavicus
metatarsus a.
atavism
atavistic epiphysis
ataxia, ataxy
acute a.
appendicular a.
Briquet a.
Bruns a.
cerebellar a.
chronic a.
a. cordis
Friedreich a.
gluten a.
hereditary cerebellar a.
hereditary spinal a.
hysterical a.
kinetic a.
Leyden a.
locomotor a.
Marie a.
motor a.
optic a.
spinocerebellar a.
a. telangiectasia
a. telangiectasia syndrome
ataxiadynamia
ataxiagram
ataxiagraph
ataxiameter
ataxiaphasia
ataxia-telangiectasia
ataxic
a. abasia
a. aphasia
a. breathing
a. dysarthria
a. gait
a. paramyotonia
a. paraplegia
ataxiophemia
ataxiophobia
ataxy (var. of ataxia)
A/T cloning
atelectasis
adhesive a.
cicatrization a.
lobar a.
passive a.
platelike a.
primary a.
round a.

rounded a.
secondary a.
subsegmental a.
atelectatic rale
ateliosis, atelia
ateliotic dwarfism
atelopidtoxin
atenolol
A2 thalassemia
athelia
atherectomy
coronary a.
directional a.
athermancy
athermanous
athermosystaltic
atheroembolism
atherogenesis
atherogenic
atheroma
atheromatous
a. degeneration
a. embolism
a. plaque
atherosclerosis
atherosclerotic aneurysm
atherosis
atherothrombosis
atherothrombotic
athetoid
athetosic
athetosis
double congenital a.
athetotic
athlete's
a. foot
a. heart
athletic
a. heart
a. therapist
a. trainer
a. training
athrepsia
athrepsy
athrocytosis
athrombia
athymia
athymism
athyrea
athyroidism
athyrosis
athyrotic

atlantad
atlantal
atlanticus
Aedes a.
atlantoaxial joint
atlantodldymus
atlantoepistrophic
atlantooccipital, atlooccipital
a. articulation
a. joint
a. membrane
atlantoodontoid
atlas
atloaxoid
atlodidymus
atloid
atlooccipital (*var. of* atlantooccipital)
atmolysis
atmometer
atmosphere
a. absolute
standard a.
atmospheric pressure
atmospherization
atom
activated a.
Bohr a.
excited a.
ionized a.
labeled a.
atomic
a. absorption spectrophotometry
a. core
a. heat
a. mass number
a. mass unit
a. theory
a. volume
a. weight (AW)
atomism
atomistic psychology
atomization
atomizer
atonia
atonic
a. bladder
a. dyspepsia
a. ectropion
a. entropion
a. epiphora
a. seizure
atonicity

NOTES

atony
    postpartum a.
    uterine a.
atopen
atopic
    a. allergy
    a. asthma
    a. cataract
    a. conjunctivitis
    a. dermatitis
    a. eczema
    a. keratoconjunctivitis
    a. reagin
atopognosia, atopognosis
atopy
atoxic
atrabiliary capsule
atraumatic
    a. needle
    a. suture
atrepsy
atresia
    anal a.
    a. ani
    aortic a.
    biliary a.
    bronchial a.
    choanal a.
    esophageal a.
    ileal a.
    intestinal a.
    laryngeal a.
    pulmonary artery a.
    pulmonic a.
    pyloric a.
    tricuspid a.
    vaginal a.
atresic teratosis
atretic
    a. corpus luteum
    a. ovarian follicle
atretoblepharia
atretocystia
atretogastria
atretopsia
atria (*pl. of* atrium)
atrial
    a. appendage
    a. artery
    a. auricle
    a. auricula
    a. bigeminy
    a. branch
    a. capture
    a. capture beat
    a. chaotic tachycardia
    a. complex
    a. deflection
    a. diastole

    a. dissociation
    a. echo
    a. extrasystole
    a. fibrillation
    a. flutter
    a. fusion beat
    a. gallop
    a. infarction
    a. kick
    a. myxoma
    a. natriuretic factor (ANF)
    a. natriuretic peptide (ANP)
    a. septal defect
    a. septostomy
    a. sound
    a. standstill
    a. synchronous pulse generator
    a. systole
    a. transport function
    a. triggered pulse generator
    a. ventricular canal defect
atriales
    arteriae a.
atrial-well technique
atrichia
atrichosis
atrichous
atriomegaly
atrionector
atriopeptin
atrioseptoplasty
atrioseptostomy
    balloon a.
atriosystolic murmur
atriotomy
atrioventricular (AV, A-V)
    a. band
    a. block
    a. bundle
    a. canal
    a. canal cushion
    a. conduction (AVC)
    a. connection
    a. dissociation (AVD)
    a. gradient
    a. groove
    a. interval
    a. junctional bigeminy
    a. junctional rhythm
    a. junctional tachycardia
    a. nodal branch
    a. nodal extrasystole
    a. node
    a. septum
    a. sulcus
    a. valve
atriplicism
atrium, pl. **atria**
    accessory a.

A

a. cordis dextrum
a. cordis sinistrum
a. dextrum cordis
a. glottidis
left a.
a. pulmonale
right a.
a. sinistrum cordis
atrophia cutis
atrophic
a. excavation
a. gastritis
a. glossitis
a. heterochromia
a. inflammation
a. kidney
a. pharyngitis
a. rhinitis
a. thrombosis
a. vaginitis
atrophica
macula a.
atrophicae
lineae a.
atrophicans
acrodermatitis chronica a.
atrophicus
lichen sclerosus et a.
atrophie blanche
atrophied
atrophoderma
follicular a.
neuritic a.
atrophodermatosis
atrophy
acute reflex bone a.
acute yellow a.
alveolar a.
arthritic a.
blue a.
brown a.
Buchwald a.
central areolar choroidal a.
cerebellar a.
choroidal vascular a.
congenital cerebellar a.
congenital microvillus a.
cyanotic a.
disuse a.
dominant optic a.
essential progressive a.
facioscapulohumeral a.

familial spinal muscular a.
fatty a.
geographic retinal a.
gingival a.
gyrate a.
Hoffmann muscular a.
horizontal a.
inactivity a.
infantile muscular a.
infantile progressive spinal
muscular a.
infantile spinal muscular a.
ischemic muscular a.
juvenile muscular a.
juvenile spinal muscular a.
Kjer optic a.
Leber hereditary optic a.
linear a.
macular a.
marantic a.
multiple system a.
muscular a.
neurotic a.
peroneal muscular a.
Pick a.
progressive choroidal a.
progressive muscular a.
spinal muscular a.
traumatic a.
tubular a.
Vulpian a.
Zimmerlin a.
atropine
a. sulfate
a. test
atropinic
atropinism
atropinization
atroscine
atrotoxin
attached
a. cranial section
a. craniotomy
a. gingiva
attachment
a. apparatus
bar clip a.
bar-sleeve a.
epithelial a.
frictional a.
internal a.

NOTES

attachment *(continued)*
    key a.
    keyway a.
attack
    anxiety a.
    apnea a.
    brain a.
    drop a.
    glottal a.
    heart a.
    incipient heart a.
    myoclonic a.
    panic a.
    a. rate
    transient ischemic a. (TIA)
attar of rose
attending
    a. physician
    a. staff
attention
    a. deficit hyperactivity disorder
    a. span
attenuant
attenuate
attenuated
    a. tuberculosis
    a. vaccine
    a. virus
attenuation
    a. compensation
    interaural a.
attenuator
attic
atticomastoid
atticotomy
attitude
    emotional a.
    fetal a.
attitudinal reflex
attorney
    durable power of a.
attraction
    capillary a.
    chemical a.
    magnetic a.
    a. sphere
attributable risk
attrition
atypical
    a. absence seizure
    a. achromatopsia
    a. antipsychotic agent
    a. endometrial hyperplasia
    a. facial neuralgia
    a. fibroxanthoma
    a. gingivitis
    a. glandular cell
    a. glandular cell of undetermined significance (AGUS)

    a. lipoma
    a. lymphocyte
    a. measles
    a. melanocytic hyperplasia
    a. mycobacteria
    a. pneumonia
    a. squamous cell
    a. squamous cell of undetermined significance (ASCUS)
    a. trigeminal neuralgia
    a. verrucous endocarditis
atypism
Au
    A. antigen
    A. blood group
Aub-DuBois table
Auberger blood group
Aubert phenomenon
Auchincloss operation
audible rhonchi
audile
audioanalgesia
audiogenic
    a. convulsion
    a. seizure
audiogram
    pure-tone a.
audiologist
audiology
audiometer
    automatic a.
    Békésy a.
audiometric
audiometrist
audiometry
    ABR a.
    auditory brainstem response a.
    automatic a.
    behavioral observation a.
    Békésy a.
    brainstem evoked response a.
    BSER a.
    cortical a.
    diagnostic a.
    electrodermal a.
audiovisual
audit
    nursing a.
audition
    chromatic a.
auditive
auditoria
    tuba a.
auditoriae
    semicanalis tubae a.
auditory
    a. agnosia
    a. alternans
    a. amnesia

a. aphasia
a. area
a. aura
a. brainstem response (ABR)
a. brainstem response audiometry
a. canal
a. capsule
a. cortex
a. defensiveness
a. fatigue
a. feedback
a. field
a. ganglion
a. hair
a. hallucination
a. hyperesthesia
a. lemniscus
a. localization
a. meatus
a. nerve
a. neuropathy
a. nucleus
a. oculogyric reflex
a. organ
a. ossicle
a. pathway
a. pit
a. placode
a. pore
a. process
a. prosthesis
a. receptor cell
a. stria
a. string
a. teeth
a. threshold
a. tract
a. tube
a. vertigo
a. vesicle
audouinii
  Microsporum a.
Auenbrugger sign
Auer
  A. body
  A. rod
Auerbach
  A. ganglion
  A. plexus
Aufrecht sign
Auger electron
augmentation mammaplasty

augmentative and alternative communication
augmented
  a. histamine test
  a. lead
augmentor
  a. fiber
  a. nerve
Aujeszky disease virus
aura, pl. **aurae**
  abdominal a.
  auditory a.
  experiential a.
  gustatory a.
  intellectual a.
  kinesthetic a.
  olfactory a.
  somatosensory a.
  visual a.
aural
  a. myiasis
  a. rehabilitation
  a. vertigo
auramine O
auranofin
aurem
  musculus attollens a.
  musculus attrahens a.
auriasis
auric
auricle
  accessory a.
  atrial a.
  cervical a.
  a. hematoma
  left a.
auricula, pl. **auriculae**
  apex auriculae
  atrial a.
auriculam
  musculus attollens a.
  musculus attrahens a.
auricular
  a. appendage
  a. appendectomy
  a. appendix
  a. arc
  a. branch
  a. canaliculus
  a. cartilage
  a. complex
  a. extrasystole

NOTES

auricular *(continued)*
    a. fibrillation
    a. fissure
    a. flutter
    a. ganglion
    a. glaucoma
    a. index
    a. ligament
    a. muscle
    a. notch
    a. point
    a. reflex
    a. standstill
    a. systole
    a. tachycardia
    a. triangle
    a. tubercle
    a. vein
auricularis
    a. anterior muscle
    a. posterior muscle
    a. superior muscle
auriculocranial
auriculoinfraorbital plane
auriculopalpebral reflex
auriculopressor reflex
auriculotemporal
    a. nerve
    a. nerve syndrome
auriculoventricular
    a. groove
    a. interval
aurid
auriform
auris
    ala a.
    a. externa
    a. interna
    a. media
aurochromoderma
auromercaptoacetanilid
auropalpebral reflex
aurotherapy
aurum
Aus antigen
ausculatory triangle
auscultate, auscult
auscultation
    direct a.
    immediate a.
    mediate a.
    percussion and a. (P&A)
    a. and percussion (A&P)
    triangle of a.
auscultatory
    a. alternans
    a. gap
    a. percussion

    a. sign
    a. sound
Auspitz sign
aussage test
Austin
    A. Flint
    A. Flint murmur
    A. Flint phenomenon
Australia antigen
Australian
    A. bat Lyssavirus
    A. Q fever
    A. tick typhus
    A. X disease
    A. X disease virus
    A. X encephalitis
autacoid substance
autecic
autecious
autemesia
authenticity
authoritarian personality
authority figure
autism
    early infantile a.
    infantile a.
autistic
    a. disorder
    a. parasite
autoactivation
autoagglutination
autoagglutinin
    anti-Pr cold a.
    cold a.
autoallergic
autoallergization
autoallergy
autoanalysis
autoanalyzer
autoanaphylaxis
autoantibody
    antiidiotype a.
    cold a.
    Donath-Landsteiner cold a.
    hemagglutinating cold a.
    idiotype a.
autoanticomplement
autoantigen
autoassay
autoaugmentation
autoblast
autocatalysis
autocatalytic
autocatheterism
autocatheterization
autochthonous
    a. idea
    a. malaria
    a. parasite

autoclasia
autoclasis
autoclave
autocoid
autocrine hypothesis
autocystoplasty
autocytolysin
autocytolysis
autocytotoxin
autodermic graft
autodigestion
autodiploid
autodrainage
autoecholalia
autoerotic asphyxia
autoeroticism
autoerotism
autoerythrocyte
    a. sensitization
    a. sensitization syndrome
autofluoroscope
autogamous
autogamy
autogeneic graft
autogenesis
autogenetic
autogenic
autogenous
    a. control
    a. graft
    a. keratoplasty
    a. union
    a. vaccine
autognosis
autograft
autografting
autogram
autographism
autohemagglutination
autohemolysin
autohemolysis test
autohexaploid
autohypnosis
autohypnotic
autohypnotism
autoimmune
    a. disease
    a. hemolytic anemia
    a. neonatal thrombocytopenia
    a. thyroiditis
autoimmunity
autoimmunization

autoimmunocytopenia
autoinfection
autoinfusion
autoinoculable
autoinoculation
autointoxicant
autointoxication
autoisolysin
autokeratoplasty
autokinesia, autokinesis
autokinetic effect
autolesion
autologous
    a. antigen
    a. fat graft
    a. protein
autolysate
autolyse
autolysin
autolysis
autolytic enzyme
autolyze
automallet
automated
    a. differential leukocyte counter
    a. lamellar keratectomy
automatic
    a. audiometer
    a. audiometry
    a. auditory brainstem response
    a. beat
    a. condenser
    a. contraction
    a. epilepsy
    a. gain control
    a. plugger
    a. speech
    a. transport ventilator
automatism
    alcohol a.
    ambulatory a.
    epileptic a.
    immediate posttraumatic a.
    postictal a.
automatograph
automixis
automnesia
automotor seizure
automysophobia
autonomic
    a. division
    a. dysreflexia

NOTES

autonomic *(continued)*
    a. epilepsy
    a. ganglion
    a. hyperreflexia
    a. imbalance
    a. motor neuron
    a. nerve
    a. nerve fiber
    a. nervous system
    a. neurogenic bladder
    a. plexus
    a. seizure
    a. visceral motor nuclei
autonomotropic
autonomous psychotherapy
autonomy
    functional a.
autooxidation
autoparenchymatous metaplasia
autopathic
auto-PEEP
autopentaploid
autopepsia
autophagia
autophagic vacuole
autophagolysosome
autophagy
autophobia
autophony
autoplastic graft
autoplasty
autoploid
autoploidy
autoplugger
autopod
autopodium
autopoisonous
autopolymerization
autopolymerizing resin
autopolymer resin
autopolyploid
autopolyploidy
auto-positive-end-expiratory-pressure
autopsy
    verbal a.
autoradiogram
autoradiograph
autoradiography
    thick-layer a.
autoreceptor
autoregulation
    heterometric a.
    homeometric a.
autoreinfection
autoreproduction
autorrhaphy
autoscopic phenomenon
autosensitize
autosepticemia

autoserotherapy
autoserum therapy
autosite
autosmia
autosomal
    a. dominant
    a. gene
    a. hereditary
    a. recessive
autosomatognosis
autosomatognostic
autosome
autosuggestibility
autosuggestion
autosynnoia
autosynthesis
autotelic
autotemnous
autotetraploid
autotherapy
autotomy
autotopagnosia
autotoxemia
autotoxic
autotoxicosis
autotoxin
autotransfusion
autotransplant
autotransplantation
autotriploid
autotroph
autotrophic
autotrophy
    carbon a.
autovaccination
autoxidation
autozygous
autumn fever
auxanogram
auxanographic method
auxanography
auxanology
auxesis
auxetic growth
auxiliary abutment
auxiliomotor
auxilytic
auxocardia
auxochrome
auxodrome
auxoflore
auxogluc
auxotonic
auxotox
auxotroph
auxotrophic
    a. mutant
    a. strain

AV, A-V
  arteriovenous
  atrioventricular
    AV block
    AV conduction
    AV difference
    AV dissociation
    AV interval
    AV junction
    AV junctional rhythm
    AV junctional tachycardia
    AV nodal extrasystole
    AV node
    AV shunt
    AV strabismus syndrome
    AV valve
available arch length
avalanche conduction
avalvular
avascularization
avascular necrosis
AVC
  atrioventricular conduction
AVD
  atrioventricular dissociation
Avellis syndrome
avenae
  farina a.
avenin
average
  a. evoked potential
  a. flow rate
  a. pulse magnitude
  pure-tone a.
avermectin
aversion therapy
aversive
  a. behavior
  a. conditioning
  a. control
  a. stimulus
  a. training
aVF lead
avian
  a. encephalomyelitis virus
  a. influenza virus
  a. leukemia-sarcoma complex
  a. leukosis-sarcoma complex
  a. leukosis-sarcoma virus
  a. lymphomatosis virus
  a. neurolymphomatosis virus
  a. pneumoencephalitis virus

  a. sarcoma
  a. viral arthritis virus
aviation medicine
aviator's disease
avidin
avidity antibody
avirulent
avis
  nidus a.
avitaminosis
  conditioned a.
avium
    Mycobacterium a.
avium-intracellulare
    Mycobacterium a.-i. (MAI)
avivement
aVL lead
Avogadro
  A. constant
  A. hypothesis
  A. law
  A. number
  A. postulate
avoidance
  a. conditioning
  a. training
avoidance-avoidance conflict
avoidant
  a. disorder of adolescence
  a. disorder of childhood
  a. personality
  a. personality disorder
avoirdupois weight
aVR lead
avulsed wound
avulsion
  a. fracture
  nerve a.
AW
  atomic weight
awareness
  kinesthetic a.
  reality a.
  sensory a.
axanthum
    Acholeplasma a.
axenic
axerophthol
axes (*pl. of* axis)
axial
  a. ametropia
  a. aneurysm

NOTES

axial *(continued)*
- a. angle
- a. cataract
- a. current
- a. filament
- a. hyperopia
- a. illumination
- a. loading
- a. muscle
- a. myopia
- a. neuritis
- a. pattern flap
- a. plane
- a. plate
- a. point
- a. projection
- a. section
- a. skeleton
- a. surface
- a. view

axialis
axifugal
axile corpuscle
axilla, pl. **axillae**
- a. thermometer

axillaris
trichomycosis a.

axillary
- a. abscess
- a. anesthesia
- a. arch
- a. arch muscle
- a. artery
- a. cavity
- a. fascia
- a. fold
- a. fossa
- a. hair
- a. line
- a. lymphatic plexus
- a. lymph node
- a. nerve
- a. region
- a. sheath
- a. space
- a. sweat gland
- a. thermometer
- a. thoracotomy
- a. triangle
- a. vein

axiobuccal
axiobuccocervical
axiobuccogingival
axiobuccolingual
axiocervical
axiodistal
axiodistocervical
axiodistogingival
axioincisal

axiolabial
axiolabiolingual plane
axiolingual
axiolinguocervical
axiolinguoclusal
axiolinguogingival
axiomesial
axiomesiocervical
axiomesiodistal plane
axiomesiogingival
axiomesioincisal
axion
axio-occlusal
axioplasm
axiopodium
axiopulpal
axioversion
axipetal
axis, pl. **axes**
- basibregmatic a.
- basicranial a.
- basifacial a.
- biauricular a.
- celiac a.
- cephalocaudal a.
- cerebrospinal a.
- condylar a.
- conjugate a.
- a. corpuscle
- craniofacial a.
- dens a.
- a. deviation
- electrical a.
- embryonic a.
- encephalomyelonic a.
- external a.
- facial a.
- axes of Fick
- hinge a.
- instantaneous electrical a.
- internal a.
- long a.
- mandibular a.
- mean electrical a.
- optic a.
- pelvic a.
- principal optic a.
- sagittal a.
- secondary a.
- a. shift
- a. traction
- transverse horizontal a.
- visual a.

axis-traction forceps
axoaxonic synapse
axodendritic synapse
axofugal
axograph
axolemma

axolysis
axon
    a. degeneration
    a. hillock
    a. loss polyneuropathy
    a. reflex
    a. terminal
axonal
    a. degeneration
    a. polyneuropathy
    a. terminal bouton
axoneme
axonography
axonopathy
axonotmesis
axopetal
axoplasm
axoplasmic transport
axopodium
axosomatic synapse
axostyle
axotomy
Ayala
    A. index
    A. quotient
Ayerza
    A. disease
    A. syndrome
Ayre brush
azacrine
azapirone
azar
    kala a.
azaribine
azaserine
azathioprine
azeotrope
    halothane-ether a.
azeotropic
azide
azidothymidine (AZT)
azin dye
azlocillin sodium

azo
    a. dye
    a. itch
azobilirubin
azocarmine
    a. B, G
    a. dye
azoic
azole
azolitmin
azoospermia
azophloxin
azoprotein
Azorean disease
azosulfamide
azotemia
azotemic
azothermia
azotobacter nuclease
azoturia
azovan blue
AZT
    azidothymidine
Aztec ear
aztreonam
azure
    a. A, B, C
    a. I, II
    a. lunule
azuresin
azurophil, azurophile
    a. granule
azurophilia
azygoesophageal recess
azygogram
azygography
azygos
    a. artery
    a. fissure
    a. lobe
    a. vein
azygous

NOTES

β (*var. of* beta)
B
    B bile
    B cell
    B cell co-receptor
    B cell differentiating factor
    B cell differentiation/growth factor
    B cell receptor
    B cell stimulatory factor 2
    B chain
    B fiber
    B lymphocyte
    B virus
    B wave
B1
    vitamin B1
B6
    B6 bronchus sign
    vitamin B6
B-100
    apolipoprotein B-100
B12
    vitamin B12
B-48
    apolipoprotein B-48
1b
    interferon beta 1b
2b
    interferon alfa 2b
b5
    cytochrome b5
B19 virus
Babbitt metal
Babcock tube
Babès
    B. node
    B. nodule
    B. tubercle
Babesia microti
babesiosis
    bovine b.
    human b.
Babinski
    B. phenomenon
    B. reflex
    B. sign
    B. syndrome
baby
    blue b.
    blueberry muffin b.
    b. bottle syndrome
    collodion b.
    test-tube b.
    b. tooth
baccate

Baccelli sign
bacciform
Bachmann bundle
Bachman-Pettit test
Bachman test
bacillar
bacillary
    b. angiomatosis
    b. dysentery
    b. layer
    b. phthisis
bacille Calmette-Guérin (BCG)
bacillemia
bacilli (*pl. of* bacillus)
bacilliform
bacilliformis
    Bartonella b.
bacillin
bacillomyxin
bacillosis
bacilluria
Bacillus
    B. anthracis
    B. brevis
    B. cereus
    B. circulans
    B. pumilis
    B. sphaericus
bacillus, pl. bacilli
    abortus b.
    acid-fast b. (AFB)
    Bang b.
    Battey b.
    blue pus b.
    Boas-Oppler b.
    Bordet-Gengou b.
    Calmette-Guérin b.
    b. Calmette-Guérin vaccine
    coliform bacilli
    comma b.
    Döderlein b.
    Ducrey b.
    dysentery b.
    Eberth b.
    Flexner b.
    Friedländer b.
    gas b.
    grass b.
    Hansen b.
    hay b.
    Hofmann b.
    influenza b.
    Kitasato b.
    Klebs-Loeffler b.
    Koch b.

B

bacillus *(continued)*
    Koch-Weeks b.
    lactic acid b.
    leprosy b.
    Loeffler b.
    Moeller grass b.
    Newcastle-Manchester b.
    Pfeiffer b.
    Shiga-Kruse b.
    Sonne b.
    tubercle b.
    typhoid b.
    Vincent b.
    Weeks b.
    Welch b.
bacitracin
back
    adolescent round b.
    b. board
    b. cross
    hollow b.
    b. mutation
    b. pressure
    b. table procedure
    b. tooth
    b. vertex power
backache
back-action plugger
back-and-forth suture
backboard splint
backbone
backcross
    double b.
back-extrapolation
backflow
    pyelorenal b.
    pyelovenous b.
background
    b. activity
    b. level
    b. radiation
    b. retinopathy
back-knee
backprojection
backscatter
backtracking
backward
    b. curvature
    b. heart failure
backwash ileitis
Bacon anoscope
bacteremia
bacteria (*pl. of* bacterium)
bacterial
    b. allergy
    b. antagonism
    b. antigen
    b. arthritis
    b. capsule

    b. cast
    b. cystitis
    b. encephalitis
    b. endarteritis
    b. endocarditis
    b. enteritis
    b. food poisoning
    b. growth
    b. hemolysin
    b. interference
    b. overgrowth syndrome
    b. peliosis
    b. pericarditis
    b. peritonitis
    b. photosynthesis
    b. plaque
    b. pneumonia
    b. toxin
    b. translocation
    b. vaginosis
    b. vegetation
    b. virus
bactericholia
bactericidal antibiotic
bactericide
bacterid
bacteriemia
bacterioagglutinin
bacteriochlorin
bacteriochlorophyll
bacteriocidal
bacteriocide
bacteriocidin
bacteriocin factor
bacteriocinogen
bacteriocinogenic plasmid
bacteriofluorescin
bacteriogenic agglutination
bacteriogenous
bacterioid
bacteriologic
bacteriological
bacteriologist
bacteriology
bacteriolysin
bacteriolysis
bacteriolytic serum
bacteriolyze
bacteriopexy
bacteriophage
    defective b.
    filamentous b.
    b. immunity
    mature b.
    b. plaque
    b. resistance
    temperate b.
    b. typing

B

vegetative b.
virulent b.
bacteriophagia
bacteriophagology
bacteriopheophorbin
bacteriophytoma
bacterioprotein
bacteriopsonin
bacteriosis
bacteriospermia
bacteriostasis
bacteriostat
bacteriostatic
 b. agent
 b. antibiotic
bacteriotoxic
bacteriotropic substance
bacteriotropin
bacteriotrypsin
bacterium, pl. **bacteria**
 blue-green b.
 cell wall–defective bacteria
 coryneform bacteria
 endoteric b.
 exoteric b.
 lysogenic b.
bacteriuria
bacteroid
Bacteroides
 B. bivius
 B. capillosus
 B. corrodens
 B. disiens
 B. distasonis
 B. fragilis
 B. furcosus
 B. melaninogenicus
 B. nodosus
 B. oralis
 B. oris
 B. splanchnicus
 B. thetaiotamicron
bacteroidosis
baculiform
baculovirus
badge
 film b.
Baehr-Lohlein lesion
Baelz disease
BAER
 brainstem auditory evoked response
Baer law

Baermann concentration
Baeyer theory
bag
 Ambu b.
 breathing b.
 colostomy b.
 Douglas b.
 Politzer b.
 reservoir b.
 b. ventilation
 b. of waters
bagassosis
Bagdad boil
Baggenstoss change
Baghdad
 bouton de B.
bag-mask device
Bagolini test
bag-valve-mask device
Baillarger
 B. band
 B. line
 B. stria
 B. stripe
Bailliart ophthalmodynamometer
Bainbridge reflex
baja
 patella b.
baked tongue
baker
 B. acid hematein
 B. cyst
 b. eczema
 b. itch
 B. pyridine extraction
baking soda
BAL
 bronchoalveolar lavage
Balamuth aqueous egg yolk infusion medium
balance
 acid-base b.
 nitrogen b.
 phonetic b.
 B. sign
 b. theory
balanced
 b. anesthesia
 b. articulation
 b. bite
 b. diet
 b. occlusion

NOTES

balanced *(continued)*
    b. polymorphism
    b. translocation
balancing
    b. contact
    b. occlusal surface
    b. side
    b. side condyle
balanic hypospadias
balanitic epispadias
balanitis
    b. circumscripta plasmacellularis
    b. diabetica
    b. xerotica obliterans
balanoplasty
balanoposthitis
balantidial dysentery
balantidiasis
Balantidium coli
balantidosis
balanus
balatus
    Acarus b.
Balbani ring
baldness
    common b.
    congenital b.
    male pattern b.
bald tongue
Balint syndrome
Balkan
    B. beam
    B. frame
    B. nephropathy
    B. splint
ball
    chondrin b.
    food b.
    fungus b.
    hair b.
    B. operation
    b. thrombus
    b. valve
    b. valve action
    b. variance
Ballance sign
ball-and-socket
    b.-a.-s. abutment
    b.-a.-s. joint
ballerina-foot pattern
ballet
    cardiac b.
ballismus, ballism
ballistocardiogram
ballistocardiograph
ballistocardiography
ballistophobia
balloon
    angioplasty b.

    b. atrioseptostomy
    b. biliary catheter
    b. cell
    b. cell nevus
    b. counter pulsation
    b. defecation
    detachable b.
    b. dilatation
    intraaortic b.
    b. septostomy
    b. sickness
    b. tamponade
ballooning
    b. degeneration
    b. mitral cusp
balloon-tip catheter
ballotable patella
ballottable
ballottement
    abdominal b.
ballpoint pen technique
ball-valve thrombus
balm of Gilead
balneotherapeutics
balneotherapy
Baló disease
balsam
    Canada b.
    Mecca b.
balsamic
BALT
    bronchus-associated lymphoid tissue
Baltic myoclonus disease
Bamberger
    B. albuminuria
    B. disease
    B. sign
Bamberger-Marie
    B.-M. disease
    B.-M. syndrome
Bamberger-Pins-Ewart sign
bamboo
    b. hair
    b. spine
bamipine
banana
    b.'s, rice cereal, applesauce, toast (BRAT)
    b. sign
bancroftian filariasis
bancroftiasis, bancroftosis
band
    A b.
    absorption b.
    amnionic b.
    amniotic b.
    anogenital b.
    anular b.
    atrioventricular b.

Baillarger b.
Bechterew b.
Broca diagonal b.
b. cell
b. centrifugation
chromosome b.
Clado b.
b. of colon
contraction b.
diagonal b.
Essick cell b.
Gennari b.
b. of Giacomini
H b.
His b.
Hunter-Schreger b.
I b.
iliotibial b.
b. of Kaes-Bechterew
Ladd b.
Lane b.
longitudinal b.
M b.
Mach b.
Maissiat b.
matrix b.
Meckel b.
moderator b.
b. neutrophil
oligoclonal b.
periosteal b.
Simonart b.
ventricular b.
Z b.
bandage
adhesive b.
Barton b.
butterfly b.
capeline b.
circular b.
compression b.
b. contact lens
cravat b.
crucial b.
demigauntlet b.
Desault b.
elastic b.
Esmarch b.
figure-of-8 b.
fixation b.
gauntlet b.
gauze b.

Gibney fixation b.
Gibson b.
hammock b.
immobilizing b.
immovable b.
Martin b.
plaster b.
pressure b.
roller b.
Scultetus b.
spica b.
spiral b.
suspensory b.
4-tailed b.
triangular b.
Velpeau b.
bandbox resonance
banding
high-resolution b.
Trusler rule for pulmonary artery b.
Bandl ring
bandpass filter
band-shaped keratopathy
bandwidth
bandy-leg
bane
leopard's b.
bang
B. bacillus
B. disease
banisterine
bank
blood b.
eye b.
Bankart lesion
banked blood
Bannister disease
Bannwarth syndrome
Banti
B. disease
B. syndrome
baptitoxine
bar
arch b.
clasp b.
b. clasp
b. clasp arm
b. clip attachment
connector b.
b. joint denture
labial b.

NOTES

bar *(continued)*
    lingual b.
    median b.
    Mercier b.
    prism b.
    terminal b.
baragnosis
Bárány
    B. caloric test
    B. sign
barba
barbae
    folliculitis b.
    tinea b.
barbaloin
barbed broach
barber
    b. itch
    b. pilonidal sinus
barbital
barbiturate
barbiturism
barbotage
barbula hirci
Barclay-Baron disease
Barcoo vomit
Barcroft-Warburg
    B.-W. apparatus
    B.-W. technique
Bardet-Biedl syndrome
Bardinet ligament
bare
    b. area
    b. lymphocyte syndrome
baresthesia
baresthesiometer
bariatric
bariatrics
baricity
baritosis
barium
    b. chloride
    b. enema
    b. hydroxide
    b. meal
    b. monoxide
    b. oxide
    b. sulfate
    b. sulfide
    b. swallow
bark
    bayberry b.
    cassia b.
    cinchona b.
    cotton-root b.
    Jesuits b.
    kurchi b.

Barkan
    B. membrane
    B. operation
Barkman reflex
Barkow ligament
Barlow
    B. disease
    B. maneuver
    B. syndrome
    B. test
Barmah Forest virus
Barnes
    B. curve
    B. zone
baroceptor
barognosis
barograph
barometric pressure
barometrograph
barophilic
baroreceptor nerve
baroreflex
baroscope
barosinusitis
barostat
barotaxis
barotitis media
barotrauma
barotropism
Barraquer
    B. disease
    B. method
    B. Roviralta
Barr chromatin body
barrel
    b. chest
    b. distortion
    b. dressing
    b. hoop sign
barrel-shaped thorax
Barré sign
Barrett
    B. epithelium
    B. esophagus
    B. metaplasia
    B. syndrome
barrier
    architectural b.
    blood-air b.
    blood-aqueous b.
    blood-brain b. (BBB)
    blood-cerebrospinal fluid b.
    blood-CSF b.
    blood-testis b.
    blood-thymus b.
    b. contraceptive
    incest b.
    placental b.
bar-sleeve attachment

Bart
    hemoglobin B.
    B. syndrome
Barth
    B. hernia
    B. syndrome
Bartholin
    B. abscess
    B. anus
    B. cyst
    B. cystectomy
    B. duct
    B. gland
bartholinitis
Barton
    B. bandage
    B. forceps
    B. fracture
Bartonella
    B. anemia
    B. *bacilliformis*
    B. *henselae*
    B. *quintana*
bartonellosis
Bartter syndrome
Baruch law
baruria
baryta water
basad
basal
    b. age
    b. anesthesia
    b. arachnoiditis
    b. body
    b. body temperature
    b. bone
    b. cell
    b. cell adenoma
    b. cell epithelioma
    b. cell hyperplasia
    b. cell layer
    b. cell nevus
    b. cell nevus syndrome
    b. cell papilloma
    b. cistern
    b. corpuscle
    b. crest
    b. diet
    b. encephalocele
    b. ganglia
    b. gland
    b. granule

    b. iridectomy
    b. joint reflex
    b. lamina
    b. laminar drusen
    b. layer
    b. linear drusen
    b. metabolic rate (BMR)
    b. metabolism
    b. nucleus
    b. ophthalmoplegia
    b. part
    b. plate
    b. pleurisy
    b. ration
    b. ridge
    b. rod
    b. seat
    b. seat area
    b. skull fracture (BSF)
    b. sphincter
    b. squamous cell carcinoma
    b. striation
    b. substantia
    b. surface
    b. tentorial branch
    b. tuberculosis
    b. vein
basale
    stratum b.
basaloid
    b. carcinoma
    b. cell
base
    acrylic resin b.
    anterior cranial b.
    Brønsted b.
    cement b.
    b. composition
    cranial b.
    b. deficit
    denture b.
    b. excess
    hexone b.
    histone b.
    b. hospital
    b. increase
    internal b.
    Lewis b.
    b. line
    b. material
    metal b.
    b. metal

B

NOTES

base *(continued)*
    methamphetamine b.
    b. pair
    b. plate
    pressor b.
    b. projection
    b. station
    b. unit
    b. view
baseball finger
basedoid
Basedow
    B. disease
    B. goiter
    B. pseudoparaplegia
basedowian
baseline
    b. fetal heart rate
    b. tonus
    b. variability
basement
    b. lamina
    b. membrane
baseplate wax
base-stacking
bas-fond
Basham mixture
basialveolar
basibregmatic axis
basic
    b. amino acid
    b. diet
    b. dye
    b. electrical rhythm
    b. esotropia
    b. exotropia
    b. fuchsin
    b. fuchsin-methylene blue stain
    b. life support (BLS)
    b. metal
    b. oxide
    b. personality
    b. personality type
    b. protein
    b. reaction
    b. salt
basicity
basicranial
    b. axis
    b. flexure
basicranium
basidium
basifacial axis
basihyal
basihyoid
basilar
    b. angle
    b. apophysis
    b. artery

    b. bone
    b. cartilage
    b. cell
    b. fibrocartilage
    b. impression
    b. index
    b. invagination
    b. lamina
    b. leptomeningitis
    b. membrane
    b. meningitis
    b. migraine
    b. papilla
    b. part
    b. pontine sulcus
    b. process
    b. prognathism
    b. sinus
    b. venous plexus
    b. vertebra
basilaris
basilateral
basilemma
basilicus
basilic vein
basin
    emesis b.
    kidney b.
basinasal line
basioccipital bone
basiocciput
basioglossus
basion
basipetal
basipharyngeal canal
basiphobia
basisphenoid
basisquamous carcinoma
basivertebral vein
basket
    b. cell
    fibrillar b.
    b. nucleus
    stone b.
basocyte
basocytopenia
basocytosis
basoerythrocyte
basoerythrocytosis
basolateral
basometachromophil,
    basometachromophile
basopenia
basophil, basophile
    b. adenoma
    b. granule
    b. substance
basophilia
    Grawitz b.

basophilic
- b. degeneration
- b. leukemia
- b. leukocyte
- b. leukocytosis
- b. leukopenia
- b. substance

basophilism
Cushing pituitary b.

basophilocytic leukemia

basoplasm

basosquamous carcinoma

Bassen-Kornzweig syndrome

Bassini
- B. herniorrhaphy
- B. operation

Bassler sign

Bassora gum

bassorin

Bastedo sign

bastokinin

batch
- b. analyzer
- b. culture

bat ear

bath
- colloid b.
- contrast b.
- douche b.
- dousing b.
- electric b.
- electrotherapeutic b.
- Greville b.
- hafussi b.
- hydroelectric b.
- immersion b.
- b. itch
- light b.
- needle b.
- b. pruritus
- sitz b.
- sponge b.

bathing trunk nevus

bathmotropic

bathochromic

bathoflore

bathophobia

bathyanesthesia

bathycardia

bathyesthesia

bathygastry

bathyhyperesthesia

bathyhypesthesia

Batista procedure

batrachotoxin

Batson plexus

Batten disease

Batten-Mayou disease

battered
- b. child syndrome
- b. spouse syndrome

battery
Halstead-Reitan b.

Battey bacillus

Battista operation

battle
- b. fatigue
- b. neurosis
- B. sign

battledore placenta

Baudelocque operation

Bauer
- B. chromic acid leucofuchsin stain
- B. syndrome

Bauer-Kirby test

Bauhin
- B. gland
- B. valve

Baumé scale

Baumès symptom

Baumgarten
- B. gland
- B. vein

bauxite pneumoconiosis

bay
- celomic b.
- lacrimal b.

bayberry bark

Bayesian hypothesis

Bayle disease

Baynton operation

bayonet
- b. apposition
- b. forceps
- b. hair

Bayou virus

Bazett formula

Bazex syndrome

Bazin disease

BBB
blood-brain barrier

BCG
bacille Calmette-Guérin
BCG vaccine

NOTES

BCR/ABL gene
B-E
    below the elbow
        B-E amputation
Bea antigen
beaded hair
beading of rib
beaked pelvis
beaker cell
beak sign
Beale cell
beam
    Balkan b.
    cantilever b.
    continuous b.
    electron b.
bean
    Calabar b.
    castor b.
bearing
    central b.
    b. down
bearing-down pain
beat
    apex b.
    atrial capture b.
    atrial fusion b.
    automatic b.
    combination b.
    coupled b.'s
    dependent b.
    Dressler b.
    dropped b.
    echo b.
    ectopic b.
    escape b.
    escaped b.
    forced b.
    fusion b.
    heart b.
    interference b.
    mixed b.
    retrograde b.
    ventricular fusion b.
beat-to-beat variability
Beau line
Bechterew
    B. band
    B. disease
    layer of B.
    line of B.
    B. nucleus
    B. sign
Bechterew-Mendel reflex
Beck
    B. method
    B. triad
Becker
    B. antigen

    B. disease
    B. muscular dystrophy
    B. nevus
    B. stain for spirochetes
Becker-type tardive muscular dystrophy
Beckmann apparatus
Beckwith-Wiedemann syndrome
Béclard
    B. anastomosis
    B. hernia
    B. triangle
beclomethasone dipropionate
becquerel
Becquerel ray
bed
    air-fluidized b.
    capillary b.
    fracture b.
    Gatch b.
    nail b.
    b. rest
bedbug
Bednar
    B. aphthae
    B. tumor
bedside
    b. radiography
    b. testing
bedsore
bed-wetting
beech oil
beer
    b. heart
    B. knife
    B. law
Beer-Lambert law
bee toxin
Beevor sign
Begg light wire differential force technique
Béguez César disease
behavior
    adaptive b.
    appetitive b.
    aversive b.
    b. chain
    coronary-prone b.
    b. disorder
    displacement b.
    health b.
    hookean b.
    hostile b.
    b. modification
    molar b.
    molecular b.
    occupational b.
    b. reflex
    b. therapy
    type A, B b.

B

behavioral
- b. epidemic
- b. genetics
- b. health
- b. immunogen
- b. manifestation
- b. medicine
- b. observation audiometry
- b. pathogen
- b. psychology
- b. science

behaviorism
behaviorist
behavioristic psychology
Behçet
- B. disease
- B. syndrome

behind-the-ear hearing aid
Behr
- B. disease
- B. syndrome

Behring law
Békésy
- B. audiometer
- B. audiometry

belching
belemnoid
Belgian Congo anemia
bell
- b. clapper deformity
- B. law
- B. muscle
- B. palsy
- B. phenomenon
- B. respiratory nerve
- b. sound
- B. spasm
- b. stage

belladonna
- b. extract
- b. tincture

belladonnine
bell-crowned
belle indifférence
Bellini
- B. duct
- B. ligament

Bell-Magendie law
bellmetal resonance
bellows murmur

bell-shaped
- b.-s. crown
- b.-s. curve

belly
- b. button
- frontal b.
- prune b.
- spider b.

bellyache
belonephobia
below
- b. the elbow (B-E)
- b. the knee (B-K)

Belsey
- B. fundoplication
- B. Mark operation
- B. procedure

belt test
Bence
- B. Jones albumin
- B. Jones cylinder
- B. Jones myeloma
- B. Jones protein
- B. Jones proteinuria
- B. Jones reaction

benchmarking
bench testing
Bender Visual Motor Gestalt test
bending fracture
beneceptor
Benedek reflex
Benedict
- B. solution
- B. test

Benedict-Hopkins-Cole reagent
Benedict-Roth
- B.-R. apparatus
- B.-R. calorimeter

Benedikt syndrome
benefit
- maximum hospital b.
- maximum medical b.

bengal
- rose b.

benign
- b. albuminuria
- b. bone aneurysm
- b. cementoblastoma
- b. childhood epilepsy
- b. coital cephalalgia
- b. congenital hypotonia
- b. cystic teratoma

NOTES

benign *(continued)*
    b. dry pleurisy
    b. dyskeratosis
    b. essential tremor
    b. exertional headache
    b. familial chorea
    b. familial chronic pemphigus
    b. familial icterus
    b. fructosuria
    b. giant lymph node hyperplasia
    b. glycosuria
    b. hypertension
    b. infantile myoclonus
    b. inoculation lymphoreticulosis
    b. inoculation reticulosis
    b. juvenile melanoma
    b. lymphadenosis
    b. lymphocytoma cutis
    b. lymphoepithelial lesion
    b. lymphoma
    b. mesothelioma
    b. migratory glossitis
    b. monoclonal gammopathy
    b. mucosal pemphigoid
    b. myalgic encephalomyelitis
    b. neonatal convulsion
    b. neoplasm
    b. nephrosclerosis
    b. paroxysmal peritonitis
    b. paroxysmal positional vertigo
    b. paroxysmal torticollis
    b. polycythemia
    b. positional nystagmus
    b. prostatic hyperplasia (BPH)
    b. prostatic hypertrophy (BPH)
    b. rheumatoid nodule
    b. stupor
    b. tertian fever
    b. tertian malaria
    b. tetanus
    b. tumor
benignum
    lymphogranuloma b.
benjamin
    gum b.
benne oil
Bennett
    B. angle
    B. fracture
    B. movement
Bennhold Congo red stain
Bensley specific granule
bentiromide test
bentonite flocculation test
benzene
    b. nucleus
    b. ring
benzeneamine
benzethonium chloride

benzidine test
benzimidazole
benzoate
    ammonium b.
    benzyl b.
    denatonium b.
    ecgonine b.
    estradiol b.
    magnesium b.
benzoic
    b. acid
    b. aldehyde
benzoin
    gum b.
benzoinated lard
benzoquinone
benzoyl
    b. chloride
    b. hydrate
    b. peroxide
benzoylecgonine
benzoylpas
    calcium b.
benzyl
    b. alcohol
    b. benzoate
benzylidene
benzyloxycarbonyl
Beradinelli syndrome
Bérard aneurysm
Berardinelli syndrome
Béraud valve
bereavement
Berger
    B. cell
    B. disease
    B. focal glomerulonephritis
    B. rhythm
    B. space
Bergmann
    B. cord
    B. fiber
Bergman sign
Bergmeister papilla
Berg stain
beri
    beri b.
beriberi, beri beri
    dry b.
    b. heart
    infantile b.
Berkefeld filter
berkelium
Berlin
    B. blue
    B. edema
berloque, berlock
    b. dermatitis

B

Bernard
  B. canal
  B. duct
  B. operation
  B. puncture
Bernard-Cannon homeostasis
Bernard-Horner syndrome
Bernard-Sergent syndrome
Bernard-Soulier
  B.-S. disease
  B.-S. syndrome
Bernays sponge
Bernhardt
  B. disease
  B. formula
Bernhardt-Roth syndrome
Bernheim syndrome
Bernoulli
  B. distribution
  B. effect
  B. law
  B. principle
  B. theorem
  B. trial
Bernstein test
berry
  b. aneurysm
  b. cell
  fish b.
  B. ligament
Berson test
Berthelot reaction
Berthollet law
Bertin
  B. bone
  B. column
  B. ligament
  B. ossicle
berylliosis
beryllium granuloma
Besnier-Boeck-Schaumann
  B.-B.-S. disease
  B.-B.-S. syndrome
Besnier prurigo
Besnoitiidae
best
  B. carmine stain
  B. disease
  b. frequency
bestiality
besylate

beta, β
  b. angle
  b. cell
  b. error
  b. fiber
  b. granule
  interferon b.
  b. particle
  b. radiation
  b. ray
  b. rhythm
  b. sheet
  B. test
  b. wave
beta-adrenergic
  b.-a. blocking agent
  b.-a. receptor
beta-blocker
betacism
betacyanin
betacyaninuria
betaine
  b. aldehyde
  glycine b.
beta-lactam antibiotic
betamethasone
beta-oxidation-condensation theory
betatron
betel
  b. cancer
  b. nut
bethanechol chloride
Bethesda
  B. classification
  B. system
  B. unit
Bethesda-Ballerup group
Betke-Kleihauer test
Bettendorff test
betula oil
Betz cell
Beuren syndrome
Bevan-Lewis cell
bevel
  cavosurface b.
bevelled anastomosis
bezoar
Bezold
  B. abscess
  B. ganglion
Bezold-Jarisch reflex
BH interval

NOTES

bi
- b. antigen
- b. bi reaction

Bial test
Bianchi nodule
biarticular
bias
- ascertainment b.
- cross-level b.
- recall b.
- reporting b.
- response b.
- sampling b.

biasterionic
biauricular axis
biaxial joint
bibasilar rhonchi
bibliomania
bibulous
bicameral abscess
bicanalicular sphincter
BICAP
- bipolar circumactive probe
- BICAP cautery

bicapsular
bicarbonate
- b. of soda
- sodium b.
- standard b.

bicardiogram
bicellular
bicephalus
biceps
- b. brachii muscle
- b. femoris muscle
- b. femoris reflex

Bichat
- B. canal
- B. fat-pad
- B. fissure
- B. foramen
- B. fossa
- B. ligament
- B. membrane
- B. protuberance
- B. tunic

bichloride
- copper b.
- mercury b.

bicipital
- b. aponeurosis
- b. fascia
- b. groove
- b. rib
- b. ridge
- b. tuberosity

bicipitalis
- aponeurosis b.

bicipitoradial bursa

Bickel ring
biclonal
- b. gammopathy
- b. peak

biclonality
bicollis
- uterus bicornis b.

bicolor
- iris b.

biconcave lens
bicondylar
- b. articulation
- b. joint

biconvex lens
bicornate, bicornous
- b. uterus

bicoudate catheter
bicron
bicuculline
bicuspid
- b. aortic valve
- b. murmur
- b. tooth

bicuspidization
bidactyly
bidirectional
- b. replication
- b. ventricular tachycardia

bidiscoidal placenta
biduous
Biebl loop
Biebrich scarlet red
Biederman sign
Bielschowsky
- B. disease
- B. sign
- B. stain

Biemond syndrome
bieneusi
- *Enterocytozoon b.*

Bier
- B. amputation
- B. block
- B. hyperemia
- B. method

Biermer
- B. anemia
- B. disease

Biernacki sign
Biesiadecki fossa
bifascicular
bifenestratus
- hymen b.

bifermentans
- *Clostridium b.*

bifid
- b. clitoris
- b. cranium
- b. epiglottis

b. foot
b. penis
b. rib
b. thumb
b. tongue
b. uterus
b. uvula
bifida
spina b.
Bifidobacterium dentium
bifidum
cranium b.
bifocal
b. lens
b. spectacles
biforate uterus
biforis
hymen b.
bifoveal fixation
bifunctional
bifurcated ligament
bifurcate ligament
bifurcation
b. of aorta
aortic b.
b. of trachea
Bigelow
B. ligament
B. septum
bigeminal
b. body
b. pulse
b. rhythm
bigeminus
pulsus b.
bigeminy
atrial b.
atrioventricular junctional b.
escape-capture b.
rule of b.
bilaminar blastoderm
bilateral
b. coordination
b. hermaphroditism
b. left-sidedness
b. medial orbital ecchymosis
b. otitis media (BOM)
b. pleurisy
b. rhonchi
b. synchrony
b. vagotomy
bilateralism

bile
A b.
b. acid
b. acid tolerance test
b. alcohol
B. antigen
B b.
C b.
b. capillary
b. cyst
b. duct
b. duct carcinoma
b. esculin test
b. gastritis
b. papilla
b. peritonitis
b. pigment
b. pigment hemoglobin
b. salt
b. salt agar
b. solubility test
b. thrombus
bi-leaflet valve
bilevel positive airway pressure
bilharzial
b. appendicitis
b. dysentery
b. granuloma
bilharziasis
bilharzioma
bilharziosis
biliaropancreatic ampulla
biliary
b. atresia
b. calculus
b. canaliculus
b. cirrhosis
b. colic
b. duct
b. ductule
b. dyskinesia
b. fistula
b. gland
b. steatorrhea
b. xanthomatosis
bilifaction
biliferous
bilification
biligenesis
biligenic
bilin, biline

NOTES

bilious
    b. cholera
    b. headache
    b. pneumonia
    b. remittent fever
    b. remittent malaria
    b. typhoid of Griesinger
    b. vomit
biliousness
bilirachia
bilirubin
    conjugated b.
    delta b.
    direct reacting b.
    b. encephalopathy
    indirect reacting b.
bilirubinemia
bilirubinglobulin
bilirubin-glucuronoside
  glucuronosyltransferase
bilirubinoid
bilirubinuria
bilitherapy
biliuria
biliverdin
biliverdine
Billings method
Bill maneuver
billowing mitral valve syndrome
Billroth
    B. cord
    B. I, II anastomosis
    B. operation I, II
biloba
    Ginkgo b.
bilobate
bilobectomy
bilobed
bilobular
bilocular
    b. femoral hernia
    b. joint
    b. stomach
biloculare
    cor b.
biloculate
bimalleolar fracture
bimanual
    b. examination
    b. palpation
    b. percussion
    b. version
bimastoid
bimaxillary
    b. dentoalveolar protrusion
    b. protrusive occlusion
bimolecular
binangle chisel

binary
    b. combination
    b. complex
    b. digit
    b. fission
    b. nomenclature
    b. process
binasal hemianopia
binaural
    b. alternate loudness balance test
    b. diplacusis
    b. stethoscope
binauricular arc
bind
    double b.
binder
    obstetrical b.
binding
    b. constant
    b. energy
Binet
    B. age
    B. scale
    B. test
Binet-Simon scale
Bingham
    B. flow
    B. model
    B. plastic
Bing reflex
biniodide
    mercury b.
binocular
    b. fixation
    b. heterochromia
    b. loupe
    b. microscope
    b. ophthalmoscope
    b. parallax
    b. rivalry
    b. vision
binomial
    b. distribution
    b. nomenclature
binotic
binovular twin
Binswanger
    B. disease
    B. encephalopathy
binuclear
binucleate
binucleolate
bioacoustics
bioactive nonnutrient
bioassay
bioastronautics
bioavailability
bioburden
biocatalyst

biocenosis
biochemical
  b. biopsy
  b. genetics
  b. metastasis
  b. modulation
  b. oxygen demand
  b. pharmacology
  b. profile
biochemistry
biochemorphic
biochrome
biocidal
bioclimatology
biocompatibility
biocybernetics
biocytin
biocytinase
biodegradable
biodegradation
biodynamic
biodynamics
bioecology
bioelectrical impedance analysis
bioelectric potential
bioelement
bioenergetics
bioengineering
biofeedback
  EMG b.
bioflavonoids
biogenesis
  mitochondrial b.
biogenetic law
biogenic amine
biogeochemistry
biogravics
bioinformatics
bioinstrument
biokinetics
biologic
  b. assay
  b. chemistry
  b. control
  b. evolution
  b. half-life
  b. hemolysis
  b. immunotherapy
  b. indicator
  b. psychiatry
  b. response modifier
  b. time

  b. valve
  b. vector
biological
  b. coefficient
  b. sampling
  b. standard unit
  b. vector
biologist
biology
  cellular b.
  molecular b.
  oral b.
  radiation b.
bioluminescence
biolysis
biolytic
biomacromolecule
biomass
biomaterial
biomechanical
  b. analysis
  b. frame of reference
biomechanics
  dental b.
biomedical
  b. engineering
  b. model
biomembrane
biometrical school
biometrician
biometry fetal
biomicroscope
biomicroscopy
Biomphalaria
Biondi-Heidenhain stain
bionecrosis
bionic
bionics
bionomics
bionomy
biophage
biophagism, biophagy
biophagous
biopharmaceutics
biophylactic
biophylaxis
biophysical profile
biophysics
  cellular b.
  dental b.
  medical b.
  molecular b.

B

NOTES

115

bioplasm
bioplasmic
biopolymer
    aperiodic b.
biopsy
    aspiration b.
    biochemical b.
    brush b.
    cervical punch b.
    chorionic villus b.
    endoscopic b.
    excision b.
    fine-needle b.
    incision b.
    needle b.
    b. needle
    open b.
    punch b.
    sentinel node b.
    shave b.
    surface b.
    wound b.
biopsychology
biopsychosocial model
biopterin
bioptome
biorbital angle
biorheology
biorhythm
biosafety
biosis
biosocial
biospectrometry
biospectroscopy
biospeleology
biosphere
biostatics
biostatistics
biosynthesis
biosynthetic
biosystem
Biot
    B. breathing
    B. breathing sign
    B. respiration
biota
biotaxis
biotechnology
biotelemetry
biotest
biotic
    b. community
    b. factor
    b. potential
biotics
biotin
biotinidase deficiency
biotinides
biotope

biotoxicology
biotoxin
biotransformation
biotype
biovar
biovular
bipalatinoid
biparasitism
biparental
biparietal
    b. diameter
    b. suture
biparous
bipartite
    b. uterus
    b. vagina
biped
bipedal
bipedicle flap
bipennate muscle
bipenniform
biperforate
biperiden
biphase
    external pin fixation, b.
biphasic
    b. insulin
    b. response
biphenotypic
biphenotypy
biphenyl
biplane angiography
bipolar
    b. cautery
    b. cell
    b. circumactive probe (BICAP)
    b. disorder
    b. lead
    b. neuron
    b. psychosis
    b. version
bipotentiality
biramous
Birbeck granule
birch
    b. tar
    b. tar oil
Bircher operation
Birch-Hirschfeld stain
bird
    b. face
    b. shot retinochoroiditis
    B. sign
    b. unit
bird-breeder's
    b.-b. disease
    b.-b. lung
bird-fancier's lung
birdseed agar

bird's nest filter
birefringence
birefringent
Birkett hernia
birotation
birth
   b. amputation
   breech b.
   b. canal
   b. certificate
   b. control
   date of b. (DOB)
   b. defect
   b. fracture
   immature b.
   live b.
   b. palsy
   partial b.
   premature b.
   b. rate
   b. trauma
   viable b.
   b. weight
birthing center
birthmark
bisacromial
bisalbuminemia
bisaxillary
Bischof myelotomy
biscuit-bake
biscuit bite
biscuit-firing
bisdequalinium chloride
bisexual libido
bisferiens
   pulsus b.
bisferient
bisferious pulse
Bishop
   B. score
   B. sphygmoscope
bishydroxycoumarin
bisiliac
Biskra
   bouton de B.
   B. button
Bismarck brown R, Y
bismuth
   b. aluminate
   b. ammonium citrate
   b. carbonate
   b. chloride oxide

   b. hydroxide
   b. iodide
   b. line
   milk of b.
   b. oxycarbonate
   b. oxychloride
bismuthosis
bismuthyl
bissac
   hernia en b.
bistoury
bistratal
bisulfate
bisulfide
   carbon b.
bisulfite
bitartrate
   levarterenol b.
bite
   b. analysis
   balanced b.
   biscuit b.
   b. block
   closed b.
   deep b.
   edge-to-edge b.
   end-to-end b.
   b. fork
   b. gauge
   jumping the b.
   locked b.
   open b.
   b. plane
   b. rim
bitemporal hemianopia
biteplane
biteplate
bitewing
   b. film
   b. radiograph
bithermal caloric test
biting
   b. louse
   b. pressure
   b. strength
Bitot spot
bitrochanteric
bitter
   b. almond oil
   b. apple
   aromatic b.
   b. orange peel

NOTES

B

bitter *(continued)*
    b. orange peel oil
    b. peptide
    b. principle
    b. tonic
    b. water
bitters
Bittner
    B. agent
    B. milk factor
    B. virus
Bittorf reaction
biundulant meningoencephalitis
biuret
    b. reaction
    b. reagent
    b. test
bivalence
bivalency
bivalent
    b. antibody
    b. chromosome
    b. gas gangrene antitoxin
bivalved
    b. incision
    b. speculum
biventer
    b. cervicis
    b. lobule
    b. mandibulae
biventral lobule
biventricular
bivia
    Prevotella b.
bivius
    Bacteroides b.
Bixler type hypertelorism
bizygomatic
Bizzozero
    B. corpuscle
    B. red cell
Bjerrum
    B. scotoma
    B. screen
    B. sign
Björk-Shiley valve
Björnstad syndrome
B-K
    below the knee
    B-K amputation
BK virus
black
    animal b.
    bone b.
    b. box
    b. braided suture
    b. cataract
    B. classification

B. Creek Canal virus
b. currant rash
b. death
b. eye
b. fever
B. formula
b. globe thermometer
b. hairy tongue
b. heel
b. imported fire ant
b. lead
b. line
b. lung
b. measles
b. mustard
b. piedra
b. plague
b. root
b. sickness
b. spore
b. tarantula
b. urine
b. vomit
black-dot ringworm
blackhead
blackout
blackwater fever
bladder
    air b.
    allantoic b.
    atonic b.
    autonomic neurogenic b.
    b. calculus
    b. compliance
    b. dome
    b. ear
    encysted b.
    gall b.
    hyperreflexic b.
    hypertonic b.
    ileal b.
    kidneys, ureters, b. (KUB)
    nervous b.
    neurogenic b.
    neuropathic b.
    b. reflex
    reflex neurogenic b.
    runner's b.
    sacculated b.
    b. schistosomiasis
    stammering b.
    b. stone
    transurethral resection of b. (TURB)
    trigone of b.
    uninhibited neurogenic b.
    urinary b.
bladderworm

blade
    b. bone
    shoulder b.
bladevent
Blagden law
Blainville ears
Blair-Brown graft
Blalock-Hanlon operation
Blalock shunt
Blalock-Taussig
    B.-T. operation
    B.-T. shunt
blanch
blanche
    atrophie b.
bland
    b. diet
    b. embolism
    b. infarct
Blandin gland
blanket
    mucus b.
    b. suture
blank hallucination
Blaschko
    line of B.
Blasius duct
blast
    b. cell
    b. chest
    b. crisis
    b. effect
    b. injury
    lung b.
    stoma b.
    b. transformation
blastema
    metanephric b.
blastemic
blastic
blastocele
blastocelic
blastocoele
blastocoelic
blastocyst
Blastocystis hominis
blastocyte
blastocytoma
blastoderm
    bilaminar b.
    embryonic b.
    extraembryonic b.

blastoderma
blastodermal
blastodermic
    b. disc
    b. layer
    b. vesicle
blastodisk
blastogenesis
blastogenetic
blastogenic
blastolysis
blastolytic
blastoma
blastomere
blastomerotomy
blastomogenic
Blastomyces dermatitidis
blastomycetic dermatitis
blastomycin
blastomycosis
    Brazilian b.
    cutaneous b.
    North American b.
    South American b.
blastoneuropore
blastophore
blastopore
blastoporic canal
blastospore
blastotomy
blastula
blastular
blastulation
Blatin syndrome
BLB
    Boothby-Lovelace-Bulbulian
    BLB mask
bleached wax
bleaching powder
blear eye
bleary eye
bleb
    filtering b.
    pulmonary b.
bleed
bleeder
bleeding
    dysfunctional uterine b.
    b. polyp
    b. time
    b. of undetermined origin (BUO)
blemish

NOTES

blending inheritance
blennadenitis
blennemesis
blennogenic
blennogenous
blennoid
blennophthalmia
blennorrhagic
blennorrhagica
    keratosis b.
blennorrhea
    b. conjunctivalis
    inclusion b.
    b. neonatorum
blennorrheal
blennostasis
blennostatic
blennuria
blepharadenitis
blepharal
blepharectomy
blepharedema
blepharitis
    ciliary b.
    demodectic b.
    marginal b.
    meibomian b.
    posterior b.
    seborrheic b.
    staphylococcal b.
blepharoadenitis
blepharoadenoma
blepharochalasis
blepharoclonus
blepharocoloboma
blepharoconjunctivitis
blepharodiastasis
blepharokeratoconjunctivitis
blepharon
blepharophimosis
blepharoplast
blepharoplastic
blepharoplasty
blepharoplegia
blepharoptosia
blepharoptosis
    b. adiposa
    false b.
blepharospasm
blepharospasmus
blepharostat
blepharostenosis
blepharosynechia
blepharotomy
blighted ovum
blind
    b. abscess
    b. boil
    b. enema

    b. fistula
    b. foramen
    b. gut
    b. headache
    b. loop syndrome
    b. nasotracheal intubation
    b. passage
    b. spot
    b. study
    b. test
blinding
    b. disease
    b. glare
blindness
    change b.
    color b.
    cortical b.
    day b.
    eclipse b.
    flash b.
    flight b.
    functional b.
    hysterical b.
    legal b.
    letter b.
    mind b.
    night b.
    snow b.
    text b.
    word b.
blink
    b. reflex
    b. response
blinking tic
blister
    b. agent
    blood b.
    fever b.
    fly b.
    fracture b.
    sucking b.
blistering
    b. collodion
    b. distal dactylitis
bloat
bloating
bloc
    en b.
Bloch reaction
Bloch-Sulzberger
    B.-S. disease
    B.-S. syndrome
block
    alveolocapillary b.
    b. anesthesia
    antegrade b.
    anterograde b.
    arborization b.
    atrioventricular b.

AV b.
Bier b.
bite b.
bone b.
bundle-branch b.
complete AV b.
conduction b.
congenital heart b.
depolarizing b.
b. design test
divisional b.
entrance b.
epidural b.
exit b.
fascicular b.
field b.
first-degree AV b.
heart b.
incomplete atrioventricular b.
interatrial b.
intraatrial b.
intraventricular b. (IVB)
I-V b.
left bundle branch b. (LBBB)
Mobitz b.
nerve b.
nondepolarizing b.
b. osteotomy
paravertebral b.
periinfarction b.
perineural b.
phase I, II b.
pupillary b.
regional b.
retrograde b.
reverse pupillary b.
S-A b.
second-degree AV b.
sinoatrial b.
sinuatrial b.
sinus b.
spinal b.
stellate b.
b. vertebra
Wenckebach b.
Wilson b.
blockade
adrenergic b.
cholinergic b.
ganglionic b.
myoneural b.
narcotic b.

blocked
b. aerogastria
b. pleurisy
b. reading frame
blocker
angiotensin receptor b.
calcium channel b.
blocking
b. activity
b. agent
alpha b.
b. antibody
block-out
Blocq disease
Blom-Singer valve
blood
b. agar
b. albumin
arterial b.
b. bank
banked b.
b. blister
b. boosting
b. calculus
b. capillary
b. cast
b. cell
b. circulation
b. clot
cord b.
b. corpuscle
b. count
b. crisis
b. crystal
b. cyst
b. disc
b. doping
b. dust
b. dyscrasia
b. fluke
b. gas
b. gas analysis
b. group
b. group agglutinin
b. group agglutinogen
b. group antibody
b. group antigen
b. group antiserum
b. grouping
b. group-specific substances A and B
b. group substance

NOTES

121

blood *(continued)*
 b. group systems
 b. island
 b. islet
 laky b.
 b. lymph
 b. mote
 occult b.
 b. pH
 b. plasma
 b. plasma fraction
 b. plastid
 b. plate
 b. poisoning
 b. pool imaging
 b. pressure (BP)
 b. relationship
 b. relative
 b. serum
 b. spot
 b. substitute
 b. sugar
 b. tumor
 b. type
 b. urea nitrogen (BUN)
 venous b.
 b. vessel
 b. volume expander
 b. volume nomogram
 whole b.
blood-air barrier
blood-aqueous barrier
blood-brain barrier (BBB)
blood-cerebrospinal fluid barrier
blood-CSF barrier
bloodless
 b. amputation
 b. decerebration
 b. operation
 b. phlebotomy
bloodletting
 general b.
 local b.
bloodshot
bloodstream
blood-testis barrier
blood-thymus barrier
blood-vascular system
bloodworm
Bloom syndrome
blot
 Western b.
blotting
 Western b.
Blount-Barber disease
Blount disease
blow-bottles
blowfly
blowing murmur

blowout
 b. fracture
 b. pipette
BLS
 basic life support
blubber finger
blue
 Alcian b.
 aniline b.
 b. atrophy
 azovan b.
 b. baby
 Berlin b.
 bromophenol b.
 bromthymol b.
 b. cone monochromatism
 b. dextran
 b. diaper syndrome
 b. disease
 b. dome cyst
 b. dot cataract
 b. dot sign
 b. edema
 Evans b.
 b. fever
 indigo b.
 isosulfan b.
 Kühne methylene b.
 leucomethylene b.
 leuco patent b.
 b. line
 Loeffler methylene b.
 Luxol fast b.
 methyl b.
 methylene b.
 b. nevus
 b. ointment
 postpartum b.'s
 Prussian b.
 b. pus
 b. pus bacillus
 b. rubber-bleb nevus
 b. sclera
 b. spot
 b. toe syndrome
 b. vision
blueberry muffin baby
blue-green
 b.-g. algae
 b.-g. bacterium
bluetongue virus
bluish
 eosin I b.
Blumberg sign
Blumenau nucleus
Blumenbach clivus
Blumer shelf
blunt
 b. affect

B

b. dissection
b. duct adenosis
blunted affect
blunt-ended DNA
blunt-end ligation
blush
  tumor b.
B-mode
BMR
  basal metabolic rate
board
  back b.
  communication b.
  conversation b.
  institutional review b.
  language b.
  spine b.
  transfer b.
Boas-Oppler bacillus
boat
  b. conformation
  b. form
bobbing
  inverse ocular b.
Bochdalek
  flower basket of B.
  B. foramen
  B. ganglion
  B. gap
  B. hernia
  B. muscle
  B. valve
Bock
  B. ganglion
  B. nerve
Bockhart impetigo
Bodansky unit
Bödecker index
Bodian copper-protargol stain
body
  acetone b.
  adrenal b.
  alcoholic hyaline b.
  Alder b.
  alveolar b.
  amygdaloid b.
  amylogenic b.
  anococcygeal b.
  anterior quadrigeminal b.
  aortic b.
  Arnold b.
  asbestos b.

Aschoff b.
asteroid b.
Auer b.
Barr chromatin b.
basal b.
bigeminal b.
brassy b.
b. burden
Cabot ring b.
Call-Exner b.
carotid b.
cavernous b.
b. cavity
cell b.
central fibrous b.
chromaffin b.
chromatin b.
ciliary b.
Civatte b.
coccygeal b.
colloid b.
compressible cavernous b.
conchoidal b.
Councilman hyaline b.
Cowdry type A, B inclusion b.
creola b.
cyanobacteriumlike b.
cytoid b.
cytoplasmic inclusion b.
Deetjen b.
demilune b.
dense b.
Döhle b.
Donovan b.
b. dysmorphic disorder
Ehrlich inner b.
elementary b.
embryoid b.
epithelial b.
fat b.
ferruginous b.
foreign b. (FB)
fruiting b.
fuchsin b.
Gamna-Favre b.
Gamna-Gandy b.
Gandy-Gamna b.
geniculate b.
glass b.
glomus b.
Golgi b.
Guarnieri b.

NOTES

body (*continued*)

Halberstaedter-Prowazek b.
Hassall b.
Hassall-Henle b.
Heinz b.
Heinz-Ehrlich b.
hematoxylin b.
hematoxyphil b.
Herring b.
Highmore b.
Howell-Jolly b.
hyaline b.
hyaloid b.
b. image
inclusion b.
infrapatellar fat b.
intercarotid b.
intermediate b.
Jaworski b.
Jolly b.
juxtaglomerular b.
juxtarestiform b.
ketone b.
Lafora b.
Lallemand b.
b. language
lateral geniculate b.
L-D b.
LE b.
Leishman-Donovan b.
Lewy b.
Lieutaud b.
Lindner b.
loose b.
Luse b.
Luys b.
Mallory b.
malpighian b.
mammillary b.
b. mass index
b. mechanics
medial geniculate b.
melon-seed b.
metachromatic b.
metallic foreign b.
Michaelis-Gutmann b.
Miyagawa b.
molluscum b.
multilamellar b.
Negri b.
Nissl b.
nuclear inclusion b.
pacchionian b.
Pappenheimer b.
paraaortic b.
parabasal b.
Pick b.
pineal b.
b. plethysmograph

polar b.
psammoma b.
restiform b.
retained foreign b.
b. righting reflex
Russell b.
b. schema
b. scheme
sclerotic b.
b. stalk
striate b.
b. substance isolation
b. surface area (BSA)
b. temperature
trachoma b.
vitreous b.
wolffian b.
Zuckerkandl b.

body-weight ratio
bodywork
Boeck

B. disease
B. and Drbohlav Locke-egg-serum medium
B. sarcoid

Boehmer hematoxylin
Boerhaave syndrome
bogbean
Bogros

B. serous membrane
B. space

Bohn nodule
Bohr

B. atom
B. effect
B. equation
B. magneton
B. theory

boil

Aleppo b.
Bagdad b.
blind b.
date b.
Delhi b.
Jericho b.
Madura b.

boilermaker's hearing loss
boiling point
Boley gauge
Bolivian

B. hemorrhagic fever
B. hemorrhagic fever virus

Boll cell
Bollinger granule
Bolognini symptom
bolometer
bolus

b. dressing

B

b. graft
intravenous b.
BOM
bilateral otitis media
bombard
Bombay
B. blood type
B. phenomenon
B. trait
bomb calorimeter
bombé
iris b.
bombesin
bond
acylmercaptan b.
apolar b.
conjugated double b.'s
coordinate covalent b.
disulfide b.
double b.
electrostatic b.
energy-rich b.
eupeptide b.
heteropolar b.
high-energy phosphate b.
hydrogen b.
hydrophobic b.
isopeptide b.
noncovalent b.
peptide b.
semipolar b.
single b.
triple b.
bonding
bone
b. abscess
b. ache
b. age
Albrecht b.
alveolar b.
alveolar supporting b.
ankle b.
b. architecture
b. ash
basal b.
basilar b.
basioccipital b.
Bertin b.
b. black
blade b.
b. block
b. block fusion

breast b.
Breschet b.
brittle b.
bundle b.
calcaneal b.
calf b., calf-bone
b. canaliculus
cancellous b.
capitate b.
carpal b.
cartilage b.
b. cell
central b.
b. charcoal
cheek b.
b. chip
coccygeal b.
collar b.
compact b.
b. conduction
convoluted b.
b. corpuscle
cortical b.
coxal b.
cranial b.
cubital b.
cuboid b.
cuneiform b.
b. cyst
b. density
dermal b.
dorsal talonavicular b.
ear b.
ectopic b.
elbow b.
endochondral b.
epactal b.
epihyal b.
epipteric b.
episternal b.
ethmoid b.
exoccipital b.
facial b.
first cuneiform b.
flank b.
b. flap
flat b.
Flower b.
foot b.
b. forceps
fourth turbinated b.
frontal b.

NOTES

bone (*continued*)
    funny b.
    Goethe b.
    b. graft
    greater horn of hyoid b.
    greater multangular b.
    hamate b.
    heel b.
    heterotopic b.
    highest turbinated b.
    hip b.
    hollow b.
    hooked b.
    hyoid b.
    iliac b.
    incarial b.
    incisive b.
    b. infarct
    inferior turbinated b.
    innominate b.
    intermaxillary b.
    intermediate cuneiform b.
    interparietal b.
    irregular b.
    ischial b.
    b. island
    jaw b.
    jugal b.
    Krause b.
    lacrimal b.
    b. lacuna
    lamella of b.
    lamellar b.
    lateral cuneiform b.
    lenticular b.
    lentiform b.
    lesser multangular b.
    lingual b.
    long b.
    lunate b.
    malar b.
    marble b.
    b. marrow
    b. marrow dose
    b. marrow embolism
    b. marrow transplantation
    mastoid b.
    b. matrix
    medial cuneiform b.
    membrane b.
    mesethmoid b.
    metacarpal b.
    metatarsal b.
    middle cuneiform b.
    middle turbinated b.
    multangular b.
    nasal b.
    navicular b.
    nonlamellar b.

    occipital b.
    palatine b.
    parietal b.
    perichondral b.
    b. phosphate
    pisiform b.
    b. plate
    pneumatic b.
    premaxillary b.
    pubic b.
    pyramidal b.
    b. resorption
    reticulated b.
    rider's b.
    b. salt
    b. scan
    scaphoid b.
    b. sclerosis
    semilunar b.
    b. sensibility
    sesamoid b.
    shin b.
    short b.
    sphenoid b.
    spongy b.
    b. spur
    sutural b.
    tarsal b.
    temporal b.
    b. tissue
    trabecular b.
    trapezium b.
    trapezoid b.
    triangular b.
    triquetral b.
    tympanic b.
    unciform b.
    b. wax
    wedge b.
    wormian b.
    woven b.
    zygomatic b.
bonelet
bone sialoprotein 1
Bonhoeffer sign
Bonner position
Bonnet capsule
Bonnet-Dechaume-Blanc syndrome
Bonney test
Bonnier syndrome
Bonwill triangle
bony
    b. ampulla
    b. ankylosis
    b. crepitus
    b. heart
    b. labyrinth
    b. nasal septum

b. palate
b. semicircular canal
Böök syndrome
BOOP
  bronchiolitis obliterans with organizing
  pneumonia
booster
  b. dose
  b. response
boosting
  blood b.
boot
  air b.
  Gibney b.
  pneumatic b.
Boothby-Lovelace-Bulbulian (BLB)
borate
  sodium b.
borborygmus
Bordeaux mixture
border
  alveolar b.
  anterior b.
  brush b.
  b. cell
  ciliary b.
  denture b.
  fibular peroneal b.
  free b.
  frontal b.
  hidden b.
  inferior b.
  inner b.
  interosseous b.
  lacrimal b.
  lambdoid b.
  lateral b.
  lower sternal b. (LSB)
  mastoid b.
  medial b.
  mesovarian b.
  b. molding
  b. seal
  striated b.
  b. tissue movement
  vermilion b.
borderline
  b. case
  b. hypertension
  b. leprosy
  b. ovarian tumor

b. personality
b. personality disorder
Bordetella
  B. bronchiseptica
  B. hinzii
  B. pertussis
Bordet-Gengou
  B.-G. bacillus
  B.-G. phenomenon
  B.-G. potato blood agar
Bordet and Gengou reaction
Borg scale
boric acid
borism
Börjeson-Forssman-Lehmann syndrome
Borna disease virus
Bornholm
  B. disease
  B. disease virus
Born method
boron
Borrel blue stain
Borrelia
  B. afzelii
  B. burgdorferi
  B. garinii
borreliosis
  Lyme b.
bosch yaw
Bose operation
Bosin disease
bosselated
bosselation
Boston
  B. exanthema
  B. opium
Botallo
  B. duct
  B. foramen
  B. ligament
botfly, pl. **botflies**
  head botflies
  human b.
bothriocephaliasis
bothropic antitoxin
Bothrops antitoxin
botryoid
  b. odontogenic cyst
  b. sarcoma
botryomycosis
botryomycotic

NOTES

Böttcher
- B. canal
- B. cell
- B. crystal
- B. ganglion
- B. space

bottle
- Mariotte b.
- Woulfe b.

2-bottle drainage system
3-bottle drainage system
botulin
botulinogenic
botulinum
- b. antitoxin
- *Clostridium b.*

botulinus toxin
botulism antitoxin
botulismotoxin
botulogenic
boubas
Bouchard disease
Bouchut tube
bougie
- b. à boule
- bulbous b.
- coudé b.
- Eder-Pustow b.
- elastic b.
- elbowed b.
- filiform b.
- following b.
- Hurst b.
- Maloney b.
- Savary b.

bougienage
Bouin fixative
boule
- bougie à b.

boulimia
boundary lamina
bounding
- b. mydriasis
- b. pupil

bound water
bouquet fever
Bourdon gauge
Bourgery ligament
Bourneville disease
Bourneville-Pringle disease
bouton
- axonal terminal b.
- b. de Baghdad
- b. de Biskra
- b. en chemise
- b. en passage
- b.'s en passage
- terminal b.'s
- b. terminaux

boutonneuse
- b. fever
- fièvre b.

boutonnière deformity
bovine
- b. antitoxin
- b. babesiosis
- b. brucellosis
- b. colloid
- b. ketosis
- b. leukemia virus
- b. leukosis virus
- b. papular stomatitis virus
- b. rhinovirus
- b. serum albumin (BSA)
- b. spongiform encephalopathy (BSE)
- b. virus diarrhea virus

bovinum
- cor b.

bovis
- *Actinomyces b.*
- *Cysticercus b.*
- *Mycobacterium b.*

bow
- Cupid's b.
- Logan b.

Bowditch
- B. effect
- B. law

bowel
- b. bypass
- b. bypass syndrome
- gangrenous b.
- greedy b.
- large b.
- b. movement
- b. sounds

Bowen
- B. disease
- B. precancerous dermatosis

bowenoid
- b. cell
- b. papulosis

Bowie stain
bowing tic
bowleg, bow-leg
bowler's thumb
Bowles type stethoscope
Bowman
- B. capsule
- B. disc
- B. gland
- B. layer
- B. membrane
- B. muscle
- B. probe
- B. space

Bowman-Birk inhibitor

B

box
  black b.
  brain b.
  CAAT b.
  Hogness b.
  b. jelly
boxer's
  b. ear
  b. fracture
boxing wax
Boyce position
Boyd communicating perforation vein
Boyden
  B. meal
  B. sphincter
boydii
  Shigella b.
Boyer
  B. bursa
  B. cyst
Boyle law
Bozeman
  B. operation
  B. position
Bozeman-Fritsch catheter
bozemanii
  Legionella b.
Bozzolo sign
BP
  blood pressure
  bronchopleural
  BP fistula
BPH
  benign prostatic hyperplasia
  benign prostatic hypertrophy
Braasch
  B. bulb
  B. catheter
brace
  cast b.
  chair-back b.
  clamshell b.
  dropfoot b.
  long leg b.
  toe drop b.
brachial
  b. amelia
  b. anesthesia
  b. artery
  b. autonomic plexus
  b. birth palsy
  b. fascia

  b. gland
  b. lymph node
  b. muscle
  b. neuritis
  b. paralysis
  b. plexitis
  b. plexus injury
  b. plexus neuropathy
  b. vein
brachialgia
brachialis muscle
brachiocephalic
  b. arterial trunk
  b. arteritis
  b. lymph node
  b. vein
brachiocrural
brachiocubital
brachiogram
brachioradial
  b. muscle
  b. reflex
brachioradialis muscle
brachium
  inferior quadrigeminal b.
Bracht maneuver
Bracht-Wächter lesion
brachybasia
brachybasocamptodactyly
brachybasophalangia
brachycardia
brachycephalic
brachycephalism
brachycephalous
brachycephaly, brachycephalia
brachycheilia, brachychilia
brachycnemic
brachycranic
brachydactylic
brachydactyly, brachydactylia
brachyesophagus
brachyfacial
brachyglossal
brachygnathia
brachygnathous
brachykerkic
brachymelia
brachymesophalangia
brachymetacarpalia
brachymetacarpalism
brachymetacarpia

NOTES

brachymetapody
brachymetatarsia
brachymorphic
brachyodont
brachyonychia
brachypellic, brachypelvic
    b. pelvis
brachyphalangia
brachypodous
brachyprosopic
brachyrhinia
brachyrhynchus
brachyskelic
brachystaphyline
brachysyndactyly
brachytelephalangia
brachytherapy
    high-dose-rate b.
    interstitial b.
    remote afterloading b.
    stereotactic b.
brachytype
Brackin anastomosis
Bradbury-Eggleston syndrome
Bradford frame
bradyarrhythmia
bradyarthria
bradycardia
    central b.
    essential b.
    fetal b.
    idiopathic b.
    marked fetal b.
    mild fetal b.
    physiologic b.
    postinfective b.
    sinoatrial b.
bradycardiac
bradycardic
bradycinesia
bradycrotic
bradydiastole
bradyesthesia
bradyglossia
bradykinesia
bradykinetic analysis
bradykininogen
bradykinin-potentiating peptide
bradykinin potentiator B
bradylalia
bradylexia
bradylogia
bradypepsia
bradyphagia
bradyphasia
bradyphemia
bradypnea
bradypsychia
bradyrhythmia

bradyspermatism
bradysphygmia
bradystalsis
bradytachycardia syndrome
bradyteleocinesia, bradyteleokinesis
bradytocia
bradyuria
bradyzoite
braided suture
braille
Brailsford-Morquio disease
brain
    b. attack
    b. box
    b. cicatrix
    b. concussion
    b. congestion
    b. contusion
    b. death
    b. edema
    b. laceration
    b. lipid
    b. mantle
    b. murmur
    b. potential
    B. reflex
    b. sand
    b. stem
    b. sugar
    b. swelling
    b. wave
    b. wave complex
    b. wave cycle
braincase
brain-heart infusion agar
brainstem, brain stem
    b. auditory evoked potential
    b. auditory evoked response
    (BAER)
    b. evoked response (BSER)
    b. evoked response audiometry
    b. glioma
    b. hemorrhage
brainwashing
brake phenomenon
braking radiation
branch
    accessory meningeal b.
    acetabular b.
    acromial b.
    anastomotic b.
    anterior auricular b.
    anterior basal b.
    anterior cutaneous b.
    anterior intercostal b.
    anterior interventricular b.
    anterior labial b.
    anterior lateral nasal b.
    anterior meningeal b.

anterior pectoral cutaneous b.
anterior septal b.
anterior temporal b.
anteromedial central b.
anteromedial frontal b.
articular b.
ascending b.
atrial b.
atrioventricular nodal b.
auricular b.
basal tentorial b.
bronchial b.
buccal b.
calcaneal b.
calcarine b.
capsular b.
carotid sinus b.
caudate b.
cavernous sinus b.
celiac b.
cervical b.
choroid b.
circumflex b.
clavicular b.
clivus b.
cochlear b.
collateral b.
communicating b.
cricothyroid b.
cutaneous b.
deep palmar b.
deep plantar b.
deltoid b.
dental b.
descending anterior b.
descending posterior b.
digastric b.
dorsal carpal b.
dorsal lingual b.
duodenal b.
epiploic b.
esophageal b.
external nasal b.
faucial b.
femoral b.
ganglionic b.
gastric b.
genital b.
glandular b.
hepatic b.
iliac b.
iliacus b.

inferior cervical cardiac b.
inferior dental b.
inferior gingival b.
inferior labial b.
inferior lingular b.
infrahyoid b.
infrapatellar b.
inguinal b.
interganglionic b.
intermediate atrial b.
intermediate temporal b.
intermediomedial frontal b.
internal nasal b.
interventricular septal b.
joint b.
labial b.
laryngopharyngeal b.
lateral atrial b.
lateral basal b.
lateral calcaneal b.
lateral costal b.
lateral cutaneous b.
lateral malleolar b.
lateral mammary b.
lateral medullary b.
lateral nasal b.
lateral sacral b.
left bundle b.
lingual b.
lumbar b.
mammary b.
marginal atrial b.
marginal mandibular b.
marginal tentorial b.
mastoid b.
medial basal b.
medial calcaneal b.
medial crural cutaneous b.
medial malleolar b.
medial mammary b.
medial medullary b.
medial nasal b.
mediastinal b.
meningeal b.
mental b.
middle lobe b.
middle meningeal b.
middle superior alveolar b.
middle temporal b.
b. migration
obturator b.
phrenicoabdominal b.

B

NOTES

branch (*continued*)
  posterior glandular b.
  posterior labial b.
  posterior temporal b.
  posterior vestibular b.
  prelaminar b.
  spinal b.
  subendocardial b.
  superficial b.
  superior vermian b.
  tentorial basal b.
branched
  b. calculus
  b. chain ketoaciduria
  b. chain ketonuria
brancher
  b. deficiency glycogenosis
  b. glycogen storage disease
branchial
  b. apparatus
  b. arch
  b. cartilage
  b. cleft
  b. cleft cyst
  b. efferent column
  b. fissure
  b. fistula
  b. groove
  b. mesoderm
  b. pouch
branching
  b. decay
  b. enzyme
  b. factor
  false b.
branchiogenic
branchiogenous
branchiomere
branchiomeric muscle
branchiomerism
branchiomotor nucleus
branchiootorenal
  b. dysplasia
  b. syndrome
Brandt-Andrews maneuver
brandy nose
Branham sign
branny desquamation
Brasdor method
brash
  water b.
brasiliensis
  Paracoccidioides b.
brass
  b. founder's ague
  b. founder's fever
brassiere-type dressing

brassy
  b. body
  b. cough
BRAT
  bananas, rice cereal, applesauce, toast
  BRAT diet
Braun anastomosis
Braune
  B. muscle
  B. valve
brawny
  b. arm
  b. edema
  b. induration
  b. scleritis
Braxton
  B. Hicks contraction
  B. Hicks sign
Brazelton Neonatal Behavioral Assessment Scale
brazilein
Brazilian
  B. blastomycosis
  B. hemorrhagic fever
  B. pemphigus
  B. purpuric fever
  B. spotted fever
braziliana
  bubas b.
braziliense
  Ancylostoma b.
braziliensis
  Leishmania braziliensis b.
Brazil wax
BRCA1 gene
BRCA2 gene
BrDu-banding
bread-and-butter pericardium
bread pill
break
  double-strand b.
  b. shock
breakaway phenomenon
breakbone fever
breakdown
  nervous b.
break-even point
breakoff phenomenon
breakpoint
breakthrough
breast
  accessory b.
  b. bone
  chicken b.
  funnel b.
  irritable b.
  male b.
  b. pang

pigeon b.
b. pump
breath
 b. analysis
 liver b.
 mandatory b.
 b. sounds
 b. test
breathe
breath-holding test
breathing
 apneustic b.
 ataxic b.
 b. bag
 Biot b.
 bronchial b.
 continuous positive-pressure b. (CPPB)
 continuous positive pressure b.
 glossopharyngeal b.
 intermittent positive pressure b. (IPPB)
 Kussmaul b.
 labored b.
 mouth-to-mouth b.
 positive-negative pressure b.
 b. reserve
 shallow b.
 work of b.
Breda disease
bredouillement
breech
 b. birth
 b. delivery
 b. extraction
 incomplete b.
 b. presentation
breeding
bregma
bregmatic fontanelle
bregmatolambdoid arc
bregmocardiac reflex
Brenner
 B. operation
 B. tumor
Breschet
 B. bone
 B. canal
 B. hiatus
 B. sinus
 B. vein
Brescia-Cimino fistula

Breslow thickness
Breus mole
breve
 Flavobacterium b.
brevicollis
brevis
 Bacillus b.
 Lactobacillus b.
Brewer infarct
brewers' yeast
brickdust deposit
Bricker operation
brickmaker's anemia
bridge
 arteriolovenular b.
 cantilever b.
 caudolenticular gray b.
 cell b.
 b. corpuscle
 crossing a b.
 cystine b.
 cytoplasmic b.
 dentin b.
 disulfide b.
 extension b.
 fixed b.
 Gaskell b.
 intercellular b.
 removable b.
 Wheatstone b.
bridgework
bridging
 b. hepatic necrosis
 myocardial b.
bridle
 b. stricture
 b. suture
brief psychotherapy
Brigg test
Bright disease
brightness difference threshold
Brill disease
Brill-Zinsser disease
Brimacombe fragment
brimstone
Brinell hardness number
Briquet
 B. ataxia
 B. disease
 B. syndrome
brisement forcé

NOTES

Brissaud
- B. disease
- B. infantilism
- B. reflex

Brissaud-Marie syndrome
bristle cell
British
- B. anti-Lewisite
- B. gum
- B. Pharmacopoeia
- B. thermal unit (BTU)

brittle
- b. bone
- b. diabetes

broach
- barbed b.

broad
- b. beta disease
- b. fascia
- b. ligament
- b. spectrum

Broadbent
- B. law
- B. sign

broad-spectrum antibiotic
Broca
- B. aphasia
- B. basilar angle
- B. center
- B. diagonal band
- B. facial angle
- B. field
- B. fissure
- B. formula
- B. parolfactory area
- B. pouch
- B. visual plane

Brock
- B. operation
- B. syndrome

Brockenbrough sign
Brödel bloodless line
Brodie
- B. abscess
- B. bursa
- B. disease
- B. fluid
- B. knee
- B. ligament

Brodmann area
Broesike fossa
bromate
bromated
bromazepam
bromcresol
- b. green
- b. purple

bromelain, bromelin
bromhidrosis

bromic
bromide
- b. acne
- calcium b.
- decamethonium b.
- demecarium b.
- domiphen b.
- ethidium b.
- hexafluorenium b.
- homidium b.
- hydrogen b.
- lithium b.
- methantheline b.
- methyl b.

bromidrosiphobia
bromidrosis
brominated
bromindione
bromine water
brominism
bromism
bromobenzylcyanide
bromocresol green
bromocriptine
bromodeoxyuridine
bromoderma
bromohyperhidrosis
bromohyperidrosis
bromophenol blue
bromosulfophthalein
bromphenol test
Brompton cocktail
bromsulfophthalein
bromsulphalein (BSP)
- b. test

bromthymol blue
bronchi (*pl. of* bronchus)
bronchia
bronchial
- b. arteriography
- b. artery
- b. asthma
- b. atresia
- b. branch
- b. breathing
- b. breath sounds
- b. brushing
- b. bud
- b. calculus
- b. carcinoid
- b. fremitus
- b. gland
- b. hygiene
- b. mucosa
- b. mucous gland adenoma
- b. obstruction
- b. pneumonia
- b. polyp
- b. provocation

b. respiration
b. stenosis
b. tube
b. vein
b. voice
bronchic cell
bronchiectasia
bronchiectasis
    congenital b.
    cylindrical b.
    cystic b.
    dry b.
bronchiectatic
bronchiloquy
bronchiogenic
bronchiolar
    b. adenocarcinoma
    b. carcinoid
    b. carcinoma
    b. exocrine cell
bronchiole
    alveolar b.
    respiratory b.
    terminal b.
bronchiolectasia
bronchiolectasis
bronchiolitis
    constrictive b.
    exudative b.
    b. fibrosa obliterans
    b. obliterans with organizing
    pneumonia (BOOP)
bronchioloalveolar
    b. adenocarcinoma
    b. carcinoma
bronchiolopulmonary
bronchiolus terminalis
bronchiostenosis
bronchiseptica
    Bordetella b.
bronchitic asthma
bronchitis
    arachidic b.
    asthmatic b.
    Castellani b.
    chronic b.
    croupous b.
    fibrinous b.
    hemorrhagic b.
    b. obliterans
    obliterative b.
    pseudomembranous b.

bronchium (*var. of* bronchus)
bronchoalveolar
    b. carcinoma
    b. fluid
    b. lavage (BAL)
bronchoaortic constriction
bronchobiliary fistula
bronchocavernous
bronchocavitary fistula
bronchocele
bronchocentric granulomatosis
bronchoconstriction
bronchoconstrictor
bronchodilation, bronchodilatation
bronchodilator
    adrenergic b.
bronchoedema
bronchoesophageal
    b. fistula
    b. muscle
bronchoesophageus muscle
bronchoesophagology
bronchoesophagoscopy
bronchofiberscope
bronchogenic
    b. carcinoma
    b. cyst
bronchogram
    air b.
bronchography
broncholith
broncholithiasis
bronchomalacia
bronchomediastinal lymphatic trunk
bronchomotor
bronchomycosis
bronchophony
    whispered b.
bronchoplasty
bronchopleural (BP)
    b. fistula
bronchopleural-cutaneous fistula
bronchopneumonia
    inhalational b.
bronchopulmonary
    b. dysplasia
    b. lymph node
    b. segment
    b. sequestration
    b. spirochetosis
bronchorrhaphy
bronchorrhea

B

NOTES

bronchoscope
bronchoscopic
    b. brush
    b. smear
bronchoscopy
bronchospasm
    exercise-induced b.
bronchospasmolytic
bronchospirochetosis
bronchospirography
bronchospirometer
bronchospirometry
bronchostaxis
bronchostenosis
bronchostomy
bronchotomy
bronchotracheal
bronchovesicular
    b. breath sounds
    b. respiration
bronchus, bronchium, pl. bronchi
    eparterial b.
    hyparterial b.
    intermediate b.
    b. intermedius
    intrasegmental b.
    left main b.
    lingular b.
    lower lobe b.
    middle lobe b.
bronchus-associated lymphoid tissue
  (BALT)
Brønsted
    B. acid
    B. base
    B. theory
brontophobia
bronze
    b. baby syndrome
    b. diabetes
bronzed
    b. diabetes
    b. disease
    b. skin
brood
    b. capsule
    b. cell
Brooke
    B. ileostomy
    B. tumor
brother complex
Broviac catheter
browlift
brown
    b. adipose tissue
    b. atrophy
    b. edema
    b. fat
    b. induration

    b. layer
    b. lung
    b. pellicle
    b. striae
    B. syndrome
    b. tumor
Brown-Adson forceps
Brown-Brenn stain
brownian
    b. motion
    b. movement
brownian-Zsigmondy movement
Browning vein
Brown-Séquard
    B.-S. paralysis
    B.-S. syndrome
brow presentation
Brucella
    B. abortus
    B. canis
    B. melitensis
    B. suis
brucella strain 19 vaccine
brucellergin
brucellin
brucellosis
    bovine b.
Bruce protocol
Bruch
    B. gland
    B. membrane
brucine
Bruck disease
Brücke
    B. muscle
    B. tunic
Brücke-Bartley phenomenon
Brudzinski sign
Brug filariasis
bruise
bruissement
bruit
    aneurysmal b.
    carotid b.
    cranial b.
    b. de tambour
    Roger b.
    thyroid b.
    Traube b.
Brunn
    B. membrane
    B. nest
    B. reaction
Brunner gland
Bruns
    B. ataxia
    B. nystagmus
Brunschwig operation

brush
  Ayre b.
  b. biopsy
  b. border
  bronchoscopic b.
  b. burn
  b. burn abrasion
  b. catheter
  denture b.
  Haidinger b.
  b. heap structure
  Kruse b.
Brushfield spot
Brushfield-Wyatt disease
brushing
  bronchial b.
brushite
Bruton agammaglobulinemia
bruxism
Bryant
  B. traction
  B. triangle
BSA
  body surface area
  bovine serum albumin
BSE
  bovine spongiform encephalopathy
BSER
  brainstem evoked response
  BSER audiometry
BSF
  basal skull fracture
BSP
  bromsulphalein
  BSP test
BTU
  British thermal unit
buba madre
bubas braziliana
bubble gum dermatitis
bubble-through humidifier
bubbling rale
bubo
  bullet b.
  chancroidal b.
  indolent b.
  malignant b.
  tropical b.
  venereal b.
bubonalgia
bubonic plague
bubonulus

bucardia
bucca
buccal
  b. angle
  b. artery
  b. branch
  b. caries
  b. cavity
  b. curve
  b. digestion
  b. embrasure
  b. fat-pad
  b. flange
  b. gingiva
  b. gland
  b. herpes
  b. lymph node
  b. mucosa
  b. nerve
  b. occlusion
  b. pit
  b. region
  b. root
  b. smear
  b. space abscess
  b. surface
  b. tablet
  b. vestibule
buccalis
  Entamoeba b.
  Leptotrichia b.
buccinator
  b. artery
  b. crest
  b. muscle
  b. nerve
  b. node
buccoaxial
buccoaxiocervical
buccoaxiogingival
buccocervical ridge
buccoclusal
buccodistal
buccogingival ridge
buccolabial
buccolingual
  b. diameter
  b. dimension
  b. relation
buccomesial
bucconasal membrane
bucconeural duct

NOTES

B

137

buccoocclusal angle
buccopharyngeal
    b. fascia
    b. membrane
buccopulpal
buccoversion
buccula
Büchner
    B. extract
    B. funnel
buchneri
    Lactobacillus b.
Buchwald atrophy
buck
    B. extension
    B. fascia
    b. tooth
    B. traction
buckbean
bucket-handle
    b.-h. incision
    b.-h. tear
buckle
    scleral b.
buckled
    b. aorta
    b. innominate artery
buckthorn polyneuropathy
Bucky diaphragm
buclosamide
bucrylate
bud
    bronchial b.
    end b.
    b. fission
    gustatory b.
    limb b.
    liver b.
    lung b.
    median tongue b.
    metanephric b.
    periosteal b.
    b. stage
    tail b.
    taste b.
    tooth b.
Budd-Chiari syndrome
buddeized milk
Budde process
budding
Budd syndrome
Budge center
Budin obstetrical joint
Buerger disease
bufadienolide
bufagenin
bufagin
bufanolide
bufatrienolide

bufenolide
buffalo
    b. hump
    b. neck
    b. type
buffer
    b. capacity
    dipolar b.
    exogenous b.
    b. index
    b. pair
    b. value
buffy
    b. coat
    b. coat concentration
bufogenin
buformin
bufotenine
bufotoxin
bug
    assassin b.
    harvest b.
Buie procedure
bulb
    aortic b.
    arterial b.
    Braasch b.
    carotid b.
    dental b.
    duodenal b.
    end b.
    hair b.
    jugular b.
    Krause end b.
    olfactory b.
    Rouget b.
    speech b.
    b. thermometer
bulbar
    b. apoplexy
    b. conjunctiva
    b. corticonuclear fiber
    b. myelitis
    b. palsy
    b. paralysis
    b. pulse
    b. ridge
    b. septum
bulbi (*pl. of* bulbus)
bulbitis
bulbocapnine
bulbocavernosus
    b. muscle
    b. reflex
bulboid corpuscle
bulbomimic reflex
bulbonuclear
bulbopontine
bulboreticulospinal tract

bulbosacral system
bulbospinal
bulbospongiosus muscle
bulbourethral gland
bulbous bougie
bulboventricular
   b. loop
   b. ridge
bulbus, pl. **bulbi**
   xanthomatosis bulbi
bulesis
bulgaricus
   Lactobacillus b.
bulging eye disease
bulimia nervosa
bulimic
bulkage
bulk modulus
bulk-producing laxative
bulky
   b. disease
   b. dressing
   b. lymphadenopathy
bulla, pl. **bullae**
   ethmoidal b.
   b. ethmoidalis
bulldog
   b. forceps
   b. head
bullectomy
bullet
   b. bubo
   b. forceps
bull neck
bullosa
   concha b.
   epidermolysis b.
   impetigo contagiosa b.
bullous
   b. congenital ichthyosiform erythroderma
   b. edema
   b. edema vesicae
   b. emphysema
   b. impetigo
   b. keratopathy
   b. myringitis
   b. pemphigoid
bull's-eye maculopathy
bumetanide
Bumke pupil

BUN
   blood urea nitrogen
bunching suture
bundle
   aberrant b.
   anterior ground b.
   Arnold b.
   atrioventricular b.
   Bachmann b.
   b. bone
   Flechsig ground b.
   Gantzer accessory b.
   Gierke respiratory b.
   ground b.
   Held b.
   Helie b.
   Helweg b.
   Helwig b.
   His b.
   Hoche b.
   Keith b.
   Kent b.
   Kent-His b.
   Killian b.
   Krause respiratory b.
   lateral ground b.
   lateral proprius b.
   Lissauer b.
   Loewenthal b.
   longitudinal pontine b.
   medial forebrain b.
   medial longitudinal b.
   Monakow b.
   neurovascular b.
   b. of Rasmussen
bundle-branch block
bungarotoxins
bungpagga
bunion
bunionectomy
   Keller b.
   Mayo b.
Bunnell suture
bunodont
bunolophodont
bunoselenodont
Bunsen
   B. burner
   B. solubility coefficient
Bunsen-Roscoe law

NOTES

Bunyamwera
  B. fever
  B. virus
bunyavirus encephalitis
BUO
  bleeding of undetermined origin
buoyant density
buphthalmia, buphthalmos, buphthalmus
bur, burr
  cross-cut b.
  b. drill
  end-cutting b.
  finishing b.
  fissure b.
  inverted cone b.
Burchard-Liebermann reaction
Burdach
  B. column
  B. fasciculus
  B. nucleus
  B. tract
burden
  body b.
  clinical b.
  genetic b.
  tumor b.
Burdwan fever
buret, burette
burgdorferi
  Borrelia b.
Bürger-Grütz
  B.-G. disease
  B.-G. syndrome
Burger triangle
Burgundy pitch
buried
  b. flap
  b. penis
  b. suture
Burkholderia
  B. cepacia
  B. mallei
  B. pseudomallei
Burkitt lymphoma
Burlew
  B. disc
  B. wheel
burn
  brush b.
  chemical b.
  first-degree b.
  flash b.
  fourth-degree b.
  full-thickness b.
  high-tension b.
  immersion b.
  mat b.
  partial-thickness b.
  powder b.

  radiation b.
  B. and Rand theory
  respiratory b.
  second-degree b.
  b. shock
  thermal b.
  third-degree b.
  b. unit
burner
  Bunsen b.
  b. syndrome
burnetii
  Coxiella b.
Burnett syndrome
burning
  b. drops sign
  b. foot syndrome
  b. mouth syndrome
  b. tongue
  b. tongue syndrome
  b. vulva syndrome
burnisher
burnout
Burns
  B. falciform process
  B. ligament
  B. space
burnt alum
Burow
  B. solution
  B. triangle
  B. vein
burr (*var. of* bur)
burrowing
  b. hair
  b. pus
bursa, pl. **bursae**
  Achilles b.
  adventitious b.
  anserine b.
  anterior tibial b.
  bicipitoradial b.
  Boyer b.
  Brodie b.
  Calori b.
  coracobrachial b.
  deep infrapatellar b.
  Fleischmann b.
  gluteofemoral b.
  gluteus medius bursae
  gluteus minimus b.
  iliac b.
  iliopectineal b.
  inferior subtendinous b.
  infracardiac b.
  infrahyoid b.
  infraspinatus b.
  intermuscular gluteal b.
  interosseous cubital b.

B

intratendinous olecranon b.
ischial b.
laryngeal b.
lateral malleolar subcutaneous b.
lateral malleolus b.
Luschka b.
medial malleolar subcutaneous b.
omental b.
pharyngeal b.
prepatellar b.
retrocalcaneal b.
retrohyoid b.
rider's b.
sciatic b.
semimembranous b.
subacromial b.
subdeltoid b.
subtendinous iliac b.
suprapatellar b.
synovial b.
b. of tendo calcaneus
bursal
b. abscess
b. cyst
b. synovitis
bursata
exostosis b.
bursectomy
bursitis
anserine b.
calcaneal b.
calcific b.
ischial b.
prepatellar b.
subacromial b.
bursolith
bursopathy
bursotomy
burst size
Burton
B. line
B. sign
Buruli ulcer
Busacca nodule
Buschke disease
Buschke-Ollendorf syndrome
buski
Fasciolopsis b.
Busquet disease
Busse-Buschke disease
busulfan, busulphan
butane

butanol-extractable
b.-e. iodine
b.-e. iodine test
butanoyl
butaperazine
butaverine
butethamate
buthionine sulfoximine
butter
cacao b.
cocoa b.
b. stool
b. yellow
butterfly
b. bandage
b. drain
b. dressing
b. eruption
b. fragment
b. lung
b. needle
b. patch
b. pattern
b. rash
b. vertebra
buttocks
button
belly b.
Biskra b.
mescal b.
Murphy b.
peritoneal b.
polyethylene collar b.
stoma b.
b. suture
buttonhole
b. deformity
b. iridectomy
b. operation
b. stenosis
buttress plate
butyl
b. alcohol
b. aminobenzoate
butylated
b. hydroxyanisole
b. hydroxytoluene
butylparaben
butyraceous
butyrate
butyrate-CoA ligase
butyric acid

NOTES

141

butyroid
butyrometer
butyrophenone
butyrous
butyryl
butyrylcholine esterase
butyryl-CoA synthetase
buyo cheek cancer
Buzzard maneuver
Bwamba
> B. fever
> B. virus

By antigen
Byars flap
Byler disease
bypass
> aortocoronary b.
> aortoiliac b.
> aortorenal b.
> bowel b.
> cardiopulmonary b.
> coronary b.
> coronary artery b.
> extraanatomic b.
> extracranial-intracranial b.
> femoropopliteal b.
> gastric b.
> jejunoileal b.
> left heart b.
> right heart b.

by-product material
byssinosis
bystander lysis
Byzantine arch palate

C

C bile
C carbohydrate antigen
C cell
C chain
C factor
C fiber
C gene
C group virus
C sliding osteotomy
C terminus
C value
C wave

C1

C1 esterase
C1 esterase inhibitor
vertebra C1

C2

vertebra C2

CA

cancer
carcinoma
CA virus

CA-125, CA125

CA-125 antigen

c-a

cardioarterial
c-a interval

CA-15-3 antigen
CA-19-9 antigen
CAAT box
caballus

Aedes c.

cabbage

c. goiter
c. tree

cable

c. graft
c. wire suture

Cabot-Locke murmur
Cabot ring body
cacao

c. butter
c. oil

CaCC

cathodal closure contraction

cachectic

c. diarrhea
c. edema
c. endocarditis
c. fever
c. pallor

cachecticorum

acne c.

cachectin
cachet
cachexia

amyotrophic c.
diabetic neuropathic c.
c. hypophyseopriva
hypophysial c.
malarial c.
pituitary c.
c. strumipriva
c. thyropriva

cachinnation
cacogeusia
cacomelia
cacoplastic
cacosmia
cactinomycin
cacumen
cacuminal
cadaver
cadaveric

c. rigidity
c. spasm

cadaverine
cadaverous
caddis worm
cade oil
cadherin
cadmium
caduca
caduceus
caecum (*var. of* cecum)
caeruleus

locus c.

caerulospinal tract
café au lait spot
cafe coronary
caffeine

c. citrate
c. hydrate
c. and sodium salicylate

caffeinism
Caffey

C. disease
C. syndrome

Caffey-Kempe syndrome
Caffey-Silverman syndrome
cage

thoracic c.

Cagot ear
CAHD

coronary arteriosclerotic heart disease
coronary atherosclerotic heart disease

Cain complex

C

caisson
- c. disease
- c. sickness

Cajal
- C. astrocyte stain
- C. cell

cajennense
- *Amblyomma c.*

cajeput oil

cajeputol, cajuputol

cajuput oil

cake
- c. alum
- c. kidney

Calabar
- C. bean
- C. swelling

calabash curare

calamine

calamus scriptorius

calcaneal
- c. anastomosis
- c. apophysitis
- c. arterial network
- c. artery
- c. bone
- c. branch
- c. bursitis
- c. gait
- c. petechia
- c. process
- c. region
- c. spur
- c. sulcus
- c. tendon
- c. tuber
- c. tubercle
- c. tuberosity

calcanean

calcaneoapophysitis

calcaneoastragaloid

calcaneocavus

calcaneocuboid
- c. joint
- c. ligament

calcaneodynia

calcaneofibular ligament

calcaneonavicular ligament

calcaneoscaphoid

calcaneotibial ligament

calcaneovalgocavus

calcaneovalgus
- talipes c.

calcaneovarus
- talipes c.

calcaneus, calcaneum
- bursa of tendo c.
- talipes c.

calcar

calcareous
- c. corpuscle
- c. degeneration
- c. infiltration
- c. metastasis
- c. pancreatitis

calcarine
- c. artery
- c. branch
- c. fissure
- c. spur
- c. sulcus

calcariuria

calcemia

calcergy

calcicosis

calcic water

calcidiol

calcifediol

calciferol

calciferous

calcific
- c. bursitis
- c. nodular aortic stenosis
- c. pancreatitis
- c. tendonitis

calcification
- dystrophic c.
- eggshell c.
- metastatic c.
- Mönckeberg c.
- pathologic c.

calcified
- c. cartilage
- c. pericardium

calcify

calcifying
- c. epithelial odontogenic tumor
- c. and keratinizing odontogenic cyst

calcigerous

calcination

calcine

calcined magnesia

calcineurin

calcinosis
- c. circumscripta
- dystrophic c.
- c., Raynaud phenomenon, esophageal motility disorder, sclerodactyly, and telangiectasia (CREST)
- reversible c.
- c. universalis

calciokinesis

calciokinetic

calciorrhachia

calciostat

calciotraumatic

calcipectic
calcipenia
calcipenic
calcipexic
calcipexis, calcipexy
calciphilia
calciphylaxis
calciprivia
calciprivic
calcis
calcite
calcitetrol
calcitonin gene-related peptide
calcitriol
calcium
    c. alginate
    c. antagonist
    c. benzoylpas
    c. bromide
    c. carbide
    c. carbonate
    c. channel blocker
    c. channel-blocking agent
    c. chloride
    docusate c.
    fenoprofen c.
    c. gluconate
    c. gout
    c. group
    c. hippurate
    c. hydroxide
    c. hypophosphite
    c. iodate
    c. iodobehenate
    c. ipodate
    c. lactate
    c. lactophosphate
    c. leucovorin
    leucovorin c.
    c. levulinate
    c. mandelate
    milk of c.
    c. monohydrogen phosphate
    c. oxalate
    c. oxide
    c. pantothenate
    c. propionate
    c. pump
    c. pyrophosphate deposition disease
      (CPPD)
    c. rigor
    c. saccharate

    c. sign
    c. stearate
calcium-45, -47
calciuria
calcoaceticus
    Acinetobacter c.
calcodynia
calcophorous
calcospherite
calculated
    c. mean organism
    c. serum osmolality
calculi (*pl. of* calculus)
calculosis
calculous anuria
calculus, pl. **calculi**
    alternating c.
    apatite c.
    arthritic c.
    biliary c.
    bladder c.
    blood c.
    branched c.
    bronchial c.
    cerebral c.
    coral c.
    cystine c.
    dendritic c.
    dental c.
    encysted c.
    fibrin c.
    gastric c.
    hematogenetic c.
    hemic c.
    infection c.
    intestinal c.
    lacrimal c.
    mammary c.
    matrix c.
    metabolic c.
    oxalate c.
    pancreatic c.
    pocketed c.
    preputial c.
    prostatic c.
    renal c.
    salivary c.
    staghorn c.
    struvite c.
    urate c.
    urinary c.

C

NOTES

calculus *(continued)*
    uterine c.
    vesical c.
Caldani ligament
Caldwell
    C. projection
    C. view
Caldwell-Luc operation
Caldwell-Moloy classification
calefacient
calf
    c. bone
    c. pump
caliber
calibrate
calibrated probe
calibration
    c. curve
    c. interval
calibrator
caliceal, calyceal
    c. diverticulum
calicectasis
calicectomy
calices (*pl. of* calix)
caliciform, calyciform
    c. cell
    c. ending
calicine, calycine
Caliciviridae
calicoplasty
calicotomy
caliculus
caliectasis
California
    C. encephalitis
    C. psychological inventory test
    C. virus
californium
calioplasty
caliorrhaphy
caliotomy
caliper micrometer
calipers
calisthenics
calix, calyx, pl. **calices**
    major c.
    minor c.
Calkins sign
Callahan method
Callander amputation
Calleja
    island of C.
Call-Exner body
Callison fluid
callosal
    c. convolution
    c. gyrus
    c. sulcus

callose
callosity
callosomarginal
    c. artery
    c. fissure
    c. sulcus
callous
callus
    central c.
    definitive c.
    ensheathing c.
    medullary c.
    permanent c.
calmative
Calmette-Guérin
    bacille C.-G. (BCG)
    C.-G. bacillus
    C.-G. vaccine
Calmette test
calmodulin
calomel electrode
calor
Calori bursa
caloric
    c. intake
    c. nystagmus
    c. stimulation
    c. test
    c. value
caloricum
    erythema c.
calorie
    gram c.
    kilogram c. (kcal)
    large c.
    mean c.
    small c.
calorific
calorigenic action
calorimeter
    Benedict-Roth c.
    bomb c.
    human c.
calorimetric
calorimetry
    direct c.
    indirect c.
caloritropic
Calot triangle
calsequestrin
calvaria
calvarial hook
Calvé-Perthes disease
calyceal (*var. of* caliceal)
calyciform (*var. of* caliciform)
calycine (*var. of* calicine)
calycle, calyculus
calyx (*var. of* calix)

CAM
computer-assisted myelography
cambium layer
camera
Anger c.
gamma c.
multiformat c.
c. oculi
c. postrema
scintillation c.
c. vitrea
camp
c. fever
c. hospital
Campbell
C. ligament
C. sound
Camper
C. chiasm
C. fascia
C. ligament
C. line
C. plane
camphor
cantharis c.
c. liniment
camphoraceous
camphorated
c. menthol
c. oil
c. phenol
campimeter
camplodactyly
cAMP receptor protein
camptocormia
camptodactyly, camptodactylia
camptomelia
camptomelic
c. dwarfism
c. syndrome
camptospasm
camptothecin
Campylobacter
C. coli
C. concisus
C. fetus
C. fetus jejuni
C. hyointestinalis
C. jejuni
C. lari
C. pylori
C. sputorum

campylobacteriosis
Canada
C. balsam
C. snakeroot
C. turpentine
canal
abdominal c.
accessory c.
adductor c.
Alcock c.
alimentary c.
alveolar c.
alveolodental c.
anal c.
anterior semicircular c.
archenteric c.
Arnold c.
arterial c.
atrioventricular c.
auditory c.
basipharyngeal c.
Bernard c.
Bichat c.
birth c.
blastoporic c.
bony semicircular c.
Böttcher c.
Breschet c.
carotid c.
carpal c.
caudal c.
central c.
cervical c.
cervicoaxillary c.
cervicouterine c.
ciliary c.
Civinini c.
Cloquet c.
cochlear c.
condylar c.
condyloid c.
Corti c.
Cotunnius c.
craniopharyngeal c.
deferent c.
dental c.
dentinal c.
diploic c.
Dorello c.
Dupuytren c.
ear c.
endocervical c.

NOTES

147

canal *(continued)*
    endodermal c.
    endometrial c.
    facial c.
    fallopian c.
    femoral c.
    Ferrein c.
    Fontana c.
    galactophorous c.
    Gartner c.
    gastric c.
    greater palatine c.
    gubernacular c.
    Guyon c.
    c. of Guyon
    gynecophoric c.
    Hannover c.
    haversian c.
    Hensen c.
    c. of Hering
    Hirschfeld c.
    Holmgrén-Golgi c.
    c. of Hovius
    Hoyer c.
    Huguier c.
    Hunter c.
    hyaloid c.
    hypoglossal c.
    incisive c.
    incisor c.
    inferior dental c.
    infraorbital c.
    inguinal c.
    interdental c.
    interfacial c.
    internal acoustic c.
    Jacobson c.
    Kürsteiner c.
    lateral semicircular c.
    Laurer c.
    Lauth c.
    Leeuwenhoek c.
    lesser palatine c.
    longitudinal c.
    Löwenberg c.
    mandibular c.
    marrow c.
    mental c.
    musculotubal c.
    nasolacrimal c.
    c. of Nuck
    nutrient c.
    obturator c.
    optic c.
    parturient c.
    portal c.
    pterygoid c.
    pterygopalatine c.
    pudendal c.

    pulp c.
    pyloric c.
    Rivinus c.
    root c.
    Rosenthal c.
    sacral c.
    Santorini c.
    Schlemm c.
    semicircular c.
    Sondermann c.
    spinal c.
    spiral c.
    Theile c.
    urogenital c.
    uterovaginal c.
    vertebral c.
    vesicourethral c.
    vestibular c.
    Wirsung c.
canalicular
    c. adenoma
    c. duct
    c. sphincter
canaliculi *(pl. of* canaliculus)
canaliculitis
canaliculization
canaliculus, pl. **canaliculi**
    auricular c.
    biliary c.
    bone c.
    c. chordae tympani
    c. cochleae
    cochlear c.
    canaliculi dentales
    intercellular c.
    intracellular c.
    lacrimal c.
    mastoid c.
    c. reuniens
    Thiersch c.
    tympanic c.
    c. tympanicus
canalization
Canavan
    C. disease
    C. sclerosis
Canavan-van Bogaert-Bertrand disease
cancellated
cancellous
    c. bone
    c. tissue
cancellus
cancer (CA)
    adenoid c.
    c. antigen 125 test
    asbestos c.
    betel c.
    buyo cheek c.
    chimney sweep's c.

colloid c.
conjugal c.
dermoid c.
c. à deux
c. en cuirasse
epidermoid c.
epithelial c.
familial c.
c. family
glandular c.
hereditary nonpolyposis colorectal c.
kang c.
kangri c.
mule-spinner's c.
smoker's c.
stump c.
ulcerated c.
withering c.
cancerophobia
cancerous
cancriform
cancroid
cancrum
candela (cd)
candicans
candicidin
Candida
C. albicans
C. glabrata
C. parapsilosis
C. tropicalis
candidemia
candidiasis
candidosis
candle-meter
candle-power
canicola fever
canine
c. adenovirus 1
c. amebiasis
c. carcinoma 1
c. distemper virus
c. eminence
c. fossa
c. leishmaniasis
c. prominence
c. spasm
c. tooth
caniniform
caninum
Ancylostoma c.
Dipylidium c.

canis
Brucella c.
Ehrlichia c.
Microsporum c.
canities
rapid c.
canker sore
cannabidiol
cannabinoid
cannabinol
cannabis
cannabism
Cannizzaro reaction
cannon
C. point
C. ring
c. sound
C. theory
c. wave
cannonball pulse
Cannon-Bard theory
cannula
Hasson c.
infusion c.
irrigation c.
Karman c.
laparoscopic c.
cannulation
cannulization
Cantelli sign
cantering rhythm
canthal hypertelorism
cantharidal collodion
cantharidate
cantharidin
cantharidis
cantharis camphor
canthectomy
canthi (*pl. of* canthus)
canthitis
cantholysis
canthomeatal plane
canthoplasty
canthorrhaphy
canthotomy
canthus, pl. **canthi**
external c.
internal c.
lateral c.
medial c.

NOTES

cantilever
  c. beam
  c. bridge
Cantor tube
CaOC
  cathodal opening contracture
cap
  acrosomal c.
  apical c.
  cervical c.
  chin c.
  cradle c.
  dental c.
  duodenal c.
  enamel c.
  head c.
  metanephric c.
  pyloric c.
  c. splint
  c. stage
capacitance
capacitation
capacitor
capacity
  aerobic c.
  buffer c.
  carrying c.
  cranial c.
  diffusing c.
  forced vital c. (FVC)
  functional residual c. (FRC)
  heat c.
  inspiratory c.
  iron-binding c. (IBC)
  maximum breathing c. (MBC)
  oxygen c.
  residual c.
  respiratory c.
  thermal c.
  total iron binding c.
  total lung c.
  vital c.
capactin
CAPD
  continuous ambulatory peritoneal dialysis
capeline bandage
Capgras
  C. phenomenon
  C. syndrome
capillarectasia
Capillaria **granuloma**
capillariasis
  intestinal c.
capillariomotor
capillarioscopy
capillaritis
capillarity
capillaron
capillaropathy

capillaroscopy
capillary
  c. angioma
  arterial c.
  c. arteriole
  c. attraction
  c. bed
  bile c.
  blood c.
  c. circulation
  continuous c.
  c. drainage
  fenestrated c.
  c. filling
  c. fracture
  c. fragility
  c. fragility test
  c. hemangioma
  c. lake
  c. lamina
  c. loop
  lymph c.
  c. nevus
  c. permeability factor
  c. pulse
  c. resistance
  c. resistance test
  c. vein
  venous c.
  c. vessel
  c. zone electrophoresis (CZE)
capillitii
  dermatitis papillaris c.
capillosus
  Bacteroides c.
Capim virus
capita (*pl. of* caput)
capital epiphysis
capitate bone
capitation
capitellum
capitis
  corona c.
  dolor c.
  tinea c.
capitopedal
capitular joint
capitulum
Caplan
  C. nodule
  C. syndrome
capnogram
capnograph
capnometer
capnometry
capon-comb unit
capon unit
capping
  direct pulp c.

indirect pulp c.
c. protein
Capps reflex
caprate
capriloquism
caprin
caprizant
caproate
caproyl
caproylate
caprylate
caprylic acid
capsaicin
capsicin
capsicum
capsid
capsomer, capsomere
capsular
c. advancement
c. ankylosis
c. antigen
c. branch
c. cataract
c. flap pyeloplasty
c. glaucoma
c. ligament
c. pattern
c. precipitation reaction
c. space
capsulata
Emmonsiella c.
capsulation
capsulatum
Histoplasma c.
capsule
acoustic c.
adipose c.
adrenal c.
articular c.
atrabiliary c.
auditory c.
bacterial c.
Bonnet c.
Bowman c.
brood c.
cartilage c.
c. cell
cricoarytenoid articular c.
cricothyroid articular c.
Crosby c.
crystalline c.
external c.

extreme c.
eye c.
fatty renal c.
fibrous articular c.
c. forceps
Gerota c.
Glisson c.
glomerular c.
internal c.
joint c.
c. of lens
lens c.
lenticular c.
malpighian c.
nasal c.
optic c.
otic c.
Tenon c.
capsulectomy
capsulitis
adhesive c.
hepatic c.
capsulolenticular cataract
capsuloplasty
capsulorrhaphy
capsulorrhexis
capsulotome
capsulotomy
capture
atrial c.
electron c.
K c.
capture-recapture method
Capuron point
caput, pl. **capita**
c. medusae
c. succedaneum
car
c. sickness
c. versus pedestrian accident
Carabelli
C. cusp
C. tubercle
Caraparu virus
carbamate kinase
carbamazepine
carbamic acid
carbamide
carbamino compound
carbaminohemoglobin
carbamoate
carbamoyl

NOTES

carbamoyltransferase
carbamoylurea
carbamyl
carbamylation
carbanion
carbapenem antibiotic
carbaril
carbarsone
carbaryl
carbazide
carbazole
carbenium
carbhemoglobin
carbide
    calcium c.
carbidopa
carbimazole
carbimide
    citrated calcium c.
carbinol
carbogen
carbohemoglobin
carbohydrate
    c. loading
    c. metabolism
    c. utilization test
carbohydrate-induced hyperlipemia
carbohydraturia
carbohydrazide
carbolate
carbolated
carbol fuchsin
carbol-fuchsin paint
carbolic acid
carbolize
carbol-thionin stain
carboluria
carbomer
carbometry
carbomycin
carbon
    anomeric c.
    c. autotrophy
    c. bisulfide
    c. dichloride
    c. dioxide (CO2)
    c. dioxide acidosis
    c. dioxide combining power
    c. dioxide content
    c. dioxide cycle
    c. dioxide electrode
    c. dioxide elimination
    c. dioxide-free water
    c. dioxide production
    c. dioxide snow
    c. disulfide
    c. disulfide poisoning
    c. monoxide (CO)
    c. monoxide hemoglobin
    c. monoxide poisoning
    c. tetrachloride
carbon-11, -12, -13, -14
carbonate
    ammonium c.
    bismuth c.
    calcium c.
    c. dehydratase
    c. dehydratase inhibitor
    lead c.
    lithium c.
    magnesium c.
carbonated water
1-carbon fragment
2-carbon fragment
carbonic
    c. acid
    c. acid gas
    c. anhydrase
    c. anhydrase II deficiency
    syndrome
    c. anhydrase inhibitor
    c. anhydride
    c. water
carbonium
carbonmonoxy myoglobin
carbonometer
carbonometry
carbonuria
carbonyl
carboplatin
carboprost tromethamine
carboxamide
carboximide
carboxycathepsin
carboxydismutase
carboxyhemoglobin
carboxyhemoglobinemia
carboxyl
carboxylase
carboxylation
carboxyltransferase
carboxypeptidase
    c. A, B, C, G
    acid c.
carboxy terminal
carbromal
carbuncle
    kidney c.
carbuncular
carbunculoid
carbunculosis
carburet
carbutamide
carcass
carcinemia
carcinoembryonic antigen (CEA)
carcinogen
    complete c.

carcinogenesis
    field c.
carcinogenic
carcinogenicity
carcinoid
    bronchial c.
    bronchiolar c.
    embryonal c.
    c. flush
    occult c.
    papillary c.
    c. syndrome
    c. tumor
carcinolytic
carcinoma (CA)
    acinar c.
    acinic cell c.
    adenoid cystic c.
    adenoid squamous cell c.
    adenosquamous c.
    adnexal c.
    adrenal cortical c.
    alveolar cell c.
    anaplastic c.
    apocrine c.
    basaloid c.
    basal squamous cell c.
    basisquamous c.
    basosquamous c.
    bile duct c.
    bronchiolar c.
    bronchioloalveolar c.
    bronchoalveolar c.
    bronchogenic c.
    clear cell c.
    cloacogenic c.
    colloid c.
    cribriform c.
    cuboidal c.
    cylindromatous c.
    cystic c.
    duct c.
    ductal c.
    embryonal c.
    endometrioid c.
    epidermoid c.
    epithelial myoepithelial c.
    fibrolamellar liver cell c.
    follicular c.
    giant cell c.
    glandular c.
    hepatocellular c.

    hilar c.
    Hürthle cell c.
    inflammatory c.
    intraductal c.
    intraepidermal c.
    intraepithelial c.
    invasive c.
    juvenile c.
    kangri burn c.
    large cell c.
    latent c.
    lateral aberrant thyroid c.
    leptomeningeal c.
    liver cell c.
    lobular c.
    medullary c.
    melanotic c.
    meningeal c.
    mesometanephric c.
    metaplastic c.
    metastatic c.
    microinvasive c.
    mucinous c.
    nasopharyngeal c.
    oat cell c.
    oncocytic c.
    oxyphilic c.
    papillary c.
    peritoneal c.
    polymorphous low-grade c.
    scar c.
    scirrhous c.
    secretory c.
    c. in situ (CIS)
    small cell c.
    spindle cell c.
    squamous cell c.
    sweat gland c.
    terminal duct c.
    transitional cell c.
    tubular c.
    urothelial c.
    villous c.
carcinomatosis
    leptomeningeal c.
    lymphangitic c.
    meningeal c.
carcinomatous
    c. encephalomyelopathy
    c. implant
    c. myelopathy
    c. myopathy

NOTES

C

carcinomatous *(continued)*
    c. neuromyopathy
    c. pericarditis
carcinophobia
carcinosarcoma
carcinosis
carcinostatic
carcoma
Carden amputation
cardenolide
cardia
    gastric c.
cardiac
    c. accident
    c. albuminuria
    c. alternation
    c. aneurysm
    c. antrum
    c. arrest
    c. arrhythmia
    c. asthma
    c. ballet
    c. care technician
    c. catheter
    c. cirrhosis
    c. competence
    c. contractility
    c. cycle
    c. decompression
    c. depressor reflex
    c. diuretic
    c. dropsy
    c. dyspnea
    c. dysrhythmia
    c. edema
    c. failure
    c. fibrous skeleton
    c. ganglion
    c. gating
    c. gland
    c. glycoside
    c. heterotaxia
    c. histiocyte
    c. hormone
    c. impulse
    c. index
    c. infarction
    c. insufficiency
    c. intensive care unit (CICU)
    c. jelly
    c. liver
    c. lung
    c. lymphatic ring
    c. mapping
    c. massage
    c. monitor
    c. murmur
    c. muscle
    c. muscle tissue

    c. muscle wrap
    c. nervous plexus
    c. neurosis
    c. notch
    c. opening
    c. orifice
    c. output
    c. plexus
    c. polyp
    c. prominence
    c. rehabilitation
    c. rescue technician
    c. reserve
    c. risk factor (CRF)
    c. segment
    c. shock
    c. souffle
    c. sound
    c. sphincter
    c. standstill
    c. syncope
    c. tamponade
    c. telemetry
    c. tube
    c. valve prosthesis
    c. valvular incompetence
    c. vein
cardiaca
    adiposis c.
cardial
    c. notch
    c. orifice
cardialgia
cardiataxia
cardiatelia
cardiectasia
cardiectomy
cardiectopia
cardinal
    c. ligament
    c. ocular movement
    c. point
    c. symptom
    c. vein
cardioaccelerator
cardioactive
cardioangiography
cardioaortic
cardioarterial (c-a)
    c. interval
cardiocele
cardiochalasia
cardiodiaphragmatic angle
cardiodiosis
cardiodynamics
cardiodynia
cardioesophageal
    c. junction
    c. relaxation

cardiofacial syndrome
cardiogenesis
cardiogenic
    c. plate
    c. shock
cardiogram
    esophageal c.
cardiograph
cardiography
    ultrasound c.
cardiohemothrombus
cardiohepatic
    c. angle
    c. triangle
cardiohepatomegaly
cardioid condenser
cardioinhibitory
cardiokymogram
cardiokymograph
cardiokymography
cardiolipin
cardiologist
cardiology intensive care unit (CICU)
cardiolysis
cardiomalacia
cardiomegaly
    glycogen c.
    glycogenic c.
cardiometry
cardiomotility
cardiomuscular
cardiomyoliposis
cardiomyopathy
    alcoholic c.
    congestive c.
    dilated c.
    familial hypertrophic c.
    hypertrophic obstructive c. (HOCM)
    idiopathic c.
cardiomyoplasty
cardiomyotomy
cardionatrin
cardionecrosis
cardionector
cardionephric
cardioneural
cardioneurosis
cardioomentopexy
cardiopaludism
cardiopath
cardiopathy
cardiopericardiopexy

cardiophobia
cardiophone
cardiophony
cardiophrenia
cardiophrenic angle
cardioplasty
cardioplegia
    antegrade c.
cardioplegic arrest
cardioprotective agent
cardioptosia
cardioptosis
cardiopulmonary
    c. arrest
    c. bypass
    c. murmur
    c. resuscitation (CPR)
    c. splanchnic nerve
    c. transplantation
cardiopyloric
cardiorenal
cardiorespiratory murmur
cardiorrhaphy
cardiorrhexis
cardioscope
cardioselective
cardioselectivity
cardiospasm
cardiosphygmograph
cardiotachometer
cardiothoracic ratio
cardiothrombus
cardiothyrotoxicosis
cardiotomy
cardiotonic
cardiotoxic myolysis
cardiotoxin
cardiovalvulitis
cardiovascular (CV)
    c. accident
    c. drift
    c. radiology
    c. renal disease
    c. syphilis
    c. system
cardiovasculare
cardiovasculorenal
cardioversion
cardiovert
cardioverter
carditis

C

NOTES

care

ambulatory c.
assumption of c.
comprehensive medical c.
custodial c.
end-of-life c.
episode of c.
extended c.
health c.
home health c.
intensive c.
managed c.
medical c.
pharmaceutical c.
point of c.
postoperative c.
prehospital c.
primary c.
respiratory c.
skilled nursing c.
tertiary c.

caregiver
Carey Coombs murmur
Carhart notch
caries

active c.
arrested dental c.
buccal c.
cemental c.
compound c.
dental c.
distal c.
fissure c.
incipient c.
interdental c.
mesial c.

carina, pl. carinae
carinal lymph node
carinate abdomen
carinatum

pectus c.

carinii

Pneumocystis c.

cariogenesis
cariogenic
cariogenicity
cariology
cariostatic
carious
carisoprodate
carisoprodol
Carlen tube
carmalum
Carman sign
carminate
carminative
carmine

indigo c.

lithium c.
Schneider c.

carminophil, carminophile,
  carminophilous
carminophilous
Carmody-Batson operation
carmustine
carnassial tooth
carnauba wax
carneous

c. degeneration
c. mole

Carnett sign
Carney complex
carnification
carnitine

c. acetyltransferase
c. deficiency
c. palmitoyltransferase

carnosinase
carnosine
carnosinemia
carnosity
Carnoy fixative
Caroli

C. disease
C. syndrome

carotene
carotenemia
carotenoderma
carotenoid
carotenoprotein
carotenosis cutis
caroticocavernous fistula
caroticoclinoid ligament
caroticotympanic

c. artery
c. nerve

carotid

c. artery
c. body
c. body tumor
c. bruit
c. bulb
c. canal
c. duct
c. endarterectomy (CEA)
c. foramen
c. ganglion
c. groove
c. pulse
c. sheath
c. shudder
c. sinus
c. sinus branch
c. sinus massage
c. sinus nerve
c. sinus reflex
c. sinus syncope

c. sinus syndrome
c. sinus test
c. sulcus
c. triangle
c. tubercle
carotid-cavernous fistula
carotidynia (*var. of* carotodynia)
carotinemia
carotinosis cutis
carotodynia, carotidynia
carpal
c. arch
c. artery
c. bone
c. canal
c. groove
c. joint
c. tendinous sheath
c. tunnel
c. tunnel syndrome
carpectomy
Carpenter syndrome
Carpentier-Edwards valve
carpi (*pl. of* carpus)
carp mouth
carpocarpal
carpometacarpal
c. joint
c. ligament
carpopedal
c. contraction
c. spasm
carpoptosia
carpoptosis
carpus, pl. **carpi**
c. curvus
carrageen, carragheen
carrageenan, carrageenin
Carrel-Lindbergh pump
Carrel treatment
carrier
amalgam c.
c. cell
convalescent c.
c. electrophoresis
genetic c.
hydrogen c.
incubatory c.
latent c.
manifesting c.
c. screening

c. state
c. strain
carrier-free
Carrington disease
Carrión disease
Carr-Price
C.-P. reaction
C.-P. test
Carr-Purcell experiment
carrying
c. angle
c. capacity
carry-over
cart
crash c.
cartesian nomogram
cartilage
accessory nasal c.
accessory quadrate c.
alisphenoid c.
anular c.
arthrodial c.
articular c.
arytenoid c.
auricular c.
basilar c.
c. bone
branchial c.
calcified c.
c. capsule
c. cell
cellular c.
ciliary c.
circumferential c.
conchal c.
connecting c.
corniculate c.
costal c.
cricoid c.
cuneiform c.
diarthrodial c.
elastic c.
ensiform c.
ensisternum c.
epiglottic c.
epiphysial c.
falciform c.
floating c.
c. forceps
greater alar c.
Huschke c.
hyaline c.

C

NOTES

cartilage *(continued)*
hypsiloid c.
interosseous c.
intervertebral c.
intraarticular c.
intrathyroid c.
investing c.
c. island
Jacobson c.
c. knife
c. lacuna
lateral c.
lesser alar c.
loose c.
Luschka c.
major alar c.
mandibular c.
c. matrix
meatal c.
Meckel c.
Meyer c.
minor alar c.
nasal septal c.
paranasal c.
permanent c.
precursory c.
Reichert c.
semilunar c.
sesamoid c.
slipping rib c.
c. space
temporary c.
thyroid c.
tracheal c.
vomerine c.
vomeronasal c.
xiphoid c.
Y c.
yellow c.
Y-shaped c.

cartilage-hair hypoplasia
cartilaginea
exostosis c.
cartilaginoid
cartilaginous
c. articulation
c. disc
c. joint
c. neurocranium
c. ossification
c. septum
c. tissue

caruncle
lacrimal c.
urethral c.

caruncula, pl. **carunculae**
hymenal c.

Carus
C. circle
C. curve
Carvallo sign
carvedilol
Casal necklace
cascade
arachidonic acid c.
c. stomach
case
borderline c.
c. control study
c. fatality rate
c. fatality ratio
index c.
c. management
c. mix
caseation necrosis
casei
Lactobacillus c.
casein
gluten c.
c. iodine
caseinate
caseinogen
caseo-iodine
caseosa
vernix c.
caseous
c. abscess
c. degeneration
c. necrosis
c. osteitis
c. pneumonia
c. rhinitis
c. tubercle
Casoni
C. antigen
C. intradermal test
C. skin test
Casselberry position
Casser
C. fontanelle
C. perforated muscle
casserian
cassette
c. mutagenesis
susceptibility c.
cassia
c. bark
c. cinnamon
c. fistula
c. oil
cast
bacterial c.
blood c.
c. brace
coma c.
decidual c.

dental c.
diagnostic c.
epithelial c.
false c.
fat c.
fatty c.
fibrinous c.
granular c.
hair c.
halo c.
hyaline c.
investment c.
master c.
short leg c.
Castellani
    C. bronchitis
    C. paint
Castile soap
casting
    centrifugal c.
    c. flask
    gold c.
    c. ring
    c. wax
Castle intrinsic factor
Castleman disease
castor
    c. bean
    c. oil
castrate
castration
    c. anxiety
    c. cell
    c. complex
    functional c.
CAT
    computerized axial tomography
catabasial
catabiotic
catabolic
catabolism
catabolite
    c. gene activator
    c. gene activator protein
    c. repression
catachronobiology
catacrotic pulse
catacrotism
catadicrotic pulse
catadicrotism
catadidymus
catadioptric

catadromous
catagen
catagenesis
catalase
catalatic reaction
catalepsy
cataleptic
cataleptoid
catalysis
    contact c.
catalyst
    inorganic c.
catalytic
    c. antibody
    c. center
catalyze
catalyzer
catamenial pneumothorax
catamnesis
catamnestic
catapasm
cataphasia
cataphora
cataphoresis
cataphoretic
cataplasia, cataplasis
cataplasm
cataplectic
cataplexy
cataract
    adolescent c.
    anular c.
    atopic c.
    axial c.
    black c.
    blue dot c.
    capsular c.
    capsulolenticular c.
    central c.
    cerulean c.
    cheesy c.
    complete c.
    complicated c.
    concussion c.
    congenital c.
    copper c.
    coralliform c.
    coronary c.
    cortical c.
    crystalline c.
    cuneiform c.
    cupuliform c.

C

NOTES

cataract *(continued)*
    cystic c.
    dendritic c.
    diabetic c.
    disc-shaped c.
    electric c.
    embryonic c.
    embryopathic c.
    fibrinous c.
    fibroid c.
    floriform c.
    furnacemen's c.
    fusiform c.
    galactose c.
    glassworker's c.
    glaucomatous c.
    gray c.
    hard c.
    hook-shaped c.
    hypermature c.
    hypocalcemic c.
    immature c.
    incipient c.
    infantile c.
    infrared c.
    intumescent c.
    juvenile c.
    lamellar c.
    c. lens
    life-belt c.
    mature c.
    membranous c.
    Morgagni c.
    c. needle
    nuclear c.
    polar c.
    progressive c.
    pyramidal c.
    ripe c.
    secondary c.
    senile c.
    siderotic c.
    c. spoon
    stellate c.
    subcapsular c.
    vascular c.
    zonular c.
cataractogenesis
cataractogenic
cataract-oligophrenia syndrome
cataractous
catarrh
catarrhal
    c. asthma
    c. fever
    c. gastritis
    c. inflammation
    c. ophthalmia

catarrhalis
    herpes c.
catastalsis
catastaltic
catastasis
catastrophe theory
catastrophic reaction
catatonia
    excited c.
catatonic, catatoniac
    c. dementia
    c. excitement
    c. pupil
    c. rigidity
    c. schizophrenia
    c. stupor
catatrichy
catatricrotic
catatricrotism
catatropic image
cat-bite
    c.-b. disease
    c.-b. fever
catchment area
cat-cry syndrome, cat's cry syndrome
catechase
catechin
catechinic acid
catecholamine
catechol oxidase
catechu nigrum
categorical trait
categorization
catelectrotonus
catenaformis
    Lactobacillus c.
catenate
catenating
catenin
catenoid
catenulate
caterpillar
    c. cell
    c. dermatitis
    dermatitis-causing c.
    c. flap
    c. rash
    saddleback c.
    stinging c.
caterpillar-hair ophthalmia
catgut
    chromic c.
    c. suture
catharsis
cathartic
cathectic
cathemoglobin
cathepsin

catheter
  acorn-tipped c.
  angiography c.
  arterial c.
  balloon biliary c.
  balloon-tip c.
  bicoudate c.
  Bozeman-Fritsch c.
  Braasch c.
  Broviac c.
  brush c.
  cardiac c.
  central venous c.
  c. coiling sign
  conical c.
  coudé c.
  c. coudé
  de Pezzer c.
  double-channel c.
  elbowed c.
  c. embolus
  eustachian c.
  female c.
  c. fever
  filiform c.
  Fogarty embolectomy c.
  Foley c.
  c. gauge
  Gouley c.
  c. guide
  Hickman c.
  indwelling c.
  intracardiac c.
  intraluminal c.
  intraperitoneal c.
  Malecot c.
  Nélaton c.
  pacing c.
  Phillips c.
  pigtail c.
  pulmonary artery c.
  self-retaining c.
  suction c.
  Swan-Ganz c.
  trocar c.
  umbilical c.
  ureteral c.
  venous c.
  vertebrated c.
  2-way c.
  winged c.

catheterization
  clean intermittent bladder c.
  hepatic vein c.
  retrourethral c.
catheterize
catheterostat
cathexis
cathodal, cathodic
  c. closure contraction (CaCC, CCC)
  c. opening contraction (COC)
  c. opening contracture (CaOC)
  c. opening tetanus (COTe)
cathode
  c. ray
  c. ray oscilloscope
  c. ray tube (CRT)
catholysis
cation
  c. exchange
  c. exchanger
cation-anion difference
cation-exchange resin
cationic detergent
cationogen
catlin, catling
catnep, catnip
catochus
catoptric
catscratch
  c. disease
  c. fever
cat's cry syndrome (*var. of* cat-cry syndrome)
cat's-eye
  c.-e. pupil
  c.-e. syndrome
cattaire
  frémissement c.
Cattell Infant Intelligence Scale
Catu virus
cauda
  c. epididymidis
  c. equina
  c. equina syndrome
caudad
caudal
  c. anesthesia
  c. canal
  c. flexure
  c. ligament
  c. neuropore

C

NOTES

caudal *(continued)*
   c. neurosecretory system
   c. pancreatic artery
   c. pharyngeal complex
   c. pontine reticular nucleus
   c. retinaculum
   c. sheath
   c. transtentorial herniation
   c. transverse fissure
caudate
   c. branch
   c. lobe
   c. nucleus
   c. process
caudatolenticular
caudatum
caudatus
   lobus c.
caudocephalad
caudolenticular gray bridge
caul
cauliflower ear
caumesthesia
causal
   c. additivity
   c. independence
   c. treatment
causalgia
causality
cause
   constitutional c.
   exciting c.
caustic
   c. alkali
   lunar c.
   c. potash
   c. soda
cauterant
cauterization
cauterize
cautery
   actual c.
   BICAP c.
   bipolar c.
   chemical c.
   cold c.
   c. conization
   electric c.
   gas c.
   c. knife
   monopolar c.
cava *(pl. of* cavum)
cavagram
caval
   c. fold
   c. opening
   c. valve

cave
   c. sickness
   trigeminal c.
caveola
caverniloquy
cavernitis
   fibrous c.
cavernositis
cavernosum
   corpus c.
cavernous
   c. angioma
   c. artery
   c. body
   c. groove
   c. hemangioma
   c. lymphangiectasis
   c. lymphangioma
   c. nerve
   c. nervous plexus
   c. rale
   c. resonance
   c. respiration
   c. rhonchi
   c. sinus
   c. sinus branch
   c. sinus syndrome
   c. space
   c. tissue
   c. transformation
   c. vascular plexus
   c. vein
   c. voice
   c. voice sound
caviae
   Nocardia c.
caviar lesion
cavitary
cavitation
cavitis
cavity
   abdominal c.
   abdominopelvic c.
   amnionic c.
   articular c.
   axillary c.
   body c.
   buccal c.
   cleavage c.
   cotyloid c.
   cranial c.
   crown c.
   ectoplacental c.
   ectotrophoblastic c.
   epamniotic c.
   epidural c.
   glenoid c.
   greater peritoneal c.
   head c.

idiopathic bone c.
inferior laryngeal c.
infraglottic c.
intermediate laryngeal c.
intracranial c.
joint c.
laryngeal c.
lesser peritoneal c.
c. line angle
c. liner
c. margin
Meckel c.
medullary c.
nasal c.
oral c.
orbital c.
pelvic c.
pericardial c.
peritoneal c.
pleural c.
pulp c.
segmentation c.
synovial c.
thoracic c.
tympanic c.
uterine c.
c. wall
cavogram
cavography
cavopulmonary
   c. anastomosis
   c. shunt
cavosurface
   c. angle
   c. bevel
cavum, pl. **cava**
   c. abdominis
   inferior vena cava (IVC)
   c. nasi
   c. oris
   superior vena cava
   c. tympani
   c. uteri
cavus
   pes c.
   talipes c.
C-banding stain
CBC
   complete blood count
CBF
   cerebral blood flow
CB lead

CC
   chief complaint
CCC
   cathodal closure contraction
CCK
   cholecystokinin
CCU
   coronary care unit
   critical care unit
CD
   cluster of differentiation
cd
   candela
     cytochrome c.
CD4 count
cDNA
   complementary DNA
     cDNA clone
     cDNA library
CEA
   carcinoembryonic antigen
   carotid endarterectomy
ceasmic teratosis
cebocephaly
ceca (*pl. of* cecum)
cecal
   c. artery
   c. fold
   c. foramen
   c. hernia
   c. recess
   c. volvulus
cecectomy
Cecil urethroplasty
cecitis
cecocentral scotoma
cecocolic intussusception
cecocolostomy
cecofixation
cecoileostomy
cecopexy
cecoplication
cecorrhaphy
cecosigmoidostomy
cecostomy
cecotomy
cecoureterocele
cecropins
cecum, caecum, pl. **ceca**
   cupular c.
   intestinal c.
   punctum c.

C

NOTES

Ceelen-Gellerstedt syndrome
ceftriaxone disodium
celenteron
celer
    pulsus c.
celery seed
celestine blue B
Celestin tube
celiac
    c. arterial trunk
    c. artery
    c. axis
    c. branch
    c. disease
    c. ganglion
    c. lymphatic plexus
    c. lymph node
    c. nervous plexus
    c. plexus
    c. plexus reflex
    c. rickets
    c. sprue
    c. syndrome
celiaca
    arteria c.
celiocentesis
celiomyalgia
celiomyositis
celioparacentesis
celiopathy
celiorrhaphy
celioscopy
celiotomy
    c. incision
    vaginal c.
    ventral c.
celitis
cell
    A c.
    absorption c.
    absorptive c.
    accessory c.
    acid c.
    acidophil c.
    acinar c.
    acinous c.
    acoustic c.
    adherent c.
    c. adhesion molecule
    adipose c.
    adventitial c.
    air c.
    albuminous c.
    algoid c.
    alpha c.
    alveolar c.
    amacrine c.
    ameboid c.
    amniogenic c.

anabiotic c.
anaplastic c.
angioblastic c.
Anitschkow c.
anterior ethmoidal air c.
anterior horn c.
antigen-presenting c.
antigen-responsive c.
antigen-sensitive c.
apolar c.
APUD c.
argentaffin c.
argyrophilic c.
Aschoff c.
Askanazy c.
astroglia c.
atypical glandular c.
atypical squamous c.
auditory receptor c.
B c.
balloon c.
band c.
basal c.
basaloid c.
basilar c.
basket c.
beaker c.
Beale c.
Berger c.
berry c.
beta c.
Betz c.
Bevan-Lewis c.
bipolar c.
Bizzozero red c.
blast c.
blood c.
c. body
Boll c.
bone c.
border c.
Böttcher c.
bowenoid c.
c. bridge
bristle c.
bronchic c.
bronchiolar exocrine c.
brood c.
C c.
Cajal c.
caliciform c.
capsule c.
carrier c.
cartilage c.
castration c.
caterpillar c.
c. center
centroacinar c.
chalice c.

chief c.
chromaffin c.
chromophobe c.
Clara c.
Clarke c.
Claudius c.
clear c.
cleavage c.
cleaved c.
clonogenic c.
clue c.
cochlear hair c.
column c.
compound granule c.
cone bipolar c.
conjunctival c.
connective tissue c.
contrasuppressor c.
cornified c.
Corti c.
crenated c.
crescent c.
c. culture
c. cycle
cytomegalic c.
cytotoxic c.
cytotrophoblastic c.
D c.
dark c.
daughter c.
Davidoff c.
decidual c.
decoy c.
deep c.
Deiters c.
delta c.
dendritic c.
c. determination
Dogiel c.
dome c.
Downey c.
dust c.
effector c.
egg c.
embryonic c.
enamel c.
end c.
endocervical c.
endodermal c.
endometrial c.
endothelial c.
enterochromaffin c.

enteroendocrine c.
entodermal c.
ependymal c.
epidermic c.
epithelial reticular c.
epithelioid c.
erythroid c.
ethmoid air c.
ethmoidal c.
external pillar c.
exudation c.
fagot c.
Fañanás c.
fasciculata c.
fat c.
fat-storing c.
Ferrata c.
flame c.
foam c.
follicular epithelial c.
follicular ovarian c.
foreign body giant c.
formative c.
foveolar c.
fuchsinophil c.
fusiform c.
c. fusion
G c.
gamma c.
ganglion c.
Gaucher c.
gemistocytic c.
germ c.
germinal c.
ghost c.
giant c.
Gierke c.
gitter c.
glia c.
glitter c.
globoid c.
glomerulosa c.
goblet c.
Golgi epithelial c.
Goormaghtigh c.
granule c.
granulosa lutein c.
great alveolar c.
guanine c.
gustatory c.
gyrochrome c.
hair c.

NOTES

cell *(continued)*
- hairy c.
- Haller c.
- heart failure c.
- HeLa c.
- helmet c.
- helper c.
- HEMPAS c.
- Hensen c.
- heteromeric c.
- hilus c.
- hobnail c.
- Hofbauer c.
- horizontal c.
- horny c.
- Hortega c.
- host c.
- Hürthle c.
- c. hybridization
- I c.
- immunologically activated c.
- immunologically competent c.
- inclusion c.
- indifferent c.
- inducer c.
- innocent bystander c.
- intercapillary c.
- interdigitating reticulum c.
- internal pillar c.
- interstitial c.
- irritation c.
- islet c.
- Ito c.
- Jurkat c.
- juvenile c.
- juxtaglomerular c.
- K c.
- karyochrome c.
- keratinized c.
- killer c.
- Kulchitsky c.
- Kupffer c.
- lacis c.
- Langerhans c.
- Langhans c.
- Langhans-type giant c.
- LE c.
- Leishman chrome c.
- lepra c.
- Leydig c.
- light c.
- c. line
- lining c.
- Lipschütz c.
- littoral c.
- Loevit c.
- lupus erythematosus c.
- luteal c.
- lutein c.
- lymph c.
- lymphoid c.
- M c.
- macroglia c.
- malpighian c.
- Marchand wandering c.
- marrow c.
- Martinotti c.
- mast c.
- mastoid air c.
- c. matrix
- c. membrane
- memory B, T c.
- Merkel tactile c.
- mesangial c.
- mesenchymal c.
- mesoglial c.
- mesothelial c.
- Mexican hat c.
- Meynert c.
- microfold c.
- microglia c., microglial c.
- middle ethmoidal air c.
- midget bipolar c.
- migratory c.
- Mikulicz c.
- mirror-image c.
- mitral c.
- monocytoid c.
- mother c.
- mucoserous c.
- mucous c.
- multipolar c.
- myoid c.
- natural killer c.
- navicular c.
- c. nest
- neurilemma c.
- neurolemma c.
- nevus c.
- Niemann-Pick c.
- NK c.
- null c.
- oat c.
- OKT c.
- olfactory receptor c.
- c. organelle
- osteoprogenitor c.
- outer hair c.
- oxyntic c.
- oxyphil c.
- packed red c.'s (PRCs)
- Paget c.
- pagetoid c.
- parafollicular c.
- parietal c.
- peptic c.
- peritubular contractile c.
- photoreceptor c.

Pick c.
plasma c.
c. plate
polychromatic c.
polychromatophil c.
prickle c.
Purkinje c.
pyramidal c.
red blood c.
Reed-Sternberg c.
Rieder c.
rod c.
c. sap
Schwann c.
segmented c.
sensitized c.
serous c.
Sertoli c.
sex c.
Sézary c.
sickle c.
signet ring c.
small c.
smudge c.
somatic c.
spindle c.
spur c.
squamous c.
stab c.
staff c.
stellate c.
stem c.
c. strain
strap c.
c. surface marker
target c.
tart c.
taste c.
T cytotoxic c.
teardrop c.
tendon c.
T helper subset 1, 2 c.
Toker c.
Touton giant c.
transducer c.
c. transformation
tubal air c.
tufted c.
vasoformative c.
virus-transformed c.
visual receptor c.
c. wall

c. wall–defective bacteria
wandering c.
white blood c.
zymogenic c.
cell-bound antibody
cell-mediated
c.-m. immunity (CMI)
c.-m. lymphocytotoxicity (CML)
c.-m. reaction
cellophane dressing
cellula, pl. **cellulae**
cellular
c. biology
c. biophysics
c. blue nevus
c. cartilage
c. embolism
c. immune theory
c. immunity
c. immunity deficiency syndrome
c. immunodeficiency
c. infiltration
c. mosaicism
c. pathology
c. polyp
c. spill
c. tenacity
c. tumor
cellularity
cellulase
cellule
cellulicidal
cellulifugal
cellulin
cellulipetal
cellulite
cellulitis
acute scalp c.
anaerobic c.
dissecting c.
eosinophilic c.
gangrenous c.
indurated c.
orbital c.
pelvic c.
periorbital c.
preseptal c.
celluloid
c. strip
c. suture
cellulosae
Cysticercus c.

NOTES

cellulosan
cellulose
    microcrystalline c.
    c. tape technique
CELO
    chicken embryo lethal orphan
    CELO virus
celom, celoma
    extraembryonic c.
celomic bay
celophlebitis
celoscope
celoscopy
celosomia
celozoic
Celsius scale
cement
    c. base
    composite dental c.
    copper phosphate c.
    c. corpuscle
    dental c.
    c. dermatitis
    c. disease
    c. dressing
    glass ionomer c.
    inorganic dental c.
    intercellular c.
    c. line
    modified zinc oxide-eugenol c.
    resin c.
cemental
    c. caries
    c. dysplasia
cementation
cementicle
cementification
cementing substance
cementoblast
cementoblastoma
    benign c.
cementoclasia
cementoclast
cementocyte
cementodentinal junction
cementoenamel junction
cementogenesis
cementoma
    gigantiform c.
cementoossifying fibroma
cementum
    afibrillar c.
    c. hyperplasia
cenesthesia
cenesthesic
cenesthetic
cenocyte
cenocytic
cenosite

cenotrope
censor
censoring
census
center
    active c.
    anospinal c.
    birthing c.
    Broca c.
    Budge c.
    catalytic c.
    cell c.
    chondrification c.
    ciliospinal c.
    dentary c.
    diaphysial c.
    epiotic c.
    expiratory c.
    feeding c.
    c. of gravity
    health c.
    inspiratory c.
    Kerckring c.
    medullary c.
    microtubule-organizing c.
    motor speech c.
    ossific c.
    c. of ossification
    respiratory c.
    sensory speech c.
    specialty referral c.
    speech c.
    trauma c.
    Wernicke c.
centesis
centibar
centigrade scale
centigram
centile
centiliter
centimeter (cm)
    cubic c.
centimeter-gram-second (CGS, cgs)
    c.-g.-s. system
    c.-g.-s. unit
centimorgan
centinormal
centipede
centipoise
centra (*pl. of* centrum)
centrad
centrage
central
    c. ageusia
    c. amputation
    c. amygdaloid nucleus
    c. angiospastic retinopathy
    c. apnea
    c. apparatus

c. areolar choroidal atrophy
c. areolar choroidal dystrophy
c. areolar choroidal sclerosis
c. auditory nervous system
c. axillary lymph node
c. bearing
c. bone
c. bradycardia
c. callus
c. canal
c. cataract
c. chromatolysis
c. cloudy corneal dystrophy
c. complex
c. cord syndrome
c. core disease
c. crystalline corneal dystrophy
c. deafness
c. dogma
C. European tick-borne encephalitis virus
C. European tick-borne fever
c. excitatory state
c. fibrous body
c. ganglioneuroma
c. gray substance
c. gyrus
c. illumination
c. implantation
c. incisor
c. inhibition
c. lacteal
c. and lateral intermediate substances
c. limit theorem
c. lobule
c. necrosis
c. nervous system (CNS)
c. neuritis
c. ossifying fibroma
c. osteitis
c. palmar space
c. paralysis
c. paraphasia
c. pit
c. placenta previa
c. pneumonia
c. pontine myelinolysis
c. retinal artery
c. retinal fovea
c. retinal vein
c. scotoma

c. serous choroidopathy
c. serous retinopathy
c. spindle
c. sulcal artery
c. sulcus
c. superior mesenteric lymph node
c. tegmental fasciculus
c. tegmental tract
c. tendon
c. terminal electrode
c. thalamic radiation
c. transactional core
c. type neurofibromatosis
c. venous catheter
c. venous pressure (CVP)
c. vision
central-bearing
  c.-b. device
  c.-b. point
  c.-b. tracing device
centralis
centralization phenomenon
centrencephalic epilepsy
centriacinar emphysema
centric
  acquired c.
  c. contact
  c. fusion
  habitual c.
  c. jaw relation
  c. occlusion
  c. position
centriciput
centrifugal
  c. casting
  c. current
  c. fast analyzer
  c. nerve
centrifugalization
centrifugalize
centrifugation
  band c.
  density gradient c.
centrifuge
centrilobular emphysema
centriole
  anterior c.
  distal c.
centripetal
  c. current
  c. nerve
centroacinar cell

NOTES

centroblast
centrocyte
centrofacial lentiginosis
centrokinesia
centrokinetic
centrolecithal
    c. egg
    c. ovum
centromedian nucleus
centromere banding stain
centromeric index
centronuclear myopathy
centroplasm
centrosome
centrosphere
centrostaltic
centrum, pl. centra
    c. ovale
    c. semiovale
centum
cenuriasis
cenuris
cenurosis
cepacia
    Burkholderia c.
cephalad
cephalalgia
    benign coital c.
    histaminic c.
    Horton c.
cephaledema
cephalemia
cephalexin
cephalhematocele
cephalhematoma
cephalhydrocele
cephalic
    c. angle
    c. curve
    c. flexure
    c. index
    c. pole
    c. presentation
    c. replacement
    c. tetanus
    c. triangle
    c. vein
    c. version
cephalitis
cephalization
cephalocaudal axis
cephalocele
cephalocentesis
cephalochord
cephalodidymus
cephalodiprosopus
cephalodynia
cephalogenesis
cephaloglycin

cephalogram
cephalogyric
cephalohematocele
cephalohematoma
cephalohemometer
cephalomedullary angle
cephalomegaly
cephalomelus
cephalomeningitis
cephalometer
cephalometric
    c. analysis
    c. radiograph
    c. tracing
cephalometrics
cephalometry
cephalomotor
cephalooculocutaneous telangiectasia
cephaloorbital index
cephalopagus
cephalopalpebral reflex
cephalopathy
cephalopelvic disproportion
cephalopelvimetry
cephalopharyngeus
cephaloridine
cephalorrhachidian
cephalosporin
    c. antibiotic
    c. C, N, P
cephalostat
cephalothin
cephalothoracic
cephalotome
cephalotomy
cephalotoxin
cephalotribe
cephalotrigeminal angiomatosis
cephamycin
cephapirin sodium
cephradine
ceptor
    chemical c.
    contact c.
    distance c.
ceraceous
ceramidase
ceramide
ceratocricoid
    c. ligament
    c. muscle
ceratoglossus muscle
cercaria
cerci (*pl. of* cercus)
cerclage
cercocystis
cercopithecrine herpesvirus
cercus, pl. cerci

cerea
  flexibilitas c.
  c. flexibilitas
cerebella (*pl. of* cerebellum)
cerebellar
  c. apoplexy
  c. artery
  c. astrocytoma
  c. ataxia
  c. atrophy
  c. cortex
  c. cyst
  c. falx
  c. fissure
  c. fossa
  c. frenulum
  c. gait
  c. hemisphere
  c. nucleus
  c. peduncle
  c. pyramid
  c. rigidity
  c. speech
  c. sulcus
  c. syndrome
  c. tentorium
  c. tonsil
  c. vein
cerebelli
  amygdala c.
  cortex c.
  falx c.
  lingua c.
  uvula c.
cerebellitis
cerebellohypothalamic fiber
cerebellolental
cerebellomedullary
  c. cistern
  c. malformation syndrome
cerebelloolivary fiber
cerebellopontine, cerebellopontile
  c. angle
  c. angle syndrome
  c. angle tumor
  c. cisternography
  c. recess
cerebellorubral tract
cerebellospinal fiber
cerebellothalamic tract
cerebellum, pl. **cerebella**
  folia of c.

cerebra (*pl. of* cerebrum)
cerebral
  c. amyloid angiopathy
  c. angiography
  c. anthrax
  c. aqueduct
  c. arterial circle
  c. arteriography
  c. artery
  c. blood flow (CBF)
  c. calculus
  c. cladosporiosis
  c. compression
  c. cortex
  c. cranium
  c. deafness
  c. death
  c. decompression
  c. decortication
  c. diataxia
  c. dominance
  c. dysplasia
  c. edema
  c. falx
  c. fissure
  c. flexure
  c. gigantism
  c. gyrus
  c. hemisphere
  c. hemorrhage
  c. hernia
  c. index
  c. lacuna
  c. leukodystrophy
  c. lipidosis
  c. lobe
  c. localization
  c. malaria
  c. pachymeningitis
  c. palsy
  c. peduncle
  c. porosis
  c. rheumatism
  c. sclerosis
  c. sinus
  c. sphingolipidosis
  c. sulcus
  c. surface
  c. tetanus
  c. thrombosis
  c. trigone
  c. tuberculosis

C

NOTES

cerebral *(continued)*
    c. vein
    c. ventricle
    c. vesicle
    c. vomiting
cerebrale
    cranium c.
cerebralis
    adiposis c.
cerebration
cerebri
    anus c.
    astrocytosis c.
    cortex c.
    epiphysis c.
    falx c.
    fungus c.
    glioblastosis c.
    hypophysis c.
    lacuna c.
    tomentum c.
cerebriform
cerebritis
cerebrohepatorenal syndrome
cerebroma
cerebromalacia
cerebromeningitis
cerebron
cerebropathia
cerebropathy
cerebrophysiology
cerebroretinal angiomatosis
cerebrosclerosis
cerebroside
    c. lipoidosis
    c. sulfatidase
cerebroside-sulfatase
cerebrosidosis
cerebrospinal
    c. axis
    c. fever
    c. fluid (CSF)
    c. fluid otorrhea
    c. fluid rhinorrhea
    c. index
    c. meningitis
    c. nematodiasis
    c. pressure
    c. system
cerebrospinalis
    liquor c.
cerebrosterol
cerebrotendinous xanthomatosis
cerebrotomy
cerebrovascular
    c. accident (CVA)
    c. disease
cerebrum, pl. **cerebra**
cerecloth

Cerenkov radiation
ceresin, cerin
cereus
    Bacillus c.
cerium oxalate
ceroid lipofuscinosis
ceroplasty
cerosin
certifiable
certificate
    birth c.
    death c.
certification
certified
    c. nurse-midwife
    c. pasteurized milk
    c. reference material
    c. registered nurse anesthetist
cerulea
    macula c.
cerulean cataract
cerulein
ceruloplasmin
cerumen
    inspissated c.
    c. inspissatum
ceruminal
ceruminolytic
ceruminoma
ceruminosis
ceruminous gland
cerveau isolé
cervical
    c. adenitis
    c. amputation
    c. anchorage
    c. anesthesia
    c. aortic knuckle
    c. auricle
    c. branch
    c. canal
    c. cap
    c. compression syndrome
    c. disc syndrome
    c. diverticulum
    c. duct
    c. dysplasia
    c. enlargement
    c. fibrositis
    c. flexure
    c. fusion syndrome
    c. gland
    c. hydrocele
    c. hygroma
    c. hyperesthesia
    c. iliocostal muscle
    c. incision
    c. interspinal muscle
    c. intraepithelial neoplasia

c. ligament
c. line
c. longissimus muscle
c. loop
c. lordosis
c. margin
c. myelogram
c. myositis
c. myospasm
c. nystagmus
c. orthosis
c. pleura
c. plexus
c. polyp
c. pregnancy
c. punch biopsy
c. rib
c. rib syndrome
c. rotator muscle
c. segment
c. sinus
c. smear
c. spine
c. splanchnic nerve
c. spondylosis
c. tension syndrome
c. triangle
c. vein
c. vertebra
c. vesicle
c. zone
cervicalis
ansa c.
costa c.
fascia c.
cervicectomy
cervices (*pl. of* cervix)
cervicis
biventer c.
lordosis c.
cervicitis
cervicoaxillary canal
cervicobrachial
cervicobuccal
cervicodynia
cervicofacial
cervicography
cervicolabial
cervicolingual
cervicolinguoaxial
cervicolumbar phenomenon
cervicooccipital

cervicooculoacoustic syndrome
cervicoplasty
cervicoscopy
cervicothoracic
c. ganglion
c. orthosis
c. transition
cervicotomy
cervicouterine canal
cervicovaginal artery
cervicovesical
cervilaxin
cervix, pl. **cervices**
double c.
incompetent c.
strawberry c.
c. uteri
cesarean
c. hysterectomy
c. operation
c. section
cesium
Cestan-Chenais syndrome
cestode, cestoid
cestodiasis
cestoid
cetyl
CF lead
CG
chorionic gonadotropin
CGS, cgs
centimeter-gram-second
CGS unit
Chaddock
C. reflex
C. sign
Chadwick sign
chaffeensis
Ehrlichia c.
Chagas-Cruz disease
Chagas disease
chagasic myocardiopathy
chagoma
Chagres virus
chain
A c.
B c.
behavior c.
C c.
cold c.
electron-transport c.
c. ganglion

NOTES

173

chain *(continued)*
    ganglionic c.
    H c.
    heavy c.
    J c.
    kinematic c.
    L c.
    light c.
    long c.
    ossicular c.
    c. reaction
    c. reflex
    side c.
    c. of survival
    c. suture
chain-compensated spirometer
chaining
chair-back brace
chair form
chakra
chalasia
chalasis
chalazion, chalaza
    acute c.
    collar-stud c.
    c. forceps
chalcosis lentis
chalice cell
chalicosis
chalk
    French c.
chalkitis
challenge diet
chalone
chalybeate water
chamber
    altitude c.
    anechoic c.
    anterior c.
    aqueous c.
    counting c.
    decompression c.
    high altitude c.
    hyperbaric c.
    ionization c.
    posterior c.
    postremal c.
    pulp c.
    vitreous c.
Chamberlain
    C. line
    C. procedure
Chamberlen forceps
chamecephalic
chamecephalous
chameprosopic
chamfer
chamomile
Champy fixative

Chance fracture
chancre
    erosive c.
    fungating c.
    hard c.
    indurated c.
    mixed c.
    c. redux
    soft c.
    sulcus c.
    tularemic c.
chancriform syndrome
chancroid
chancroidal bubo
chancrous
chandelier
    favic c.'s
    c. sign
Chandler syndrome
change
    Armanni-Ebstein c.
    Baggenstoss c.
    c. blindness
    Crooke hyaline c.
    E-to-A c.'s
    fatty c.
    c. of life
    mitral valve prolapse, aortic
      anomalies, skeletal and skin c.'s
      (MASS)
    QRS c.
    QRST c.
    reactive c.
    ST-segment c.
    T-wave c.
changer
    film c.
channel
    ion c.
    ligand-gated c.
channelopathies
Chantemesse reaction
chaos
    mathematical c.
    c. theory
chaotic
    c. heart
    c. rhythm
chaotropic
chaotropism
chappa
Chaput operation
character
    acquired c.
    c. analysis
    c. armor
    classifiable c.
    compound c.
    denumerable c.

discrete c.
c. disorder
dominant c.
inherited c.
mendelian c.
c. neurosis
primary sex c.
recessive c.
secondary sex c.
sex-linked c.
characteristic
c. curve
c. emission
c. frequency
c. radiation
c. symptom
characterization
denture c.
characterizing group
charas
charcoal
activated c.
animal c.
bone c.
medicinal c.
Charcot
C. artery
C. disease
C. gait
C. intermittent fever
C. joint
C. syndrome
C. triad
C. vertigo
Charcot-Böttcher crystalloid
Charcot-Bouchard aneurysm
Charcot-Leyden crystal
Charcot-Marie-Tooth disease
Charcot-Neumann crystal
Charcot-Robin crystal
Charcot-Weiss-Baker syndrome
Chargaff rule
charlatan
charlatanism
Charles law
charley horse
Charnley hip arthroplasty
Charrière scale
chart
Amsler c.
chromatic c.
color c.

isometric c.
Levey-Jennings c.
Pickles c.
quality control c.
Tanner growth c.
Walker c.
Charters method
charting
Chassaignac
C. space
C. tubercle
chattoni
Entamoeba c.
Chauffard syndrome
chaulmoogra oil
Chaussier
C. line
C. sign
Chayes method
Cheadle disease
Cheatle slit
check
delta c.
c. ligament
checkbite
checkerberry oil
Chédiak-Higashi
C.-H. disease
C.-H. syndrome
Chédiak-Steinbrinck-Higashi
C.-S.-H. anomaly
C.-S.-H. syndrome
cheek
c. bone
c. muscle
c. tooth
cheese
c. maggot
c. worker's lung
cheesy
c. abscess
c. cataract
c. necrosis
c. pus
cheilalgia
cheilectomy
cheilectropion
cheilion
cheilitis
actinic c.
angular c.
commissural c.

NOTES

175

cheilitis *(continued)*
  contact c.
  c. glandularis
  c. granulomatosa
  impetiginous c.
  solar c.
  Volkmann c.
cheilognathoglossoschisis
cheilognathopalatoschisis
cheilognathouranoschisis
cheilophagia
cheiloplasty
cheilorrhaphy
cheilosis
cheilotomy
cheiralgia paresthetica
cheirarthritis
cheirognostic
cheirokinesthesia
cheirokinesthetic
cheirology
cheiromegaly
cheiroplasty
cheiropodalgia
cheiropompholyx
cheirospasm
chelate
chelation
cheloid
chelonae
  Mycobacterium c.
chemexfoliation
chemical
  c. abuse
  c. antidote
  c. attraction
  c. burn
  c. cautery
  c. ceptor
  c. complexity
  c. conjunctivitis
  c. depilatory
  c. dermatitis
  c. diabetes
  c. energy
  c. equation
  c. evolution
  c. formula
  c. hysterectomy
  c. kinetics
  c. knife
  c. modification
  c. peeling
  c. peritonitis
  c. pneumonia
  c. potential
  c. pregnancy
  c. prophylaxis
  c. ray

  c. repair
  c. sampling
  c. shift
  c. shift artifact
  c. solution
  c. sympathectomy
  c. taxonomy
chemically cured resin
chemicocautery
chemiluminescence immunoassay
chemiosmotic theory
chemiotaxis
chemise
  bouton en c.
chemistry
  analytic c.
  biologic c.
  clinical c.
  ecologic c.
  epithermal c.
  inorganic c.
  macromolecular c.
  medicinal c.
  organic c.
  physiologic c.
chemoattractant
chemoattractants
chemoautotroph
chemoautotrophic
chemobiodynamics
chemocautery
chemoceptor
chemodectoma
chemodectomatosis
chemodifferentiation
chemoheterotroph
chemoheterotrophic
chemoimmunology
chemokine
chemokinesis
chemokinetic
chemolithotroph
chemolithotrophic
chemolithotrophy
chemoluminescence
chemolysis
chemonucleolysis
chemoorganotroph
chemoorganotrophic
chemopallidectomy
chemopallidothalamectomy
chemopallidotomy
chemoprevention
chemoprophylaxis
chemoreception
chemoreceptive
chemoreceptor
  medullary c.
chemoreflex

chemoresistance
chemoresponse
chemosensation
chemosensitive
chemoserotherapy
chemosis
chemosmosis
chemostat
chemosurgery
    Mohs c.
chemosynthesis
chemotactic
chemotaxis
chemothalamectomy
chemothalamotomy
chemotherapeutic
    c. agent
    c. index
chemotherapeutics
chemotherapy
    adjuvant c.
    combination c.
    consolidation c.
    cytostatic c.
    cytotoxic c.
    induction c.
    intensification c.
chemotic
chemotransmitter
chemotroph
chemotropism
Cheney syndrome
chenodiol
chenopodium
cherry
    c. angioma
    c. juice
cherry-red
    c.-r. spot
    c.-r. spot myoclonus syndrome
cherubic facies
cherubism
Chesapeake
    hemoglobin C. (HbChesapeake)
chest
    alar c.
    barrel c.
    blast c.
    emphysematous c.
    flail c.
    flat c.
    foveated c.

    funnel c.
    hourglass c.
    c. index
    keeled c.
    c. lead
    c. radiology
    stove-in c.
    c. tube
    c. wall
    c. wall compliance
Chevalier-Jackson dilator
chevron
    c. incision
    c. osteotomy
chevron-shaped incision
chewing
    c. cycle
    c. force
    c. louse
Cheyne operation
Cheyne-Stokes
    C.-S. psychosis
    C.-S. respiration
CHI
    closed head injury
chi
    c. sequence
    c. structure
Chiari
    C. disease
    C. II syndrome
    C. net
Chiari-Budd syndrome
Chiari-Frommel syndrome
chiasm
    Camper c.
    optic c.
chiasmapexy
chiasma syndrome
chiasmatic
    c. cistern
    c. groove
    c. sulcus
Chicago disease
chicken
    c. breast
    c. embryo lethal orphan (CELO)
    c. fat clot
chickenpox
    c. immune globulin human
    c. immunoglobulin
    c. virus

C

NOTES

Chick-Martin test
chief
  c. agglutinin
  c. cell
  c. complaint (CC)
Chievitz
  C. layer
  C. organ
chigger dermatitis
chigoe
Chilaiditi syndrome
chilalgia
chilblain
  c. lupus
  c. lupus erythematosus
CHILD
  congenital hemidysplasia with
  ichthyosiform erythroderma and limb
  defects
    CHILD syndrome
child, pl. children
  c. abuse
  linear IgA bullous disease in
  children
  c. psychiatry
  c. psychology
childbearing age
childbed fever
childbirth
childhood
  c. absence epilepsy
  c. apraxia
  avoidant disorder of c.
  c. hypophosphatasia
  c. muscular dystrophy
  c. schizophrenia
  c. type tuberculosis
children (*pl. of* child)
chilectomy
chilectropion
chilitis
chilomastigiasis
chilomastosis
chilophagia
chiloplasty
chilopodiasis
chilosis
chimera
chimeric
  c. antibody
  c. molecule
chimerism
chimney sweep's cancer
chimpanzee coryza agent
chin
  c. cap
  double c.
  c. jerk

  c. muscle
  c. reflex
Chinese
  C. cinnamon
  C. ginger
  C. restaurant syndrome
  C. wax
chip
  bone c.
  c. graft
  c. syringe
chip-blower
chiral crystal
chirality
chirarthritis
chirognostic
chirokinesthesia
chirology
chiromegaly
chiroplasty
chiropodalgia
chiropodist
chiropody
chiropompholyx
chiropractic
chiropractor
chiroscope
chirospasm
chisel
  binangle c.
chi-square
  c.-s. distribution
  c.-s. test
chitin
chitinous
CHL
  crown-heel length
Chlamydia
  C. pneumoniae
  C. psittaci
  C. trachomatis
chlamydial
chlamydiosis
chlamydoconidium
chloasma
chloracne
chloral
  amylene c.
  anhydrous c.
chloralism
chlorambucil
chloramine B, T
chloramphenicol acetyl transferase
chlorate
chloremia
chlorhydria
chloride
  acetyl c.
  acetylcholine c.

ambenonium c.
ammoniated mercuric c.
ammonium c.
antimony c.
barium c.
benzethonium c.
benzoyl c.
bethanechol c.
bisdequalinium c.
calcium c.
cobaltous c.
copper c.
corrosive mercury c.
cupric c.
cyanogen c.
dequalinium c.
dodecarbonium c.
doxacurium c.
edrophonium c.
ferric c.
ferriheme c.
ferriporphyrin c.
hematin c.
hydrogen c.
indium-111 c.
magnesium c.
mercurous c.
methacholine c.
methyl c.
c. shift
chloridimetry
chloridometer
chloriduria
chlorinated
c. lime
c. paraffin
chlorindanol
chlorine
c. acne
c. group
c. water
chloriodized oil
chloriodoquin
chlorite
chloroanemia
chloroazodin
chloroform
chloroformism
chloroleukemia
chloroma
chloromethane
chlorometry

chloromyeloma
chloropenia
chloropercha method
chlorophenol
chlorophenothane
chlorophyll
c. a, b, c, d
c. esterase
c. unit
chlorophyllase
chlorophyllide, chlorophyllid
chloropsia
chlorotic anemia
chlorotriazine dye
chloruresis
chloruretic
chloruria
choana, pl. **choanae**
choanal
c. atresia
c. polyp
choanate
choanoflagellate
choanoid
choanomastigote
chocolate
c. agar
c. cyst
Chodzko reflex
choice
embarrassment of c.'s
object c.
choked disc
cholagogue, cholagogic
cholaneresis
cholangeitis
cholangiectasis
cholangiocarcinoma
cholangioenterostomy
cholangiofibrosis
cholangiogastrostomy
cholangiogram
intravenous c. (IVC)
cholangiography
cystic duct c.
intravenous c.
percutaneous transhepatic c.
cholangiole
cholangiolitic
c. cirrhosis
c. hepatitis
cholangiolitis

C

NOTES

cholangioma
cholangiopancreatography
    endoscopic retrograde c. (ERCP)
cholangioscopy
cholangiostomy
cholangiotomy
cholangitic abscess
cholangitis
    ascending c.
cholanopoiesis
cholanopoietic
cholanthrene
cholascos
cholate
cholecalciferol
cholechromopoiesis
cholecyst
cholecystagogic
cholecystagogue
cholecystatony
cholecystectasia
cholecystectomy
cholecystenterostomy
cholecystenterotomy
cholecystic
cholecystis
cholecystitis
    acute c.
    chronic c.
    emphysematous c.
cholecystocolostomy
cholecystoduodenal fistula
cholecystoduodenostomy
cholecystogastrostomy
cholecystogram
cholecystography
cholecystoileostomy
cholecystojejunostomy
cholecystokinase
cholecystokinetic
cholecystokinin (CCK)
cholecystolithiasis
cholecystolithotripsy
cholecystomy
cholecystopaque
cholecystopathy
cholecystopexy
cholecystorrhaphy
cholecystosonography
cholecystostomy
cholecystotomy
    laparoscopic c.
choledochal
    c. cyst
    c. sphincter
choledoch duct
choledochectomy
choledochendysis
choledochiarctia

choledochitis
choledochocholedochostomy
choledochoduodenal junction
choledochoduodenostomy
choledochoenterostomy
choledochojejunostomy
choledocholith
choledocholithiasis
choledocholithotomy
choledocholithotripsy
choledochoplasty
choledochorrhaphy
choledochostomy
choledochotomy
choledochous
choledochus
choleglobin
cholehematin
cholehemia
choleic acid
cholelith
cholelithiasis
cholelithotomy
cholelithotripsy
cholelithotrity
cholemesis
cholemia
    familial c.
cholemic
choleperitoneum
choleperitonitis
cholepoiesis
cholepoietic
cholera
    Asiatic c.
    bilious c.
    c. toxin
    c. vaccine
cholerae
    Vibrio c.
choleraesuis
    Salmonella enterica c.
choleragen
choleraic diarrhea
choleraphage
choleresis
choleretic
cholerheic
choleric jaundice
choleriform
cholerigenic
cholerigenous
cholerine
choleroid
cholerrhagia
cholerrhagic
cholescintigraphy
cholestane
cholestanol

cholestanone
cholestasia
cholestasis
    intrahepatic c.
cholestatic
    c. hepatitis
    c. jaundice
cholesteatoma
    paranasal sinus c.
    primary acquired c.
    secondary acquired c.
cholesteatomatous
cholesteremia
cholesterinemia
cholesterinized antigen
cholesterinosis
cholesterinuria
cholesterol
    c. cleft
    c. embolism
    c. ester storage disease
    c. ester transport protein
    c. granuloma
cholesterolemia
cholesterologenesis
cholesterolosis
cholesteroluria
cholesterosis
cholesteryl ester storage disease
cholestyramine resin
choleuria
cholic acid
choline
    c. acetyltransferase
    activated c.
    c. esterase I, II
    c. kinase
    c. phosphatase
    c. phosphokinase
    c. salicylate
    c. theophyllinate
cholinephosphotransferase
cholinergic
    c. agent
    c. agonist
    c. blockade
    c. fiber
    c. neurotransmitter
    c. receptor
    c. urticaria

cholinesterase
    c. inhibitor
    c. reactivator
cholineter
cholinoceptive
cholinolytic
cholinomimetic
cholinoreactive
cholinoreceptor
chololithiasis
choloplania
cholopoiesis
cholorrhea
choloscopy
cholothorax
choloyl
choluria
cholyl-coenzyme A synthetase
chondral fracture
chondralgia
chondralloplasia
chondrectomy
chondrification center
chondrify
chondrin ball
chondritis
    costal c.
chondroblast
chondroblastoma
chondrocalcin
chondrocalcinosis
    articular c.
chondroclast
chondrocostal
chondrocranium
chondrocyte
    isogenous c.
chondrodynia
chondrodysplasia
    c. calcificans congenita
    Nance-Sweeney c.
chondrodystrophia
chondrodystrophic dwarfism
chondrodystrophy
    asphyxiating thoracic c.
    asymmetric c.
    hereditary deforming c.
    hypoplastic fetal c.
    myotonic c.
chondroectodermal dysplasia
chondrofibroma
chondrogenesis

NOTES

chondroglossus muscle
chondroid
 c. syringoma
 c. tissue
chondroitin sulfate A, B, C
chondrology
chondrolysis
chondroma
 extraskeletal c.
 juxtacortical c.
chondromalacia
 generalized c.
 c. patellae
chondromatosis
chondromatous
chondrome
chondromere
chondromyxoid fibroma
chondromyxoma
chondronectin
chondroosseous
chondroosteodystrophy
chondropathy
chondrophyte
chondroplast
chondroplasty
chondroporosis
chondrosarcoma
chondrosin
chondrosine
chondrosis
chondroskeleton
chondrosternal
chondrosternoplasty
chondrotome
chondrotomy
chondrotrophic
chondroxiphoid ligament
Chopart
 C. amputation
 C. joint
chorda, pl. **chordae**
 chordae tendineae
 chordae tendineae cordis
 c. tympani
chordal
chordalis
 endocarditis c.
chordate
chordee
chorditis
chordoma
chordoskeleton
chordotomy
chorea
 acanthocytosis with c.
 acute c.
 benign familial c.

chronic progressive c.
dancing c.
degenerative c.
electric c.
fibrillary c.
c. gravidarum
habit c.
hemilateral c.
Henoch c.
hereditary c.
Huntington c.
hysterical c.
juvenile c.
laryngeal c.
c. minor
Morvan c.
Sydenham c.
choreal
choreic
 c. abasia
 c. movement
choreiform, choreoid
choreoathetoid
choreoathetosis
 congenital c.
choreoid (*var. of* choreiform)
choreophrasia
chorioadenoma
chorioallantoic
 c. graft
 c. membrane
 c. placenta
chorioallantois
chorioamnionic placenta
chorioamnionitis
chorioangioma
chorioangiomatosis
chorioangiosis
choriocapillaris
choriocapillary layer
choriocarcinoma
choriocele
chorioepithelioma
choriogonadotropin
choriomammotropin
choriomeningitis
 lymphocytic c.
chorion
chorionic
 c. ectoderm
 c. epithelioma
 c. gonadotrophic hormone
 c. gonadotropic hormone
 c. gonadotropin (CG)
 c. gonadotropin unit
 c. growth hormone-prolactin
 c. plate
 c. sac

c. villus
c. villus biopsy
chorioretinal
chorioretinitis
chorioretinopathy
chorista
choristoblastoma
choristoma
choroid
c. blood vessel
c. branch
c. capillary layer
c. enlargement
c. fissure
c. glomus
c. line
c. membrane
c. plexus
c. skein
c. vein
choroidal
c. fissure
c. neovascularization
c. ring
c. vascular atrophy
choroideremia
choroiditis
anterior c.
areolar c.
diffuse c.
disseminated c.
exudative c.
juxtapupillary c.
metastatic c.
vitiliginous c.
choroidocyclitis
choroidopathy
areolar c.
central serous c.
Doyne honeycomb c.
geographic c.
helicoid c.
choroidoretinitis
choroidosis
choroplethic map
Chotzen syndrome
Chra antigen
Christchurch chromosome
Christensen-Krabbe disease
Christian
C. disease
C. syndrome

Christison formula
Christmas
C. disease
C. factor
chromaffin
c. body
c. cell
c. reaction
c. system
c. tissue
c. tumor
chromaffinoma
chromaffinopathy
chroman, chromane
chromanol
chromaphil
chromate
c. dermatitis
lead c.
c. stain
chromatic
c. aberration
c. apparatus
c. audition
c. chart
c. fiber
c. figure
c. granule
c. spectrum
c. vision
chromatid
chromatin
c. body
heteropyknotic c.
c. network
c. nucleolus
c. particle
sex c.
chromatinolysis
chromatinorrhexis
chromatism
chromatogenous
chromatogram
chromatograph
chromatographic
chromatography
absorption c.
adsorption c.
affinity c.
column c.
electric c.
fast protein liquid c. (FPLC)

C

NOTES

chromatography *(continued)*
    gas c.
    gas-liquid c. (GLC)
    gel filtration c.
    high-performance liquid c.
    high-pressure liquid c. (HPLC)
    ion exchange c.
    liquid-liquid c.
    paper c.
    c. paper
    partition c.
    thin-layer c.
chromatoid
chromatokinesis
chromatolysis
    central c.
chromatolytic
chromatometer
chromatopectic
chromatopexis
chromatophil
chromatophilia
chromatophilic, chromatophilous
chromatophobia
chromatophore
chromatophorotropic
chromatoplasm
chromatopsia
chromatosome
chromatotropism
chromaturia
chrome alum
chromesthesia
chromhidrosis, chromidrosis
    apocrine c.
chromic
    c. catgut
    c. catgut suture
chromidial
    c. apparatus
    c. net
    c. substance
chromidiation
chromidiosis
chromidrosis *(var. of* chromhidrosis)
chromium
    c. picolinate
    c. trioxide
chromoblast
chromoblastomycosis
chromocenter
chromocystoscopy
chromocyte
chromogen
chromogenesis
chromogenic
chromogranin
chromoisomerism
chromolipid

chromolysis
chromomere
chromometer
chromomycosis
chromonema
chromonychia
chromopectic
chromopexis
chromophil, chromophile
    c. adenoma
    c. granule
    c. substance
chromophilia
chromophilic
chromophilous
chromophobe
    c. adenoma
    c. cell
    c. granule
chromophobia
chromophobic adenoma
chromophore
chromophoric
chromophorous
chromophototherapy
chromoplast
chromoplastid
chromoprotein
chromoscopy
    gastric c.
chromosomal
    c. breakage syndrome
    c. deletion
    c. gap
    c. instability syndrome
    c. map
    c. region
    c. RNA
    c. trait
chromosome
    c. aberration
    accessory c.
    acentric c.
    acrocentric c.
    c. band
    bivalent c.
    Christchurch c.
    derivative c.
    dicentric c.
    double minute c.'s
    duplication of c.'s
    fragile X c.
    giant c.
    heterotypical c.
    homologous c.
    lampbrush c.
    late replicating c.
    c. map
    c. mapping

marker c.
metacentric c.
mitochondrial c.
c. mosaicism
c. pair
c. pairing
Philadelphia c.
c. puff
reduction of c.'s
ring c.
c. satellite
sex c.
c. walking
X c.
Y c.
chromotherapy
chromotoxic
chromotrichia
chromotrichial
chromotrope
chronaxie, chronaxia, chronaxy
chronaximeter
chronaximetry
chronaxis
chronaxy (*var. of* chronaxie)
chronic
    c. abscess
    c. absorptive arthritis
    c. acholuric jaundice
    c. actinic keratopathy
    c. active hepatitis
    c. active inflammation
    c. active liver disease
    c. adrenocortical insufficiency
    c. African sleeping sickness
    c. alcoholism
    c. allograft rejection
    c. amyloidosis
    c. anaphylaxis
    c. anterior poliomyelitis
    c. appendicitis
    c. ataxia
    c. atrophic polychondritis
    c. atrophic thyroiditis
    c. atrophic vulvitis
    c. bacillary diarrhea
    c. brain syndrome
    c. bronchitis
    c. cholecystitis
    c. cicatrizing enteritis
    c. conjunctivitis
    c. constrictive pericarditis

c. cutaneous leishmaniasis
c. cystic mastitis
c. desquamative gingivitis
c. diffuse sclerosing osteomyelitis
c. discoid lupus erythematosus
c. eczema
c. endemic fluorosis
c. eosinophilic pneumonia
c. erythremic myelosis
c. familial icterus
c. familial jaundice
c. familial polyneuritis
c. fatigue syndrome
c. fibrosing alveolitis
c. fibrosing pancreatitis
c. fibrous thyroiditis
c. focal sclerosing osteomyelitis
c. follicular conjunctivitis
c. glaucoma
c. glomerulonephritis
c. granulocytic leukemia
c. granulomatous disease
c. hemorrhagic villous synovitis
c. hypertensive disease
c. hypertrophic vulvitis
c. hyperventilation syndrome
c. idiopathic jaundice
c. idiopathic xanthomatosis
c. inflammatory demyelinating
  polyneuropathy (CIDP)
c. interstitial hepatitis
c. interstitial salpingitis
c. lymphadenoid thyroiditis
c. lymphocytic lymphoma
c. lymphocytic thyroiditis
c. malaria
c. mediastinal histoplasmosis
c. mountain sickness
c. myelocytic leukemia
c. myelogenous leukemia (CML)
c. myeloid leukemia
c. myocarditis
c. necrotizing aspergillosis
c. nephritis
c. nephrosis
c. nonleukemic myelosis
c. obstructive pulmonary disease
  (COPD)
c. persistent hepatitis
c. persisting hepatitis
c. pleurisy
c. posterior laryngitis

NOTES

chronic *(continued)*
    c. progressive chorea
    c. progressive external
      ophthalmoplegia (CPEO)
    c. pyelonephritis
    c. relapsing pancreatitis
    c. rheumatism
    c. rhinitis
    c. shock
    c. soroche
    c. subglottic laryngitis
    c. tamponade
    c. trypanosomiasis
    c. ulcer
    c. ulcerative proctitis
    c. urticaria
    c. vertigo
chronicity
chronicus
    lichen simplex c.
chronobiology
chronognosis
chronograph
chronologic age
chronometry
    mental c.
chronopharmacology
chronophobia
chronophotograph
chronotaraxis
chronotherapy
chronotropic
chronotropism
chrysiasis
chrysocyanosis
chrysoderma
chrysoidin
chrysotherapy
Churg-Strauss syndrome
Chvostek sign
chylangioma
chylaqueous
chyle
    c. cistern
    c. corpuscle
    c. cyst
    c. fistula
    c. peritonitis
    c. vessel
chylemia
chylidrosis
chylifaction
chylifactive
chyliferous
chylification
chyliform ascites
chylocele
chylocyst
chyloderma

chylomediastinum
chylomicronemia
chylomicron retention disease
chylopericardium
chyloperitoneum
chylophoric
chylopleura
chylopneumothorax
chylopoiesis
chylopoietic
chylorrhea
chylosis
chylosus
    ascites c.
chylothorax
chylous
    c. arthritis
    c. ascites
    c. hydrothorax
    c. peritonitis
    c. urine
chyluria
chymase
chyme, chymus
chymification
chymopapain
chymopoiesis
chymorrhea
chymosin
chymosinogen
chymostatin
chymotropic pigment
chymotrypsin
chymotrypsinogen
chymous
chymus *(var. of* chyme)
Ciaccio
    C. gland
    C. stain
Cianca syndrome
cibophobia
cicatrectomy
cicatricial
    c. alopecia
    c. conjunctivitis
    c. ectropion
    c. entropion
    c. horn
    c. pemphigoid
    c. scoliosis
cicatricotomy
cicatrisotomy
cicatrix
    brain c.
    filtering c.
cicatrizant
cicatrization atelectasis
ciclopiroxolamine

CICU
    cardiac intensive care unit
    cardiology intensive care unit
    coronary intensive care unit
cicutoxin
CIDP
    chronic inflammatory demyelinating
    polyneuropathy
cigarette drain
cigarette-paper scar
ciguatera
ciguatoxin
cilastatin sodium
cilia (*pl. of* cilium)
ciliaris
    acne c.
    anulus c.
    corona c.
    orbiculus c.
ciliary
    c. blepharitis
    c. body
    c. border
    c. canal
    c. cartilage
    c. crown
    c. disc
    c. dysentery
    c. dyskinesis
    c. fold
    c. ganglion
    c. ganglionic plexus
    c. gland
    c. ligament
    c. margin
    c. movement
    c. muscle
    c. poliosis
    c. process
    c. ring
    c. staphyloma
    c. vein
    c. wreath
    c. zone
    c. zonule
ciliastatic
ciliated epithelium
ciliectomy
ciliocytophthoria
ciliogenesis
cilioretinal

cilioscleral
ciliospinal
    c. center
    c. reflex
ciliotoxicity
cilium, pl. **cilia**
cinaedi
    Helicobacter c.
cinanesthesia
cinchona bark
cinchonic
cinchonine
cinchonism
cinchophen
cinclisis
cineangiocardiography
cinefluorography
cinefluoroscopy
cinegastroscopy
cinematic amputation
cinematics
cineole, cineol
cinephotomicrography
cineplastic amputation
cineplastics
cineradiography
cinerea
cinereal
cinereus
    locus c.
cineritious
cineroentgenography
cineseismography
cinetoplasm, cinetoplasma
cingula (*pl. of* cingulum)
cingulate
    c. convolution
    c. gyrus
    c. herniation
    c. sulcus
cingulectomy
cingulotomy
cingulum, pl. **cingula**
cinnamon
    cassia c.
    Chinese c.
    c. oil
circadian rhythm
Circe effect
circellus
circhoral

C

NOTES

circinata
  impetigo c.
  tinea c.
circinate
  c. psoriasis
  c. retinitis
  c. retinopathy
circle
  c. absorption anesthesia
  arterial c.
  articular vascular c.
  Carus c.
  cerebral arterial c.
  closed c.
  defensive c.
  greater arterial c.
  Haller c.
  Huguier c.
  least confusion c.
  lesser arterial c.
  major arterial c.
  minor arterial c.
  Pagenstecher c.
  vascular c.
  vicious c.
  Vieth-Müller c.
  c. of Willis
circuit
  anesthetic c.
  c. resistance training
  signal-processing c.
  c. weight training
circulans
  Bacillus c.
circular
  c. amputation
  c. bandage
  c. dichroism
  c. fiber
  c. fold
  c. layer
  c. reaction
  c. sinus
  c. sulcus
circulation
  assisted c.
  blood c.
  capillary c.
  collateral c.
  compensatory c.
  cross c.
  embryonic c.
  enterohepatic c.
  extracorporeal c.
  fetal c.
  greater c.
  hypophysial portal c.
  hypothalamohypophysial portal c.
  lesser c.

  lymph c.
  placental c.
  portal hypophysial c.
  pulmonary c.
  systemic c.
  c. time
circulatory
  c. arrest
  c. collapse
  c. overload
  c. system
circulus, pl. circuli
circumalveolar fixation
circumanal gland
circumareolar incision
circumarticular
circumaxillary
circumbulbar
circumcise
circumcision
  female c.
  c. incision
  c. suture
circumcorneal
circumduction gait
circumference
  articular c.
circumferential
  c. cartilage
  c. clasp
  c. clasp arm
  c. fibrocartilage
  c. implantation
  c. incision
  c. lamella
  c. wiring
circumflex
  c. branch
  c. femoral artery
  c. fibular artery
  c. humeral artery
  c. iliac artery
  c. nerve
  c. scapular artery
  c. scapular vein
circumgemmal
circumintestinal
circumlental
circumlimbal incision
circummandibular fixation
circumnuclear
circumocular
circumoral
circumorbital
circumrenal
circumscribed
  c. craniomalacia
  c. myxedema
  c. peritonitis

c. posterior keratoconus
c. pyocephalus
circumscribing incision
circumscripta
alopecia c.
calcinosis c.
lipoatrophia c.
circumscriptus
circumsporozoite protein
circumstantiality
circumvallata
placenta c.
circumvallate papillae
circumvascular
circumventricular organ
circumvolute
circumzygomatic
c. fixation
c. wiring
circus
c. movement
c. rhythm
cirrhogenic
cirrhogenous
cirrhonosus
cirrhosis
alcoholic c.
biliary c.
cardiac c.
cholangiolitic c.
congestive c.
cryptogenic c.
fatty c.
Glisson c.
Hanot c.
juvenile c.
Laënnec c.
necrotic c.
posthepatitic c.
postnecrotic c.
toxic c.
cirrhotic
cirri (*pl. of* cirrus)
cirrose
cirrous
cirrus, pl. **cirri**
cirsoid
c. aneurysm
c. varix
cirsomphalos
cirsophthalmia

CIS
carcinoma in situ
cis-aconitic acid
cistern
ambient c.
basal c.
cerebellomedullary c.
chiasmatic c.
chyle c.
interpeduncular c.
lateral cerebellomedullary c.
lumbar c.
cisternal puncture
cisternography
cerebellopontine c.
cistron
citrate
bismuth ammonium c.
caffeine c.
copper c.
cupric c.
deptropine c.
effervescent lithium c.
effervescent magnesium c.
effervescent potassium c.
ethoheptazine c.
fentanyl c.
ferric ammonium c.
ferrous c.
lithium c.
magnesium c.
citrate-cleavage enzyme
citrated calcium carbimide
citric
c. acid
c. acid cycle
citrine skin
Citrobacter
C. amalonatica
C. diversus
C. freundii
C. koseri
citrovorum factor
citrulline
citrullinemia
citrullinuria
Civatte body
Civinini
C. canal
C. ligament
C. process

NOTES

CK
  creatine kinase
cladiosis
Clado
  C. anastomosis
  C. band
  C. ligament
  C. point
cladosporiosis
  cerebral c.
Clagett procedure
clairvoyance
Claisen condensation
clamp
  anastomosis c.
  c. connection
  Cope c.
  cord c.
  Crafoord c.
  Crile c.
  fenestrated c.
  Fogarty c.
  c. forceps
  Gant c.
  Gaskell c.
  gingival c.
  hemostatic c.
  Kelly c.
  Kocher c.
  liver-shod c.
  Mikulicz c.
  Mixter c.
  Mogen c.
  mosquito c.
  Payr c.
  pedicle c.
  penile c.
  Potts c.
  Rankin c.
  rubber-shod c.
  towel c.
clamshell
  c. brace
  c. incision
  c. thoracotomy
clang association
clapotage
clapotement
Clapton line
Clara cell
clarificant
Clark
  C. electrode
  C. level
  C. weight rule
Clarke
  C. cell
  C. column
  C. nucleus

Clarke-Hadfield syndrome
clasmatocyte
clasmatosis
clasp
  c. arm
  bar c.
  c. bar
  circumferential c.
  continuous c.
  extended c.
  c. guideline
clasping reflex
clasp-knife
  c.-k. effect
  c.-k. rigidity
  c.-k. spasticity
class
  c. I, II, III antigen
  c. I, II molecule
  c. switch
  c. switching
classic
  c. cervical rib syndrome
  c. choroidal neovascularization
  c. hemophilia
  c. migraine
classical
  c. cesarean section
  c. conditioning
  c. genetics
classifiable character
classification
  adansonian c.
  Angle c.
  Arneth c.
  Astler-Coller c.
  Bethesda c.
  Black c.
  Caldwell-Moloy c.
  Cummer c.
  DeBakey c.
  Denver c.
  Dukes c.
  FAB c.
  French-American-British c.
  Gell and Coombs C.
  Jansky c.
  Kennedy c.
  Kiel c.
  Lancefield c.
  Lennert c.
  Lukes-Collins c.
  New York Heart Association c.
  REAL c.
  Runyon c.
clastic anatomy
clastogen
clastogenic
clastothrix

clathrate crystal
clathrin
Clauberg
    C. test
    C. unit
Claude syndrome
claudication
    intermittent c.
    neurogenic c.
    venous c.
claudicatory
Claudius
    C. cell
    C. fossa
clause
    Delaney c.
claustral layer
claustrophobia
claustrophobic
claustrum
claval
clavatus
    Aspergillus c.
clavi (*pl. of* clavus)
clavicle
clavicular
    c. articular facet
    c. branch
    c. head
    c. notch
    c. percussion
clavipectoral
    c. fascia
    c. triangle
clavus, pl. clavi
clawfoot, claw foot
clawhand, claw hand
Claybrook sign
clay shoveler's fracture
clean intermittent bladder
  catheterization
cleansing
    c. cream
    c. enema
clear
    c. to auscultation and percussion
    (CTAP)
    c. cell
    c. cell acanthoma
    c. cell adenocarcinoma
    c. cell carcinoma
    c. cell hidradenoma

    c. layer
    c. liquid diet
clearance
    creatinine c.
    endogenous creatinine c.
    exogenous creatinine c.
    free water c.
    interocclusal c.
    inulin c.
    isotope c.
    maximum urea c.
    mucociliary c.
    urea c.
clearing
    c. factor
    c. medium
cleavage
    adequal c.
    c. cavity
    c. cell
    complete c.
    determinate c.
    discoidal c.
    c. division
    enamel c.
    equal c.
    equatorial c.
    holoblastic c.
    hydrolytic c.
    incomplete c.
    indeterminate c.
    c. line
    meridional c.
    meroblastic c.
    c. product
    c. site
    c. spindle
cleaved cell
cleaver
    enamel c.
cleft
    anal c.
    branchial c.
    cholesterol c.
    complete posterior laryngeal c.
    craniofacial c.
    facial c.
    first visceral c.
    c. foot
    gill c.
    gingival c.
    gluteal c.

NOTES

cleft (*continued*)
    c. hand
    hyobranchial c.
    hyomandibular c.
    intergluteal c.
    interneuromeric c.
    Larrey c.
    laryngotracheoesophageal c.
    c. lip
    Maurer c.
    median maxillary anterior
      alveolar c.
    c. nose
    occult posterior laryngeal c.
    orbitonasal c.
    c. palate
    partial cricoid c.
    partial posterior laryngeal c.
    pharyngeal c.
    posterior laryngeal c.
    pudendal c.
    c. spine
    submucous laryngeal c.
    synaptic c.
    c. tongue
    total cricoid c.
    tubotympanic c.
    c. uvula
    visceral c.
cleidagra
cleidal
cleidocostal
cleidocranial
    c. dysostosis
    c. dysplasia
cleidotomy
cleistothecium
Cleland
    C. nomenclature
    C. reagent
clemastine
clenched fist sign
cleoid
cleptoparasite
clergyman's sore throat
Clevenger fissure
click
    ejection c.
    mitral c.
    c. syndrome
clicking
    c. pneumothorax
    c. rale
    c. tinnitus
clidagra
clidal
clidocostal

clidocranial
    c. dysostosis
    c. dysplasia
client-centered therapy
climacophobia
climacteric syndrome
climacterium
climatic droplike keratopathy
climatology
climatotherapy
climbing fiber
climograph
clinica
    corona c.
clinical
    c. anatomy
    c. burden
    c. chemistry
    c. crown
    c. depression
    c. diagnosis
    c. end point
    c. epidemiology
    c. eruption
    c. fitness
    c. genetics
    c. indicator
    c. lethal
    c. medicine
    c. path
    c. pathology
    c. practice guideline
    c. psychology
    c. recording
    c. root
    c. sensitivity
    c. spectrometry
    c. spectroscopy
    c. thermometer
    c. trial
clinicopathologic
clinocephalic
clinocephalous
clinocephaly
clinodactyly
clinography
clinoid process
clip
    c. forceps
    skin c.
    towel c.
    wound c.
clipped speech
clithrophobia
clitoral
    c. engorgement syndrome
    c. recession
clitoridean
clitoridectomy

clitorides (*pl. of* clitoris)
clitoridis
    glans c.
clitoriditis
clitoris, pl. **clitorides**
    bifid c.
clitorism
clitoritis
clitoromegaly
clitoroplasty
clival
clivus, pl. **clivi**
    Blumenbach c.
    c. branch
CL lead
cloaca
    ectodermal c.
    endodermal c.
    persistent c.
cloacae
    Enterobacter c.
cloacal
    c. exstrophy
    c. membrane
    c. plate
    c. theory
cloacogenic carcinoma
clock
    lens c.
clonal
    c. aging
    c. deletion theory
    c. expansion
    c. selection theory
clone
    cDNA c.
    genomic c.
clonic
    c. convulsion
    c. seizure
    c. spasm
    c. state
clonicity
clonicotonic
clonidine growth hormone stimulation test
cloning
    A/T c.
    c. vector
clonism

clonogenic
    c. assay
    c. cell
clonograph
clonorchiasis
clonorchiosis
clonospasm
clonus
    ankle c.
Cloquet
    C. canal
    C. hernia
    node of C.
    C. septum
    C. space
closed
    c. anesthesia
    c. bite
    c. chain compound
    c. chest massage
    c. circle
    c. comedo
    c. dislocation
    c. drainage
    c. head injury (CHI)
    c. hospital
    c. laparoscopy
    c. loop obstruction
    c. reading frame
    c. reduction
    c. skull fracture
    c. surgery
    c. water-seal drainage system
closed-angle glaucoma
closed-circuit
    c.-c. helium dilution
    c.-c. method
    c.-c. spirometry
close-packed position
closing
    c. contraction
    c. membrane
    c. snap
    c. volume
clostridial
Clostridium
    C. bifermentans
    C. botulinum
    C. difficile
    C. histolyticum
    C. nigrificans
    C. novyi

NOTES

C

Clostridium (continued)
    C. parabotulinum
    C. perfringens
    C. sordellii
    C. tetani
    C. welchii
closure
    flask c.
    c. principle
    visual c.
clot
    agonal c.
    antemortem c.
    blood c.
    chicken fat c.
    currant jelly c.
    c.'s and debris
    laminated c.
    passive c.
    c. retraction time
clotting
    c. factor
    c. time
clouding of consciousness
Cloudman melanoma
cloudy
    c. swelling
    c. urine
clove oil
cloverleaf
    c. model
    c. skull
    c. skull syndrome
club
    c. foot
    c. hair
    c. hand
    c. moss
clubbed
    c. digit
    c. finger
    c. penis
clubbing
    hereditary c.
clubfoot
clubhand
clue cell
clumping
cluneal
clunes
cluster
    c. analysis
    c. of differentiation (CD)
    c. of differentiation antigen
    egg c.
    c. headache
    c. sample
cluster-of-grapes appearance
cluttering

Clutton joint
clysis
cm
    centimeter
CMG
    cystometrogram
CMI
    cell-mediated immunity
CML
    cell-mediated lymphocytotoxicity
    chronic myelogenous leukemia
CMV
    controlled mechanical ventilation
    Cytomegalovirus
cnemial
cnemis
cnida
cnidocyst
CNS
    central nervous system
CO
    carbon monoxide
CO2
    carbon dioxide
    CO2 analyzer
    CO2 narcosis
CO2-withdrawal seizure test
CoA
    coenzyme A
    CoA transferase
coacervate
coacervation
coadaptation
coagglutination
coagglutinin
coagulable
coagulant
coagulate
coagulation
    disseminated intravascular c. (DIC)
    c. factor
    c. necrosis
    c. time
    c. vitamin
coagulative
coagulopathy
    consumption c.
coagulum
coal
    c. oil
    c. tar
    c. tar naphtha
    c. worker's pneumoconiosis
coalescence
coaptation
    c. splint
    c. suture
coarct
coarctate

coarctation
- aortic c.
- reversed c.

coarctectomy

coarctotomy

coarse
- c. dispersion
- c. gravel
- c. material
- c. rhonchi
- c. tremor

coat
- buffy c.
- muscular c.

coated
- c. pit
- c. tongue
- c. vesicle

coating
- antireflection c.

Coats disease

cobalamin

cobalt

cobalt-57, -58, -60

cobaltous chloride

Cobb
- C. method
- C. syndrome

cobbler's suture

cobra
- c. hemotoxin
- c. toxin
- c. venom cofactor
- c. venom factor

cobrotoxin

COC
- cathodal opening contraction

cocaine
- crack c.
- c. hydrochloride

cocainization

cocarcinogen

cocarde reaction

coccal

cocci (*pl. of* coccus)

coccidial

coccidioidal granuloma

coccidioidin test

coccidioidoma

coccidioidomycosis
- disseminated c.
- subclinical c.

coccidiosis

coccidiostat

coccidium

coccinella

coccinellin

coccobacillary

coccobacillus

coccoid

cocculin

coccus, pl. **cocci**

coccyalgia

coccycephaly

coccydynia

coccygeal
- c. body
- c. bone
- c. cornu
- c. dimple
- c. fistula
- c. foveola
- c. ganglion
- c. gland
- c. horn
- c. joint
- c. ligament
- c. muscle
- c. nerve
- c. plexus
- c. sinus
- c. vertebra
- c. whorl

coccygectomy

coccyges (*pl. of* coccyx)

coccygeus muscle

coccygodynia

coccygotomy

coccyodynia

coccyx, pl. **coccyges**

cochineal

cochlea, pl. **cochleae**
- canaliculus cochleae
- columella cochleae
- fenestra cochleae
- membranous c.

cochlear
- c. aqueduct
- c. area
- c. branch
- c. canal
- c. canaliculus
- c. cupula
- c. drill-out

C

NOTES

195

cochlear *(continued)*
    c. duct
    c. dysplasia
    c. ganglion
    c. hair cell
    c. implant
    c. joint
    c. labyrinth
    c. microphonic
    c. nerve
    c. potential
    c. prosthesis
    c. recess
    c. root
    c. window
cochleitis
cochleo-orbicular reflex
cochleopalpebral reflex
cochleopupillary reflex
cochleosacculotomy
cochleostapedial reflex
cochleotopic
cochleovestibular
Cochrane collaboration
cocillana
cockade reaction
Cockayne
    C. disease
    C. syndrome
Cockett communicating perforating vein
cocktail
    Brompton c.
    Rivers c.
cocoa butter
coconsciousness
cocontraction
coconut sound
coconversion
cocoon dressing
coctolabile
coctostabile, coctostable
code
    genetic c.
codeine
    c. phosphate
    c. sulfate
codfish vertebra
coding
    place c.
    c. sequence
    c. strand
cod liver oil
Codman
    C. triangle
    C. tumor
codogenic
codominant
    c. allele
    c. gene

    c. inheritance
    c. trait
codon
    amber c.
    initiating c.
    initiation c.
    ochre c.
    opal c.
    termination c.
coefficient
    absorption c.
    activity c.
    biological c.
    Bunsen solubility c.
    c. of consanguinity
    correlation c.
    creatinine c.
    diffusion c.
    distribution c.
    economic c.
    extinction c.
    extraction c.
    filtration c.
    Hill c.
    hygienic laboratory c.
    c. of inbreeding
    isotonic c.
    c. of kinship
    lethal c.
    linear absorption c.
    molar absorption c.
    molar extinction c.
    Ostwald solubility c.
    permeability c.
    phenol c.
    Poiseuille viscosity c.
    reflection c.
    c. of relationship
    Rideal-Walker c.
    sedimentation c.
    selection c.
    specific absorption c.
    c. of variation (CV)
    c. of viscosity
Coelenterata
coelenterate
coenesthesia
coenocyte
coenocytic
coenurosis
coenzyme
    c. A (CoA)
    c. F
    c. factor
    c. Q (CoQ)
    c. R
coeur en sabot
Coe virus
coevolution

cofactor
    cobra venom c.
    molybdenum c.
coffee-ground vomit
Coffey
    C. anastomosis
    C. suspension
Coffin-Lowry syndrome
Coffin-Siris syndrome
Cogan
    C. dystrophy
    C. syndrome
Cogan-Reese syndrome
cognition
cognitive
    c. development
    c. dissonance
    c. dissonance theory
    c. laterality quotient
    c. psychology
    c. therapy
cogwheel
    c. gait
    c. ocular movement
    c. phenomenon
    c. respiration
    c. rigidity
cohesion
cohesive gold
Cohnheim
    C. area
    C. field
cohort study
coil
    detector c.
    c. gland
    surface c.
coiled
    c. artery
    c. position
coin
    c. lesion
    c. test
coincidental evolution
coin-counting
coinosite
cointegrate structure
coital headache
Coiter muscle
coition
coitophobia

coitus
    c. interruptus
    c. reservatus
colchicine
cold
    c. abscess
    c. agglutination
    c. agglutinin
    c. agglutinin syndrome
    c. allergy
    c. antibody
    c. autoagglutinin
    c. autoantibody
    c. bend test
    c. cautery
    c. chain
    c. cream
    c. cure resin
    c. diuresis
    c. erythema
    c. gangrene
    head c.
    c. hemagglutinin disease
    c. hemolysin
    c. knife conization
    c. light
    c. nodule
    c. pack
    c. pressor test
    c. snare
    c. sore
    c. stage
    c. therapy
    c. ulcer
    c. urticaria
    c. virus
cold-curing resin
cold-reactive antibody
cold-rigor point
cold-sensitive
    c.-s. enzyme
    c.-s. mutant
Cole-Cecil murmur
colectasia
colectomy
coleoptosis
coleotomy
colestipol
coli
    adenomatous polyposis c.
    Balantidium c.
    Campylobacter c.

NOTES

coli *(continued)*
    Entamoeba c.
    enterohemorrhagic *Escherichia c.*
    enteroinvasive *Escherichia c.*
    Escherichia c.
    familial polyposis c.
    haustra c.
    melanosis c.
colibacillosis
colic
    appendicular c.
    c. artery
    biliary c.
    copper c.
    Devonshire c.
    gallstone c.
    gastric c.
    hepatic c.
    c. impression
    infantile c.
    c. intussusception
    lead c.
    c. lymph node
    meconial c.
    menstrual c.
    saburral c.
    c. sphincter
    stercoral c.
    c. surface
    c. teniae
    c. vein
    verminous c.
colicin
colicinogeny
colicky
colicoplegia
coliform bacilli
colimycin
colinearity
colipase
coliphage
coliplication
colipuncture
colistimethate sodium
colitic arthritis
colitis
    amebic c.
    collagenous c.
    granulomatous c.
    hemorrhagic c.
    mucous c.
    myxomembranous c.
    pseudomembranous c.
    ulcerative c.
collaboration
    Cochrane c.
collagen
    c. disease
    c. fiber

    c. fibril
    c. helix
    c. implantation
    c. injection
    c. suture
collagenase
    c. A, I
    microbial c.
collagenation
collagenic
collagenization
collagenolytic
collagenosis
collagenous
    c. colitis
    c. fiber
    c. plaque
    c. pneumoconiosis
collagen-vascular disease
collapse
    absorption c.
    circulatory c.
    massive c.
    pulmonary c.
collar
    c. bone
    c. dressing
    c. incision
collar-button abscess
collared flagellate
collarette
collar-stud chalazion
collateral
    c. branch
    c. circulation
    c. digital artery
    c. eminence
    c. fissure
    c. hyperemia
    c. inheritance
    c. ligament
    c. sulcus
    c. trigone
    c. vessel
collecting system
collective unconscious
collector
    fraction c.
Colles
    C. fascia
    C. fracture
    C. ligament
    C. space
Collet-Sicard syndrome
colli
    cystitis c.
    fibromatosis c.
    lordosis c.
    melanoleukoderma c.

collicular artery
colliculectomy
colliculitis
colliculus, pl. colliculi
    facial c.
    inferior nasal c.
    seminal c.
    c. seminalis
    c. urethralis
Collier
    C. tract
    C. tucked lid sign
collier's lung
colligation
colligative
collimation
collimator
colliotomy
colliquation
colliquative
    c. albuminuria
    c. diarrhea
    c. necrosis
Collis-Belsey
    C.-B. fundoplication
    C.-B. procedure
Collis gastroplasty
collision tumor
Collis-Nissen fundoplication
collodion, collodium
    c. baby
    blistering c.
    cantharidal c.
    c. dressing
    flexible c.
    hemostatic c.
    iodized c.
    c. vesicans
colloid
    c. acne
    c. adenoma
    c. bath
    c. body
    bovine c.
    c. cancer
    c. carcinoma
    c. corpuscle
    c. cyst
    c. degeneration
    dispersion c.
    emulsion c.
    c. goiter

    hydrophil c.
    hydrophilic c.
    hydrophobic c.
    irreversible c.
    lyophilic c.
    lyophobic c.
    c. milium
    c. pseudomilium
    c. system
colloidal
    c. dispersion
    c. gel
    c. gold reaction
    c. gold test
    c. metal
    c. radioactive gold
    c. silicon dioxide
    c. silver iodide
    c. solution
colloidin
colloidoclasia, colloidoclasis
colloidoclastic
colloidogen
colloxylin
collum
collyrium
coloboma
    Fuchs c.
    macular c.
colobomatous microphthalmia
colocentesis
colocholecystostomy
colocolic intussusception
colocolostomy
colocutaneous fistula
colocynth
colocystoplasty
coloenteritis
colohepatopexy
coloileal fistula
cololysis
colon
    ascending c.
    band of c.
    c. cutoff sign
    c. descendens
    descending c.
    giant c.
    iliac c.
    irritable c.
    lead-pipe c.
    sigmoid c.

NOTES

C

colon *(continued)*
    spastic c.
    transverse c.
colonalgia
colonic
    c. diverticulum
    c. fistula
    c. smear
colonization
    genetic c.
colonogram
colonometer
colonopathy
    fibrosing c.
colonorrhagia
colonorrhea
colonoscope
colonoscopy
colony
    daughter c.
    filamentous c.
    H c.
    lenticular c.
colony-forming unit
colony-stimulating factor (CSF)
colopathy
colopexostomy
colopexotomy
colopexy
colophony
coloplication
coloproctitis
coloproctostomy
coloptosia
coloptosis
colopuncture
color
    c. aberration
    c. agnosia
    c. blindness
    c. chart
    c. constancy
    extrinsic c.
    c. hearing
    intrinsic c.
    c. match
    c. radical
    saturated c.
    c. scotoma
    c. sense
    c. solid
    c. spectrum
    c. taste
    c. triangle
Colorado
    C. tick fever
    C. tick fever virus
color-contrast microscope
colorectal

colorectitis
colorectostomy
colored vision
colorimeter
    Duboscq c.
colorimetric titration
colorimetry
colorrhagia
colorrhaphy
colorrhea
coloscopy
colosigmoidostomy
colostomy
    c. bag
    end c.
    ileotransverse c.
colostric
colostrorrhea
colostrous
colostrum corpuscle
colotomy
colovaginal fistula
colovesical fistula
colpatresia
colpectasis, colpectasia
colpectomy
colpocele
colpocleisis
colpocystocele
colpocystoplasty
colpocystotomy
colpocystoureterotomy
colpodynia
colpohysterectomy
colpohysteropexy
colpohysterotomy
colpomicroscope
colpomicroscopy
colpomycosis
colpomyomectomy
colpoperineoplasty
colpoperineorrhaphy
colpopexy
colpoplasty
colpopoiesis
colpoptosis, colpoptosia
colporectopexy
colporrhagia
colporrhaphy
colporrhexis
colposcope
colposcopy
colpospasm
colpostat
colpostenosis
colpostenotomy
colposuspension
colpotomy
colpoureterotomy

colpoxerosis
columbium
columella, pl. **columellae**
    c. cochleae
    c. nasi
column
    affinity c.
    anal c.
    anterior c.
    anterior gray c.
    anterolateral c.
    Bertin c.
    branchial efferent c.
    Burdach c.
    c. cell
    c. chromatography
    Clarke c.
    dorsal c.
    c. of fornix
    general somatic afferent c.
    general somatic efferent c.
    general visceral afferent c.
    general visceral efferent c.
    Goll c.
    Gowers c.
    gray c.
    intermediate c.
    intermediolateral cell c.
    lateral c.
    Lissauer c.
    Morgagni c.
    posterior c.
    rectal c.
    renal c.
    spinal c.
    c. of Spitzka-Lissauer
    vertebral c.
columnar epithelium
columnella
coma
    c. aberration
    c. cast
    delayed c.
    diabetic c.
    hepatic c.
    hyperosmolar nonketotic c.
    hypoglycemic c.
    hypoventilation c.
    Kussmaul c.
    metabolic c.
    c. scale

    uremic c.
    c. vigil
comatosa
    malaria c.
comatose
combat neurosis
combesi
    Eubacterium c.
combination
    c. beat
    binary c.
    c. chemotherapy
    c. oral contraceptive
    c. restoration
combined
    c. approach mastoidectomy
    c. glaucoma
    c. hemorrhoid
    c. immunodeficiency
    c. immunodeficiency syndrome
    c. methods
    c. pregnancy
    c. sclerosis
    c. system disease
    c. version
combining weight
comblike septum
combustible
combustion equivalent
Comby sign
comedo
    closed c.
    c. nevus
    open c.
    solar c.
comedocarcinoma
comedogenic
comedonecrosis
comedonicus
    nevus c.
comet tail sign
comfort zone
comitance
comitant
    c. artery
    c. strabismus
comitantes
    venae c.
comma
    c. bacillus
    c. bundle of Schultze
    c. tract of Schultze

NOTES

command hallucination
commando
    c. operation
    c. procedure
commemorative sign
commensalism
    epizoic c.
commensal parasite
comminuted skull fracture
comminution
commissural
    c. cheilitis
    c. fiber
    c. myelotomy
    c. pit
commissure
    anterior gray c.
    anterior labial c.
    anterior white c.
    dorsal supraoptic c.
    Ganser c.
    gray c.
    Gudden c.
    habenular c.
    hippocampal c.
    labial c.
    c. laryngoscope
    lateral palpebral c.
    medial palpebral c.
    Meynert c.
    posterior cerebral c.
    posterior labial c.
    supraoptic c.
commissurotomy
    mitral c.
common
    c. acne
    c. antigen
    c. baldness
    c. basal vein
    c. bile duct
    c. cardinal vein
    c. carotid artery
    c. carotid nervous plexus
    c. cochlear artery
    c. cold virus
    c. facial vein
    c. fibular nerve
    c. flexor sheath
    c. hepatic artery
    c. hepatic duct
    c. iliac artery
    c. iliac lymph node
    c. iliac vein
    c. interosseous artery
    c. migraine
    c. modiolar vein
    c. palmar digital artery
    c. palmar digital nerve

    c. peroneal nerve
    c. peroneal tendon sheath
    c. plantar digital artery
    c. plantar digital nerve
    c. tendinous ring
    c. variable immunodeficiency
    c. vehicle spread
    c. wart
commune
    integumentum c.
communicable disease
communicantes
    gray ramus c.
communicating
    c. artery
    c. branch
    c. hematoma
    c. hydrocele
    c. hydrocephalus
    c. junction
    c. ramus
communication
    augmentative and alternative c.
    c. board
    c. disorder
    facilitated c.
    human c.
    nonoral c.
    nonverbal c.
    simultaneous c.
    total c.
communicative disorder
community
    biotic c.
    c. dentistry
community-acquired pneumonia
Comolli sign
comorbidity
compact
    c. bone
    c. osteoma
    c. substance
compactum
    stratum c.
companionship
    human c.
companion vein
comparascope
comparative
    c. anatomy
    c. pathology
comparator microscope
compartment
    adductor c.
    dorsiflexor c.
    extensor c.
    fibular c.
    flexor c.
    lateral c.

medial c.
posterior c.
c. syndrome
compensated
    c. glaucoma
    c. metabolic alkalosis
    c. respiratory acidosis
    c. respiratory alkalosis
compensating
    c. curve
    c. emphysema
    c. ocular
compensation
    attenuation c.
    depth c.
    gene dosage c.
    c. neurosis
compensatory
    c. circulation
    c. emphysema
    c. hypertrophy
    c. movement
    c. pause
    c. polycythemia
competence
    cardiac c.
    immunologic c.
    c. testing
competing risk
competition
    antigenic c.
competitive
    c. antagonist
    c. binding assay
    c. inhibition
competitor DNA
complaint
    chief c. (CC)
complement
    c. binding assay
    c. chemotactic factor
    component of c.
    c. factor I
    c. fixation
    heparin c.
    c. pathway
    c. system
    c. unit
complemental air
complementarity determining region
complementary
    c. air

c. DNA (cDNA)
c. hypertrophy
c. medicine
c. ribonucleic acid (cRNA)
c. role
c. strand
c. structures
complementation
    intergenic c.
    intragenic c.
complement-fixation
    c.-f. reaction
    c.-f. test
complement-fixing antibody
complete
    c. abortion
    c. achromatopsia
    c. amelia
    c. androgen insensitivity syndrome
    c. antibody
    c. antigen
    c. ascertainment
    c. atrioventricular dissociation
    c. AV block
    c. AV dissociation
    c. blood count (CBC)
    c. carcinogen
    c. cataract
    c. cleavage
    c. denture
    c. denture impression
    c. disinfectant
    c. fistula
    c. hemianopia
    c. hernia
    c. iridoplegia
    c. laryngotomy
    c. mastoidectomy
    c. medium
    c. metamorphosis
    c. posterior laryngeal cleft
    c. tetanus
    c. transduction
complex
    aberrant c.
    AIDS dementia c. (ADC)
    AIDS-related c. (ARC)
    amygdaloid c.
    anomalous c.
    antigen-antibody c.
    antigenic c.
    apical c.

C

NOTES

complex *(continued)*
    atrial c.
    auricular c.
    avian leukemia-sarcoma c.
    avian leukosis-sarcoma c.
    binary c.
    brain wave c.
    brother c.
    Cain c.
    Carney c.
    castration c.
    caudal pharyngeal c.
    central c.
    Diana c.
    diphasic c.
    EAHF c.
    Eisenmenger c.
    Electra c.
    electrocardiographic c.
    c. endometrial hyperplasia
    enzyme-substrate c.
    equiphasic c.
    father c.
    fatty acid synthase c.
    c. febrile convulsion
    femininity c.
    c. fracture
    Ghon c.
    glycine cleavage c.
    Golgi c.
    H-2 c.
    histocompatibility c.
    HLA c.
    immune c.
    inferiority c.
    inferior olivary c.
    iron-dextran c.
    isodiphasic c.
    Jocasta c.
    c. joint
    junctional c.
    juxtaglomerular c.
    K c.
    knee c.
    Lear c.
    c. learning process
    c. locus
    major histocompatibility c.
    mediator c.
    membrane attack c.
    Meyenburg c.
    Michaelis c.
    minor histocompatibility c.
    c. motor seizure
    Mycobacterium avium-
      intracellulare c.
    c. odontoma
    Oedipus c.
    c. partial seizure

    c. pleural effusion
    c. precipitated epilepsy
    primary c.
    QRS c.
    Shone c.
    shoulder c.
    sicca c.
    c. sound
    spike and wave c.
    superiority c.
    symptom c.
    synaptinemal c.
    ventricular c.
    vitamin B c.
complexity
    chemical c.
compliance
    bladder c.
    chest wall c.
    detrusor c.
    dynamic c.
    lung c.
    respiratory c.
    respiratory system c.
    static c.
complicated
    c. cataract
    c. migraine
    c. pneumoconiosis
complication
component
    c. of complement
    c. management
    performance c.
composite
    c. dental cement
    c. flap
    c. graft
    c. joint
    c. resin
composition
    base c.
    modeling c.
compos mentis
compound
    acetone c.
    c. action potential
    acyclic c.
    addition c.
    alicyclic c.
    aliphatic c.
    c. aneurysm
    aromatic c.
    c. articulation
    carbamino c.
    c. caries
    c. character
    closed chain c.
    condensation c.

conjugated c.
cyclic c.
c. cyst
c. dislocation
c. dressing
c. eye
c. flap
genetic c.
c. gland
glycosyl c.
c. granule cell
heterocyclic c.
c. heterozygote
high-energy c.
homocyclic c.
c. hyperopic astigmatism
impression c.
inclusion c.
inorganic c.
isocyclic c.
c. joint
Kendall c.
c. lens
c. lipids
meso c.
methonium c.
c. microscope
modeling c.
c. myopic astigmatism
c. nevus
c. odontoma
open chain c.
organic c.
c. pregnancy
c. presentation
c. protein
c. restoration
c. skull fracture
c. suture
comprehension
comprehensive
c. discharge planning
c. medical care
compress
graduated c.
compressed
c. sponge
c. tablet
c. yeast
compressible
c. cavernous body
c. volume

compression
c. anesthesia
c. bandage
cerebral c.
c. cyanosis
c. dressing
c. fracture
intermittent c.
c. limiting
c. molding
c. neuropathy
c. paralysis
c. plate
c. plating
c. retinopathy
c. syndrome
c. therapy
c. thrombosis
wide dynamic range c.
compressive
c. myelopathy
c. nystagmus
c. strength
compressor urethra muscle
Compton
C. effect
C. scatter
C. scattering
compulsion neurosis
compulsive
c. act
c. idea
c. neurosis
c. personality
computed
c. perimetry
c. radiography (CR)
c. tomography (CT)
computer
c. model
c. simulation
computer-assisted myelography (CAM)
computer-based patient record
computerized axial tomography (CAT)
conalbumin
conanine
conarium
conation
conative
concameration
concanavalin A
concatamer

NOTES

concatenate
Concato disease
concave
    c. lens
    c. mirror
concavity
concavoconcave lens
concavoconvex lens
concealed
    c. conduction
    c. hemorrhage
    c. hernia
    c. penis
concentrate
    mixed tocopherols c.
concentrated human red blood
  corpuscle
concentration
    Baermann c.
    buffy coat c.
    critical micelle c.
    fecal c.
    formalin-ether sedimentation c.
    formalin-ethyl acetate
      sedimentation c.
    c. gradient
    gravity c.
    M c.
    mean corpuscular hemoglobin c.
      (MCHC)
    microhematocrit c.
    minimal alveolar c.
    minimal anesthetic c.
    minimal inhibitory c. (MIC)
    molar c.
    normal c.
    zinc sulfate flotation c.
concentrator
    oxygen c.
concentric
    c. contraction
    c. fibroma
    c. hypertrophy
    c. lamella
concept
    c. formation
    self c.
conception
    imperative c.
    retained products of c.
conceptual
conceptus
concerted
    c. evolution
    c. model
concha, pl. **conchae**
    c. bullosa
    highest c.
    inferior nasal c.

    middle nasal c.
    Santorini c.
    sphenoidal conchae
    superior nasal c.
    supreme nasal c.
conchal
    c. cartilage
    c. crest
conchoidal body
concisus
    Campylobacter c.
concomitance
concomitant
    c. immunity
    c. strabismus
    c. symptom
concordance rate
concordant
    c. alternans
    c. alternation
    c. atrioventricular connection
    c. change electrocardiogram
concrement
concrescence
concrete
    c. operation
    c. thinking
concretio cordis
concretion
concretization
concurrent
    c. disinfection
    c. validity
concussion
    brain c.
    c. cataract
    c. myelitis
    spinal cord c.
condensation
    aldol c.
    Claisen c.
    c. compound
condensed milk
condenser
    automatic c.
    cardioid c.
    dark-field c.
condensing
    c. enzyme
    c. osteitis
condition
    fibrocystic c.
conditional-lethal mutant
conditionally lethal mutant
conditional probability
conditioned
    c. avitaminosis
    c. hemolysis
    c. insomnia

c. reflex
c. response
c. stimulus
conditioning
assertive c.
aversive c.
avoidance c.
classical c.
escape c.
higher order c.
instrumental c.
physical c.
reinforcement c.
c. therapy
condom
conductance
conduct disorder
conducting airway
conduction
aberrant ventricular c.
accelerated c.
air c.
c. analgesia
c. anesthesia
anomalous c.
antegrade c.
anterograde c.
c. aphasia
atrioventricular c. (AVC)
AV c.
avalanche c.
c. block
bone c.
concealed c.
c. deafness
decremental c.
delayed c.
forward c.
intraatrial c.
intraventricular c.
nerve c.
retrograde VA c.
saltatory c.
synaptic c.
ventricular c.
conductive
c. deafness
c. hearing impairment
c. hearing loss
c. heat
conductivity
hydraulic c.

conductor
conduit
apical-aortic c.
ileal c.
conduplicate
condylar
c. articulation
c. axis
c. canal
c. emissary vein
c. fossa
c. guidance
c. guidance inclination
c. guide
c. hinge position
c. joint
c. process
condylarthrosis
condyle
balancing side c.
c. cord
lateral c.
mandibular c.
medial c.
c. path
condylectomy
condylion
condyloid
c. canal
c. process
condyloma
c. acuminatum
flat c.
giant c.
c. latum
pointed c.
condylomatous
condylotomy
condylus
cone
antipodal c.
arterial c.
c. bipolar cell
c. degeneration
c. disc
c. down
c. dystrophy
elastic c.
c. fiber
c. granule
gutta-percha c.
Haller c.

NOTES

cone *(continued)*
    implantation c.
    c. of light
    medullary c.
    Politzer luminous c.
    retinal c.
    c. vision
cone-rod retinal dystrophy
confabulation
confidence interval
confidentiality
configuration
confinement
    estimated date of c. (EDC)
conflict
    approach-approach c.
    approach-avoidance c.
    avoidance-avoidance c.
    c. of interest
    interpersonal c.
    intrapersonal c.
confluence of sinus
confluent
    c. articulation
    c. smallpox
confocal microscope
conformation
    boat c.
    envelope c.
conformational map
confounding
confrontation method
congener
congenic strain
congenita
    amyoplasia c.
    amyotonia c.
    aplasia cutis c.
    arthrogryposis multiplex c.
    chondrodysplasia calcificans c.
    cutis marmorata telangiectatica c.
    dyskeratosis c.
    ectopia pupillae c.
    hyperkeratosis c.
    ichthyosis c.
    myatonia c.
    myotonia c.
    osteogenesis imperfecta c.
    paramyotonia c.
    spondyloepiphyseal dysplasia c.
congenital
    c. afibrinogenemia
    c. alopecia
    c. amputation
    c. aplasia
    c. aplastic anemia
    c. atonic pseudoparalysis
    c. baldness
    c. bronchiectasis

c. cataract
c. cerebellar atrophy
c. cerebral aneurysm
c. choreoathetosis
c. conus
c. deafness
c. diaphragmatic hernia
c. dyserythropoietic anemia
c. dysphagocytosis
c. dysplastic angiectasia
c. dysplastic angiomatosis
c. ectodermal defect
c. ectodermal dysplasia
c. elephantiasis
c. epulis of newborn
c. erythropoietic porphyria
c. facial diplegia
c. fibrosis
c. generalized fibromatosis
c. generalized muscular hypoplasia
c. glaucoma
c. heart block
c. Heinz body hemolytic anemia
c. hemidysplasia with ichthyosiform erythroderma and limb defects (CHILD)
c. hemolytic icterus
c. hemolytic jaundice
c. hereditary endothelial dystrophy
c. hip dysplasia
c. hydrocele
c. hydrocephalus
c. hypophosphatasia
c. hypoplastic anemia
c. hypothyroidism
c. ichthyosiform erythroderma
c. leukopathia
c. lobar emphysema
c. lymphedema
c. megacolon
c. methemoglobinemia
c. microvillus atrophy
c. myxedema
c. nephrosis
c. neutropenia
c. nevus
c. nonregenerative anemia
c. nystagmus
c. ophthalmoplegia
c. ossicular absence
c. pancytopenia
c. paramyotonia
c. pneumonia
c. pulmonary arteriovenous fistula
c. pyloric stenosis
c. rubella syndrome
c. spastic paraplegia
c. stridor
c. sutural alopecia

c. syphilis
c. torticollis
c. total lipodystrophy
c. toxoplasmosis
c. valve
c. virilizing adrenal hyperplasia

congenitale
P c.

congenitalis
alopecia c.
alopecia triangularis c.

congenitum
megacolon c.

congested

congestion
active c.
brain c.
functional c.
hypostatic c.
nasal c.
orthostatic c.
passive c.
physiologic c.

congestive
c. cardiomyopathy
c. cirrhosis
c. heart failure
c. splenomegaly

conglobata
acne c.

conglobate

conglomerate

conglomeratus
Micrococcus c.

conglutinant

conglutination

conglutinin

congolensis
Dermatophilus c.

Congolian red fever

congophilic angiopathy

Congo red

congruent
c. affect
c. point

congruous hemianopia

conical
c. catheter
c. cornea
c. lobule
c. papilla

conidial

conidiogenous

conidiophore

conidium

coniofibrosis

coniolymphstasis

coniometer

coniophage

coniosis

coniotomy

conium

conization
cautery c.
cold knife c.

conjoined
c. anastomosis
c. asymmetric twins
c. equal twins
c. symmetric twins
c. tendon
c. twins
c. unequal twins

conjoint
c. tendon
c. therapy

conjugal cancer

conjugant

conjugate
c. acid
c. acid-base pair
anatomic c.
anatomical c.
c. axis
c. deviation
diagonal c.
c. diameter
c. division
effective c.
external c.
false c.
c. foci
folic acid c.
c. foramen
c. gaze
internal c.
median c.
c. movement
c. nystagmus
obstetric c.
c. point

conjugated
c. antigen
c. bilirubin

NOTES

conjugated *(continued)*
    c. compound
    c. double bonds
    c. estrogen
    c. hapten
    c. protein
conjugation
conjugative plasmid
conjunctiva, pl. **conjunctivae**
    anulus conjunctivae
    bulbar c.
    Dirofilaria conjunctivae
    lithiasis conjunctivae
conjunctival
    c. artery
    c. cell
    c. cul-de-sac
    c. fornix
    c. gland
    c. layer
    c. reflex
    c. ring
    c. sac
    c. varix
    c. vein
conjunctivalis
    blennorrhea c.
conjunctiviplasty
conjunctivitis
    actinic c.
    acute contagious c.
    acute epidemic c.
    acute hemorrhagic c.
    acute viral c.
    allergic c.
    angular c.
    arc-flash c.
    atopic c.
    chemical c.
    chronic c.
    chronic follicular c.
    cicatricial c.
    diphtheritic c.
    eczematous c.
    follicular c.
    giant papillary c.
    gonococcal c.
    gonorrheal c.
    granular c.
    hyperacute purulent c.
    inclusion c.
    infantile purulent c.
    larval c.
    ligneous c.
    membranous c.
    molluscum c.
    Parinaud c.
    spring c.
    swimming pool c.

    trachomatous c.
    vernal c.
    viral c.
conjunctivochalasis
conjunctivodacryocystorhinostomy
conjunctivodacryocystostomy
conjunctivoplasty
conjunctivorhinostomy
connectin
connecting
    c. cartilage
    c. stalk
    c. tubule
connection
    ambiguous atrioventricular c.
    anomalous pulmonary venous c.
    atrioventricular c.
    clamp c.
    concordant atrioventricular c.
    discordant atrioventricular c.
    double inlet atrioventricular c.
    intertendinous c.
    marrow-mesenchyme c.
    partial anomalous pulmonary
      venous c.
connective
    c. tissue
    c. tissue cell
    c. tissue group
    c. tumor
connective-tissue disease
connector
    c. bar
    major c.
    minor c.
    nonrigid c.
    rigid c.
    stress-broken c.
Connell suture
connexus
Conn syndrome
conoid
    c. ligament
    c. process
    Sturm c.
    c. tubercle
Conradi
    C. disease
    C. line
Conradi-Hünermann
    C.-H. disease
    C.-H. syndrome
consanguineous
consanguinity
    coefficient of c.
conscious
consciousness
    clouding of c.
    double c.

field of c.
level of c.
consecutive
    c. amputation
    c. aneurysm
    c. angiitis
    c. esotropia
    c. symptom
consensual
    c. light reflex
    c. reaction
    c. validation
consent
    informed c.
conservation of energy
conservative
    c. mastoidectomy
    c. replication
    c. surgery
    c. treatment
consistency
    doughy c.
    c. principle
consolidant
consolidation chemotherapy
consonating rale
conspecific
conspicuity
constancy
    color c.
    form c.
    c. phenomenon
constant
    association c.
    Avogadro c.
    binding c.
    c. coupling
    decay c.
    diffusion c.
    disintegration c.
    dissociation c.
    equilibrium c.
    Faraday c.
    c. field equation
    flotation c.
    gas c.
    Hill c.
    c. infusion pump
    Michaelis c.
    Michaelis-Menten c.
    permeability c.
    Planck c.

radioactive c.
rate c.'s
c. region
sedimentation c.
constellation of symptoms
constipate
constipated
constipation
constitution
constitutional
    c. cause
    c. formula
    c. hepatic dysfunction
    c. hirsutism
    c. hyperbilirubinemia
    c. jaundice
    c. psychology
    c. reaction
    c. symptom
    c. thrombopathy
constitutive
    c. enzyme
    c. heterochromatin
constriction
    bronchoaortic c.
    diaphragmatic c.
    esophageal c.
    c. hyperemia
    inferior esophageal c.
    middle esophageal c.
    pyloric c.
    c. ring
constrictive
    c. bronchiolitis
    c. endocarditis
    c. pericarditis
constrictor
constructional
    c. agraphia
    c. apraxia
construct validity
consultand
    dummy c.
consultant
consultation
consulting staff
consumption
    c. coagulopathy
    maximal oxygen c.
    myocardial oxygen c.
    oxygen c.
consumptive

NOTES

contact
    c. allergy
    c. area
    c. area zone
    balancing c.
    c. catalysis
    centric c.
    c. ceptor
    c. cheilitis
    deflective occlusal c.
    c. dermatitis
    c. hypersensitivity
    c. hysteroscope
    c. illumination
    c. inhibition
    initial c.
    interceptive occlusal c.
    c. lens
    c. metastasis
    c. point
    c. splint
    c. surface
    c. ulcer
    c. with reality
contactant
contact-type dermatitis
contagion
contagiosa
    impetigo c.
contagiosum
    molluscum c.
contagious
    c. disease
    c. ecthyma
contagiousness
contagium
contained disc herniation
containment
contaminant
contaminate
contamination
content
    c. analysis
    carbon dioxide c.
    latent c.
    manifest c.
    oxygen c.
    c. validity
context
    performance c.
contig map
contiguity
    law of c.
    solution of c.
contiguous
contiguum
    per c.
continence
    fecal c.

contingency table
continua
    acrodermatitis c.
continued fever
continuity
    amputation in c.
    solution of c.
continuous
    c. ambulatory peritoneal dialysis (CAPD)
    c. arrhythmia
    c. bar retainer
    c. beam
    c. capillary
    c. clasp
    c. culture
    c. epidural anesthesia
    c. eruption
    c. flow analyzer
    c. interleaved sampling
    c. loop wiring
    c. murmur
    c. otoacoustic emission
    c. passive motion (CPM)
    c. phase
    c. positive airway pressure (CPAP)
    c. positive-pressure breathing (CPPB)
    c. positive pressure breathing
    c. positive pressure ventilation (CPPV)
    c. random variable
    c. spectrum
    c. spinal anesthesia
    c. suction drainage system
    c. suture
    c. training
    c. tremor
    c. variation
    c. wave laser
continuum
    per c.
contortum
    Eubacterium c.
contour
    flange c.
    gingival c.
    gum c.
    height of c.
    c. line of Owen
    c. retractor
    ventricular c.
contraangle
contraaperture
contrabevel
contraception
    emergency hormonal c.
    postcoital c.

contraceptive
    barrier c.
    combination oral c.
    c. device
    oral c.
    c. sponge
contracted
    c. foot
    c. kidney
    c. pelvis
contractile
    c. stricture
    c. vacuole
contractility
    cardiac c.
contraction
    anodal closure c. (ACC, AnCC)
    anodal opening c. (AnOC, AOC)
    automatic c.
    c. band
    c. band necrosis
    Braxton Hicks c.
    carpopedal c.
    cathodal closure c. (CaCC, CCC)
    cathodal opening c. (COC)
    closing c.
    concentric c.
    eccentric c.
    escape c.
    escape ventricular c.
    fibrillary c.
    front-tap c.
    Gowers c.
    hourglass c.
    hunger c.
    idiomuscular c.
    isometric c.
    isotonic c.
    myotatic c.
    paradoxical c.
    postural c.
    c. stress test
    tonic c.
    uterine c.
contractual
    c. psychiatry
    c. psychotherapy
contractural diathesis
contracture
    cathodal opening c. (CaOC)
    c. deformity
    Dupuytren c.

    fixed c.
    functional c.
    ischemic c.
    organic c.
    Volkmann c.
contrafissura
contraindicant
contraindication
contralateral
    c. hemiplegia
    c. partner
    c. reflex
    c. routing
    c. sign
contrast
    c. agent
    c. bath
    c. echocardiography
    c. enema
    c. enhancement
    c. material
    c. medium
    radiographic c.
    c. sensitivity
    c. sensitivity testing
    c. stain
contrasuppressor cell
contrecoup
    fracture by c.
    c. injury
contributory cause of death
control
    c. animal
    autogenous c.
    automatic gain c.
    aversive c.
    biologic c.
    birth c.
    delusion of c.
    direct medical c.
    c. experiment
    c. gene
    c. group
    idiodynamic c.
    locus of c.
    quality c.
    c. release suture
    stimulus c.
    c. syringe
controlled
    delusion of being c.
    c. hypotension

NOTES

controlled *(continued)*
    c. mechanical ventilation (CMV)
    c. respiration
    c. substance
contusion
    brain c.
conular
conus
    c. arteriosus
    congenital c.
    distraction c.
    c. elasticus
    c. medullaris
convalescence
convalescent
    c. carrier
    c. serum
convallaria
convection
convective heat
convenience form
conventional
    c. animal
    c. sign
    c. thoracoplasty
    c. tomography
convergence
    accommodative c.
    amplitude of c.
    angle of c.
    c. excess
    far point of c.
    c. insufficiency
    negative c.
    positive c.
convergence-accommodation
    accommodative c.-a. (AC/A)
convergence-retraction nystagmus
convergent
    c. evolution
    c. squint
    c. strabismus
converging meniscus
conversation board
conversion
    c. disorder
    c. electron
    c. hysteria
    c. hysteria neurosis
    c. reaction
    c. symptom
conversive heat
convertase
convertin
convex
    high c.
    c. lens
    low c.
    c. mirror

convexity
    cortical c.
convexobasia
convexoconcave lens
convexoconvex lens
convolute
convoluted
    c. bone
    c. gland
    c. seminiferous tubule
convolution
    angular c.
    anterior central c.
    ascending frontal c.
    ascending parietal c.
    callosal c.
    cingulate c.
    first temporal c.
    hippocampal c.
    inferior frontal c.
    inferior temporal c.
    middle frontal c.
    middle temporal c.
convulsant threshold
convulsion
    audiogenic c.
    benign neonatal c.
    clonic c.
    complex febrile c.
    febrile c.
    hysterical c.
    hysteroid c.
    immediate posttraumatic c.
    infantile c.
    mimetic c.
    tonic c.
    traumatic c.
    uremic c.
convulsive
    c. seizure
    c. state
    c. therapy
    c. tic
cooing murmur
Cooke speculum
cool-down
    active c.-d.
cooled-knife method
Cooley anemia
Coolidge tube
Coombs
    C. murmur
    C. serum
    C. test
Cooper
    C. fascia
    C. hernia
    C. herniotome
    C. ligament

cooperative enzyme
cooperativity model
Cooper-Rand artificial larynx
coordinate covalent bond
coordination
    bilateral c.
co-ossification
co-ossify
COPD
    chronic obstructive pulmonary disease
Cope
    C. clamp
    C. sign
copepod
copolymer-1
copolymer resin
copper
    c. arsenite
    c. bichloride
    c. cataract
    c. chloride
    c. citrate
    c. colic
    c. dichloride
    c. nose
    c. phosphate cement
    c. protein
    c. sulfate
    c. sulfate method
    c. sulphate
copper-64, -67
copperhead
Coppet law
copra itch
coprecipitation
copremesis
coproantibody
coprolagnia
coprolalia
coprolith
coprology
coproma
coprophagia
coprophagous
coprophagy
coprophil, coprophilic
coprophile
coprophilia
coprophilic (*var. of* coprophil)
coprophobia
coprophrasia
coproplanesia

coproporphyria
    hereditary c.
coproporphyrin
coproporphyrinogen oxidase
coprostasis
copula
    His c.
copulation
CoQ
    coenzyme Q
cor
    c. adiposum
    c. biloculare
    c. bovinum
    c. mobile
    c. pendulum
    c. pulmonale
    c. triatriatum
    c. triloculare
coracoacromial
    c. arch
    c. ligament
coracobrachial
    c. bursa
    c. muscle
coracobrachialis muscle
coracoclavicular ligament
coracohumeral ligament
coracoid
    c. notch
    c. process
    c. tuberosity
coral calculus
coralliform cataract
corallin
cord
    Bergmann c.
    Billroth c.
    c. blood
    c. clamp
    condyle c.
    dental c.
    false tendinous c.
    false vocal c.
    Ferrein c.
    ganglionated c.
    genital c.
    germinal c.
    gonadal c.
    gubernacular c.
    hepatic c.
    c. hydrocele

NOTES

cord *(continued)*
    lateral c.
    lymph c.
    medial c.
    medullary c.
    nephrogenic c.
    nuchal c.
    posterior c.
    prolapse of umbilical c.
    spermatic c.
    spinal c.
    tendinous c.
    testicular c.
    true vocal c.
    umbilical c.
    Willis c.
cordate pelvis
cordatum
    Diphyllobothrium c.
cordectomy
cordial
cordianine
cordiform
    c. pelvis
    c. uterus
cordis
    accretio c.
    ataxia c.
    atrium dextrum c.
    atrium sinistrum c.
    chordae tendineae c.
    concretio c.
    delirium c.
    diastasis c.
    ectasia c.
    ectopia c.
    hypodynamia c.
    ictus c.
    theca c.
    trepidatio c.
cordocentesis
cordon sanitaire
cordopexy
cordotomy
    anterolateral c.
cordylobiasis
cordy pulse
core
    atomic c.
    central transactional c.
    c. particle
    c. pneumonia
    c. temperature
co-receptor
    B cell c.-r.
corectopia
corelysis
coremium
coreoplasty

corepexy
corepraxy
    laser c.
    mechanical c.
corepressor
Cori
    C. cycle
    C. disease
    C. ester
coria (*pl. of* corium)
coriander
corii
    rete cutaneum c.
corium, pl. **coria**
corkscrew vessel
corn
    c. ergot
    hard c.
    c. oil
    c. smut
    soft c.
    c. sugar
cornea
    conical c.
    floury c.
    c. plana
    c. urica
    c. verticillata
corneae
    dystrophia epithelialis c.
    herpes c.
    lamina limitans anterior c.
    lamina limitans posterior c.
    macula c.
corneal
    c. abrasion
    c. astigmatism
    c. corpuscle
    c. decompensation
    c. dystrophy
    c. dystrophy of Snyder
    c. ectasia
    c. endothelial polymorphism
    c. facet
    c. fissure
    c. graft
    c. implant
    c. layer
    c. lens
    c. limbus
    c. margin
    c. pannus
    c. reflex
    c. space
    c. spot
    c. staphyloma
    c. transplantation
    c. trepanation
    c. vertex

cornealis
    arcus c.
Cornelia de Lange syndrome
corneoblepharon
corneocyte envelope
corncosclera
corneoscleral
    c. incision
    c. junction
    c. scissors
corneous
Corner-Allen
    C.-A. test
    C.-A. unit
Corner tampon
corniculate
    c. cartilage
    c. tubercle
corniculopharyngeal ligament
corniculum
cornification
cornified cell
cornmeal agar
cornoid lamella
cornsilk
cornu, pl. **cornua**
    coccygeal c.
    c. posterius
cornual pregnancy
corona
    c. capitis
    c. ciliaris
    c. clinica
    c. dentis
    c. radiata
    c. seborrheica
    c. veneris
coronad
coronal
    c. epispadias
    c. hypospadias
    c. plane
    c. pulp
    c. section
    c. suture
coronarism
coronaritis
coronary
    c. angiography
    c. arteriosclerosis
    c. arteriosclerotic heart disease
    (CAHD)

    c. arteritis
    c. artery
    c. artery aneurysm
    c. artery bypass
    c. artery disease
    c. atherectomy
    c. atherosclerotic heart disease
    (CAHD)
    c. blood flow
    c. bypass
    cafe c.
    c. care unit (CCU)
    c. cataract
    c. endarterectomy
    c. failure
    c. groove
    c. heart disease
    c. insufficiency
    c. intensive care unit (CICU)
    c. ligament
    c. nodal rhythm
    c. node
    c. occlusion
    c. ostial stenosis
    c. perfusion pressure
    c. plexus
    c. sinus
    c. sinus rhythm
    c. steal
    c. sulcus
    c. tendon
    c. thrombosis
    c. valve
    c. vein
coronary-prone behavior
coronata
    Entomophthora c.
coronion
coronoid
    c. fossa
    c. process
coronoidectomy
corpora (*pl. of* corpus)
corporeal
corporis
    tinea c.
corps
    medical c.
corpulence
corpulency
corpulent
corpus, pl. **corpora**

NOTES

corpus *(continued)*
    c. adiposum
    c. albicans
    c. amylaceum
    corpora arenacea
    c. cavernosum
    c. epididymidis
    c. fimbriatum
    c. hemorrhagicum
    corpora lutea cyst
    c. luteum cyst
    c. luteum hormone
    corpora quadrigemina
    c. spongiosum urethrae muliebris
corpuscle
    amnionic c.
    amylaceous c.
    amyloid c.
    articular c.
    axile c.
    axis c.
    basal c.
    Bizzozero c.
    blood c.
    bone c.
    bridge c.
    bulboid c.
    calcareous c.
    cement c.
    chyle c.
    colloid c.
    colostrum c.
    concentrated human red blood c.
    corneal c.
    Dogiel c.
    Donné c.
    dust c.
    Eichhorst c.
    exudation c.
    genital c.
    ghost c.
    Gluge c.
    Golgi c.
    Golgi-Mazzoni c.
    Hassall concentric c.
    inflammatory c.
    lamellated c.
    lymph c.
    lymphatic c.
    lymphoid c.
    malpighian c.
    Mazzoni c.
    Meissner c.
    Merkel c.
    Mexican hat c.
    milk c.
    molluscum c.
    Norris c.
    pacinian c.

    phantom c.
    Purkinje c.
    Rainey c.
    red c.
    renal c.
    Ruffini c.
    tactile c.
    thymic c.
    Traube c.
    white c.
corpuscular
    c. lymph
    c. radiation
corpusculum renis
corrected dextrocardia
corrective emotional experience
corrector
    function c.
correlational method
correlation coefficient
correlative differentiation
Correra line
correspondence
    anomalous retinal c.
    dysharmonious retinal c.
    harmonious retinal c.
Corrigan
    C. disease
    C. pulse
    C. sign
corrigent
corrin
corrodens
    Bacteroides c.
    Eikenella c.
corrosion preparation
corrosive
    c. mercury chloride
    c. poison
    c. sublimate
corrugator
    c. cutis muscle
    c. supercilii muscle
cortex, pl. **cortices**
    adrenal c.
    agranular c.
    association c.
    auditory c.
    cerebellar c.
    c. cerebelli
    cerebral c.
    c. cerebri
    deep c.
    dysgranular c.
    fetal adrenal c.
    frontal c.
    granular c.
    heterotypic c.
    homotypic c.

insular c.
laminated c.
c. lentis
mastoid c.
motor c.
premotor c.
renal c.
c. renalis
sensory c.
somatic sensory c.
somatosensory c.
suprarenal c.
c. thymi
visual c.

Corti
C. arch
C. auditory teeth
C. canal
C. cell
C. ganglion
C. membrane
C. organ
C. pillar
C. rod
C. tunnel

cortical
c. amygdaloid nucleus
c. apraxia
c. arch
c. audiometry
c. blindness
c. bone
c. cataract
c. convexity
c. deafness
c. dysgenesis
c. dysplasia
c. epilepsy
c. fracture
c. hormone
c. implantation
c. lobule
c. mastoidectomy
c. osteitis
c. part
c. radiate artery
c. sensibility
c. substance

corticale
Cryptostroma c.
corticalization
corticalosteotomy

corticectomy
cortices (*pl. of* cortex)
corticifugal
corticipetal
corticoafferent
cortlcobasal degeneration
corticobulbar
c. fiber
c. tract
corticocerebellum
corticoefferent
corticofugal
corticoid
corticomedial
corticomesencephalic fiber
corticonuclear fiber
corticopontine
c. fiber
c. tract
corticoreticular fiber
corticorubral fiber
corticospinal
c. fiber
c. tract
corticosteroid-binding
c.-b. globulin
c.-b. protein
corticosteroid-induced glaucoma
corticosterone
corticothalamic fiber
corticotroph
corticotropic hormone
corticotropin
corticotropin-like intermediate-lobe peptide
corticotropin-releasing
c.-r. factor (CRF)
c.-r. hormone (CRH)
corticotropin-zinc hydroxide
cortilymph
cortisol acetate
cortisone
Corvisart facies
corymbiform
corynebacteriophage
Corynebacterium
C. acnes
C. amycolatum
C. diphtheriae
C. equi
C. glucuronolyticum
C. haemolyticum

NOTES

Corynebacterium (continued)
    C. hofmannii
    C. jeikeium
    C. matruchotii
    C. minutissimum
    C. parvum
    C. pseudodiphtheriticum
    C. striatum
    C. xerosis
coryneform bacteria
coryza
    allergic c.
Cos
    Hippocrates of C.
cosmesis
cosmetic
    c. dermatitis
    c. surgery
cosmetica
    acne c.
cosmic ray
cosmopolitan
costa
    c. cervicalis
    c. lumbalis
    c. prima
costal
    c. angle
    c. arch
    c. arch reflex
    c. cartilage
    c. chondritis
    c. facet
    c. fringe
    c. groove
    c. line
    c. margin
    c. notch
    c. pleura
    c. pleurisy
    c. process
    c. respiration
    c. surface
    c. tuberosity
costalgia
costectomy
Costen syndrome
costicartilage
costiform
costimulatory molecule
costive
costiveness
costoaxillary vein
costocervical
    c. arterial trunk
    c. artery
costochondral
    c. joint

    c. junction
    c. syndrome
costochondritis
costoclavicular
    c. ligament
    c. line
    c. syndrome
costocolic ligament
costocoracoid
costodiaphragmatic recess
costogenic
costoinferior
costomediastinal
    c. recess
    c. sinus
costopectoral reflex
costophrenic
    c. angle
    c. septal line
    c. sulcus
costoscapular
costosternal
costosternoplasty
costosuperior
costotome
costotomy
costotransverse
    c. foramen
    c. joint
    c. ligament
costotransversectomy
costovertebral
    c. angle (CVA)
    c. angle tenderness (CVAT)
    c. joint
costoxiphoid
    c. angle
    c. ligament
cosubstrate
cosyntropin
Cotard syndrome
cotarnine
cot death
COTe
    cathodal opening tetanus
Côte-d'Ivoire
    Ebola virus C.-d.
    C.-d. virus
cothromboplastin
cotranslational
cotransport
Cotte operation
Cotting operation
cotton
    absorbent c.
    C. effect
cotton-dust asthma
cotton-fiber embolism
cotton-mill fever

cottonpox
cotton-root bark
cottonseed oil
cotton-wool
    c.-w. patch
    c.-w. spot
cotunnii
    liquor c.
Cotunnius
    C. aqueduct
    C. canal
    C. liquid
    C. space
cotyle
cotyledon
    fetal c.
    maternal c.
cotyledonary placenta
cotyloid
    c. cavity
    c. joint
    c. ligament
    c. notch
coudé
    c. bougie
    catheter c.
    c. catheter
cough
    aneurysmal c.
    brassy c.
    dry c.
    c. fracture
    habit c.
    productive c.
    c. reflex
    reflex c.
    c. resonance
    whooping c.
coulomb
coulometry
coumaranone
coumaric anhydride
coumarin
Coumel tachycardia
coumetarol
Councilman hyaline body
counseling
    genetic c.
    marital c.
    c. psychology
count
    Addis c.

    Arneth c.
    blood c.
    CD4 c.
    complete blood c. (CBC)
    c. density
    differential white blood c.
    epidermal ridge c.
    filament-nonfilament c.
    c.'s per minute (cpm)
    Schilling blood c.
counter
    automated differential leukocyte c.
    electronic cell c.
    Geiger-Müller c.
    scintillation c.
    c. transference
    whole-body c.
counterbalancing
counterconditioning
countercurrent
    c. distribution
    c. exchanger
    c. mechanism
    c. multiplier
counterextension
counterimmunoelectrophoresis
counterincision
counterinvestment
counterirritant
counterirritation
counteropening
counterphobic
counterpulsation
    intraaortic balloon c.
counterpuncture
countershock, counter-shock
counterstain
countertraction
countertransference
countertransport
counting chamber
coup
    c. de glotte
    c. de sabre
    c. injury
coupled
    c. beats
    c. pulse
    c. rhythm
coupling
    constant c.
    c. defect

C

NOTES

221

coupling *(continued)*
    c. factor
    fixed c.
    c. interval
    c. phase
Cournand dip
course
    postoperative c.
Courvoisier
    C. gallbladder
    C. law
    C. sign
couvade
Couvelaire uterus
couvercle
covalent modification
cove plane
cover
    c. glass
    c. test
coverslip
covert sensitization
cover-uncover test
cow
    c. face
    c. kidney
    c. milk anemia
Cowden disease
Cowdry type A, B inclusion body
Cowling rule
cowl muscle
Cowper
    C. cyst
    C. gland
    C. ligament
cowperian
cowperitis
cowpox virus
coxa
    c. adducta
    c. magna
    c. plana
    c. valga
    c. vara
coxal bone
coxalgia
Coxiella burnetii
coxitic scoliosis
coxitis
coxodynia
coxofemoral
coxotuberculosis
coxsackie
    c. encephalitis
    c. virus
coxsackievirus, coxsackie virus
CPAP
    continuous positive airway pressure

CPEO
    chronic progressive external
      ophthalmoplegia
C-peptide
CPK
    creatine phosphokinase
CPM
    continuous passive motion
cpm
    counts per minute
CPPB
    continuous positive-pressure breathing
CPPD
    calcium pyrophosphate deposition disease
CPPV
    continuous positive pressure ventilation
CPR
    cardiopulmonary resuscitation
cps
    cycles per second
CR
    computed radiography
    CR lead
crab hand
Crabtree effect
crack
    c. cocaine
    lacquer c.
cracked heel
cracked-pot
    c.-p. resonance
    c.-p. sound
crackle
crackling
    c. jaw
    c. rale
cradle cap
Crafoord clamp
Cramer wire splint
cramp
    heat c.'s
    intermittent c.
    miner's c.'s
Crampton
    C. line
    C. muscle
    C. test
Crandall syndrome
crania *(pl. of* cranium*)*
craniad
cranial
    c. arachnoid mater
    c. arteritis
    c. base
    c. bone
    c. bruit
    c. capacity
    c. cavity
    c. dura mater

c. dystonia
c. extradural space
c. flexure
c. fontanelle
c. index
c. nerve
c. neuralgia
c. neuropore
c. pia mater
c. polyneuritis
c. root
c. sinus
c. suture
c. synchondrosis
c. synovial joint
c. vault
c. vertebra
cranialis
dura mater c.
craniamphitomy
craniectomy
linear c.
cranio-aural
craniocardiac reflex
craniocarpotarsal
c. dysplasia
c. dystrophy
craniocele
craniocerebral
cranioclasia
cranioclasis
cranioclast
craniocleidodysostosis
craniodiaphysial dysplasia
craniodidymus
craniofacial
c. angle
c. appliance
c. axis
c. cleft
c. dysjunction fracture
c. dysostosis
c. fixation
c. hypoplasia
c. surgery
c. suspension wiring
craniofenestria
craniognomy
craniograph
craniography
craniolacunia
craniology

craniomalacia
circumscribed c.
craniomeningocele
craniometaphysial dysplasia
craniometer
craniometric point
craniometry
craniopathy
metabolic c.
craniopharyngeal
c. canal
c. duct
craniopharyngioma
ameloblastomatous c.
cystic papillomatous c.
craniophore
cranioplasty
craniopuncture
craniorrhachidian
craniorrhachischisis
craniosacral
c. division
c. nervous system
c. therapy
cranioschisis
craniosclerosis
cranioscopy
craniospinal sensory ganglion
craniostenosis
craniostosis
craniosynostosis
craniotabes
craniotome
craniotomy
attached c.
detached c.
c. scissors
craniotonoscopy
craniotrypesis
craniotympanic
cranium, pl. **crania**
bifid c.
c. bifidum
cerebral c.
c. cerebrale
c. viscerale
crank test
crapulent
crapulous
crash cart
crassamentum

NOTES

223

crassus
  pannus c.
crater arc
crateriform
craterization
cravat bandage
craw-craw
crazing
C-reactive protein
cream
  cleansing c.
  cold c.
  greaseless c.
  leukocyte c.
  lubricating c.
  c. of tartar
crease
  digital flexion c.
  ear lobe c.
  flexion c.
  c. wound
creatinase
creatine
  c. kinase (CK)
  c. kinase isoenzyme
  c. phosphate
  c. phosphokinase (CPK)
creatinemia
creatininase
creatinine
  c. clearance
  c. coefficient
creatinuria
creative thinking
Credé
  C. maneuver
  C. method
credentialing
creeping
  c. eruption
  c. thrombosis
creep recovery
cremasteric
  c. artery
  c. fascia
  c. reflex
cremaster muscle
cremnocele
cremnophobia
crena, pl. **crenae**
crenate
crenated cell
crenation
crenocyte
crenocytosis
creola body
creophagism
creophagy
creosol

creosote
crepitant rale
crepitation
crepitus
  articular c.
  bony c.
crescendo
  c. angina
  c. murmur
crescent
  articular c.
  c. cell
  c. cell anemia
  Giannuzzi c.
  glomerular c.
  Heidenhain c.
  c. incision
  malarial c.
  myopic c.
  scleral c.
  c. sign
crescentic lobule
crescograph
cresolase
cresol red
CREST
  calcinosis, Raynaud phenomenon,
    esophageal motility disorder,
    sclerodactyly, and telangiectasia
    CREST syndrome
crest
  acoustic c.
  alveolar c.
  ampullary c.
  anterior lacrimal c.
  arched c.
  arcuate c.
  articular c.
  basal c.
  buccinator c.
  conchal c.
  deltoid c.
  dental c.
  ethmoidal c.
  external occipital c.
  falciform c.
  frontal c.
  ganglionic c.
  gingival c.
  gluteal c.
  iliac c.
  incisor c.
  infratemporal c.
  inguinal c.
  intermediate sacral c.
  internal occipital c.
  interosseous c.
  intertrochanteric c.
  interureteric c.

lateral epicondylar c.
lateral sacral c.
lateral supracondylar c.
marginal c.
medial epicondylar c.
medial supracondylar c.
median sacral c.
nasal c.
neural c.
obturator c.
palatine c.
posterior lacrimal c.
pubic c.
sacral c.
sphenoid c.
supramastoid c.
supraventricular c.
urethral c.
vestibular c.
Cresylecht violet stain
cretin
cretinism
cretinistic
cretinoid
cretinous
Creutzfeldt-Jakob disease
crevice
gingival c.
crevicular
c. epithelium
c. fluid
CRF
cardiac risk factor
corticotropin-releasing factor
CRH
corticotropin-releasing hormone
crib
c. death
tongue c.
crib-biting
criblé
état c.
cribra (*pl. of* cribrum)
cribrate
cribration
cribriform
c. area
c. carcinoma
c. fascia
c. foramen
c. hymen
c. plate

cribrous lamina
cribrum, pl. **cribra**
cricoarytenoid
c. articular capsule
c. articulation
c. joint
c. ligament
cricoesophageal tendon
cricoid
c. cartilage
c. split operation
cricoidynia
cricopharyngeal
c. achalasia
c. ligament
c. myotomy
cricopharyngeus muscle
cricosantorinian ligament
cricothyroid
c. artery
c. articular capsule
c. articulation
c. branch
c. joint
c. membrane
c. muscle
cricothyroideus
cricothyroidotomy
cricothyrotomy
cricotomy
cricotracheal
c. ligament
c. membrane
cricovocal membrane
cri-du-chat syndrome, cri du chat syndrome
Crigler-Najjar
C.-N. disease
C.-N. syndrome
Crile clamp
Crile-Matas operation
Crimean-Congo
C.-C. hemorrhagic fever
C.-C. hemorrhagic fever virus
Crimean fever
criminal
c. abortion
c. anthropology
c. hygiene
c. insanity
c. irresponsibility
c. psychology

NOTES

criminology
crinin
crinium
    fragilitas c.
crinogenic
crinophagy
crippled
crisis, pl. crises
    addisonian c.
    adolescent c.
    adrenal c.
    anaphylactoid c.
    blast c.
    blood c.
    Dietl c.
    ego c.
    febrile c.
    gastric c.
    gender c.
    glaucomatocyclitic c.
    hemolytic c.
    hypertensive c.
    identity c.
    c. intervention
    laryngeal c.
    midlife c.
    otolithic c.
    sexual c.
    sickle cell c.
    therapeutic c.
    thyroid c.
    thyrotoxic c.
crispation
crispatum
    Eubacterium c.
crispatus
    Lactobacillus c.
crisscross heart
criteria, sing. criterion
    Amsel c.
    Hill c.
    Jones c.
    Spiegelberg c.
criterion-related validity
critical
    c. angle
    c. appraisal
    c. care unit (CCU)
    c. flicker fusion frequency
    c. illness polyneuropathy
    c. illumination
    c. incident stress management
    c. limit
    c. micelle concentration
    c. organ
    c. pathway
    c. period
    c. pH
    c. point

    c. pressure
    c. rate
    c. temperature
CRL
    crown-rump length
CRM
    cross-reacting material
cRNA
    complementary ribonucleic acid
crocodile
    c. tears
    c. tears syndrome
Crocq disease
Crohn disease
cromolyn sodium
Cronkhite-Canada syndrome
Crooke
    C. granule
    C. hyaline change
    C. hyaline degeneration
Crookes glass
Crookes-Hittorf tube
Crosby capsule
cross
    c. agglutination
    back c.
    c. circulation
    c. flap
    c. hybridization
    c. infection
    maltese c.
    c. mating
    c. section
    c. tolerance
crossbite tooth
crossbreed
cross-cultural psychiatry
cross-cut bur
cross-dressing
crossed
    c. adductor jerk
    c. adductor reflex
    c. amblyopia
    c. anesthesia
    c. aphasia
    c. cylinder
    c. diplopia
    c. embolism
    c. extension reflex
    c. eyes
    c. fixation
    c. hemianesthesia
    c. hemianopia
    c. hemiplegia
    c. immunoelectrophoresis
    c. knee jerk
    c. knee reflex
    c. laterality
    c. paralysis

c. pyramidal tract
c. renal ectopia
c. spino-adductor reflex
c. testicular ectopia

cross-eye
cross-hybridisation
crossing a bridge
crossing-over
somatic c.-o.
cross-level bias
cross-link
cross-linked
c.-l. polymer
c.-l. resin
cross-matching
crossover study
cross-reacting
c.-r. agglutinin
c.-r. antibody
c.-r. material (CRM)
cross-reaction
cross-section
cross-sectional
c.-s. echocardiography
c.-s. method
c.-s. study
cross-table lateral projection
cross-taper
crossway
crotalaria poisoning
crotalin
crotalism
Crotalus
C. antitoxin
C. toxin
crotamiton
crotaphion
crotonase
croton oil
crotonyl-ACP reductase
crotoxin
crottle
croup
croup-associated virus
croupous
c. bronchitis
c. laryngitis
c. lymph
c. membrane
croupy

Crouzon
C. disease
C. syndrome
crowding phenomenon
Crowe-Davis mouth gag
Crow-Fukase syndrome
crowing inspiration
crown
anatomic c.
anatomical c.
artificial c.
bell-shaped c.
c. cavity
ciliary c.
clinical c.
c. flask
c. glass
jacket c.
c. pulp
radiate c.
c. saw
c. tubercle
crown-heel length (CHL)
crowning
crown-rump length (CRL)
CRT
cathode ray tube
cruces (*pl. of* crux)
crucial
c. anastomosis
c. bandage
c. ligament
cruciate
c. anastomosis
c. eminence
c. incision
c. ligament
c. muscle
crucible
cruciform
c. eminence
c. ligament
c. loops
c. pulley
c. suture
crude
c. calcium sulfide
c. death rate
c. drug
c. urine
crufomate

NOTES

crunch
    mediastinal c.
crura (*pl. of* crus)
crural
    c. arch
    c. fascia
    c. fossa
    c. hernia
    c. interosseous nerve
    c. ligament
    c. ring
    c. septum
    c. sheath
    c. triangle
crureus
cruris
    angina c.
    fascia c.
    tinea c.
crus, pl. **crura**
    ampullary c.
    lateral c.
    medial c.
    c. penis
crush
    c. kidney
    c. syndrome
crusotomy
crust
    milk c.
crusta lactea
crusted
    c. ringworm
    c. scabies
crutch
    c. palsy
    c. paralysis
Cruveilhier
    C. disease
    C. fascia
    C. fossa
    C. joint
    C. ligament
    C. plexus
    C. ulcer
Cruveilhier-Baumgarten
    C.-B. disease
    C.-B. murmur
    C.-B. sign
    C.-B. syndrome
crux, pl. **cruces**
    cruces pilorum
Cruz trypanosomiasis
cryalgesia
cryanesthesia
cryesthesia
cry for help
crymodynia
crymophilic

crymophylactic
cryoanesthesia
cryobiology
cryocautery
cryoconization
cryoextraction
cryoextractor
cryofibrinogen
cryofibrinogenemia
cryofluorane
cryofracture
cryogen
cryogenic
cryogenics
cryoglobulin
cryoglobulinemia
cryohydrate
cryohypophysectomy
cryokinetics
cryolysis
cryometer
cryopallidectomy
cryopathy
cryopexy
cryophilic
cryophylactic
cryoprecipitability
cryoprecipitate
cryoprecipitation
cryopreservation
cryoprobe
cryoprostatectomy
cryoprotein
cryopulvinectomy
cryoscope
cryoscopy
cryospasm
cryostat
cryosurgery
cryothalamectomy
cryotherapy
cryotolerant
crypt
    c. abscess
    anal c.
    dental c.
    enamel c.
    c. of Lieberkühn
    lingual c.
    synovial c.
    tonsillar c.
cryptectomy
cryptic
cryptitis
cryptochrome
cryptococcoma
cryptococcosis
Cryptococcus
cryptocrystalline

cryptodidymus
cryptogenic
    c. cirrhosis
    c. epilepsy
    c. fibrosing alveolitis
    c. infection
    c. pyemia
    c. septicemia
cryptolith
cryptomenorrhea
cryptophthalmia
cryptophthalmus syndrome
cryptopodia
cryptopyrrole
cryptorchidism
cryptorchidopexy
cryptorchid testis
cryptorchism
cryptoscope
cryptosporidiosis
Cryptosporidium parvum
Cryptostroma corticale
cryptotia
cryptoxanthin
cryptozoite
cryptozygous
crystal
    asthma c.
    blood c.
    Böttcher c.
    Charcot-Leyden c.
    Charcot-Neumann c.
    Charcot-Robin c.
    chiral c.
    clathrate c.
    ear c.
    Florence c.
    hematoidin c.
    hydrate c.
    knife-rest c.
    Leyden c.
    Lubarsch c.
    c. rash
    c. structure
    Teichmann c.
    c. violet
    c. violet vaccine
crystallin
    gamma c.
crystallina
    miliaria c.

crystalline
    c. capsule
    c. cataract
    c. digitalin
    c. insulin zinc suspension
    c. interface
    c. lens
crystallization
crystallized trypsin
crystallogram
crystallography
crystalloid
    Charcot-Böttcher c.
crystallophobia
crystalluria
C&S
    culture and sensitivity
C-section
CSF
    cerebrospinal fluid
    colony-stimulating factor
CT
    computed tomography
        dynamic CT
        helical CT
        CT number
        CT pelvimetry
        CT scan
        CT unit
CTAP
    clear to auscultation and percussion
Cuban itch
cube pessary
cubic
    c. centimeter
    c. niter
cubital
    c. anastomosis
    c. bone
    c. fossa
    c. joint
    c. lymph node
    c. nerve
    c. tunnel syndrome
cubitus
    c. valgus
    c. varus
cuboidal
    c. articular surface
    c. carcinoma
    c. epithelium
cuboid bone

NOTES

C

cuboideonavicular
>   c. joint
>   c. ligament

cuboidodigital reflex

cudbear

cued speech

cuff
>   rotator c.
>   vaginal c.

cuffing

cuirass
>   analgesic c.
>   c. respirator
>   c. ventilator

cuirasse
>   cancer en c.

cul-de-sac
>   conjunctival c.-d.-s.
>   Douglas c.-d.-s.
>   greater c.-d.-s.
>   Gruber c.-d.-s.
>   lesser c.-d.-s.
>   c.-d.-s. smear

culdocentesis

culdoplasty

culdoscope

culdoscopy

culdotomy

Culex
>   *C. nigripalpus*
>   *C. restuans*
>   *C. salinarius*

culicidal

culicide

culicifuge

Cullen sign

culmen, pl. **culmina**

Culp pyeloplasty

cultivated yeast

cultivation

cultural
>   c. anthropology
>   c. diversity
>   c. shock

culture
>   batch c.
>   cell c.
>   continuous c.
>   discontinuous c.
>   elective c.
>   enrichment c.
>   hanging-block c.
>   Harada-Mori filter paper strip c.
>   c. medium
>   mixed lymphocyte c.
>   monoxenic c.
>   organ c.
>   Petri dish c.
>   plastic envelope c.

>   pouch c.
>   pure c.
>   c. and sensitivity (C&S)
>   slant c.
>   smear c.
>   stab c.
>   stock c.
>   streak c.
>   tissue c.
>   type c.
>   xenic c.

Culver root

cumarin

cumetharol

Cummer
>   C. classification
>   C. guideline

cumulative
>   c. action
>   c. dose
>   c. effect
>   C. Index Medicus
>   c. trauma disorder

cuneate
>   c. fasciculus
>   c. funiculus
>   c. nucleus
>   c. tubercle

cuneiform
>   c. bone
>   c. cartilage
>   c. cataract
>   c. lobe
>   c. nucleus
>   c. part
>   c. tubercle

cuneocerebellar
>   c. fiber
>   c. tract

cuneocuboid
>   c. interosseous ligament
>   c. joint

cuneometatarsal
>   c. interosseous ligament
>   c. joint

cuneonavicular
>   c. articulation
>   c. joint
>   c. ligament

cuneoscaphoid

cuneospinal fiber

cuneus

cuniculatum
>   epithelioma c.

cuniculi
>   *Encephalitozoon c.*

cuniculus

cunnilingus

cup
 acetabular c.
 c. biopsy forceps
 dry c.
 eye c.
 glaucomatous c.
 optic c.
cup:disc ratio
Cupid's bow
cupola
cupping glass
cupric
 c. acetate
 c. acetate normal
 c. arsenite
 c. chloride
 c. citrate
 c. sulfate
cupriuresis
cupula, pl. **cupulae**
 ampullary c.
 cochlear c.
cupular
 c. blind sac
 c. cecum
cupulate
cupuliform cataract
cupulogram
cupulolithiasis
curage
curantur
 similia similibus c.
curare
 calabash c.
curariform
curarimimetic
curarine
curarization
curative dose
curb tenotomy
curcumin
curd soap
curdy pus
curet (*var. of* curette)
curetment
curettage
 diagnostic dilatation and c.
 dilatation and c. (D&C)
 dilation and c. (D&C)
 fractional dilatation and c.
 periapical c.

 subgingival c.
 suction dilatation and c.
curette, curet
 Hartmann c.
curettement
curie
curing
 dental c.
curium
curlicue ureter
Curling ulcer
currant
 c. jelly clot
 c. jelly stool
 c. jelly thrombus
currens
 larva c.
current
 action c.
 alternating c.
 anodal c.
 ascending c.
 axial c.
 centrifugal c.
 centripetal c.
 d'Arsonval c.
 demarcation c.
 descending c.
 direct c. (DC)
 electrotonic c.
 galvanic c.
 high-frequency c.
 c. of injury
 labile c.
Curschmann spiral
curse
 Ondine c.
curtain
 aortic c.
curvature
 c. aberration
 angular c.
 anterior c.
 backward c.
 gingival c.
 greater c.
 c. hyperopia
 lateral c.
 lesser c.
 c. myopia
 Pott c.
 spinal c.

NOTES

C

231

curvatus
  Lactobacillus c.
curve
  active length-tension c.
  alignment c.
  anti-Monson c.
  Barnes c.
  bell-shaped c.
  buccal c.
  calibration c.
  Carus c.
  cephalic c.
  characteristic c.
  compensating c.
  distribution c.
  dose-response c.
  dye-dilution c.
  epidemic c.
  flow-volume c.
  force-velocity c.
  Frank-Starling c.
  frequency c.
  Friedman c.
  gaussian c.
  growth c.
  H and D c.
  Heidelberger c.
  Hunter and Driffield c.
  indicator-dilution c.
  intracardiac pressure c.
  isovolume pressure-flow c.
  labor c.
  logistic c.
  milled-in c.
  c. of occlusion
  oxyhemoglobin dissociation c.
  Price-Jones c.
  c. of Spee
  Starling c.
  tension c.
  Traube-Hering c.
  tuning c.
  von Spee c.
  c. of Wilson
curvus
  carpus c.
Cushing
  C. disease
  C. effect
  C. phenomenon
  C. pituitary basophilism
  C. response
  C. suture
  C. syndrome
  C. syndrome medicamentosus
  C. ulcer
cushingoid appearance
cushion
  anal c.

  atrioventricular canal c.
  endocardial c.
  eustachian c.
  hemorrhoidal c.
  levator c.
cusp
  c. angle
  anterior c.
  ballooning mitral c.
  Carabelli c.
  c. and groove pattern
  c. height
  c. ridge
  supporting c.
cuspad
cuspal interference
cuspidate tooth
cuspid tooth
custodial care
cutaneomeningospinal angiomatosis
cutaneomucosal
cutaneomucouveal syndrome
cutaneous
  c. absorption
  c. albinism
  c. ancylostomiasis
  c. anergy
  c. anthrax
  c. blastomycosis
  c. branch
  c. cervical nerve
  c. diphtheria
  c. emphysema
  c. focal mucinosis
  c. gangrene
  c. gland
  c. graft versus host reaction
  c. hemorrhoid
  c. horn
  c. larva migrans
  c. leishmaniasis
  c. leishmaniasis granuloma
  c. leprosy
  c. loop ureterostomy
  c. lupus erythematosus
  c. meningioma
  c. muscle
  c. pseudolymphoma
  c. pupil reflex
  c. schistosomiasis japonica
  c. suture
  c. tuberculin test
  c. tuberculosis
  c. vasculitis
  c. vein
  c. vesicostomy
cutaneous-pupillary reflex
cutdown

cuticle
    acquired enamel c.
    dental c.
    enamel c.
cuticula, pl. **cuticulae**
cuticular
    c. drusen
    c. suture
cutireaction
cutis
    amebiasis c.
    amyloidosis c.
    c. anserina
    asteatosis c.
    atrophia c.
    benign lymphocytoma c.
    carotenosis c.
    carotinosis c.
    leiomyoma c.
    leukemia c.
    c. marmorata
    c. marmorata telangiectatica
      congenita
    neuroma c.
    osteoma c.
    osteosis c.
    c. plate
    c. rhomboidalis nuchae
    c. vera
cutization
cutpoint
cutting
    c. edge
    c. forceps
    c. loop
    c. needle
    c. teeth
cuttlefish disc
cuvet, cuvette
    c. oximeter
Cuvier
    C. duct
    C. vein
CV
    cardiovascular
    coefficient of variation
CVA
    cerebrovascular accident
    costovertebral angle
CVAT
    costovertebral angle tenderness

CVP
    central venous pressure
cyanalcohol
cyanamide
cyanate
cyanemia
cyanide
    hydrogen c.
    c. methemoglobin
    c. poisoning
cyanide-nitroprusside test
cyanidenon
cyanin
    alizarin c.
cyaniventris
    Dermatobia c.
cyanmethemoglobin
Cyanobacteria
cyanobacteriumlike body
cyanochrous
cyanocobalamin
cyanogen chloride
cyanogenic glycoside
cyanohydrin
cyanophil, cyanophile
cyanophilous
cyanopia
cyanopsia
cyanosed
cyanose tardive
cyanosis
    compression c.
    enterogenous c.
    false c.
    hereditary methemoglobinemic c.
    late c.
    tardive c.
cyanotic
    c. asphyxia
    c. atrophy
    c. induration
cyanuria
cyanuric acid
cybernetics
cybrid
cyclamate
cyclamide
cyclandelate
cyclarthrodial
cyclarthrosis

NOTES

cyclase
    adenyl c.
    adenylate c.
cycle
    alanine-glucose c.
    anovulatory c.
    brain wave c.
    carbon dioxide c.
    cardiac c.
    cell c.
    chewing c.
    citric acid c.
    Cori c.
    dicarboxylic acid c.
    duty c.
    endogenous c.
    erythrocytic c.
    estrous c.
    exoerythrocytic c.
    exogenous c.
    fatty acid oxidation c.
    forced c.
    futile c.
    glycine-succinate c.
    glyoxylic acid c.
    gonadotrophic c.
    hair c.
    heterogonic life c.
    homogonic life c.
    Krebs-Henseleit c.
    Krebs-Kornberg c.
    Krebs ornithine c.
    Krebs urea c.
    c. length alternans
    life c.
    masticating c.
    menstrual c.
    mitotic c.
    nitrogen c.
    ovarian c.
    pain-spasm-ischemia c.
    pain-spasm-pain c.
    c.'s per second (cps)
    reproductive c.
    tricarboxylic acid c.
    urea c.
cyclectomy
cyclencephalia
cyclencephaly
cycle-specific agent
cyclic
    c. AMP
    c. compound
    c. vomiting
cyclin D
cyclist's
    c. nipples
    c. palsy

cyclitis
    Fuchs heterochromic c.
    heterochromic c.
cyclocephalia
cyclocephaly
cyclochoroiditis
cyclocryotherapy
cyclocumarol
cyclodestructive
cyclodialysis
cyclodiathermy
cycloduction
cycloguanil pamoate
cycloheximide
cycloid
cyclopeptide
cyclophorase
cyclophoria
cyclophotocoagulation
cyclopia
cyclopian eye
cycloplegia
cycloplegic
cyclopropane
cyclops
cycloserine
cyclosis
cyclosporin A
cyclosporine effect
cyclothiazide
cyclothymia
cyclothymiac
cyclothymic
    c. personality
    c. personality disorder
cyclotomy
cyclotorsion
cyclotron
cyclotropia
cyclozoonosis
cyesis
cylinder
    Bence Jones c.
    crossed c.
    Külz c.
    c. retinoscopy
cylindraxis
cylindrical
    c. bronchiectasis
    c. epithelium
    c. joint
    c. lens
cylindroadenoma
cylindroid aneurysm
cylindroma
cylindromatous carcinoma
cylindruria
cyllosoma
cymarin

cymbocephalic
cymbocephalous
cymbocephaly
cynanthropy
cynic spasm
cynocephaly
cynodont
cynophobia
Cyon nerve
cypionate
  estradiol c.
cypridophobia
cyst
  adventitious c.
  allantoic c.
  alveolar hydatid c.
  aneurysmal bone c.
  angioblastic c.
  apical periodontal c.
  apoplectic c.
  arachnoid c.
  Baker c.
  Bartholin c.
  bile c.
  blood c.
  blue dome c.
  bone c.
  botryoid odontogenic c.
  Boyer c.
  branchial cleft c.
  bronchogenic c.
  bursal c.
  calcifying and keratinizing
    odontogenic c.
  cerebellar c.
  chocolate c.
  choledochal c.
  chyle c.
  colloid c.
  compound c.
  corpora lutea c.
  corpus luteum c.
  Cowper c.
  daughter c.
  dentigerous c.
  dentinal lamina c.
  dermoid c.
  distention c.
  duplication c.
  Echinococcus c.
  endodermal c.
  endometrial c.

  endothelial c.
  enterogenous c.
  ependymal c.
  epidermal c.
  epidermoid c.
  epithelial c.
  eruption c.
  extravasation c.
  exudation c.
  false c.
  fissural c.
  follicular c.
  ganglion c.
  Gartner c.
  gas c.
  gingival c.
  globulomaxillary c.
  glomerular c.
  Gorlin c.
  granddaughter c.
  hemorrhagic c.
  hepatic c.
  heterotrophic oral gastrointestinal c.
  hydatid c.
  hymenal c.
  implantation c.
  incisive canal c.
  inclusion c.
  junctional c.
  keratinizing odontogenic c.
  keratinous c.
  Klestadt c.
  lacteal c.
  lateral periodontal c.
  leptomeningeal c.
  lymphoepithelial c.
  median anterior maxillary c.
  median palatal c.
  median raphe c.
  meibomian c.
  milk c.
  morgagnian c.
  mother c.
  mucous c.
  multilocular c.
  myxoid c.
  nabothian c.
  nasoalveolar c.
  nasopalatine c.
  neurenteric c.
  odontogenic c.
  osseous hydatid c.

NOTES

cyst *(continued)*
ovarian c.
parasitic c.
parent c.
pericardial c.
pilar c.
pilonidal c.
radicular c.
Rathke cleft c.
retention c.
sebaceous c.
serous c.
solitary bone c.
sterile c.
sublingual c.
sudoriferous c.
synovial c.
Tarlov c.
tarry c.
tarsal c.
Tornwaldt c.
tubular c.
unicameral bone c.
unilocular c.
vitellointestinal c.
wolffian c.
cystacanth
cystadenocarcinoma
cystadenoma
pseudomucinous c.
serous c.
cystalgia
cystamine
cystathionase
cystathionine
cysteamine
cystectasia
cystectasy
cystectomy
Bartholin c.
cysteic acid
cysteine
cystic
c. acne
c. adenomatoid malformation
c. artery
c. bronchiectasis
c. carcinoma
c. cataract
c. diathesis
c. disease
c. duct cholangiography
c. emphysema
c. fibrosis
c. gall duct
c. goiter
c. hygroma
c. kidney
c. lung

c. lymphangiectasis
c. lymph node
c. mastitis
c. medial necrosis
c. mole
c. node
c. papillomatous craniopharyngioma
c. polyp
c. prostatic hyperplasia
c. teratoma
c. vein
cystica
cystitis c.
osteitis fibrosa c.
spina bifida c.
cysticercoid
cysticercosis
Cysticercus
C. bovis
C. cellulosae
cysticercus disease
cysticum
epithelioma adenoides c.
cystiform
cystine
c. bridge
c. calculus
half c.
c. lyase
c. storage disease
cystinemia
cystinosis
cystinotic leukocyte
cystinuria
cystinyl
cystistaxis
cystitis
allergic c.
bacterial c.
c. colli
c. cystica
emphysematous c.
eosinophilic c.
follicular c.
gangrenous c.
c. glandularis
hemorrhagic c.
incrusted c.
interstitial c.
papillary c.
subacute c.
submucous c.
cystoadenoma
cystocarcinoma
cystocele
cystochromoscopy
cystoduodenal ligament
cystoduodenostomy
pancreatic c.

cystoenterocele
cystoenterostomy
cystoepiplocele
cystoepithelioma
cystofibroma
cystogastrostomy
cystogram
    excretory c.
    gravity c.
    voiding c.
cystography
    antegrade c.
cystohepatic triangle
cystoid
    c. macular edema
    c. maculopathy
cystojejunostomy
cystolith
cystolithiasis
cystolithic
cystolitholapaxy
cystolithotomy
cystoma
cystometer
cystometrogram (CMG)
cystometrography
cystometry
cystomorphous
cystomyoma
cystomyxoadenoma
cystomyxoma
cystopanendoscopy
cystoparalysis
cystopexy
cystophotography
cystoplasty
cystoplegia
cystoprostatectomy
cystoptosia
cystoptosis
cystopyelitis
cystopyelonephritis
cystorectostomy
cystorrhaphy
cystorrhea
cystosarcoma phyllodes
cystoscope
cystoscopic urography
cystoscopy
cystospasm
cystostomy
cystotome

cystotomy
    suprapubic c.
cystoureteritis
cystoureterogram
cystoureterography
cystourethritis
cystourethrocele
cystourethrogram
    micturating c.
    retrograde c.
    voiding c.
cystourethrography
cystourethroscope
cytapheresis
cytarabine
cytase
cythemolytic icterus
cytidine
cytidylic acid
cytisine
cytoanalyzer
cytoarchitectonics
cytoarchitectural
cytoarchitecture
cytobiology
cytobiotaxis
cytocentrum
cytochalasin
cytochemistry
cytochrome
    c. aa3
    c. b
    c. b5
    c. b5 reductase
    c. c
    c. cd
    c. c3 hydrogenase
    c. c oxidase
    c. c reductase
    c. c2 reductase
    c. oxidase *Pseudomonas*
    c. P-450 system
cytochylema
cytocidal
cytocide
cytoclasis
cytoclastic
cytoclesis
cytocrine secretion
cytocuprein
cytocyst
cytodiagnosis

C

NOTES

cytodieresis
cytogene
cytogenesis
cytogeneticist
cytogenetic map
cytogenetics
cytogenic reproduction
cytogenous
cytoglucopenia
cytoid body
cytokeratin filament
cytokine network
cytokinesis
cytolemma
cytolipin
cytologic
    c. examination
    c. filter preparation
    c. screening
    c. smear
    c. specimen
cytologist
cytology
    exfoliative c.
cytolysin
cytolysis
cytolysosome
cytolytic
cytomatrix
cytomegalic
    c. cell
    c. inclusion disease
Cytomegalovirus (CMV)
cytomegalovirus disease
cytomembrane
cytomere
cytometaplasia
cytometer
    image c.
cytometry
    Feulgen c.
    flow c.
cytomicrosome
cytomorphology
cytomorphosis
cytopathic effect
cytopathogenic virus
cytopathologic
cytopathological
cytopathologist
cytopathology
cytopathy
cytopempsis
cytopenia
cytophagic histiocytic panniculitis
cytophagous
cytophagy
cytophanere
cytopharynx

cytophil group
cytophilic antibody
cytophotometry
    flow c.
cytophylactic
cytophylaxis
cytophyletic
cytopipette
cytoplasm
    ground-glass c.
cytoplasmic
    c. bridge
    c. inclusion body
    c. inheritance
    c. matrix
cytoplasmon
cytoplast
cytopoiesis
cytopreparation
cytoprotective agent
cytopyge
cytoreductive therapy
cytoryctes, cytorrhyctes
cytoscreener
cytosides
cytosine
    c. arabinoside
    c. ribonucleoside
cytosis
cytoskeleton
cytosmear
cytosol
cytosolic
cytosome
cytostasis
cytostatic chemotherapy
cytostome
cytotactic
cytotaxia
cytotaxis
cytotechnologist
cytothesis
cytotonic enterotoxin
cytotoxic
    c. cell
    c. chemotherapy
    c. reaction
cytotoxicity
    antibody-dependent cell-mediated c.
    lymphocyte-mediated c.
cytotoxin
    vero c.
cytotrophoblast
cytotrophoblastic
    c. cell
    c. shell
cytotropic
    c. antibody
    c. antibody test

cytotropism
cytozoic
cytozoon
cyturia
Czapek-Dox medium
Czapek solution agar

CZE
    capillary zone electrophoresis
Czerny
    C. operation
    C. suture
Czerny-Lembert suture

NOTES

C

δ (*var. of* delta)
D
    D antigen
    D cell
    D enzyme
    D loop
    D wave
D2
    vitamin D2
D3
    vitamin D3
Daae disease
dacarbazine
    Adriamycin, bleomycin, vinblastine,
      and d. (ABVD)
dacryadenitis
dacryoadenitis
dacryoblennorrhea
dacryocele
dacryocyst
dacryocystalgia
dacryocystectomy
dacryocystitis
dacryocystocele
dacryocystogram
dacryocystography
dacryocystorhinostomy
dacryocystotomy
dacryocyte
dacryohemorrhea
dacryolith
    Desmarres d.
dacryolithiasis
dacryon
dacryops
dacryopyorrhea
dacryorrhea
dacryostenosis
dactinomycin
dactyl
dactylalgia
Dactylaria
dactylitis
    blistering distal d.
dactylocampsis
dactylocampsodynia
dactylodynia
dactylogryposis
dactylology
dactylomegaly
dactyloscopy
dactylospasm
dactylus
dacuronium
Da Fano stain

dahlia
dahlin
dahllite
daily dose
Dakin
    D. fluid
    D. solution
Dakin-Carrel treatment
Dale-Feldberg law
Dalen-Fuchs nodule
Dale reaction
Dalgarno
Dalrymple sign
dalton
Dalton-Henry law
daltonian
daltonism
Dalton law
DALY
    disability-adjusted life year
dam
    d. methylase
    D. unit
damage
    diffuse alveolar d.
dammar
dAMP
    deoxyadenylic acid
d-amphetamine
    d-a. phosphate
    d-a. sulfate
damping
dampness
Damus-Kaye-Stancel procedure
Damus-Stancel-Kaye anastomosis
Dana operation
danazol
dance
    hilar d.
    Saint Anthony d.
    Saint John d.
    Saint Vitus d.
    D. sign
dancing chorea
dander
dandruff
dandy
    d. fever
    D. operation
Dandy-Walker syndrome
Dane
    D. particle
    D. stain
Danforth sign
dangle foot

D

Danielssen-Boeck disease
Danielssen disease
dantrolene sodium
Danubian endemic familial nephropathy
Danysz phenomenon
DA pregnancy test
dapsone neuropathy
d'Arcet metal
Darier
> D. disease
> D. sign

dark
> d. adaptation
> d. cell
> d. reaction

dark-adapted eye
dark-field
> d.-f. condenser
> d.-f. illumination
> d.-f. microscope

dark-ground illumination
Darling disease
Darrow red
d'Arsonval
> d. current
> d. galvanometer

dartoic tissue
dartoid
dartos
> d. fascia
> d. muliebris
> d. muscle

darwinian
> d. ear
> d. evolution
> d. reflex
> d. theory
> d. tubercle

data
> d. dictionary
> objective assessment d.
> d. processing
> subjective assessment d.

date
> d. of birth (DOB)
> d. boil
> d. of death (DOD)
> d. fever

datum plane
Datura
> D. metel
> D. poisoning
> D. stramonium

daturine
Daubenton
> D. angle
> D. line
> D. plane

daughter
> d. cell
> d. colony
> d. cyst
> DES d.
> diethylstilbestrol d.
> d. isotope
> d. star

daunomycin
daunorubicin
David
> lyre of D.

Davidoff cell
Davidson syringe
Daviel
> D. operation
> D. spoon

Davies disease
Davis
> D. graft
> D. interlocking sound

dawn phenomenon
Dawson encephalitis
day
> d. blindness
> d. hospital
> d. residue
> d. sight
> d. surgery
> D. test

5-day fever
3-day measles
dazzling glare
dB
> decibel

DC
> direct current

D&C
> dilatation and curettage
> dilation and curettage

d-digitoxose
d-dimer
D-dimer test
D&E
> dilatation and evacuation
> dilation and evacuation

de
> d. Clerambault syndrome
> d. Lange syndrome
> D. Morgan spot
> d. Morsier syndrome
> d. Musset sign
> d. novo
> d. Pezzer catheter
> d. Quervain disease
> d. Quervain tenosynovitis
> d. Quervain thyroiditis
> D. Sanctis-Cacchione syndrome
> d. Wecker scissors

deacetylase
  acetylornithine d.
deacidification
deactivation
deacylase
dead
  d. arm syndrome
  d. fetus syndrome
  d. finger
  d. nerve
  d. on arrival (DOA)
  d. pulp
  d. space
  d. tooth
  d. tract
dead-end host
dead-in-bed syndrome
deadly
  d. agaric
  d. nightshade
deafferentation
deafmutism
deafness
  central d.
  cerebral d.
  conduction d.
  conductive d.
  congenital d.
  cortical d.
  functional d.
  genetic d.
  hereditary d.
  labyrinthine d.
  lentigines, electrocardiographic
    abnormalities, ocular hypertelorism,
    pulmonary stenosis, abnormalities
    of genitalia, retardation of
    growth, and d. (LEOPARD)
  perceptive d.
  psychogenic d.
  sensorineural d.
  sudden d.
  toxic d.
  word d.
dealbation
dealcoholization
deallergize
deamidase
deamidation
deamidization
deamidize
deamidizing enzyme

deaminase
  adenine d.
  adenosine d.
  adenosine monophosphate d.
  AMP d.
  guanine d.
  homoserine d.
deaminating enzyme
deamination
deaminization
deaminize
Dean fluorosis index
deanol acetamidobenzoate
dearterialization
dearth
  d. of evidence
  d. of findings
  d. of symptoms
death
  black d.
  brain d.
  cerebral d.
  d. certificate
  contributory cause of d.
  cot d.
  crib d.
  date of d. (DOD)
  fetal d.
  genetic d.
  infant d.
  d. instinct
  intrauterine fetal d.
  local d.
  maternal d.
  d. rate
  somatic d.
  sudden d.
  systemic d.
  d. trance
  underlying cause of d.
death-rattle
Deaver
  D. incision
  D. method
DeBakey
  D. classification
  D. forceps
debanding
debilitant
debilitating illness
debility
  profound d.

D

NOTES

243

debond
debouch
débouchement
debrancher deficiency
debranching
    d. deficiency limit dextrinosis
    d. enzyme
    d. factor
Debré phenomenon
Debré-Sémélaigne syndrome
débridement
debris
    clots and d.
    particulate wear d.
    purulent d.
    stonelike d.
debrisoquine sulfate
debt
    alactic oxygen d.
    lactacid oxygen d.
    lactic acid oxygen d.
    oxygen d.
debulking operation
decagram
decalcification
decalcify
decalcifying
decaliter
decalvans
    folliculitis d.
decalvant
decameter
decamethonium bromide
decamine
decannulation
decanoin
decanormal
decant
decantation
decapacitation factor
decapeptide
decapitate
decapitation
decapsulation of kidney
decarbonization
decarboxylase
    amine precursor uptake, d. (APUD)
    aromatic d-amino acid d.
    dopa d.
    histidine d.
    hydroxytryptophan d.
    lysine d.
decarboxylated dopa
decarboxylation
decay
    branching d.
    d. constant

free induction d. (FID)
    d. theory
decayed, missing, and filled surface
    (DMFS)
deceleration
    early d.
    late d.
decentered lens
decentration
decerebrate
    d. rigidity
    d. state
decerebration
    bloodless d.
decerebrize
dechloridation
dechlorination
dechloruration
decholesterolization
decibel (dB)
decidua
    ectopic d.
    membrana d.
    d. menstrualis
    d. parietalis
    d. polyposa
    d. reflexa
    d. serotina
    d. spongiosa
    d. vera
decidual
    d. cast
    d. cell
    d. endometritis
    d. fissure
    d. reaction
deciduate placenta
deciduation
deciduitis
deciduoma
    Loeb d.
deciduous
    d. dentition
    d. membrane
    d. skin
    d. tooth
deciduus
    dens d.
decigram
deciliter
decimeter
decimorgan
decinormal
decision
    d. analysis
    limiting d.
    d. tree

declamping
    d. phenomenon
    d. shock
declination
declinator
declive
declivis
decoction
décollement
decompensation
    corneal d.
decompose
decomposition of movement
decompression
    cardiac d.
    cerebral d.
    d. chamber
    d. disease
    explosive d.
    internal d.
    nerve d.
    d. operation
    pericardial d.
    d. sickness
    spinal d.
decongestant
decongestive
decontamination
deconvolution
decorticate
    d. rigidity
    d. state
decortication
    cerebral d.
decoy cell
decrement
decremental conduction
decrepitation
decrudescence
decubital gangrene
decubitus
    Andral d.
    angina d.
    d. film
    d. projection
    d. radiograph
    d. ulcer
decurrent
decussate
decussatio lemniscorum
decussation
    anterior tegmental d.

    dorsal tegmental d.
    Forel d.
    fountain d.
    Held d.
    Meynert d.
    motor d.
    optic d.
    pyramidal d.
    rubrospinal d.
    tegmental d.
dedentition
dedifferentiation
dedolation
deduction
deefferentation
deemetinized ipecacuanha
deep
    d. abdominal reflex
    d. anterior cervical lymph node
    d. auricular artery
    d. bite
    d. brachial artery
    d. cardiac plexus
    d. cell
    d. cervical artery
    d. cervical fascia
    d. cervical vein
    d. circumflex iliac artery
    d. circumflex iliac vein
    d. cortex
    d. crural arch
    d. dorsal sacrococcygeal ligament
    d. dorsal vein
    d. epigastric artery
    d. epigastric vein
    d. facial vein
    d. femoral vein
    d. fibular nerve
    d. flexor muscle
    d. hypothermic arrest
    d. infrapatellar bursa
    d. inguinal lymph node
    d. inguinal ring
    d. lamina
    d. lateral cervical lymph node
    d. layer
    d. lingual artery
    d. lingual vein
    d. lymph vessel
    d. middle cerebral vein
    d. palmar arterial arch
    d. palmar branch

D

NOTES

deep *(continued)*
 d. palmar venous arch
 d. parotid lymph node
 d. percussion
 d. perineal fascia
 d. perineal pouch
 d. perineal space
 d. peroneal nerve
 d. petrosal nerve
 d. place
 d. plantar arterial arch
 d. plantar artery
 d. plantar branch
 d. posterior sacrococcygeal ligament
 d. punctate keratitis
 d. scleritis
 d. sensibility
 d. temporal artery
 d. temporal nerve
 d. temporal vein
 d. tendon reflex (DTR)
 d. tissue massage
 d. transitional gyrus
 d. transverse metacarpal ligament
 d. transverse metatarsal ligament
 d. transverse perineal muscle
 d. venous thrombosis
deepicardialization
deer-fly
 d.-f. disease
 d.-f. fever
Deetjen body
defatigation
defecate
defecation
 balloon d.
defecography
defect
 aorticopulmonary septal d.
 aortic septal d.
 atrial septal d.
 atrial ventricular canal d.
 birth d.
 congenital ectodermal d.
 congenital hemidysplasia with
  ichthyosiform erythroderma and
  limb d.'s (CHILD)
 coupling d.
 Eisenmenger d.
 endocardial cushion d.
 fibrous cortical d.
 filling d.
 Gerbode d.
 iodide transport d.
 iodotyrosine deiodinase d.
 luteal phase d.
 metaphysial fibrous cortical d.
 obstructive ventilatory d.
 restrictive ventilatory d.

 septal d.
 ventricular septal d.
defective
 d. bacteriophage
 d. interfering particle
 d. organism
 d. phage
 d. probacteriophage
 d. prophage
 d. virus
defemination
defense
 insanity d.
 d. mechanism
 d. reflex
defensins
defensive
 d. circle
 d. medicine
defensiveness
 auditory d.
 oral d.
 tactile d.
deferens
 ductus d.
 vas d.
deferent
 d. canal
 d. duct
deferentectomy
deferential
 d. artery
 d. nervous plexus
deferentitis
deferoxamine mesylate
deferred shock
defervescence
defervescent stage
defibrillation
defibrillator
 external d.
defibrination
deficiency
 adult lactase d.
 d. anemia
 antitrypsin d.
 1-antitrypsin d.
 arch length d.
 arylsulfatase A, B d.
 biotinidase d.
 carnitine d.
 debrancher d.
 d. disease
 familial high density lipoprotein d.
 fructokinase d.
 galactokinase d.
 immune d.
 immunity d.
 immunoglobulin G subclass d.

immunologic d.
LCAT d.
leukocyte adhesion d.
luteal phase d.
medium-chain acyl-CoA
 dehydrogenase d.
mental d.
d. mutant
d. symptom
deficit
base d.
oxygen d.
pulse d.
sleep d.
definition
definitive
d. callus
d. host
d. lysosome
d. method
d. prosthesis
deflection
atrial d.
His bundle d.
intrinsic d.
intrinsicoid d.
QRS d.
deflective occlusal contact
deflexion
deflorescence
defluoridation
defluvium
defluxion
deformability
deformans
arthritis d.
dystonia musculorum d.
endarteritis d.
osteitis d.
spondylitis d.
deformation
deforming
deformity
Åkerlund d.
Arnold-Chiari d.
bell clapper d.
boutonnière d.
buttonhole d.
contracture d.
Erlenmeyer flask d.
gooseneck d.
gunstock d.

Haglund d.
J-sella d.
keyhole d.
lobster-claw d.
Madelung d.
nasal d.
reduction d.
silver-fork d.
Sprengel d.
torsional d.
ulnar drift d.
valgus d.
varus d.
defurfuration
deganglionate
degeneracy
degenerate
degeneratio
degeneration
adipose d.
adiposogenital d.
age-related macular d.
amyloid d.
angiolithic d.
ascending d.
atheromatous d.
axon d.
axonal d.
ballooning d.
basophilic d.
calcareous d.
carneous d.
caseous d.
colloid d.
cone d.
corticobasal d.
Crooke hyaline d.
descending d.
disciform macular d.
ectatic marginal d.
elastoid d.
elastotic d.
familial pseudoinflammatory
 macular d.
fascicular d.
fatty d.
fibrinoid d.
fibrinous d.
fibrous d.
granular d.
granulovacuolar d.
gray d.

D

NOTES

degeneration *(continued)*
    hepatolenticular d.
    hyaline d.
    hyaloideoretinal d.
    hydropic d.
    infantile neuronal d.
    lattice d.
    liquefaction d.
    macular d.
    Mönckeberg d.
    mucoid d.
    orthograde d.
    parenchymatous d.
    pellucid marginal corneal d.
    reticular d.
    Salzmann nodular corneal d.
    secondary d.
    snail track d.
    Sorsby macular d.
    subacute combined d.
    Terrien marginal d.
    transsynaptic d.
    Türck d.
    wallerian d.
    waxy d.
    Zenker d.
degenerative
    d. arthritis
    d. chorea
    d. hysteria
    d. index
    d. inflammation
    d. joint disease
    d. myopia
    d. tic
degloving injury
deglutition
    d. apnea
    d. pneumonia
    d. reflex
    d. syncope
deglutitive
Degos
    D. disease
    D. syndrome
degradation
degranulation
degree
    d.'s of freedom
    d. of kindred
degustation
dehalogenase
Dehio test
dehiscence
    iris d.
dehumanization
dehydrase

dehydratase
    carbonate d.
    homoserine d.
dehydrate
dehydrated alcohol
dehydration
    absolute d.
    d. fever
dehydroacetic acid
dehydrobilirubin
dehydrocholate test
dehydrocholic acid
dehydroemetine
dehydroepiandrosterone (DHEA)
    sulfate salt of d. (DHEAS)
dehydrogenase
    acyl-ACP d.
    acyl-CoA d.
    aerobic d.
    alcohol d.
    amino acid d.
    anaerobic d.
    dihydrolipoamide d.
    glucose d.
    glycine d.
    hydrogen d.
    isocitrate d.
    isocitric acid d.
    lactate d.
    lactic acid d.
    lipoamide d.
    lipoyl d.
    malate d.
    malic acid d.
    medium-chain acyl-CoA d.
    retinol d.
dehydrogenate
dehydrogenation
dehydroretinol
dehydrosugar
dehypnotize
deiminase
    allantoate d.
    arginine d.
deinstitutionalization
deiodase
    iodotyrosine d.
deionization
deionized water
deiterospinal tract
Deiters
    D. cell
    D. nucleus
    D. terminal frame
DEJ
    dentinoenamel junction
déjà
    d. voulu

d. vu
d. vu phenomenon
dejection
Dejerine
D. disease
D. hand phenomenon
D. reflex
D. sign
Dejerine-Klumpke
D.-K. palsy
D.-K. syndrome
Dejerine-Roussy syndrome
Dejerine-Sottas disease
Delafield hematoxylin
delamination
Delaney clause
delayed
d. allergy
d. coma
d. conduction
d. dentition
d. eruption
d. flap
d. graft
d. hypersensitivity
d. onset muscle soreness
d. puberty
d. reaction
d. reaction experiment
d. reflex
d. sensation
d. shock
d. suture
d. symptom
delayed-type hypersensitivity (DTH)
Delbet sign
delbrueckii
Lactobacillus d.
Del Castillo syndrome
de-lead
deleterious effect
deletion
chromosomal d.
gene d.
interstitial d.
d. mutation
Delhi
D. boil
D. sore
delimitation
delimiting keratotomy

delinquent
juvenile d.
deliquesce
deliquescence
deliquescent
delirious
delirium
acute d.
alcohol withdrawal d.
anxious d.
d. cordis
posttraumatic d.
d. tremens (DT, DTs)
delitescence
deliver
delivery
assisted cephalic d.
breech d.
forceps d.
high forceps d.
low forceps d.
midforceps d.
outlet forceps d.
postmortem d.
premature d.
delomorphous
delouse
delphian node
delphinine
Delphinium ajacis
delta, δ
d. agent
d. antigen
d. bilirubin
d. cell
d. check
d. fiber
d. fornicis
Galton d.
d. granule
d. hepatitis
d. mesoscapulae
d. rhythm
d. virus
d. wave
deltoid
d. branch
d. crest
d. eminence
d. impression
d. ligament
d. muscle

NOTES

deltoid *(continued)*
 d. region
 d. tubercle
 d. tuberosity
deltoideopectoral
 d. triangle
 d. trigone
deltoideum
 ligamentum d.
deltopectoral
 d. flap
 d. triangle
delusion
 d. of being controlled
 d. of control
 encapsulated d.
 expansive d.
 d. of grandeur
 grandiose d.
 d. of negation
 organic d.
 d. of passivity
 d. of persecution
 persecutory d.
 d. of reference
 somatic d.
 systematized d.
 unsystematized d.
delusional disorder
demand
 biochemical oxygen d.
 d. oxygen delivery device
 d. pacemaker
 d. pulse generator
demarcation
 d. current
 line of d.
 d. line
 d. potential
Demarquay sign
demasculinizing
Dematiaceae
dematiaceous fungus
demecarium bromide
demeclocycline
demecolcine
demented
dementia
 AIDS d.
 alcoholic d.
 Alzheimer d.
 catatonic d.
 dialysis d.
 epileptic d.
 hebephrenic d.
 Lewy body d.
 paralytic d.
 d. paralytica
 paretic d.

posttraumatic d.
 d. praecox
 presenile d.
 d. presenilis
 primary d.
 primary senile d.
 secondary d.
 senile d.
 terminal d.
 vascular d.
demethylase
demethylation
demigauntlet bandage
demilune
 Heidenhain d.
demilune body
demineralization
demipenniform
demodectic
 d. blepharitis
 d. mange
Demodex folliculorum
demodicosis
demography
 dynamic d.
Demoivre formula
demoniac
demonstration ophthalmoscope
demonstrator
demorphinization
demucosation
demulcent
demyelinated myelitis
demyelinating
 d. disease
 d. encephalopathy
 d. polyneuropathy
demyelination
demyelinization
denarcotize
denarcotized opium
denatonium benzoate
denaturation temperature of DNA
denatured
 d. alcohol
 d. protein
dendriform keratitis
dendrite
 apical d.
dendritic
 d. calculus
 d. cataract
 d. cell
 d. corneal ulcer
 d. depolarization
 d. keratitis
 d. process
 d. spine
 d. thorn

dendriticum
    Diphyllobothrium d.
dendrogram
dendroid
dendron
denervate
denervation
dengue
    hemorrhagic d.
    d. hemorrhagic fever
    d. shock syndrome
    d. virus
denial
denidation
Denis
    D. Browne pouch
    D. Browne splint
denitration
denitrificans
    Jonesia d.
    Listeria d.
denitrification
denitrify
denitrogenation
Dennie line
Dennie-Morgan fold
denominator
Denonvilliers
    D. aponeurosis
    D. ligament
dens
    d. angularis
    d. axis
    d. deciduus
    d. in dente
    d. molaris
densa
    macula d.
dense body
dense-deposit disease
densimeter
densitometer
densitometry
density
    bone d.
    buoyant d.
    count d.
    flux d.
    d. gradient
    d. gradient centrifugation
    incidence d.
    optic d.

    optical d.
    radiographic d.
    spin d.
dental
    d. abscess
    d. acquired pellicle
    d. anatomy
    d. anesthesia
    d. ankylosis
    d. anthropology
    d. apparatus
    d. arch
    d. articulation
    d. assistant
    d. biomechanics
    d. biophysics
    d. branch
    d. bulb
    d. calculus
    d. canal
    d. cap
    d. caries
    d. cast
    d. cement
    d. cord
    d. crest
    d. crypt
    d. curing
    d. cuticle
    d. drill
    d. dysfunction
    d. engine
    d. engineering
    d. fiber
    d. fistula
    d. floss
    d. follicle
    d. forceps
    d. formula
    d. furnace
    d. geriatrics
    d. germ
    d. granuloma
    d. groove
    d. hygienist
    d. impaction
    d. implant
    d. index (DI)
    d. jurisprudence
    d. lamina
    d. ledge
    d. lever

NOTES

dental *(continued)*
    d. lymph
    d. material
    d. neck
    d. nerve
    d. organ
    d. orthopedics
    d. osteoma
    d. papilla
    d. pathology
    d. plaque
    d. polyp
    d. process
    d. prophylaxis
    d. prosthesis
    d. prosthetic
    d. public health
    d. pulp
    d. pump
    d. ramus
    d. ridge
    d. sac
    d. sealant
    d. senescence
    d. shelf
    d. surgeon
    d. syringe
    d. tubercle
    d. tubule
    d. ulcer
    d. wedge
dentales
    canaliculi d.
dentalgia
dentalis
    alveolus d.
dentary center
dentata
    vertebra d.
dentate
    d. fascia
    d. fissure
    d. fracture
    d. gyrus
    d. ligament
    d. line
    d. nucleus
    d. suture
dentatectomy
dentatorubral fiber
dentatothalamic
    d. fiber
    d. tract
dentatum
dente
    dens in d.
denticle
denticola
    Prevotella d.

denticulate
    d. hymen
    d. ligament
denticulated
dentiform
dentifrice
dentigerous cyst
dentilabial
dentilingual
dentin
    d. bridge
    d. dysplasia
    d. globule
    hereditary opalescent d.
    hypersensitive d.
    interglobular d.
    irregular d.
    irritation d.
    opalescent d.
    primary d.
    reparative d.
    sclerotic d.
    secondary d.
    tertiary d.
    transparent d.
dentinal
    d. canal
    d. fiber
    d. fluid
    d. lamina cyst
    d. papilla
    d. pulp
    d. sheath
    d. tubule
dentinalgia
dentine
dentinocemental junction
dentinoenamel junction (DEJ)
dentinogenesis imperfecta
dentinoid
dentinoma
dentinum
dentiparous
dentis
    apex radicis d.
    corona d.
    gubernaculum d.
dentist
    pediatric d.
dentistry
    community d.
    esthetic d.
    forensic d.
    legal d.
    pediatric d.
    preventive d.
    restorative d.
dentition
    artificial d.

deciduous d.
delayed d.
first d.
mandibular d.
maxillary d.
milk d.
permanent d.
primary d.
retarded d.
secondary d.
transitional d.
dentium
    Bifidobacterium d.
dentoalveolar
    d. abscess
    d. joint
dentode
dentofacial zone
dentogingival lamina
dentoid
dentolegal
dentoliva
dentulous
denture
    bar joint d.
    d. basal surface
    d. base
    d. border
    d. brush
    d. characterization
    complete d.
    design d.
    d. edge
    d. esthetics
    fixed partial d.
    d. flange
    d. flask
    d. foundation
    d. foundation area
    d. foundation surface
    full d.
    d. hyperplasia
    immediate insertion d.
    implant d.
    d. impression surface
    interim d.
    d. occlusal surface
    overlay d.
    d. packing
    partial d.
    d. polished surface
    d. prognosis

removable partial d.
d. retention
d. service
d. sore mouth
d. space
d. stability
temporary d.
transitional d.
trial d.
denture-bearing area
denture-supporting
    d.-s. area
    d.-s. structure
denturist
Denucé ligament
denucleated
denudation
denude
denumerable character
Denver
    D. classification
    D. Developmental Screening Test
    D. shunt
Denys-Drash syndrome
Denys-Leclef phenomenon
deodorant
deodorize
deodorized opium
deodorizer
deontology
deorsumduction
deossification
deoxidation
deoxidize
deoxyadenosine methylase
deoxyadenylic acid (dAMP)
deoxybarbiturate
deoxycholate
deoxycholic acid
deoxycoformycin
deoxycorticosterone acetate
deoxycortone
deoxycytidine
deoxycytidylic acid
deoxyepinephrine
deoxyguanosine
deoxyguanylic acid
deoxyhemoglobin
deoxyhexose
deoxynucleoside
deoxynucleotide
deoxypentose

D

NOTES

deoxyriboaldolase
deoxyribodipyrimidine photolyase
deoxyribonuclease (DNAse, DNAase, DNase)
    acid d.
    d. I, II
    d. S1
deoxyribonucleic acid (DNA)
deoxyribonucleoprotein
deoxyribonucleoside
deoxyribonucleotide
    adenine d.
    guanine d.
deoxyribose phosphate
deoxyribosephosphate aldolase
deoxyriboside
deoxyribosyl
deoxyribosyltransferases
deoxyribotide
deoxyribovirus
deoxy sugar
deoxythymidine
deoxythymidylic acid
deoxyuridine
deozonize
Depage position
department
    imaging d.
dependence
    anchorage d.
    substance d.
dependency
dependent
    d. beat
    d. drainage
    d. edema
    d. personality
    d. personality disorder
    d. variable
depersonalization
    d. disorder
    d. syndrome
dephasing
dephosphorylation
depigmentation
depilate
depilation
depilatory
    chemical d.
depletional hyponatremia
depletion response
depolarization
    alternating, failure of response, mechanical, to electrical d. (AFORMED)
    dendritic d.
depolarize

depolarizing
    d. block
    d. relaxant
depolymerase
depolymerization
deposit
    brickdust d.
depot
    d. injection
    d. reaction
    d. therapy
depravation
depraved
depravity
deprenyl
depressant
depressed skull fracture
depression
    agitated d.
    anaclitic d.
    clinical d.
    endogenous d.
    exogenous d.
    involutional d.
    lingual salivary gland d.
    major d.
    postpartum d.
    reactive d.
depressive
    d. neurosis
    d. psychosis
    d. reaction
    d. stupor
    d. syndrome
depressor
    d. anguli oris muscle
    d. fiber
    d. labii inferioris muscle
    d. nerve
    d. reflex
    d. septi muscle
    d. supercilii muscle
deprivation
    d. amblyopia
    androgen d.
    d. dwarfism
    emotional d.
    sensory d.
depsipeptide
depth
    anesthetic d.
    d. compensation
    d. dose
    focal d.
    d. of focus
    d. perception
    d. psychology
    d. recording
deptropine citrate

depulization
depurant
depuration
depurative
dequalinium
    d. acetate
    d. chloride
deradelphus
derailment
deranencephalia
deranencephaly
derangement
derby hat fracture
Dercum disease
derealization
dereism
dereistic
derencephalia
derencephalocele
derencephaly
derepression
derivation
derivative
    d. chromosome
    indanedione d.'s
    purified protein d. (PPD)
derived protein
dermabrader
dermabrasion
Dermacentor
    D. albopictus
    D. andersoni
    D. marginatus
    D. occidentalis
    D. reticulatus
    D. variabilis
dermad
dermal
    d. bone
    d. duct tumor
    d. graft
    d. leishmanoid
    d. papilla
    d. ridge
    d. sinus
dermal-fat graft
Dermanyssus gallinae
dermatalgia
dermatan sulfate
dermatic

dermatitidis
    Blastomyces d.
dermatitis, pl. dermatitides
    actinic d.
    allergic contact d.
    ashy d.
    atopic d.
    berloque d.
    blastomycetic d.
    bubble gum d.
    caterpillar d.
    cement d.
    chemical d.
    chigger d.
    chromate d.
    contact d.
    contact-type d.
    cosmetic d.
    diaper d.
    d. exfoliativa infantum
    d. exfoliativa neonatorum
    exfoliative d.
    factitial d.
    d. gangrenosa infantum
    d. herpetiformis
    infectious eczematoid d.
    irritant contact d.
    livedoid d.
    mango d.
    meadow grass d.
    d. medicamentosa
    d. papillaris capillitii
    radiation d.
    d. repens
    rhus d.
    schistosomal d.
    seborrheic d.
    d. seborrheica
    stasis d.
dermatitis-arthritis-tenosynovitis syndrome
dermatitis-causing caterpillar
dermatoarthritis
    lipoid d.
Dermatobia
    D. cyaniventris
    D. hominis
dermatobiasis
dermatocellulitis
dermatochalasis
dermatoconiosis
dermatocyst

D

NOTES

dermatodynia
dermatofibroma
dermatogenic torticollis
dermatoglyphics
dermatograph
dermatographism
dermatoid
dermatologic paste
dermatologist
dermatology
dermatolysis
dermatoma
dermatomal distribution
dermatome
dermatomegaly
dermatomere
dermatomic area
dermatomycosis pedis
dermatomyoma
dermatomyositis
dermatoneurosis
dermatonosology
dermatopathia
dermatopathic
    d. lymphadenitis
    d. lymphadenopathy
dermatopathology
dermatopathy
Dermatophagoides pteronyssinus
dermatophilosis
Dermatophilus congolensis
dermatophobia
dermatophylaxis
dermatophyte
dermatophytid
dermatophytosis
dermatoplasty
dermatopolyneuritis
dermatorrhagia
dermatorrhea
dermatorrhexis
dermatosclerosis
dermatoscopy
dermatosis, pl. dermatoses
    acute febrile neutrophilic d.
    angioneurotic d.
    ashy d.
    Bowen precancerous d.
    dermolytic bullous d.
    digitate d.
    juvenile plantar d.
    lichenoid d.
    d. medicamentosa
    menstrual d.
    neutrophilic d.
    precancerous d.
    radiation d.
    seborrheic d.

    stasis d.
    transient acantholytic d.
dermatotherapy
dermatothlasia
dermatotropic
dermatozoon
dermatozoonosis
dermatrophia
dermatrophy
dermenchysis
dermic
dermis
    adventitial d.
dermoblast
dermocyma
dermoepidermal interface
dermographia
dermographism
dermography
dermoid
    d. cancer
    d. cyst
    inclusion d.
    d. tumor
dermoidectomy
dermolysis
dermolytic bullous dermatosis
dermonecrotic
dermopathy
    diabetic d.
dermophlebitis
dermoplasty
dermoskeleton
dermostenosis
dermotoxin
dermotropic
dermotuberculin reaction
dermovascular
derodidymus
derotation
DES
    diethylstilbestrol
    DES daughter
desamidize
desaturate
desaturation
Desault bandage
Descartes law
descemetitis
Descemet membrane
descemetocele
descendens
    colon d.
descending
    d. anterior branch
    d. colon
    d. current
    d. degeneration
    d. genicular artery

left anterior d. (LAD)
d. mesocolon
d. neuritis
d. nucleus
d. palatine artery
d. posterior branch
d. scapular artery
d. thoracic aorta
d. tract
d. urography
descensus
descent
arrest of d.
homozygous by d.
Deschamps needle
descriptive
d. anatomy
d. myology
d. psychiatry
d. statistics
desensitization
heterologous d.
homologous d.
desensitize
desensitizing paste
deserpidine
desert
d. fever
d. sore
deserted place
desetope
desferrioxamine mesylate
desflurane
deshydremia
desiccans
glossitis d.
desiccant
desiccate
desiccated
d. liver
d. pituitary
desiccation
desiccative
desiccator
designation
design denture
deslanoside
Desmarres
D. dacryolith
D. retractor
desmin
desmitis

desmocranium
desmodentium
desmodontium
desmogenous
desmography
desmoid
extraabdominal d.
d. tumor
desmolase
desmology
desmopathy
desmoplasia
desmoplastic
d. cerebral astrocytoma
d. fibroma
d. malignant melanoma
d. medulloblastoma
d. small cell tumor
d. trichoepithelioma
desmopressin acetate
desmosine
desmosome
desmosterol
desmoteric medicine
desonide
desoximetasone
desoxycorticosterone
desoxycortone
desoxy sugar
despeciated antitoxin
despeciation
D'Espine sign
despumation
desquamate
desquamation
branny d.
desquamative
d. inflammatory vaginitis
d. interstitial pneumonia
d. pneumonia
desquamativum
erythroderma d.
desthiobiotin
destructive distillation
destrudo
desulfhydrase
desulfinase
Desulfotomaculum nigrificans
desulfurase
desynchronous
detachable balloon

D

NOTES

detached
    d. cranial section
    d. craniotomy
    d. retina
detachment
    exudative retinal d.
    d. of retina
    retinal d.
    vitreous d.
detail
    recorded d.
detailed physical examination
detection
detector
    d. coil
    lie d.
detergent
    cationic d.
deterioration
    alcoholic d.
determinant
    allotypic d.
    antigenic d.
    genetic d.
    d. group
    idiotypic antigenic d.
    isoallotypic d.
    mathematical d.
determinant
    disease d.
determinate cleavage
determination
    cell d.
    sex d.
determinism
detersive
detoxicate
detoxication
    ammonia d.
detoxification
detoxify
detraining
detrition
detritus
detrusor
    d. areflexia
    d. compliance
    d. hyperreflexia
    d. instability
    d. muscle
    d. pressure
    d. sphincter dyssynergia
    d. stability
detrusorrhaphy
detumescence
deturgescence
deutencephalon
deuteranomaly
deuteranope

deuteranopia
deuterium oxide
deuteromycetes
Deuteromycota
deuteron
deuteropathic
deuteropathy
deuteroplasm
deuteroporphyrin
deuterosome
deuterotocia
deuterotoky
deutogenic
deutoiodide
    mercury d.
deutomerite
deuton
deutonymph
deutoplasm
deutoplasmic
deutoplasmigenon
deutoplasmolysis
Deutschländer disease
deux
    cancer à d.
    folie à d.
devascularization
development
    cognitive d.
    lifespan d.
    psychosexual d.
developmental
    d. age
    d. anatomy
    d. anomaly
    d. apraxia
    d. disability
    d. dyspraxia
    d. groove
    d. hip dysplasia
    d. line
    d. milestone
    d. psychology
Deventer pelvis
deviance
deviant
deviated nasal septum
deviation
    angle of d.
    axis d.
    conjugate d.
    dissociated horizontal d.
    dissociated vertical d.
    immune d.
    d. to the left
    left axis d.
    primary d.
    d. to the right

secondary d.
standard d.
deviational nystagmus
Devic disease
device
assistive listening d.
bag-mask d.
bag-valve-mask d.
central-bearing d.
central-bearing tracing d.
contraceptive d.
demand oxygen delivery d.
hot-wire flow-measuring d.
intrauterine d. (IUD)
intrauterine contraceptive d. (IUCD)
left-ventricular assist d.
left ventricular assist d. (LVAD)
reservoir oxygen-conserving d.
ventricular assist d.
devil grip
deviometer
devitalization
devitalize
devitalized tooth
devolution
Devonshire colic
Dewar flask
dew point
dexamethasone suppression test
dexamphetamine sodium phosphate
dexbrompheniramine maleate
dexchlorpheniramine maleate
dexiocardia
dexpanthenol
dexter
dextra
hemicardia d.
dextrad
dextral
dextrality
dextran
d. 40, 70, 75, 110
acid d.
animal d.
blue d.
d. sulfate
dextranase
dextrin d.
dextransucrase
dextrase
dextriferron

dextrin
acid d.
d. dextranase
d. limit
d. transglycosylase
dextrinase
dextrinogenic
dextrinosis
debranching deficiency limit d.
dextrinuria
dextroamphetamine
d. phosphate
d. sulfate
dextrocardia
corrected d.
false d.
isolated d.
mirror image d.
d. with situs inversus
dextrocardiogram
dextrocerebral
dextrocular
dextrocycloduction
dextroduction
dextrogastria
dextroglucose
dextrogram
dextrogyration
dextromanual
dextromethorphan hydrobromide
dextropedal
dextroposition of heart
dextrorotation
dextrorotatory
dextrose
dextrosinistral
dextrothyroxine sodium
dextrotorsion
dextrotropic
dextroversion of heart
dextrum
atrium cordis d.
d-galacturonic acid
d-glucuronolactone
d-glyceric aciduria
d-glycogenous
Dharmendra antigen
DHEA
dehydroepiandrosterone
DHEAS
sulfate salt of dehydroepiandrosterone
d'Herelle phenomenon

NOTES

DI
  dental index
Di
  D. antigen
  D. blood group
  D. Ferrante syndrome
  D. Guglielmo disease
  D. Guglielmo syndrome
diabetes
  adult-onset d.
  alimentary d.
  alloxan d.
  brittle d.
  bronze d.
  bronzed d.
  chemical d.
  galactose d.
  gestational d.
  growth-onset d.
  d. innocens
  d. insipidus
  insulinopenic d.
  d. intermittens
  juvenile d.
  juvenile-onset d.
  ketosis-prone d.
  ketosis-resistant d.
  latent d.
  lipoatrophic d.
  lipogenous d.
  maturity-onset d.
  d. mellitus (DM)
  metahypophysial d.
  phosphate d.
  starvation d.
  subclinical d.
  type 1, 2 d.
  type I, II d.
diabetic
  d. acidosis
  d. amaurosis
  d. amyotrophy
  d. arthropathy
  d. cataract
  d. coma
  d. dermopathy
  d. diet
  d. fetopathy
  d. gangrene
  d. gingivitis
  d. glomerulosclerosis
  d. iritis
  d. ketoacidosis (DKA)
  d. lipemia
  d. myelopathy
  d. nephropathy
  d. neuropathic cachexia
  d. neuropathy
  d. ophthalmoplegia

  d. polyneuropathy
  d. polyradiculopathy
  d. puncture
  d. retinitis
  d. retinopathy
  d. thoracic radiculopathy
diabetica
  balanitis d.
  rubeosis iridis d.
diabeticorum
  gastroparesis d.
diabetogenic factor
diabetogenous
diabetology
diacele
diacetal
diacetate
  diflorasone d.
diacetemia
diacetic acid
diacetonuria
diaceturia
diacetyl
diacetylcholine
diacetylmonoxime
diacetylmorphine
diacetyltannic acid
diachronic study
diacid
diaclasia
diaclasis
diacrinous
diacrisis
diacritic
diacritical
diactinic
diacylglycerol lipase
diad
diadochokinesia, diadochocinesia
diadochokinesis
diadochokinetic
diagnosis
  admitting d. (AD)
  antenatal d.
  clinical d.
  differential d.
  d. by exclusion
  laboratory d.
  neonatal d.
  nursing d.
  pathologic d.
  physical d.
  prenatal d.
  principal d.
  provocative d.
diagnosis-related group (DRG)
diagnostic
  d. anesthesia
  d. audiometry

d. cast
d. dilatation and curettage
d. diphtheria toxin
DNA d.'s
d. radiology
d. sensitivity
d. specificity
d. ultrasound
diagnostician
diagonal
d. band
d. conjugate
d. conjugate diameter
d. section
diagonalis stria
diagram
Dieuaide d.
flow d.
diakinesis
dial
astigmatic d.
d. manometer
diallyl
dialysance
dialysate
dialysis
continuous ambulatory peritoneal d. (CAPD)
d. dementia
d. disequilibrium syndrome
d. encephalopathy syndrome
equilibrium d.
extracorporeal d.
peritoneal d.
d. retinae
d. shunt
dialyze
dialyzer
diamagnetic
diamagnetism
di-amelia
diameter
anteroposterior d.
biparietal d.
buccolingual d.
conjugate d.
diagonal conjugate d.
external conjugate d.
oblique d.
occipitofrontal d.
occipitomental d.
posterior sagittal d.

suboccipitobregmatic d.
total end-diastolic d.
total end-systolic d.
trachelobregmatic d.
transverse d.
diamide
diamidine
diamine oxidase
diamniotic
diamond
d. cutting instrument
d. disc
d. fuchsin
Diamond-Blackfan
D.-B. anemia
D.-B. syndrome
diamond-shaped murmur
Diana complex
diandria
diandry
dianoetic
diapause
embryonic d.
diapedesis
diaper
d. dermatitis
d. rash
diaphanography
diaphanoscope
diaphanoscopy
diaphemetric
diaphorase
diaphoresis
diaphoretic
diaphragm
aperture d.
Bucky d.
eventration of d.
pelvic d.
d. pessary
Potter-Bucky d.
d. sellae
urogenital d.
diaphragmalgia
diaphragmatic
d. constriction
d. flutter
d. hernia
d. ligament
d. myocardial infarction
d. pacemaker
d. peritonitis

NOTES

diaphragmatic *(continued)*
   d. pleura
   d. pleurisy
   d. surface
diaphragmatocele
diaphragmodynia
diaphysectomy
diaphysial, diaphyseal
   d. center
   d. dysplasia
diaphysis
diaphysitis
diapiresis
diaplacental
diaplexus
diapnoic
diapnotic
diapophysis
Diaptomus
diarrhea
   cachectic d.
   choleraic d.
   chronic bacillary d.
   colliquative d.
   dientamoeba d.
   dysenteric d.
   fatty d.
   flagellate d.
   gastrogenous d.
   lienteric d.
   nausea, vomiting, and d. (NVD)
   d. pancreatica
   summer d.
   traveler's d.
   tropical d.
diarrheal
diarrheic
diarrhetic
diarthric
diarthrodial
   d. cartilage
   d. joint
diarthrosis
diarticular
diaschisis
diascope
diascopy
diastalsis
diastaltic
diastase
diastasis
   d. cordis
   d. recti
diastasuria
diastatic skull fracture
diastema
diastematocrania
diastematomyelia
diaster

diastereoisomer
diastole
   atrial d.
   electrical d.
   gastric d.
   late d.
diastolic
   d. afterpotential
   d. murmur (DM)
   d. pressure
   d. shock
   d. thrill
diastology
diastrophic
   d. dwarfism
   d. dysplasia
diastrophism
diataxia
   cerebral d.
diatela
diathermal
diathermancy
diathermanous
diathermic therapy
diathermocoagulation
diathermy
   medical d.
   surgical d.
   ultrashortwave d.
diathesis
   contractural d.
   cystic d.
   gouty d.
diathetic
diatom
diatomaceous earth
diatomic
diatoric
diatrizoate
diazepam
diazine
diazinon
diazo
   d. reaction
   d. reagent
   d. stain for argentaffin granule
diazonium salt
diazotize
diazoxide
dibasic amino acid
dibenamine
dibrachius
   acephalus d.
dibromsalan
dibucaine number
DIC
   disseminated intravascular coagulation
dicarboxylic acid cycle
dicelous

dicentric chromosome
dicephalous
dicheilia
dicheiria
Dichelobacter nodosus
dichilia
dichiria
dichloride
    carbon d.
    copper d.
dichlorisone
dichlorophen
dichlorovos
dichlorphenamide
dichlorvos
dichorial twin
dichorionic diamnionic placenta
dichotic
dichotomous
dichotomy
dichroic
dichroism
    circular d.
dichromat
dichromate
dichromatic
dichromatism
dichromatopsia
dichromic
dichromophil, dichromophile
Dick
    D. method
    D. test
    D. test toxin
Dickens shunt
diclofenac
dicloxacillin sodium
dicophane
dicoria
dicotyledon
dicrocoeliosis
dicrotic
    d. notch
    d. pulse
    d. wave
dicrotism
dictionary
    data d.
dictyoma
dictyosome
dictyotene
dicumarol resistance

dicysteine
didactic analysis
didactylism
didelphic
didelphys
    uterus d.
dideoxy
    d. procedure
    d. sequencing
didymus
diecious
Diego blood group
dieldrin
dielectrography
dielectrolysis
Diels hydrocarbon
diencephalic
    d. epilepsy
    d. syndrome
diencephalohypophysial
diencephalon
dienestrol
dientamoeba diarrhea
Dientamoeba fragilis
dieresis
dieretic
diesterase
diestrous
diestrus
diet
    acid-ash d.
    alkaline-ash d.
    balanced d.
    basal d.
    basic d.
    bland d.
    BRAT d.
    challenge d.
    clear liquid d.
    diabetic d.
    elimination d.
    full liquid d.
    Giordano-Giovannetti d.
    Giovannetti d.
    gluten-free d.
    gout d.
    high-calorie d.
    high-fat d.
    high-fiber d.
    Kempner d.
    ketogenic d.
    low-calorie d.

D

NOTES

diet *(continued)*
   low-fat d.
   low-purine d.
   low-residue d.
   low-salt d.
   macrobiotic d.
   Meulengracht d.
   Minot-Murphy d.
   d. quality index
   smooth d.
   soft d.
dietary
   d. amenorrhea
   d. fiber
Dieterle stain
dietetic
   d. albuminuria
   d. treatment
dietetics
diethadione
diethanolamine
diethazine
diethenoid fatty acid
diethyl ether
diethylstilbestrol (DES)
   d. daughter
dieting
   yo-yo d.
dietitian
Dietl crisis
Dieuaide diagram
Dieulafoy
   D. erosion
   D. lesion
   D. ulcer
difarnesyl group
difenoxin
difenoxylic acid
difference
   A-aO2 d.
   alveolar-arterial oxygen tension d.
   arteriovenous carbon dioxide d.
   arteriovenous oxygen d.
   AV d.
   cation-anion d.
   individual d.'s
   light d.
   d. limen
   masking level d.
   standard error of d.
differens
   pulsus d.
differential
   d. blood pressure
   d. diagnosis
   d. display
   d. gene expression
   d. growth

   d. manometer
   d. renal function test
   d. spinal anesthesia
   d. stain
   d. stethoscope
   d. thermometer
   d. threshold
   d. ureteral catheterization test
   d. white blood count
differentiated teratoma
differentiation
   cluster of d. (CD)
   correlative d.
   echocardiographic d.
   invisible d.
   pressure pulse d.
difficile
   Clostridium d.
diffluence
diffraction grating
diffusa
   encephalitis periaxialis d.
diffusate
diffuse
   d. abscess
   d. alveolar damage
   d. aneurysm
   d. angiokeratoma
   d. arterial ectasia
   d. choroiditis
   d. cutaneous leishmaniasis
   d. cutaneous mastocytosis
   d. deep keratitis
   d. esophageal spasm
   d. ganglion
   d. glomerulonephritis
   d. goiter
   d. hyperkeratosis
   d. idiopathic skeletal hyperostosis (DISH)
   d. infantile familial sclerosis
   d. injuries
   d. lesion
   d. Lewy body disease
   d. mesangial proliferation
   d. obstructive emphysema
   d. panbronchiolitis
   d. peritonitis
   d. pleurisy
   d. rhonchi
   d. small cleaved cell lymphoma
   d. unilateral subacute neuroretinitis (DUSN)
   d. waxy spleen
diffused
   d. psoriasis
   d. reflex
diffusible stimulant

diffusing
- d. capacity
- d. factor

diffusion
- d. anoxia
- d. cocfficient
- d. constant
- facilitated d.
- Fick laws of d.
- gel d.
- d. hypoxia
- d. method
- d. respiration
- d. shell

diflorasone diacetate
diflucortolone
diflunisal
digametic
digastric
- d. branch
- d. fossa
- d. groove
- d. muscle
- d. notch
- d. triangle

digastricus
digenesis
digenetic
DiGeorge syndrome
digest
digestant
digestion
- buccal d.
- duodenal d.
- gastric d.
- intercellular d.
- intestinal d.
- intracellular d.
- pancreatic d.
- peptic d.
- primary d.
- salivary d.
- secondary d.

digestive
- d. apparatus
- d. enzyme
- d. fever
- d. glycosuria
- d. leukocytosis
- d. system
- d. tract

- d. tube
- d. vacuole

digit
- binary d.
- clubbed d.

digital
- d. collateral artery
- d. dilatation
- d. fibromatosis
- d. flexion crease
- d. fossa
- d. furrow
- d. gray scale
- d. hearing aid
- d. joint
- d. plethysmograph
- d. pulp
- d. radiography (DR)
- d. reflex
- d. subtraction angiography (DSA)
- d. vein
- d. whorl

digitalin
- crystalline d.

digitalis
- d. effect
- herpes d.
- d. tincture
- d. unit

digitalism
digitalization
digitatae
- impressiones d.

digitate
- d. dermatosis
- d. impression
- d. wart

digitation
digitin
digitonin reaction
digitoxigenin
digitoxin
digitoxose
diglossia
diglyceride lipase
dignathus
digoxigenin
digoxin
digyny, digynia
diheterozygote
dihybrid
dihydralazine

D

NOTES

dihydrate
dihydrazone
dihydric alcohol
dihydroascorbic acid
dihydrobiopterin reductase
dihydrocodeine tartrate
dihydrocodeinone
dihydrocortisone
dihydroergocornine
dihydroergocristine
dihydroergocryptine
dihydroergotamine
dihydroergotoxine mesylate
dihydrofolate reductase
dihydrogen phosphate
dihydrolipoamide dehydrogenase
dihydropteroic acid
dihydrouridine
dihydroxyacetone
diiodide
diiodotyrosine
diketone
diketopiperazines
dilaceration
Dilantin gingivitis
dilatancy
dilatation
    balloon d.
    d. and curettage (D&C)
    digital d.
    d. and evacuation (D&E)
dilatator
dilate
dilated
    d. cardiomyopathy
    fixed and d. (F&D)
    d. pore
dilation
    d. and curettage (D&C)
    d. and evacuation (D&E)
    d. and extraction
    d. and suction
    d. thrombosis
dilator
    Chevalier-Jackson d.
    esophageal d.
    Hanks d.
    Hegar d.
    hydrostatic d.
    Kollmann d.
    pneumatic d.
    d. pupillae muscle
    Walther d.
dildo, dildoe
dilemma
    masking d.
dileptic seizure
dill oil
diloxanide furoate

diluent
dilute
    d. alcohol
    d. phosphoric acid
    d. Russell's viper venom test
diluted
    d. acetic acid
    d. hydrochloric acid
dilution
    d. anemia
    closed-circuit helium d.
    serial d.
dilutional hyponatremia
dimazon
dimelia
dimenhydrinate
dimension
    buccolingual d.
    double gel diffusion precipitin test
    in 1 d.
    double gel diffusion precipitin test
    in 2 d.'s
dimensional stability
2-dimensional echocardiography
2-dimension–3-dimension phenomenon
dimer
dimercaprol
dimercurion
dimeric
dimerous
dimethadione
dimethicone
dimethyl
    d. iminodiacetic acid (HIDA)
    d. ketone
    d. sulfoxide
dimetria
dimidiate hermaphroditism
Dimmer keratitis
dimorphic anemia
dimorphism
    sexual d.
dimorphous leprosy
dimple
    coccygeal d.
    d. sign
dimpling
dineric
dinitrate
    isosorbide d.
dinitrocellulose
dinitrogen monoxide
dinitrophenylhydrazine test
dinner pad
dinoflagellate toxin
dinoprostone
dinucleotide
    d. domain

flavin adenine d.
d. fold
nicotinamide adenine d.
dioctophymiasis
diodoquin
diolamine
diopter
prism d.
dioptric aberration
dioptrics
dioscin
diose
diosgenin
diotic
diovular twins
diovulatory
dioxane
dioxide
activated carbon d.
active carbon d.
carbon d. (CO2)
colloidal silicon d.
hydrogen d.
silicon d.
dioxin
dioxybenzone
dioxygenase
DIP
distal interphalangeal
DIP joint
dip
Cournand d.
d. phenomenon
dipeptidase
methionyl d.
proline d.
prolyl d.
dipeptide
dipeptidyl
d. peptidase
d. transferase
Dipetalonema
D. reconditum
D. streptocerca
diphallus
diphasic
d. complex
d. milk fever
diphemanil methylsulfate
diphemethoxidine
diphenadione
diphenan

diphenidol
diphenyl
diphenylhydantoin gingivitis
diphenylmethane
d. dye
d. laxative
diphosgene
diphosphatase
inorganic d.
diphosphate
adenosine d.
5′-diphosphate
adenosine 5′-d. (ADP)
diphosphopyridine nucleotide
diphtheria
d. antitoxin
d. antitoxin unit
cutaneous d.
false d.
faucial d.
laryngeal d.
laryngotracheal d.
d., tetanus, and acellular pertussis
(DTaP)
d. toxin
d. toxoid, tetanus toxoid, and
pertussis vaccine (DTP)
diphtheriae
Corynebacterium d.
diphtherial
diphtheria-pertussis-tetanus (DPT)
diphtheric
diphtheritic
d. conjunctivitis
d. enteritis
d. membrane
d. neuropathy
d. paralysis
d. ulcer
diphtheroid
diphtherotoxin
diphyllobothriasis
Diphyllobothrium
D. cordatum
D. dendriticum
D. hians
D. houghtoni
D. latum
D. linguloides
D. mansoni
D. mansonoides
D. nihonkaiense

D

NOTES

Diphyllobothrium *(continued)*
    D. orcini
    D. pacificum
    D. scoticum
diphyllobothrium anemia
diphyodont
dipiproverine
diplacusis
    binaural d.
diplegia
    congenital facial d.
    facial d.
    infantile d.
    masticatory d.
    spastic d.
diploalbuminuria
diplobacillus
diplobacteria
diploblastic
diplocardia
diplocephalus
diplocheiria
diplochiria
diplococcemia
diplococcin
diplococcus
diplocoria
diplogenesis
diploic
    d. canal
    d. vein
diploid nucleus
diplokaryon
diplomelituria
diplomyelia
diplon
diplonema
diploneural
diplopagus
diplophonia
diplopia
    crossed d.
    heteronymous d.
    homonymous d.
    monocular d.
    paradoxical d.
diplopodia
diplosome
diplosomia
diplotene
dipodia
dipolar
    d. buffer
    d. ions
dipole
    d. moment
    d. theory
dipotassium phosphate
diprenorphine

dipropionate
    beclomethasone d.
    estradiol d.
dipropyltryptamine
diprosopus
dipsesis
dipsogen
dipsomania
dipsosis
dipsotherapy
dipstick
dipteran
dipterous
dipus
    acephalus d.
dipylidiasis
Dipylidium caninum
dipyridamole
dipyrimidine photolyase
dipyrine
dipyrone
direct
    d. acrylic restoration
    d. auscultation
    d. bone impression
    d. calorimetry
    d. composite resin restoration
    d. Coombs test
    d. current (DC)
    d. diuretic
    d. embolism
    d. filling resin
    d. flap
    d. fluorescent antibody test
    d. fracture
    d. illumination
    d. image
    d. immunofluorescence
    d. inguinal hernia
    d. laryngoscopy
    d. lateral vein
    d. lead
    d. medical control
    d. nuclear division
    d. ophthalmoscope
    d. ophthalmoscopy
    d. oxidase
    d. percussion
    d. pulp capping
    d. pyramidal tract
    d. ray
    d. reacting bilirubin
    d. retainer
    d. retention
    d. symptom
    d. technique
    d. transfusion
    d. vision
    d. vision spectroscope

d. wet mount examination
d. zoonosis
direction
pelvic d.
directional
d. atherectomy
d. preponderance
d. weakness
directive
advance d. (AD)
d. psychotherapy
directly observed therapy
director
medical d.
dire straits
Dirofilaria
D. conjunctivae
D. immitis
dirofilariasis
dirt-eating
disability
developmental d.
learning d.
disability-adjusted life year (DALY)
disaccharidases
disaccharide
disaggregation
disappearing bone disease
disarticulation
disassimilation
disassociation
disc, disk
A d.
acromioclavicular d.
Airy d.
anisotropic d.
articular d.
blastodermic d.
blood d.
Bowman d.
Burlew d.
cartilaginous d.
choked d.
ciliary d.
cone d.
cuttlefish d.
diamond d.
d. electrophoresis
embryonic d.
emery d.
germ d.
germinal d.

H d.
hair d.
Hensen d.
herniated d.
d. herniation
I d.
intercalated d.
intermediate d.
interpubic d.
intervertebral d.
isotropic d.
d. kidney
mandibular d.
Merkel tactile d.
Newton d.
optic d.
Placido da Costa d.
protruded d.
ruptured d.
d. sensitivity method
d. space
d. syndrome
d. valve prosthesis
discectomy
discharge
early d.
discharging tubule
Dische
D. reaction
D. reagent
Dische-Schwarz reagent
dischronation
disciform
d. keratitis
d. macular degeneration
disciformis
keratitis d.
discission needle
discitis, discitis
disclosing
d. agent
d. solution
discoblastic
discoblastula
discogastrula
discogenic
discogram
discography
discoid
d. aortic prosthesis
d. lupus
d. lupus erythematosus

NOTES

discoidal cleavage
disconjugate movement
disconnection syndrome
discontinuation test
discontinuous
    d. culture
    d. phase
    d. sterilization
discopathy
    traumatic d.
discoplacenta
discordance
discordant
    d. alternans
    d. alternation
    d. atrioventricular connection
    d. change electrocardiogram
discotomy
discrete
    d. activity
    d. analyzer
    d. character
    d. disease
    d. mass
    d. narrowing
    d. nodule
    d. organ enlargement
    d. random variable
    d. smallpox
discriminant
    d. analysis
    d. function
    d. stimulus
discrimination
    right-left d.
    d. score
disc-shaped cataract
disdiaclast
disease
    ABO hemolytic d.
    accumulation d.
    Acosta d.
    acute cardiovascular d. (ACVD)
    acute respiratory d. (ARD)
    Adams-Stokes d.
    adaptation d.
    Addison d.
    Addison-Biermer d.
    akamushi d.
    Albers-Schönberg d.
    Albright d.
    Alexander d.
    Almeida d.
    Alpers d.
    altitude d.
    Alzheimer d.
    anarthritic rheumatoid d.
    Anders d.
    Andersen d.

    antibody deficiency d.
    aortoiliac occlusive d.
    Aran-Duchenne d.
    arteriosclerotic cardiovascular d.
     (ACVD)
    Australian X d.
    autoimmune d.
    aviator's d.
    Ayerza d.
    Azorean d.
    Baelz d.
    Baló d.
    Baltic myoclonus d.
    Bamberger d.
    Bamberger-Marie d.
    Bang d.
    Bannister d.
    Banti d.
    Barclay-Baron d.
    Barlow d.
    Barraquer d.
    Basedow d.
    Batten d.
    Batten-Mayou d.
    Bayle d.
    Bazin d.
    Bechterew d.
    Becker d.
    Béguez César d.
    Behçet d.
    Behr d.
    Berger d.
    Bernard-Soulier d.
    Bernhardt d.
    Besnier-Boeck-Schaumann d.
    Best d.
    Bielschowsky d.
    Biermer d.
    Binswanger d.
    bird-breeder's d.
    blinding d.
    Bloch-Sulzberger d.
    Blocq d.
    Blount d.
    Blount-Barber d.
    blue d.
    Boeck d.
    Bornholm d.
    Bosin d.
    Bouchard d.
    Bourneville d.
    Bourneville-Pringle d.
    Bowen d.
    Brailsford-Morquio d.
    brancher glycogen storage d.
    Breda d.
    Bright d.
    Brill d.
    Brill-Zinsser d.

Briquet d.
Brissaud d.
broad beta d.
Brodie d.
bronzed d.
Bruck d.
Brushfield-Wyatt d.
Buerger d.
bulging eye d.
bulky d.
Bürger-Grütz d.
Buschke d.
Busquet d.
Busse-Buschke d.
Byler d.
Caffey d.
caisson d.
calcium pyrophosphate deposition d. (CPPD)
Calvé-Perthes d.
Canavan d.
Canavan-van Bogaert-Bertrand d.
cardiovascular renal d.
Caroli d.
Carrington d.
Carrión d.
Castleman d.
cat-bite d.
catscratch d.
celiac d.
cement d.
central core d.
cerebrovascular d.
Chagas d.
Chagas-Cruz d.
Charcot d.
Charcot-Marie-Tooth d.
Cheadle d.
Chédiak-Higashi d.
Chiari d.
Chicago d.
cholesterol ester storage d.
cholesteryl ester storage d.
Christensen-Krabbe d.
Christian d.
Christmas d.
chronic active liver d.
chronic granulomatous d.
chronic hypertensive d.
chronic obstructive pulmonary d. (COPD)
chylomicron retention d.

Coats d.
Cockayne d.
cold hemagglutinin d.
collagen d.
collagen-vascular d.
combined system d.
communicable d.
Concato d.
connective-tissue d.
Conradi d.
Conradi-Hünermann d.
contagious d.
Cori d.
coronary arteriosclerotic heart d. (CAHD)
coronary artery d.
coronary atherosclerotic heart d. (CAHD)
coronary heart d.
Corrigan d.
Cowden d.
Creutzfeldt-Jakob d.
Crigler-Najjar d.
Crocq d.
Crohn d.
Crouzon d.
Cruveilhier d.
Cruveilhier-Baumgarten d.
Cushing d.
cystic d.
cysticercus d.
cystine storage d.
cytomegalic inclusion d.
cytomegalovirus d.
Daae d.
Danielssen d.
Danielssen-Boeck d.
Darier d.
Darling d.
Davies d.
decompression d.
deer-fly d.
deficiency d.
degenerative joint d.
Degos d.
Dejerine d.
Dejerine-Sottas d.
demyelinating d.
dense-deposit d.
de Quervain d.
Dercum d.
d. determinant

D

NOTES

disease *(continued)*

Deutschländer d.
Devic d.
diffuse Lewy body d.
Di Guglielmo d.
disappearing bone d.
discrete d.
diverticular d.
dog d.
dominantly inherited Lévi d.
drug-induced d.
Dubois d.
Duchenne d.
Duchenne-Aran d.
Duhring d.
Dukes d.
Duncan d.
Dupuytren d.
Duroziez d.
Dutton d.
Eales d.
Ebstein d.
Echinococcus d.
Eisenmenger d.
elephant man's d.
elevator d.
emotional d.
endemic d.
end-stage renal d. (ESRD)
Engelmann d.
English sweating d.
eosinophilic endomyocardial d.
epidemic d.
Epstein d.
Erb d.
Erb-Charcot d.
Erdheim d.
ergot alkaloid-associated heart d.
Eulenburg d.
exanthematous d.
extramammary Paget d.
extrapyramidal motor system d.
Fabry d.
Fahr d.
Farber d.
Favre-Durand-Nicholas d.
Favre-Racouchot d.
Fazio-Londe d.
Feer d.
femoropopliteal occlusive d.
fibrocystic d.
fibromuscular d.
fifth d.
Filatov d.
Filatov-Dukes d.
fish eye d.
flax-dresser's d.
Flegel d.
flight into d.

flint d.
focal metastatic d.
Folling d.
foot-and-mouth d. (FMD)
Forbes d.
Fordyce d.
Forestier d.
Fothergill d.
Fournier d.
fourth d.
Fox-Fordyce d.
Franklin d.
Freiberg d.
Friend d.
functional cardiovascular d.
fusospirochetal d.
Gairdner d.
Gamna d.
Gandy-Nanta d.
garapata d.
Garré d.
gastroesophageal reflux d. (GERD)
Gaucher d.
Gerhardt-Mitchell d.
Gerlier d.
gestational trophoblastic d.
Gierke d.
Gilbert d.
Gilchrist d.
Gilles de la Tourette d.
Glanzmann d.
global burden of d.
glycogen-storage d.
Goldflam d.
Gorham d.
Gougerot and Blum d.
Gougerot-Sjögren d.
Gowers d.
G protein d.
graft versus host d.
granulomatous d.
Graves d.
Griesinger d.
Grover d.
GVH d.
Haff d.
Haglund d.
Hailey-Hailey d.
Hallervorden-Spatz d.
Hallopeau d.
Hamman d.
Hamman-Rich d.
Hammond d.
hand-foot-and-mouth d.
Hand-Schüller-Christian d.
Hansen d.
Harada d.
Hartnup d.
Hashimoto d.

heart d.
heavy chain d.
Heck d.
Heerfordt d.
hemoglobin C d.
hemoglobin H d.
hemolytic d.
hemorrhagic d.
herring-worm d.
Hers d.
Hirschsprung d.
Hodgkin d.
Hodgson d.
holoendemic d.
hookworm d.
Huntington d.
Hurler d.
Hurst d.
Hutchinson-Gilford d.
hyaline membrane d.
hydatid d.
hyperendemic d.
hypertensive renal d.
hypertensive vascular d.
Iceland d.
I-cell d.
idiopathic d.
immune complex d.
immunoproliferative small
  intestinal d.
inborn lysosomal d.
inclusion body d.
inclusion cell d.
industrial d.
infantile celiac d.
infectious d.
infective d.
intercurrent d.
interstitial d.
iron-storage d.
ischemic heart d.
island d.
Itai-Itai d.
Jaffe-Lichtenstein d.
Jansky-Bielschowsky d.
Jensen d.
jumper d.
jumping d.
Jüngling d.
Kashin-Bek d.
Katayama d.
Kawasaki d.

Kennedy d.
Kienböck d.
Kikuchi d.
Kimmelstiel-Wilson d.
Kimura d.
kinky-hair d.
Köhler d.
Krabbe d.
Kufs d.
Kugelberg-Welander d.
Kussmaul d.
Kyasanur Forest d.
Kyrle d.
Lafora body d.
Lane d.
Larson-Johansson d.
L-chain d.
Legg d.
Legg-Calvé-Perthes d.
Legg-Perthes d.
Legionnaires d.
Leigh d.
Leiner d.
Lenègre d.
lenticular progressive d.
Leri-Weill d.
Letterer-Siwe d.
Lev d.
Lindau d.
Little d.
Lobo d.
Löffler d.
Lorain d.
Lou Gehrig d.
Luft d.
lung fluke d.
Lutz-Splendore-Almeida d.
Lyell d.
Lyme d.
lysosomal d.
Machado-Joseph d.
mad cow d.
Madelung d.
Manson d.
maple bark d.
maple syrup urine d.
marble bone d.
Marburg virus d.
Marchiafava-Bignami d.
Marfan d.
margarine d.
Marie-Strümpell d.

D

NOTES

273

disease *(continued)*

Marion d.
Martin d.
McArdle d.
McArdle-Schmid-Pearson d.
mechanobullous d.
Meige d.
Ménétrier d.
Ménière d.
mental d.
Merzbacher-Pelizaeus d.
metabolic d.
Meyenburg d.
Meyer-Betz d.
Mibelli d.
microcystic d.
micrometastatic d.
microvillus inclusion d.
Mikulicz d.
Milroy d.
Minamata d.
miner's d.
minimal-change d.
Mitchell d.
mixed connective-tissue d.
molecular d.
Mondor d.
Monge d.
Morgagni d.
Morvan d.
motor neuron d. (MND)
multisystem d.
myocardial d.
Niemann-Pick C1 d.
no evidence of recurrent d.
Norrie d.
nosocomial d.
notifiable d.
occupational d.
Ofuji d.
Oguchi d.
Oppenheim d.
organic d.
Ormond d.
orphan d.
Osgood-Schlatter d.
Osler d.
Osler-Vaquez d.
Otto d.
Owren d.
Paas d.
Paget d.
Panner d.
paper mill worker's d.
Parkinson d.
Parrot d.
Parry d.
Pel-Ebstein d.
Pellegrini d.

pelvic inflammatory d. (PID)
periodic d.
periodontal d.
Peyronie d.
Pick d.
pink d.
polycystic d.
Pompe d.
posttransplant lymphoproliferative d.
Pott d.
primary d.
pulseless d.
reactive airways d.
recalcitrant d.
Recklinghausen d.
Refsum d.
reportable d.
rheumatic heart d.
Roger d.
Rokitansky d.
Rosai-Dorfman d.
salivary gland d.
Sandhoff d.
Schenck d.
Scheuermann d.
Schilder d.
Schlatter d.
Schlatter-Osgood d.
secondary d.
serum d.
Sever d.
sexually transmitted d.
sickle cell d.
sickle cell C d.
Simmonds d.
sixth d.
slow virus d.
Stargardt d.
startle d.
Still d.
storage d.
Strümpell d.
Sutton d.
Swift d.
Sylvest d.
Taylor d.
Tay-Sachs d.
third d.
Thomsen d.
thromboembolic d. (TED)
thyrocardiac d.
Tommaselli d.
Tourette d.
tropical d.
tsutsugamushi d.
Unna d.
Unverricht d.
upper respiratory d.
vagabond's d.

vagrant's d.
Vaquez d.
venereal d.
venoocclusive d.
Vincent d.
Voltolini d.
von Gierke d.
von Willebrand d.
Weil d.
Werlhof d.
Westphal-Strümpell d.
Whipple d.
white matter d.
Wilson d.
Wolman d.
disease-modifying antirheumatic drug (DMARD)
disengagement
disequilibrium
genetic d.
linkage d.
disfluency
disfluent
disgerminoma
DISH
diffuse idiopathic skeletal hyperostosis
disharmony
maxillomandibular d.
dish face
dishpan fracture
disiens
Bacteroides d.
disimpaction
disinfect
disinfectant
complete d.
incomplete d.
disinfection
concurrent d.
terminal d.
disinfestation
disinhibition
disinsection
disinsectization
disintegration constant
disinvagination
disjoined pyeloplasty
disjunction
disjunctive absorption
disk (*var. of* disc)
dislocate

dislocation
arytenoid d.
closed d.
compound d.
divergent d.
fracture d.
d. fracture
Kienböck d.
d. of lens
open d.
simple d.
subcoracoid d.
subglenoid d.
dismember
dismembered pyeloplasty
dismutase
superoxide d.
dismutation
disobliteration
disodium
ceftriaxone d.
edetate calcium d.
d. phosphate
disofenin
disomic
disomy
disopromine
disorder
adjustment d.
affective d.
antisocial personality d.
anxiety d.
articulation d.
Asperger d.
asthenic personality d.
attention deficit hyperactivity d.
autistic d.
avoidant personality d.
behavior d.
bipolar d.
body dysmorphic d.
borderline personality d.
character d.
communication d.
communicative d.
conduct d.
conversion d.
cumulative trauma d.
cyclothymic personality d.
delusional d.
dependent personality d.
depersonalization d.

D

NOTES

disorder *(continued)*
    dissociative identity d.
    dysthymic d.
    eating d.
    emotional d.
    erotomanic d.
    factitious d.
    familial bipolar mood d.
    functional d.
    gender identity d.
    generalized anxiety d.
    histrionic personality d.
    hysterical personality d.
    identity d.
    immune complex d.
    immunoproliferative d.
    impulse control d.
    induced psychotic d.
    intermittent explosive d.
    internet addiction d.
    ion channel d.
    isolated explosive d.
    late luteal phase dysphoric d.
    LDL receptor d.
    lymphoplasmacellular d.
    major depressive d.
    major mood d.
    manic-depressive d.
    mental d.
    mitochondrial d.
    neuropsychologic d.
    neurotic d.
    obsessive-compulsive d.
    oppositional defiant d.
    organic mental d.
    overanxious d.
    panic d.
    personality d.
    pervasive developmental d.
    posttraumatic stress d.
    premenstrual dysphoric d.
    psychogenic pain d.
    psychophysiologic d.
    psychosomatic d.
    psychotic d.
    regulatory d.
    repetitive strain d.
    schizoid personality d.
    schizotypal personality d.
    seasonal affective d.
    seizure d.
    sexual d.
    somatization d.
    somatoform d.
    stress d.
    substance abuse d.
    substance dependence d.
    temporomandibular d.

    thought d.
    triple repeat d.
disorganization
disorganized schizophrenia
disorientation
dispar
    Entamoeba d.
disparate
disparity
    d. angle
    fixation d.
dispensary
dispense
dispensing tablet
dispermy, dispermia
dispersal
    flash d.
dispersed phase
disperse placenta
dispersing electrode
dispersion
    coarse d.
    d. colloid
    colloidal d.
    d. medium
    molecular d.
    optic rotatory d.
    d. phase
dispersity
dispersoid
dispireme
displaceability
displaced fracture
displacement
    affect d.
    d. analysis
    d. behavior
    d. loop
    mesial d.
    d. osteotomy
    d. threshold
display
    affect d.
    differential d.
disposable sigmoidoscope
disposition
disproportion
    cephalopelvic d.
disproportionate dwarfism
disproportionating enzyme
disputed neurogenic thoracic outlet syndrome
dissecans
    endometritis d.
    osteochondritis d.
dissect
dissecting
    d. aneurysm
    d. cellulitis

d. forceps
d. microscope

dissection
aortic d.
blunt d.
functional neck d.
limited neck d.
radical neck d.
sharp d.
supraomohyoid neck d.
d. tubercle

dissector

disseminata
leiomyomatosis peritonealis d.

disseminated
d. aspergillosis
d. choroiditis
d. coccidioidomycosis
d. cutaneous gangrene
d. cutaneous leishmaniasis
d. gonococcal infection
d. histoplasmosis
d. intravascular coagulation (DIC)
d. lesion
d. lipogranulomatosis
d. lupus erythematosus
d. sclerosis
d. tuberculosis

disseminatum
keratoma d.
xanthoma d.

dissepiment

Disse space

dissimilar twin

dissimilation

dissimulation

dissociated
d. anesthesia
d. horizontal deviation
d. nystagmus
d. vertical deviation

dissociation
albuminocytologic d.
atrial d.
atrioventricular d. (AVD)
AV d.
complete atrioventricular d.
complete AV d.
d. constant
electromechanical d.
incomplete atrioventricular d.
incomplete AV d.

d. by interference
interference d.
isorhythmic d.
light-near d.
longitudinal d.
d. movement
d. sensibility
visual-kinetic d.

dissociative
d. anesthesia
d. hysteria
d. identity disorder
d. reaction

dissolve

dissonance
cognitive d.

dissymmetry

distad

distal
d. angle
d. caries
d. centriole
d. end
d. ileitis
d. interphalangeal (DIP)
d. interphalangeal joint
d. intestinal obstructive syndrome
d. medial striate artery
d. myopathy
d. occlusion
d. part
d. phalanx
d. radioulnar articulation
d. radioulnar joint
d. spiral septum
d. splenorenal shunt
d. surface of tooth
d. tibiofibular joint
d. tingling on percussion

distalis

distance
d. ceptor
focal d.
focal-film d.
infinite d.
interarch d.
interocclusal d.
interridge d.
large interarch d.
map d.
pupillary d.
source-to-image d.

D

NOTES

distant flap
distasonis
    Bacteroides d.
distemper virus
distensibility
distention, distension
    d. cyst
    jugular venous d. (JVD)
    d. ulcer
distichiasis
distill
distillate
distillation
    destructive d.
    dry d.
    fractional d.
    molecular d.
distilled water
distobuccal
distobuccoocclusal
distobuccopulpal
distocervical
distoclusal
distoclusion
distogingival
distoincisal
distolabial
distolabiopulpal
distolingual
distolinguo-occlusal
distomatosis
distomiasis
    hemic d.
distomolar
distoocclusal
distoplacement
distopulpal
distortion
    d. aberration
    barrel d.
    parataxic d.
    pincushion d.
    radiologic d.
distortion-product otoacoustic emission
distoversion
distractibility
distraction
    d. conus
    d. osteogenesis
distress
    acute respiratory d. (ARD)
    fetal d.
distributed effort
distributing artery
distribution
    Bernoulli d.
    binomial d.
    chi-square d.
    d. coefficient

    countercurrent d.
    d. curve
    dermatomal d.
    epidemiological d.
    exponential d.
    f d.
    frequency d.
    gaussian d.
    d. leukocytosis
    lognormal d.
    nitrogen d.
    normal d.
    d. volume
distributive analysis
districhiasis
distrix
distropin
disturbance
    emotional d.
    mental d.
disulfamide
disulfate
disulfide
    asymmetric d.
    d. bond
    d. bridge
    carbon d.
    lipoamide d.
disulfiduria
    mercaptolactate-cysteine d.
disulfiram
disuse atrophy
diterpene
dithiazanine iodide
dithiothreitol
dithranol
Dittrich
    D. plug
    D. stenosis
diuresis
    alcohol d.
    cold d.
    osmotic d.
    tubular d.
    water d.
diuretic
    cardiac d.
    direct d.
    d. effect
    indirect d.
    loop d.
    mercurial d.
    osmotic d.
    potassium sparing d.
diurnal
    d. enuresis
    d. periodicity
    d. rhythm
divalence

D

divalency
divalent
divalproex sodium
divarication
divergence
    d. excess exotropia
    d. insufficiency
    d. insufficiency exotropia
    d. paresis
divergent
    d. dislocation
    d. evolution
    d. squint
    d. strabismus
diverging meniscus
diver's
    d. palsy
    d. paralysis
    d. spectacles
diversion
diversity
    cultural d.
diversus
    Citrobacter d.
diverticula (*pl. of* diverticulum)
diverticular
    d. disease
    d. hernia
diverticulectomy
diverticulitis
diverticuloma
diverticulopexy
diverticulosis
diverticulum, pl. **diverticula**
    allantoenteric d.
    allantoic d.
    caliceal d.
    cervical d.
    colonic d.
    ductus d.
    duodenal d.
    epiphrenic d.
    false d.
    Heister d.
    hepatic d.
    hypopharyngeal d.
    Kommerell d.
    laryngotracheal d.
    Meckel d.
    metanephric d.
    Pertik d.
    pharyngoesophageal d.

    pituitary d.
    pulsion d.
    supradiaphragmatic d.
    traction d.
    true d.
    vesical d.
    Zenker d.
divicine
divided
    d. dose
    d. spectacles
diving
    d. goiter
    d. reflex
division
    autonomic d.
    cleavage d.
    conjugate d.
    craniosacral d.
    direct nuclear d.
    equatorial d.
    indirect nuclear d.
    lateral d.
    left lateral d.
    left medial d.
    meiotic d.
    mitotic d.
    multiplicative d.
    Remak nuclear d.
    right lateral d.
    right medial d.
divisional block
divulse
divulsion
divulsor
Dix-Hallpike maneuver
dixyrazine
dizygotic twin
dizygous
dizziness
djenkolic acid
djenkol poisoning
DKA
    diabetic ketoacidosis
DM
    diabetes mellitus
    diastolic murmur
DMARD
    disease-modifying antirheumatic drug
DMFS
    decayed, missing, and filled surface
      DMFS caries index

NOTES

DNA
    deoxyribonucleic acid
      antisense DNA
      blunt-ended DNA
      competitor DNA
      complementary DNA (cDNA)
      denaturation temperature of DNA
      DNA diagnostics
      extrachromosomal DNA
      DNA fingerprinting
      DNA gap
      genomic DNA
      DNA helix
      DNA homology
      DNA hybridization
      junk DNA
      DNA ligase
      linker DNA
      DNA marker
      DNA nucleotidylexotransferase
      DNA polymerase
      DNA polymorphism
      DNA profiling
      recombinant DNA
      selfish DNA
      sticky-ended DNA
      DNA typing
      DNA virus
DNA-RNA hybrid
DNAse, DNAase, DNase
    deoxyribonuclease
      DNAse I, II
DNR
    do not resuscitate
DOA
    dead on arrival
DOB
    date of birth
dobutamine
d'Ocagne nomogram
docking protein
doctrine
    humoral d.
    Monro d.
docusate
    d. calcium
    d. sodium
DOD
    date of death
dodecane
dodecanoyl-CoA synthetase
dodecarbonium chloride
dodecyl
    d. gallate
    d. sulfate
Döderlein bacillus
DOE
    dyspnea on exertion
Doerfler-Stewart test

dog
    d. disease
    d. distemper virus
    d. ear
    d. nose
    scotty d.
    d. unit
Dogiel
    D. cell
    D. corpuscle
dogma
    central d.
dogmatic school
dogmatist
Döhle
    D. body
    D. inclusion
Dohlman operation
dolichocephalic
dolichocephalism
dolichocephalous
dolichocephaly
dolichocolon
dolichocranial
dolichoectatic artery
dolichofacial
dolichol phosphate
dolichopellic, dolichopelvic
    d. pelvis
dolichoprosopic
dolichoprosopous
dolichostenomelia
dolichouranic
dolichuranic
doll's
    d. eye sign
    d. head maneuver
dolor capitis
dolorific
dolorimetry
dolorogenic zone
dolorology
dolorosa
    adiposis d.
    analgesia d.
    anesthesia d.
dolorosus
    hallux d.
domain
    dinucleotide d.
    frequency d.
    immunoglobulin d.
Dombrock blood group
dome
    bladder d.
    d. cell
    dysfunctional uterine d.
    d. of pleura

domestic
 d. soap
 d. violence
domiciliated
dominance
 cerebral d.
 false d.
 genetic d.
 d. hierarchy
 d. of traits
dominant
 autosomal d.
 d. character
 d. eye
 d. frequency
 d. gene
 d. hemisphere
 d. hereditary
 d. idea
 d. inheritance
 d. lethal trait
 d. optic atrophy
dominantly inherited Lévi disease
domiodol
domiphen bromide
domperidone
Donath-Landsteiner
 D.-L. antibody
 D.-L. cold autoantibody
 D.-L. phenomenon
 D.-L. rest
 D.-L. syndrome
Donders
 D. law
 D. pressure
Don Juanism
Donnan equilibrium
Donné corpuscle
Donohue syndrome
donor
 hydrogen d.
 d. insemination
 universal d.
do not resuscitate (DNR)
Donovan body
donovani
 Leishmania d.
donovanosis
Doose syndrome
dopa
 alpha methyl d.
 d. decarboxylase

decarboxylated d.
 d. oxidase
 d. quinone
 d. reaction
dopamine
dopaminergic
doping
 blood d.
Doppler
 D. color flow
 D. echocardiography
 D. effect
 D. phenomenon
 D. shift
 D. ultrasonography
Dor
 D. fundoplication
 D. procedure
d'orange
 peau d.
doraphobia
Dorello canal
Dorendorf sign
Dorfman-Chanarin syndrome
dornase
doromania
dorsabdominal
dorsad
dorsal
 d. accessory olivary nucleus
 d. calcaneocuboid ligament
 d. callosal vein
 d. carpal arterial arch
 d. carpal branch
 d. carpal ligament
 d. carpal network
 d. carpal tendinous sheath
 d. carpometacarpal ligament
 d. column
 d. column stimulation
 d. cuboideonavicular ligament
 d. cuneocuboid ligament
 d. cuneonavicular ligament
 d. decubitus position
 d. digital artery
 d. digital nerve
 d. digital vein
 d. elevated position
 d. fascia
 d. flexure
 d. funiculus
 d. hood

D

NOTES

dorsal *(continued)*
  d. hypothalamic area
  d. hypothalamic region
  d. intercuneiform ligament
  d. intermediate sulcus
  d. interossei interosseous muscle
  d. interosseous artery
  d. interosseous nerve
  d. lateral cutaneous nerve
  d. lateral geniculate nucleus
  d. lingual branch
  d. lingual vein
  d. lithotomy position
  d. longitudinal fasciculus
  d. medial cutaneous nerve
  d. median sulcus
  d. mesocardium
  d. mesogastrium
  d. metacarpal artery
  d. metacarpal ligament
  d. metacarpal vein
  d. metatarsal artery
  d. metatarsal ligament
  d. metatarsal vein
  d. midbrain syndrome
  d. nasal artery
  d. pallidum
  d. pancreas
  d. pancreatic artery
  d. part
  d. plate
  d. premammillary nucleus
  d. primary ramus
  d. radiocarpal ligament
  d. recumbent position
  d. reflex
  d. rigid position
  d. root
  d. root ganglion
  d. sacrococcygeal muscle
  d. sacroiliac ligament
  d. scapular artery
  d. scapular nerve
  d. scapular vein
  d. septal nucleus
  d. spine
  d. spinocerebellar tract
  d. striatum
  d. supraoptic commissure
  d. surface
  d. talonavicular bone
  d. tarsal ligament
  d. tarsometatarsal ligament
  d. tegmental decussation
  d. thalamus
  d. thoracic artery
  d. thoracic nucleus
  d. trigeminothalamic tract
  d. tubercle

  d. vagal nucleus
  d. venous arch
  d. venous network
  d. vertebra
dorsalgia
dorsalis
  Aedes d.
  funiculus d.
  d. pedis artery
  tabes d.
Dorset culture egg medium
dorsi *(pl. of* dorsum)
dorsiduct
dorsiflexion
dorsiflexor compartment
dorsiscapular
dorsispinal vein
dorsocephalad
dorsolateral
  d. fasciculus
  d. incision
  d. nucleus
  d. plate
  d. sulcus
  d. tract
dorsolumbar
dorsomedial hypothalamic nucleus
dorsosacral position
dorsoventrad
dorsum, pl. **dorsi**
  d. nasi
  d. pedis
  d. pedis reflex
  d. penis
  d. scapulae
  d. sellae
dosage
dose
  absorbed d.
  air d.
  bone marrow d.
  booster d.
  cumulative d.
  curative d.
  daily d.
  depth d.
  divided d.
  effective d. (ED)
  effective median d. (ED_{50})
  epilation d.
  equianalgesic d.
  equivalent d.
  d. equivalent limit
  erythema d.
  exit d.
  exposure d.
  fractional d.
  gonad d.
  gonadal d.

initial d.
integral d.
L d.
L+ d.
lethal d.
Lf d.
Lo d.
loading d.
Lr d.
maintenance d.
maximal permissible d.
maximum permissible d.
maximum tolerated d.
median effective d.
minimal infecting d. (MID)
minimal lethal d. (MLD, mld)
minimal reacting d.
optimum d.
skin d.
tolerance d.
dose-response
d.-r. curve
d.-r. relationship
dosimeter
pocket d.
thermoluminescent d.
dosimetry
dot
Gunn d.
Horner-Trantas d.
Maurer d.
Mittendorf d.
Schüffner d.
Trantas d.
Ziemann d.
dotage
dotted tongue
double
d. antibody immunoassay
d. antibody method
d. antibody precipitation
d. antibody sandwich assay
d. aorta
d. aortic arch
d. aortic stenosis
d. backcross
d. bind
d. bond
d. bubble sign
d. cervix
d. chin
d. compartment hydrocephalus

d. concave lens
d. congenital athetosis
d. consciousness
d. contrast enema
d. convex lens
d. displacement mechanism
d. elevator palsy
d. enterostomy
d. flap amputation
d. fracture
d. gel diffusion precipitin test in 1 dimension
d. gel diffusion precipitin test in 2 dimensions
d. helix
d. hemiplegia
illusion of d.'s
d. image
d. immunodiffusion
d. inlet atrioventricular connection
d. intussusception
d. lip
d. loop hernia
d. membrane
d. minute chromosomes
d. outlet right ventricle
d. pedicle flap
d. pleurisy
d. pneumonia
d. product
d. protrusion
d. quartan
d. quotidian fever
d. refraction
d. ring sign
d. salt
d. stain
d. tachycardia
d. tertian
d. tertian malaria
d. track sign
d. ureter
d. vision
double-blind
d.-b. clinical trial
d.-b. experiment
d.-b. study
d.-b. test
double-button suture
double-channel catheter
double-emulsion adjuvant
double-masked experiment

NOTES

double-mouthed uterus
double-point threshold
double-reciprocal plot
double-shock sound
double-strand break
doublet
    Wollaston d.
doubling time
doubly
    d. armed suture
    d. heterozygous
douche bath
doughnut
    d. lesion
    d. pessary
doughy
    d. abdomen
    d. consistency
Douglas
    D. abscess
    D. bag
    D. cul-de-sac
    D. fold
    D. line
    D. mechanism
    D. pouch
douloureux
    tic d.
dousing bath
doute
    folie du d.
dovetail stress-broken abutment
dowager hump
dowel graft
down
    bearing d.
    cone d.
    D. syndrome
downbeat nystagmus
Downey cell
downgrowth
    epithelial d.
down-regulation
Downs analysis
downward drainage
downy hair
doxacurium chloride
doxophylline
doxorubicin
doxycycline
Doyère eminence
Doyle operation
Doyne honeycomb choroidopathy
DPT
    diphtheria-pertussis-tetanus
DR
    digital radiography
Drabkin reagent
drachm

dracunculiasis
dracunculosis
Dracunculus
    D. lova
    D. medinensis
    D. oculi
    D. persarum
draft
dragée
Dragendorff
    D. reagent
    D. test
Dräger respirometer
dragon pyelogram
drain
    butterfly d.
    cigarette d.
    Mikulicz d.
    Penrose d.
    quarantine d.
    stab d.
    sump d.
drainage
    capillary d.
    closed d.
    dependent d.
    downward d.
    infusion-aspiration d.
    lymph d.
    manual lymph d.
    open d.
    postural d.
    suction d.
    through d.
    tidal d.
    d. tube
drain-trap stomach
dram
draped
    prepped and d.
Draper law
draught
drawer
    d. sign
    d. test
draw-sheet
dream
    anxiety d.
    d. associations
dream-work
dreamy state
Drechslera
drepanidium
drepanocyte
drepanocytic anemia
dressing
    absorbable d.
    adhesive absorbent d.
    anorectal d.

antiseptic d.
barrel d.
bolus d.
brassiere-type d.
bulky d.
butterfly d.
cellophane d.
cement d.
cocoon d.
collar d.
collodion d.
compound d.
compression d.
dry d.
felt d.
fine mesh d.
fixed d.
fluffy compression d.
foam rubber d.
d. forceps
impregnated d.
Lister d.
many-tailed d.
mustache d.
occlusive d.
patch d.
petrolatum gauze d.
pressure d.
stent d.
stockinette d.
4-tailed d.
wet-to-dry d.

Dressler
D. beat
D. syndrome
Dreyer formula
DRG
diagnosis-related group
dried
d. alum
d. ferrous sulfate
d. human albumin
d. human plasma protein fraction
d. human serum
d. yeast
drift
antigenic d.
cardiovascular d.
genetic d.
d. movement
ulnar d.
drifting

drill
bur d.
dental d.
intramedullary d.
mirror d.
drill-out
cochlear d.-o.
Drinker respirator
drip
alkaline milk d.
intravenous d.
Murphy d.
d. phleboclysis
postnasal d.
d. transfusion
drive
acquired d.
exploratory d.
learned d.
meiotic d.
physiological d.
secondary d.
driving
photic d.
dromograph
dromomania
dromostanolone propionate
dromotropic
dronabinol
drooping lily sign
drop
d. attack
enamel d.
eye d.
d. finger
d. hand
hanging d.
d. heart
knock-out d.
droperidol
dropfoot, drop foot
d. brace
droplet
d. infection
d. nucleus
dropped beat
dropper
dropsical
dropsy
abdominal d.
cardiac d.
epidemic d.

D

NOTES

285

dropsy *(continued)*
    famine d.
    d. of pericardium
drowning
    dry d.
drowsiness
drug
    d. abuse
    addictive d.
    d. allergy
    antisense d.
    crude d.
    disease-modifying antirheumatic d.
      (DMARD)
    d. eruption
    d. fever
    d. holiday
    d. interaction
    nonsteroidal antiinflammatory d.
      (NSAID)
    orphan d.
    d. pathogenesis
    d. psychosis
    d. rash
    d. resistance
    street d.
    d. tetanus
    therapeutic d.
    d. use evaluation
    d. utilization review
drug-fast
druggist
drug-induced
    d.-i. disease
    d.-i. hepatitis
    d.-i. lupus
drumhead
drum membrane
Drummond-Morison operation
Drummond sign
drumstick
    d. appendage
    d. finger
drunkenness
drusen
    basal laminar d.
    basal linear d.
    cuticular d.
    exudative d.
    hard d.
    intrapapillary d.
    macular d.
    soft d.
    typical d.
dry
    d. abscess
    d. amputation
    d. beriberi
    d. bronchiectasis

    d. cough
    d. cup
    d. cutaneous leishmaniasis
    d. distillation
    d. dressing
    d. drowning
    d. eye syndrome
    d. gangrene
    d. hernia
    d. ice
    d. joint
    d. labor
    d. leprosy
    d. nurse
    d. pack
    d. pericarditis
    d. pleurisy
    d. rale
    d. socket
    d. synovitis
    d. vomiting
    d. weight
DSA
    digital subtraction angiography
DT, DTs
    delirium tremens
DTaP
    diphtheria, tetanus, and acellular pertussis
DTH
    delayed-type hypersensitivity
DTP
    diphtheria toxoid, tetanus toxoid, and
      pertussis vaccine
DTR
    deep tendon reflex
DTs *(var. of* DT*)*
dual
    d. personality
    d. relationships
dual-cure resin
dualism
Duane syndrome
Dubin-Johnson syndrome
Dubois
    D. abscess
    D. disease
DuBois formula
duboisine
Duboscq colorimeter
Dubowitz score
Dubreuil-Chambardel syndrome
Duchenne
    D. disease
    D. dystrophy
    D. sign
Duchenne-Aran disease
Duchenne-Erb paralysis
duck
    d. embryo origin vaccine

d. hepatitis virus
d. influenza virus
d. plague virus
duckbill speculum
Duckworth phenomenon
Ducrey
    D. bacillus
    D. test
ducreyi
    Haemophilus d.
duct
    aberrant bile d.
    accessory pancreatic d.
    alveolar d.
    amnionic d.
    anal d.
    arterial d.
    Bartholin d.
    Bellini d.
    Bernard d.
    bile d.
    biliary d.
    Blasius d.
    Botallo d.
    bucconeural d.
    canalicular d.
    d. carcinoma
    carotid d.
    cervical d.
    choledoch d.
    cochlear d.
    common bile d.
    common hepatic d.
    craniopharyngeal d.
    Cuvier d.
    cystic gall d.
    deferent d.
    efferent d.
    ejaculatory d.
    endolymphatic d.
    excretory d.
    frontonasal d.
    galactophorous d.
    gall d.
    Gartner d.
    genital d.
    guttural d.
    hemithoracic d.
    Hensen d.
    hepatic d.
    hepatocystic d.
    Hoffmann d.

hypophysial d.
incisive d.
intercalated d.
interlobar d.
interlobular d.
intralobular d.
jugular d.
lacrimal d.
lactiferous d.
left hepatic d.
longitudinal d.
Luschka d.
lymphatic d.
major sublingual d.
mammary d.
mammillary d.
mesonephric d.
metanephric d.
milk d.
minor sublingual d.
Müller d.
müllerian d.
nasolacrimal d.
omphalomesenteric d.
pancreatic d.
d. papilloma
paramesonephric d.
paraurethral d.
parotid d.
perilymphatic d.
prostatic d.
right hepatic d.
right lymphatic d.
Rivinus d.
Santorini d.
semicircular d.
seminal d.
d. of Skene gland
spermatic d.
Steno d.
Stensen d.
striated d.
submandibular d.
thoracic d.
Walther d.
Wharton d.
Wirsung d.
wolffian d.
ductal
    d. aneurysm
    d. carcinoma
    d. hyperplasia

NOTES

ductile
duction
    forced d.
ductless gland
ductular
ductule
    aberrant d.
    biliary d.
    efferent d.
    inferior aberrant d.
    interlobular d.
    prostatic d.
ductus
    d. aberrantes
    d. arteriosus
    d. deferens
    d. diverticulum
    d. venosus
Duddell membrane
Duffy
    D. antigen
    D. blood group
Dugas test
Duhring disease
Dührssen incision
Duke bleeding time test
Dukes
    D. classification
    D. disease
dulcin
dulcite
dulcitol
dulcose
dullness
Dulong-Petit law
dumbbell ganglioneuroma
dumb rabies
Dumdum fever
dummy consultand
dumoffii
    Legionella d.
Dumontpallier pessary
dumping
    d. stomach
    d. syndrome
Duncan
    D. disease
    D. fold
    D. mechanism
    D. placenta
    D. position
    D. syndrome
    D. ventricle
duocrinin
duodena (*pl. of* duodenum)
duodenal
    d. ampulla
    d. branch
    d. bulb

    d. cap
    d. digestion
    d. diverticulum
    d. fistula
    d. fossa
    d. gland
    d. ileus
    d. impression on liver
    d. obstruction
    d. smear
    d. sphincter
duodenale
    Ancylostoma d.
duodenectomy
duodenitis
duodenocholangitis
duodenocholecystostomy
duodenocholedochotomy
duodenocystostomy
duodenoenterostomy
duodenojejunal
    d. angle
    d. flexure
    d. fold
    d. fossa
    d. hernia
    d. junction
    d. recess
    d. sphincter
duodenojejunostomy
duodenolysis
duodenomesocolic fold
duodenorenal ligament
duodenorrhaphy
duodenoscopy
duodenostomy
duodenotomy
duodenum, pl. duodena
duovirus
duplex
    d. Doppler scan
    ileum d.
    d. kidney
    d. transmission
    d. ultrasonography
    d. uterus
duplication
    d. of chromosomes
    d. cyst
    gene d.
duplicity theory of vision
Dupré muscle
Dupuy-Dutemps operation
Dupuytren
    D. amputation
    D. canal
    D. contracture
    D. disease
    D. fascia

D. fracture
D. hydrocele
D. sign
D. suture
D. tourniquet
dura
d. mater
d. mater cranialis
d. mater encephali
d. mater spinalis
durable power of attorney
duraencephalosynangiosis
dural
d. cavernous sinus fistula
d. forceps
d. hook
d. sheath
d. venous sinus
duramatral
Duran-Reynals
D.-R. permeability factor
D.-R. spreading factor
duraplasty
duration
half amplitude pulse d.
pulse wave d.
d. tetany
Dürck node
Duret
D. hemorrhage
D. lesion
Durham
D. rule
D. tube
Duroziez
D. disease
D. murmur
D. sign
durum
heloma d.
DUSN
diffuse unilateral subacute neuroretinitis
dust
d. asthma
blood d.
d. cell
d. corpuscle
Dutton
D. disease
D. relapsing fever
duty cycle
Duvenhage virus

Duverney
D. fissure
D. gland
D. muscle
dwarf
hypophysial d
hypothyroid d.
d. pelvis
dwarfed enamel
dwarfism
achondroplastic d.
acromelic d.
acromesomelic d.
aortic d.
asexual d.
ateliotic d.
camptomelic d.
chondrodystrophic d.
deprivation d.
diastrophic d.
disproportionate d.
Fröhlich d.
Hunter-Thompson d.
hypothyroid d.
infantile d.
Laron-type d.
lethal d.
Lorain-Lévi d.
mesomelic d.
metatropic d.
micromelic d.
pituitary d.
proportionate d.
rhizomelic d.
Dwyer osteotomy
dyad
dyadic
d. psychotherapy
d. symbiosis
dydrogesterone
dye
acidic d.
acridine d.
azin d.
azo d.
azocarmine d.
basic d.
chlorotriazine d.
diphenylmethane d.
d. disappearance test
d. exclusion test
ketonimine d.

D

NOTES

dye *(continued)*
    natural d.
    oxazin d.
    thiazin d.
    xanthene d.
dye-dilution curve
Dyggve-Melchior-Clausen syndrome
dynamic
    d. aorta
    d. compliance
    d. computed tomography
    d. constant external resistance
      training
    d. CT
    d. demography
    d. equilibrium
    d. force
    d. friction
    group d.'s
    d. ileus
    d. movement
    d. murmur
    d. posturography
    d. psychiatry
    d. psychology
    d. psychotherapy
    d. refraction
    d. relations
    d. school
    d. splint
    d. viscosity
dynamogenesis
dynamogenic
dynamogeny
dynamograph
dynamometer
dynamoscope
dynamoscopy
dynatherm
dyne
dynein arm
dynorphin
dyphylline
dysacusis, dysacousia, dysacusia
dysadaptation
dysantigraphia
dysaphia
dysaphic
dysarteriotony
dysarthria
    ataxic d.
    flaccid d.
    hyperkinetic d.
    hypokinetic d.
    lower motor neuron d.
    parkinsonian d.
    spastic d.
dysarthria–clumsy hand syndrome
dysarthric

dysarthrosis
dysautonomia
    familial d.
dysbarism
dysbasia
    d. angiosclerotica
    d. angiospastica
    d. lordotica progressiva
dysbetalipoproteinemia
dysbolism
dysbulia
dysbulic
dyscalculia
dyscephalia mandibulo-oculofacialis
dyscephaly
dyscheiral, dyschiral
dyscheiria, dyschiria
dyschezia
dyschiral *(var. of* dyscheiral*)*
dyschondrogenesis
dyschondroplasia with hemangioma
dyschondrosteosis
dyschroia, dyschroa
dyschromatopsia
dyschromatosis
dyschromia
dyscinesia *(var. of* dyskinesia*)*
dysconjugate gaze
dyscontrol
dyscoria
dyscrasia
    blood d.
dyscrasic
dyscratic
dysdiadochokinesia, dysdiadochocinesia
dysdiadochokinesis
dysembryoplastic neuroepithelial tumor
dysemia
dysenteriae
    Shigella d.
dysenteric
    d. algid malaria
    d. diarrhea
dysentery
    amebic d.
    d. antitoxin
    bacillary d.
    d. bacillus
    balantidial d.
    bilharzial d.
    ciliary d.
    fulminating d.
    helminthic d.
    malignant d.
    sporadic d.
    viral d.
dyserethism
dysergia
dysesthesia

dysfibrinogenemia
dysfluency
dysfunction
    constitutional hepatic d.
    dental d.
    minimal brain d.
    myocardial d.
    psychosexual d.
    sensorineural d.
    sexual d.
    sphincter of Oddi d.
    temporomandibular joint d.
dysfunctional
    d. uterine bleeding
    d. uterine dome
dysgammaglobulinemia
dysgenesis
    cortical d.
    gonadal d.
    iridocorneal mesenchymal d.
    seminiferous tubule d.
dysgenic
dysgerminoma
dysgeusia
dysgnathia
dysgnathic
dysgnosia
dysgonic
dysgranular cortex
dysgraphia
dysharmonious retinal correspondence
dyshematopoiesis
dyshematopoietic
dyshemopoiesis
dyshemopoietic anemia
dyshidria
dyshidrosis
dyshidrotic eczema
dysjunction
    Le Fort III craniofacial d.
dysjunctive nystagmus
dyskaryosis
dyskaryotic
dyskeratoma
dyskeratosis
    benign d.
    d. congenita
    intraepithelial d.
    malignant d.
dyskeratotic
dyskinesia, dyscinesia
    d. algera

    biliary d.
    extrapyramidal d.
    d. intermittens
    lingual-facial-buccal d.
    d. syndrome
dyskinesis
    ciliary d.
dyskinetic
dyslexia
dyslexic
dyslogia
dysmasesis
dysmature
dysmaturity
dysmelia
dysmenorrhea
    essential d.
    functional d.
    intrinsic d.
    mechanical d.
    membranous d.
    obstructive d.
    primary d.
    secondary d.
    spasmodic d.
dysmenorrheal membrane
dysmetria
dysmnesic syndrome
dysmorphia
dysmorphism
dysmorphogenesis
dysmorphology
dysmorphophobia
dysmyelination
dysmyotonia
dysnystaxis
dysodontiasis
dysontogenesis
dysontogenetic
dysorexia
dysosmia
dysosteogenesis
dysostosis
    acrofacial d.
    cleidocranial d.
    clidocranial d.
    craniofacial d.
    mandibuloacral d.
    mandibulofacial d.
    metaphysial d.
    d. multiplex
    orodigitofacial d.

D

NOTES

dyspallia
dyspareunia
dyspepsia
    acid d.
    adhesion d.
    atonic d.
    fermentative d.
    flatulent d.
    functional d.
dyspeptic
dysphagia, dysphagy
dysphagocytosis
    congenital d.
dysphasia
dysphasic
dysphemia
dysphonia
    abductor spasmodic d.
    adductor spasmodic d.
    spasmodic d.
    spastic d.
dysphoria
    late luteal phase d.
dysphrasia
dyspigmentation
dyspinealism
dyspituitarism
dysplasia
    anhidrotic ectodermal d.
    anterofacial d.
    anteroposterior d.
    anteroposterior facial d.
    arteriohepatic d.
    asphyxiating thoracic d.
    branchiootorenal d.
    bronchopulmonary d.
    cemental d.
    cerebral d.
    cervical d.
    chondroectodermal d.
    cleidocranial d.
    clidocranial d.
    cochlear d.
    congenital ectodermal d.
    congenital hip d.
    cortical d.
    craniocarpotarsal d.
    craniodiaphysial d.
    craniometaphysial d.
    dentin d.
    developmental hip d.
    diaphysial d.
    diastrophic d.
    ectodermal d.
    enamel d.
    d. epiphysialis hemimelia
    d. epiphysialis multiplex
    d. epiphysialis punctata
    epithelial d.

    faciodigitogenital d.
    familial white folded d.
    fibromuscular d.
    fibrous d.
    florid osseous d.
    hidrotic ectodermal d.
    hypohidrotic ectodermal d.
    mandibuloacral d.
    mandibulofacial d.
    McKusick metaphysial d.
    metaphysial d.
    Mondini d.
    multiple epiphysial d.
    otospondylomegaepiphyseal d.
    periapical cemental d.
    septooptic d.
    skeletal d.
    spondyloepiphyseal d.
dysplastic
    d. nevus
    d. nevus syndrome
dyspnea
    cardiac d.
    exertional d.
    expiratory d.
    functional d.
    nocturnal d.
    d. on exertion (DOE)
    orthostatic d.
    paroxysmal nocturnal d. (PND)
dyspneic
dyspraxia
    developmental d.
    verbal d.
dysprosium
dysproteinemia
    angioimmunoblastic
      lymphadenopathy with d.
dysproteinemic retinopathy
dysraphia
dysraphism
    spinal d.
dysreflexia
    autonomic d.
dysrhythmia
    cardiac d.
    electroencephalographic d.
    esophageal d.
dyssebacia
dyssomnia
dysspermatogenic sterility
dysspondylism
dysstasia
dysstatic
dyssyllabia
dyssynergia
    d. cerebellaris myoclonica
    detrusor sphincter d.
dystasia

dystelephalangy
dysthymia
dysthymic disorder
dysthyroid
    d. myopathy
    d. orbitopathy
dysthyroidal infantilism
dystocia
    fetal d.
    maternal d.
    placental d.
    shoulder d.
dystonia
    cranial d.
    d. lenticularis
    d. musculorum deformans
dystonic
    d. reaction
    d. torticollis
dystopia
    pituitary d.
dystopic
dystrophia
    d. adiposogenitalis
    d. epithelialis corneae
    d. unguium
dystrophic
    d. calcification
    d. calcinosis
dystrophin
dystrophy
    adiposogenital d.
    adult foveomacular retinal d.
    adult pseudohypertrophic
      muscular d.
    anterior corneal d.
    asphyxiating thoracic d.
    Becker muscular d.
    Becker-type tardive muscular d.
    central areolar choroidal d.
    central cloudy corneal d.
    central crystalline corneal d.
    childhood muscular d.
    Cogan d.
    cone d.
    cone-rod retinal d.
    congenital hereditary endothelial d.
    corneal d.

craniocarpotarsal d.
Duchenne d.
Emery-Dreifuss muscular d.
endothelial d.
epithelial d.
facioscapulohumeral muscular d.
Favre d.
fingerprint d.
fleck d.
Fuchs endothelial d.
Fuchs epithelial d.
gelatinous droplike corneal d.
granular corneal d.
Groenouw corneal d.
gutter d.
hereditary epithelial d.
hypertrophic d.
infantile neuroaxonal d.
Landouzy-Dejerine d.
lattice corneal d.
Leyden-Möbius muscular d.
limb-girdle muscular d.
macular corneal d.
macular retinal d.
map-dot-fingerprint d.
Meesman d.
microcystic epithelial d.
muscular d.
myotonic d.
oculopharyngeal d.
pattern retinal d.
posterior polymorphous corneal d.
pre-Descemet corneal d.
progressive tapetochoroidal d.
reflex sympathetic d.
Reis-Bücklers corneal d.
reticular d.
ringlike corneal d.
stromal corneal d.
vitelliform retinal d.
vitreotapetoretinal d.
vortex corneal d.
dystropin
dystropy
dysuria, dysury
dysuric
dysversion

D

NOTES

EAC
EAC rosette
EAC rosette assay
Eadie-Hofstee plot
EAE
experimental allergic encephalitis
Eagle
E. basal medium
E. minimum essential medium
Eagle-Barrett syndrome
Eagleton operation
EAHF
eczema, asthma, hay fever
EAHF complex
Eales disease
ear
Aztec e.
bat e.
bladder e.
Blainville e.'s
e. bone
boxer's e.
Cagot e.
e. canal
cauliflower e.
e. crystal
darwinian e.
dog e.
external e.
glue e.
internal e.
e. lobe
e. lobe crease
middle e.
Morel e.
e.'s, nose, and throat (ENT)
outstanding e.
protruding e.
Stahl e.
swimmer's e.
telephone e.
e. wax
Wildermuth e.
earache
eardrum
Earle
E. L fibrosarcoma
E. solution
early
e. deceleration
e. diastolic murmur
e. discharge
e. dumping syndrome
e. infantile autism
e. latent syphilis

e. posttraumatic epilepsy
e. reaction
e. receptor potential (ERP)
e. seizure
early-phase response
earpiece
earplug
earth
alkaline e.'s
diatomaceous e.
fuller's e.
e. wax
earthy water
East
E. African sleeping sickness
E. African trypanosomiasis
eastern
e. equine encephalomyelitis (EEE)
e. equine encephalomyelitis virus
eating
e. disorder
e. epilepsy
eating-right pyramid
Eaton agent
Eaton-Lambert syndrome
EB
Epstein-Barr
EB virus
Ebbinghaus test
Eberth
E. bacillus
E. line
E. perithelium
Ebner
E. gland
E. reticulum
Ebola
E. hemorrhagic fever
E. virus
E. virus Côte-d'Ivoire
E. virus Reston
E. virus Sudan
E. virus Zaire
ebonation
ébranlement
Ebstein
E. anomaly
E. disease
E. sign
EBT
electron beam tomography
ebullism
eburnation
eburneous
eburnitis

E

EBV
Epstein-Barr virus
E-cadherin
écarteur
ecaudate
ecboline
eccentric
e. amputation
e. contraction
e. fixation
e. hypertrophy
e. implantation
e. occlusion
e. position
e. relation
eccentricity
angle of e.
eccentrochondroplasia
eccentropiesis
ecchondroma
ecchondrosis
ecchordosis physaliphora
ecchymoma
ecchymosed
ecchymosis
bilateral medial orbital e.
Tardieu e.
ecchymotic mask
eccrine
e. acrospiroma
e. gland
e. poroma
e. spiradenoma
eccrinology
eccrisis
eccritic
eccyesis
ecdemic
ecdysial gland
ecdysiasm
ecdysis
ecdysist
ECF
extended care facility
extracellular fluid
ECFV
extracellular fluid volume
ECG
electrocardiogram
ECG trigger
ecgonine benzoate
echidninus
Laelaps e.
Echidnophaga gallinacea
echinate
Echinochasmus
echinococciasis
echinococcosis

Echinococcus
E. cyst
E. disease
E. granulosus
E. multilocularis
E. vogeli
echinocyte
echinoderm
Echinodermata
Echinorhynchus
echinosis
Echinostoma
E. ilocanum
E. malayanum
echinostomiasis
echinulate
echo
atrial e.
e. beat
navigator e.
e. planar
e. reaction
e. sign
e. speech
spin e.
echoacousia
echoaortography
echocardiogram
echocardiographic differentiation
echocardiography
contrast e.
cross-sectional e.
2-dimensional e.
Doppler e.
M-mode e.
real-time e.
sector e.
transesophageal e.
echoencephalography
echo-free
echogenic
echogram
echographer
echographia
echography
echolalia
echolocation
echomimia
echomotism
echopathy
echophonia
echophony
echophrasia
echopraxia
echoscope
echothiophate iodide
echovirus
Ecker fissure
Eck fistula

eclabium
eclampsia
    puerperal e.
eclamptic
eclamptogenic
eclamptogenous
eclectic
eclecticism
eclipse
    e. blindness
    e. period
    e. phase
ecoendocrinology
ECoG
    electrocorticography
ecologic
    e. chemistry
    e. study
ecological
    e. ectocrine
    e. fallacy
    e. system
ecology
    human e.
    landscape e.
econazole
economic coefficient
economy
    exercise e.
    movement e.
ecospecies
ecosystem
ecotaxis
ecotropic virus
écouvillon
ecphyma
ecstrophe
ECT
    electroconvulsive therapy
ectad
ectal
ectasia
    annuloaortic e.
    aortoannular e.
    e. cordis
    corneal e.
    diffuse arterial e.
    familial aortic e.
    hypostatic e.
    mammary duct e.
ectasis

ectatic
    e. aneurysm
    e. emphysema
    e. marginal degeneration
ectental
ectethmoid
ecthyma
    contagious e.
    e. gangrenosum
ectiris
ectoantigen
ectoblast
ectocardia
ectocervical smear
ectochoroidea
ectocornea
ectocrine
    ecological e.
ectocyst
ectoderm
    amnionic e.
    chorionic e.
    epithelial e.
    extraembryonic e.
ectodermal
    e. cloaca
    e. dysplasia
ectodermatosis
ectodermic
ectodermosis
ectoentad
ectoental
ectoenzyme
ectoethmoid
ectogenic teratosis
ectogenous
ectoglobular
ectohormone
ectomere
ectomerogony
ectomesenchyme
ectomorph
ectomorphic
ectopagus
ectoparasite
ectoparasiticide
ectoparasitism
ectoperitonitis
ectophyte
ectopia
    e. cordis
    crossed renal e.

E

NOTES

ectopia *(continued)*
    crossed testicular e.
    e. lentis
    e. pupillae congenita
    e. testis
    ureteral e.
ectopic
    e. ACTH syndrome
    e. beat
    e. bone
    e. decidua
    e. eyelash
    e. hormone
    e. impulse
    e. ossification
    e. pacemaker
    e. pinealoma
    e. pregnancy
    e. rhythm
    e. schistosomiasis
    e. tachycardia
    e. teratosis
    e. testis
    e. ureter
    e. ureterocele
ectoplacental cavity
ectoplasm
ectoplasmatic
ectopy
ectoretina
ectosarc
ectoscopy
ectosteal
ectostosis
ectothrix
ectotoxin
ectotrophoblastic cavity
ectozoon
ectrocheiry
ectrochiry
ectrodactyly, ectrodactylia, ectrodactylism
ectrodactyly–ectodermal dysplasia–clefting
    syndrome
ectrogenic
ectrogeny
ectromelia virus
ectromelic
ectropion, ectropium
    atonic e.
    cicatricial e.
    flaccid e.
    e. uveae
ectropody
ectrosyndactyly
ectylurea
ectype
ecuresis
eczema
    allergic e.

    e., asthma, hay fever (EAHF)
    atopic e.
    baker e.
    chronic e.
    dyshidrotic e.
    e. erythematosum
    flexural e.
    hand e.
    e. herpeticum
    infantile e.
    e. intertrigo
    lichenoid e.
    e. marginatum
    nummular e.
    e. papulosum
    e. parasiticum
    pustular e.
    e. pustulosum
    stasis e.
    e. tyloticum
    e. verrucosum
    e. vesiculosum
eczematization
eczematoid seborrhea
eczematous conjunctivitis
ED
    effective dose
ED$_{50}$
    effective median dose
edathamil
EDC
    estimated date of confinement
eddy sound
edea
edema
    alveolar e.
    ambulant e.
    angioneurotic e.
    Berlin e.
    blue e.
    brain e.
    brawny e.
    brown e.
    bullous e.
    cachectic e.
    cardiac e.
    cerebral e.
    cystoid macular e.
    dependent e.
    gestational e.
    e. glottidis
    heat e.
    hereditary angioneurotic e. (HANE)
    hydremic e.
    infantile acute hemorrhagic e.
    inflammatory e.
    interstitial e.
    lymphatic e.
    marantic e.

menstrual e.
e. neonatorum
nonpitting e.
pitting e.
pulmonary e.
subpleural e.

edematization
edematous
edentate
edentulous
Eder-Pustow bougie
edestin
edetate calcium disodium
edetic acid
edge

cutting e.
denture e.
e. enhancement
incisal e.
leading e.

edge-to-edge

e.-t.-e. bite
e.-t.-e. occlusion

edgewise appliance
Edinger-Westphal nucleus
Edison effect
edisylate
Edlefsen reagent
Edman

E. method
E. reagent

Edridge-Green lamp
edrophonium chloride
EDS

Ehlers-Danlos syndrome

education

health e.

educational psychology
educt
edulcorant
edulcorate
Edwardsiella
Edwards syndrome
EEE

eastern equine encephalomyelitis
EEE virus

EEG

electroencephalogram
EEG activation

eel

vinegar e.

EENT

eye, ear, nose, and throat

effacement
effect

abscopal e.
additive e.
adverse e.
Anrep e.
Arias-Stella e.
autokinetic e.
Bernoulli e.
blast e.
Bohr e.
Bowditch e.
Circe e.
clasp-knife e.
Compton e.
Cotton e.
Crabtree e.
cumulative e.
Cushing e.
cyclosporine e.
cytopathic e.
deleterious e.
digitalis e.
diuretic e.
Doppler e.
Edison e.
electrophonic e.
estrogen e.
experimenter e.'s
Fahraeus-Lindqvist e.
Fenn e.
first-pass e.
flash-lag e.
founder e.
gene dosage e.
generation e.
Haldane e.
halo e.
Hawthorne e.
healthy worker e.
hyperchromic e.
hypochromic e.
Mach e.
e. modifier
Pasteur e.
position e.
quantal e.
side e.
Somogyi e.

E

NOTES

effective
  e. conjugate
  e. dose (ED)
  e. half-life
  e. median dose (ED$_{50}$)
  e. osmotic pressure
  e. refractory period
  e. renal blood flow (ERBF)
  e. renal plasma flow (ERPF)
  e. stroke
  e. temperature
  e. temperature index
effectiveness
  relative biologic e.
effector cell
effemination
efferent
  e. duct
  e. ductule
  e. fiber
  gamma e.
  e. glomerular arteriole
  e. loop
  e. lymphatic
  e. nerve
  e. vessel
effervesce
effervescent
  e. lithium citrate
  e. magnesium citrate
  e. magnesium sulfate
  e. potassium citrate
  e. salt
  e. sodium phosphate
efficacy
efficiency
  mechanical e.
effleurage
effloresce
efflorescent
effluvium
  anagen e.
  telogen e.
effort
  angina of e.
  distributed e.
effort-induced thrombosis
effuse
effusion
  complex pleural e.
  joint e.
  loculated pleural e.
  middle-ear e.
  pericardial e.
  pericarditis with e.
  pleural e.
EGD
  esophagogastroduodenoscopy
egesta

EGF
  epidermal growth factor
EGFR
  epidermal growth factor receptor
egg
  e. albumin
  e. cell
  centrolecithal e.
  e. cluster
  homolecithal e.
  isolecithal e.
  e. membrane
  microlecithal e.
  e. shell nail
Egger line
Eggleston method
eggshell
  e. appearance
  e. calcification
egg-white
  e.-w. injury
  e.-w. syndrome
eglandulous
Eglis gland
ego
  e. analysis
  e. crisis
  e. ideal
  e. identity
  e. instinct
  e. libido
ego-alien
egobronchophony
egocentric
egocentricity
ego-dystonic homosexuality
ego-ideal
egomania
egophonic
egophony
ego-syntonic
egotropic
Egyptian
  E. hematuria
  E. ophthalmia
  E. splenomegaly
Ehlers-Danlos syndrome (EDS)
Ehrenritter ganglion
Ehret phenomenon
Ehrlich
  E. acid hematoxylin stain
  E. anemia
  E. aniline crystal violet stain
  E. benzaldehyde reaction
  E. diazo reaction
  E. diazo reagent
  E. inner body
  E. phenomenon
  E. postulate

E. theory
E. triacid stain
E. triple stain
Ehrlichia
E. *canis*
E. *chaffeensis*
E. *equi*
E. *phagocytophilia*
E. *risticii*
E. *sennetsu*
ehrlichiosis
human e.
human granulocytic e. (HGE)
human monocytic e. (HME)
Ehrlich-Türk line
Eichhorst
E. corpuscle
E. neuritis
Eicken method
eicosanoid
eidetic image
eighth
e. cranial nerve
e. nerve tumor
Eikenella corrodens
eikonometer
eiloid
Einarson gallocyanin-chrome alum stain
einstein
einsteinium
Einthoven
E. equation
E. law
E. string galvanometer
E. triangle
Eisenmenger
E. complex
E. defect
E. disease
E. syndrome
E. tetralogy
eisodic
ejaculate
ejaculation
premature e.
retrograde e.
ejaculatory duct
ejecta
ejection
e. click
e. fraction
e. murmur

e. period
e. sound
ejector
EJP
excitatory junction potential
Ejrup maneuver
Ekbom syndrome
Ekehorn operation
EKG
electrocardiogram
EKG trigger
ekiri
ektoplasmic
ektoplastic
EKY
electrokymogram
elaboration
Elaeophora schneideri
elaidic acid
elaiopathia
elapid
elastance
elastase
elastic
e. artery
e. bandage
e. band fixation
e. bougie
e. cartilage
e. cone
e. fiber
intermaxillary e.
e. lamella
e. lamina
e. layer
e. ligature
e. limit
e. membrane
e. skin
e. suture
e. tissue
e. traction
elastica
elasticin
elasticity
elasticum
pseudoxanthoma e.
elasticus
conus e.
elastin
Weigert stain for e.
elastofibroma

NOTES

E

elastoid degeneration
elastoidin
elastolysis
    generalized e.
elastoma
    juvenile e.
    Miescher e.
elastometer
elastomucin
elastorrhexis
elastosis
    solar e.
elastotic degeneration
elation
elaunin
Elaut triangle
elbow
    above e. (A-E)
    below the e. (B-E)
    e. bone
    e. jerk
    e. joint
    Little League e.
    Little Leaguer's e.
    miner's e.
    nursemaid's e.
    e. reflex
    tennis e.
elbowed
    e. bougie
    e. catheter
elder
    e. abuse
    e. flower
elderly primigravida
elective
    e. abortion
    e. amnesia
    e. culture
    e. mutism
    e. surgery
Electra complex
electric
    e. anesthesia
    e. bath
    e. cardiac pacemaker
    e. cataract
    e. cautery
    e. chorea
    e. chromatography
    e. irritability
    e. retinopathy
    e. shock
    e. sleep
electrical
    e. alternans
    e. alternation
    e. axis
    e. diastole

    e. failure
    e. formula
    e. heart position
    e. systole
electricity
electroacupuncture
electroanalgesia
electroanalysis
electroanesthesia
electroaxonography
electrobioscopy
electrocardiogram (ECG, EKG)
    concordant change e.
    discordant change e.
electrocardiograph
electrocardiographic
    e. complex
    e. wave
electrocardiography
    fetal e.
electrocardiophonogram
electrocardiophonography
electrocauterization
electrocautery
electrocerebral
    e. inactivity
    e. silence
electrochemical gradient
electrocoagulation
electrocochleogram
electrocochleography
electrocontractility
electroconvulsive therapy (ECT)
electrocorticogram
electrocorticography (ECoG)
electrocute
electrocution
electrocystography
electrode
    active e.
    calomel e.
    carbon dioxide e.
    e. catheter ablation
    central terminal e.
    Clark e.
    dispersing e.
    exciting e.
    exploring e.
    glass e.
    hydrogen e.
    indifferent e.
    ion-selective e.
    e. knife
    localizing e.
    negative e.
    resectoscope e.
    rollerball e.
electrodermal audiometry
electrodermatome

electrodesiccation
electrodiagnosis
electrodiagnostic medicine
electrodialysis
electroencephalogram (EEG)
    flat e.
    isoelectric e.
electroencephalograph
electroencephalographic dysrhythmia
electroencephalography
electroendosmosis
electrofocusing
electrogastrogram
electrogastrograph
electrogastrography
electrogram
    His bundle e. (HBE)
electrographic seizure
electrohemostasis
electrohydraulic shock wave lithotripsy
electrohysterograph
electroimmunodiffusion
electrokymogram (EKY)
electrokymograph
electrolarynx
electrolysis
electrolyte
    amphoteric e.
    e. metabolism
electrolytic
electrolyze
electrolyzer
electromagnet
electromagnetic
    e. flowmeter
    e. induction
    e. radiation
    e. spectrum
    e. unit
electromassage
electromechanical
    e. dissociation
    e. systole
electromicturation
electromorph
electromotility
electromotive force
electromuscular sensibility
electromyogram (EMG)
electromyograph
electromyography
    evoked e.

electron
    Auger e.
    e. beam
    e. beam tomography (EBT)
    e. capture
    conversion e.
    emission e.
    e. interferometer
    e. interferometry
    internal conversion e.
    e. magneton
    e. micrograph
    e. microscope
    e. microscopy
    e. paramagnetic resonance (EPR)
    e. radiography
    e. resonance absorption
    e. spin resonance
    e. transfer flavin
    e. transport particle (ETP)
electronarcosis
electronegative element
electroneurography
electroneurolysis
electroneuromyography
electronic
    e. cell counter
    e. fetal monitor
    e. number
    e. pacemaker
    e. pacemaker load
electron-transport
    e.-t. chain
    e.-t. system
electron-volt
    1 million e.-v.'s (Mev)
electronystagmography (ENG)
electrooculogram
electrooculography (EOG)
electroolfactogram
electro-osmosis
electroparacentesis
electropherogram
electrophil, electrophile
electrophilic
electrophobia
electrophonic effect
electrophoresis
    capillary zone e. (CZE)
    carrier e.
    disc e.
    free e.

E

NOTES

electrophoresis *(continued)*
    gel e.
    isoenzyme e.
    lipoprotein e.
    polyacrylamide gel e.
    pulse-field gel e.
electrophoretic
electrophoretogram
electrophrenic respiration
electrophysiology
electroporation
electropositive element
electropuncture
electroradiology
electroradiometer
electroretinogram (ERG)
electroretinography
electroscission
electroscope
electroshock therapy
electrosol
electrospectrography
electrospinogram
electrospinography
electrostatic
    e. bond
    e. unit
electrostenolysis
electrostethograph
electrostriction
electrosurgery
electrosurgical needle
electrotaxis
electrothanasia
electrotherapeutic
    e. bath
    e. sleep
    e. sleep therapy
electrotherapeutics
electrotherapy
electrotherm
electrotome
electrotomy
electrotonic
    e. current
    e. junction
    e. synapse
electrotonus
electrotropism
electuary
eledoisin
eleidin
element
    actinide e.
    alkaline earth e.
    amphoteric e.
    anatomical e.
    electronegative e.
    electropositive e.

    extrachromosomal e.
    extrachromosomal genetic e.
    fold-back e.
    labile e.
    long interspersed e.
    trace e.
    transposable e.
elementary
    e. body
    e. granule
    e. particle
5-element theory
eleoma
eleometer
eleopathy
eleostearic acid
eleotherapy
elephant
    e. leg
    e. man's disease
elephantiac
elephantiasic
elephantiasis
    congenital e.
    gingival e.
    e. neuromatosa
    e. scroti
    e. telangiectodes
    e. vulvae
elephantoid fever
elevator
    e. disease
    joker e.
    e. muscle
    palatal e.
    periosteal e.
eleventh cranial nerve
elfin
    e. facies
    e. facies syndrome
eliminant
eliminase
    heparin e.
elimination
    carbon dioxide e.
    e. diet
    immune e.
elinguation
elinin
ELISA
    enzyme-linked immunosorbent assay
elixir
Ellik evacuator
Elliot
    E. operation
    E. position
Elliott law
ellipsis
ellipsoidal joint

elliptical
  e. amputation
  e. anastomosis
  e. recess
elliptocytary anemia
elliptocyte
elliptocytosis
elliptocytotic anemia
Ellis-van Creveld syndrome
Ellsworth-Howard test
Eloesser
  E. flap
  E. procedure
elongation factor
Elschnig
  E. pearl
  E. spot
Elsner asthma
El Tor vibrio
eluant
eluate
eluent
elusive ulcer
elutant
elute
elution
  gradient e.
elutriate
elutriation
E-M
  eosinophilia-myalgia
  E-M syndrome
EMA
  epithelial membrane antigen
emaciation
emaculation
emanation
  actinium e.
emanatorium
emancipation
emanon
emanotherapy
emarginate
emargination
emasculation
embalm
embarrassment
  e. of choices
  e. of riches
Embden ester
Embden-Meyerhof-Parnas pathway
Embden-Meyerhof pathway

embed
embedded tooth
embedding agent
embelin
emboitement
embole
embolectomy
embolemia
embolia
embolic
  e. abscess
  e. aneurysm
  e. gangrene
  e. infarct
  e. necrosis
  e. pneumonia
emboliform nucleus
embolism
  air e.
  amnionic fluid e.
  atheromatous e.
  bland e.
  bone marrow e.
  cellular e.
  cholesterol e.
  cotton-fiber e.
  crossed e.
  direct e.
  fat e.
  gas e.
  hematogenous e.
  infective e.
  lymph e.
  lymphogenous e.
  miliary e.
  obturating e.
  paradoxical e.
  pulmonary e.
  pyemic e.
  retrograde e.
  venous e.
embolization
embololalia
embolomycotic aneurysm
embolophrasia
embolotherapy
embolus
  catheter e.
emboly
embouchement
embrasure
  buccal e.

E

NOTES

embrasure *(continued)*
    gingival e.
    incisal e.
    labial e.
    lingual e.
embrocation
embryo
    heterogametic e.
    hexacanth e.
    homogametic e.
    e. transfer
embryoblast
embryocardia
embryogenesis
embryogenetic
embryogenic
embryogeny
embryoid body
embryologist
embryology
embryoma
embryomorphous
embryonal
    e. adenoma
    e. area
    e. carcinoid
    e. carcinoma
    e. inducer
    e. leukemia
    e. medulloepithelioma
    e. rhabdomyosarcoma
    e. tumor
embryonate
embryonic
    e. anideus
    e. area
    e. axis
    e. blastoderm
    e. cataract
    e. cell
    e. circulation
    e. diapause
    e. disc
    e. hemoglobin
    e. membrane
    e. shield
    e. tumor
embryoniform
embryonization
embryonoid
embryony
embryopathic cataract
embryopathy
embryophore
embryoplastic
embryotomy
embryotoxicity

embryotoxon
    anterior e.
    posterior e.
embryotroph
embryotrophic
embryotrophy
emedullate
emeiocytosis
emergence
emergency
    e. hormonal contraception
    e. medical service (EMS)
    e. medical technician (EMT)
    e. theory
emergent evolution
emerging virus
emery disc
Emery-Dreifuss muscular dystrophy
emesis basin
emetic
emetine
emetocathartic
emetogenic
emetogenicity
EMG
    electromyogram
    EMG biofeedback
    EMG examination
    EMG syndrome
emiction
emigration
eminence
    abducens e.
    arcuate e.
    articular e.
    canine e.
    collateral e.
    cruciate e.
    cruciform e.
    deltoid e.
    Doyère e.
    facial e.
    forebrain e.
    frontal e.
    genital e.
    hypobranchial e.
    hypoglossal e.
    hypothenar e.
    ileocecal e.
    iliopectineal e.
    iliopubic e.
    intercondylar e.
    intercondyloid e.
    maxillary e.
    medial e.
    median e.
    thenar e.
emiocytosis

emissary
    e. foramen
    e. vein
emission
    e. angiography
    characteristic e.
    continuous otoacoustic e.
    distortion-product otoacoustic e.
    e. electron
    evoked otoacoustic e.
    nasal e.
    otoacoustic e.
    thermionic e.
    transient evoked otoacoustic e.
emissivity
EMIT
    enzyme-multiplied immunoassay
    technique
emmenia
emmenic
emmeniopathy
Emmet
    E. needle
    E. operation
emmetropia
emmetropic
emmetropization
Emmonsiella capsulata
emodin
emollient laxative
emotional
    e. age
    e. amenorrhea
    e. amnesia
    e. attitude
    e. deprivation
    e. disease
    e. disorder
    e. disturbance
    e. lability
    e. leukocytosis
    e. overlay
    e. tone
emotiovascular
empasm, empasma
empathic index
empathize
empathy
    generative e.
emperipolesis
emphraxis

emphysema
    alveolar duct e.
    bullous e.
    centriacinar e.
    centrilobular e.
    compensating e.
    compensatory e.
    congenital lobar e.
    cutaneous e.
    cystic e.
    diffuse obstructive e.
    ectatic e.
    familial e.
    gangrenous e.
    generalized e.
    increased markings e.
    interlobular e.
    interstitial e.
    intestinal e.
    irregular e.
    lobar e.
    mediastinal e.
    panlobular e.
    paracicatricial e.
    pulmonary e.
    subcutaneous e.
    surgical e.
    unilateral lobar e.
    vesicular e.
emphysematous
    e. chest
    e. cholecystitis
    e. cystitis
    e. gangrene
empiric
    e. risk
    e. treatment
empirical
    e. formula
    e. horopter
empiricism
emporiatrics
emprosthotonos position
empty sella
empyectomy
empyema
    latent e.
    loculated e.
    mastoid e.
    pulsating e.
    e. tube
empyemic scoliosis

E

NOTES

empyesis
empyocele
empyreuma
EMS
    emergency medical service
      EMS system
EMT
    emergency medical technician
emu
emulgent
emulsifier
emulsify
emulsifying wax
emulsin
emulsion colloid
emulsive
emulsoid
emuresis
emylcamate
en
    e. bloc
    e. grappe
    e. thyrse
enalaprilat
enalapril maleate
enamel
    e. cap
    e. cell
    e. cleavage
    e. cleaver
    e. crypt
    e. cuticle
    e. drop
    dwarfed e.
    e. dysplasia
    e. epithelium
    e. fiber
    e. fissure
    e. germ
    e. hypocalcification
    e. hypoplasia
    interrod e.
    e. lamella
    e. layer
    e. ledge
    e. membrane
    mottled e.
    e. niche
    e. nodule
    e. organ
    e. pearl
    e. prism
    e. projection
    e. pulp
    e. rod
    e. rod inclination
    e. rod sheath
    e. tuft
    e. wall

enamelin
enameloblast
enamelogenesis imperfecta
enameloma
enamelum
enanthal
enanthate
enanthem, enanthema
enanthematous
enanthesis
enantiomer
enantiomeric
enantiomerism
enantiomorph
enantiomorphic
enantiomorphism
enantiomorphous
enarthrodial joint
enarthrosis
encapsulated
    e. abscess
    e. delusion
encapsulation
encapsuled
encarditis
enceliitis
encelitis
encephalalgia
encephalatrophic
encephalatrophy
encéphale isolé
encephalemia
encephali
    arachnoidea mater e.
    dura mater e.
encephalic vesicle
encephalithogenic protein
encephalitic
encephalitis
    acute hemorrhagic e.
    acute inclusion body e.
    acute necrotizing e.
    Australian X e.
    bacterial e.
    bunyavirus e.
    California e.
    coxsackie e.
    Dawson e.
    epidemic e.
    equine e.
    experimental allergic e. (EAE)
    Far East Russian e.
    herpes simplex e.
    hyperergic e.
    Ilhéus e.
    inclusion body e.
    Japanese B e.
    lead e.
    Mengo e.

Murray Valley e.
e. periaxialis diffusa
Powassan e.
Rasmussen e.
secondary e.
varicella e.
e. virus
encephalitogen
encephalitogenic
Encephalitozoon
    E. cuniculi
    E. hellem
    E. intestinale
    E. intestinalis
encephalization
encephalocele
basal e.
encephaloclastic microcephaly
encephalocraniocutaneous lipomatosis
encephalocystocele
encephaloduroarteriosynangiosis
encephalodynia
encephalodysplasia
encephalogram
encephalography
gamma e.
encephaloid
encephalolith
encephalology
encephaloma
encephalomalacia
encephalomeningitis
encephalomeningocele
encephalomeningopathy
encephalomere
encephalometer
encephalomyelitis
acute disseminated e.
acute necrotizing hemorrhagic e.
benign myalgic e.
eastern equine e. (EEE)
epidemic myalgic e.
equine e.
experimental allergic e.
granulomatous e.
herpes B e.
myalgic e.
postvaccinal e.
western equine e.
encephalomyelocele
encephalomyeloneuropathy
encephalomyelonic axis

encephalomyelopathy
carcinomatous e.
epidemic myalgic e.
paraneoplastic e.
encephalomyeloradiculitis
encephalomyeloradiculopathy
encephalomyocarditis virus
encephalon
encephalopathia
encephalopathy
bilirubin e.
Binswanger e.
bovine spongiform e. (BSE)
demyelinating e.
hepatic e.
HIV e.
hypernatremic e.
hypertensive e.
hypoxic-hypercarbic e.
hypoxic ischemic e.
lead e.
metabolic e.
portal-systemic e.
spongiform e.
subacute spongiform e.
traumatic e.
viral spongiform e.
Wernicke-Korsakoff e.
encephalopyosis
encephalorrhachidian
encephaloschisis
encephalosclerosis
encephaloscope
encephaloscopy
encephalosis
encephalospinal
encephalotome
encephalotomy
encephalotrigeminal
e. angiomatosis
e. vascular syndrome
enchondral
enchondroma
enchondromatosis
enchondromatous
enclave
enclosed space
encoding
frequency e.
gradient e.
encopresis
encounter group

E

NOTES

encranial
encranius
encu
    equivalent normal child unit
      encu method
encysted
    e. abscess
    e. bladder
    e. calculus
    e. hernia
    e. hydrocele
    e. pleurisy
encystment
end
    acromial e.
    e. artery
    e. bud
    e. bulb
    e. cell
    e. colostomy
    distal e.
    fixed e.
    mobile e.
    e. organ
    e. oxidation
    e. piece
    e. plate
    e. point
    e. product
    e. product inhibition
    e. product repression
    e. stage
    e. tracheostome
endadelphos
endangeitis
endangiitis
endaortitis
endarterectomy
    carotid e. (CEA)
    coronary e.
endarteritis
    bacterial e.
    e. deformans
    e. obliterans
    obliterating e.
    e. proliferans
    proliferating e.
endaural incision
endbrain
end-brush
end-bulb
end-cutting bur
end-diastolic volume
endectocide
endemia
endemic
    e. disease
    e. funiculitis
    e. goiter

    e. hematuria
    e. hemoptysis
    e. hypertrophy
    e. index
    e. influenza
    e. neuritis
    e. nonbacterial infantile
      gastroenteritis
    e. osteoarthritis
    e. paralytic vertigo
    e. stability
    e. syphilis
    e. typhus
    e. urticaria
endemica
    urticaria e.
endemoepidemic
endergonic
endermatic
endermic
endermosis
end-feel
end-feet
endgut
ending
    annulospiral e.
    caliciform e.
    epilemmal e.
    flower-spray e.
    free nerve e.
    grape e.
    hederiform e.
Endo
    E. agar
    E. medium
endoabdominal fascia
endoamylase
endoaneurysmoplasty
endoaneurysmorrhaphy
endoangiitis
endo-aortitis
endoappendicitis
endoarteritis
endoauscultation
endobag
endobasion
endobiotic
endoblast
endobronchial tube
endocardiac
endocardial
    e. cushion
    e. cushion defect
    e. fibroelastosis
    e. fibrosis
    e. murmur
    e. sclerosis
    e. tube
endocardiography

endocarditic
endocarditis
    abacterial thrombotic e.
    acute bacterial e.
    atypical verrucous e.
    bacterial e.
    cachectic e.
    e. chordalis
    constrictive e.
    fungal e.
    gonococcal e.
    infectious e.
    infective e.
    isolated parietal e.
    Libman-Sacks e.
    Löffler parietal fibroplastic e.
    malignant e.
    marantic e.
    mural e.
    nonbacterial verrucous e.
    prosthetic valve e.
    rheumatic e.
    subacute bacterial e.
    syphilitic e.
    valvular e.
    vegetative e.
    verrucous e.
endocardium
endoceliac
endocervical
    e. canal
    e. cell
    e. polyp
    e. sinus tumor
    e. smear
endocervicitis
endocervix
endochondral
    e. bone
    e. ossification
    e. osteogenesis
endocoagulation
endocochlear potential
endocolitis
endocranial
endocranium
endocrine
    e. exophthalmos
    e. gland
    e. hormone
    e. myopathy

    e. ophthalmopathy
    e. system
endocrinologist
endocrinology
endocrinoma
endocrinopathic
endocrinopathy
endocrinotherapy
endocyclic
endocyst
endocystitis
endocytosis
endoderm
endodermal
    e. canal
    e. cell
    e. cloaca
    e. cyst
    e. pouch
    e. sinus tumor
endodiascope
endodiascopy
endodontia
endodontic
    e. stabilizer
    e. treatment
endodontics
endodontist
endodontologist
endodontology
endodyocyte
endodyogeny
endoenteritis
endoenzyme
endoesophagitis
endofaradism
end-of-life care
endogalvanism
endogamy
endogastric
endogastritis
endogenic toxicosis
endogenote
endogenous
    e. aneurysm
    e. creatinine clearance
    e. cycle
    e. depression
    e. fiber
    e. hyperglyceridemia
    e. infection
    e. pyrogen

E

NOTES

endoglin
endognathion
endoherniotomy
endointoxication
endolaryngeal
endolemniscal nucleus
endolith
endolymph
endolympha
endolymphatic
    e. duct
    e. hydrops
    e. sac
    e. sac surgery
    e. shunt operation
    e. space
endolymphic
endomembrane system
endomerogony
endometrial
    e. ablation
    e. canal
    e. cell
    e. cyst
    e. gland
    e. hyperplasia
    e. implant
    e. polyp
    e. smear
    e. stromal sarcoma
endometrioid
    e. carcinoma
    e. tumor
endometrioma
endometriosis
endometritis
    decidual e.
    e. dissecans
endometrium
endometropic
endomitosis
endomorph
endomorphic
endomotorsonde
endomyocardial
    e. fibroelastosis
    e. fibrosis
endomyocarditis
endomyometritis
endomysium
endoneurium
end-on mattress suture
endonuclease
    micrococcal e.
    restriction e.
    e. S1 *Aspergillus*
    e. *Serratia marcescens*
endonucleolus
endo-osseous implant

endoparasite
endopeduncular nucleus
endopelvic fascia
endopeptidase
endoperiarteritis
endopericardiac
endopericarditis
endoperimyocarditis
endoperitonitis
endoperoxide
endophlebitis
endophthalmitis
    granulomatous e.
    e. ophthalmia nodosa
    e. phacoanaphylactica
endophthalmodonesis
endophyte
endophytic
endoplasm
endoplasmic reticulum
endoplast
endoplastic
endopolygeny
endopolyploid
endopolyploidy
endorectal pull-through procedure
endoreduplication
endorphin
endorphinergic
endorrhachis
endosac
endosalpingiosis
endosalpingitis
endosalpinx
endosarc
endoscope
    flexible e.
endoscopic
    e. biopsy
    e. retrograde cholangiopancreatography (ERCP)
endoscopist
endoscopy
    flexible e.
    peroral e.
    virtual e.
endoskeleton
endosome
endosonography
endosonoscopy
endosperm
endospore
endosteal, endosseous
    e. implant
    e. lamella
endosteitis
endosteoma
endostethoscope
endosteum

endostitis
endostoma
endotendineum
endoteric bacterium
endothelial
    e. cell
    e. cyst
    e. dystrophy
    e. leukocyte
    e. myeloma
    e. relaxing factor
    e. tuberculosis
endothelial-leukocyte adhesion molecule
endothelin
endotheliochorial placenta
endotheliocyte
endothelio-endothelial placenta
endothelioid
endothelioma
endotheliosis
endothelium
    vascular e.
endothelium-derived relaxing factor
endothermic
endothoracic fascia
endothrix
endothyropexy
endotoxemia
endotoxic
endotoxicosis
endotoxin shock
endotracheal
    e. anesthesia
    e. intubation
    e. stylet
    e. tube
endotrachelitis
endourology
endovaccination
endovaginal ultrasonography
endovasculitis
    hemorrhagic e.
endovenous septum
end-piece
endplate, end-plate, end plate
    motor e.
end-point
    e.-p. measurement
    e.-p. nystagmus
end-stage
    e.-s. lung
    e.-s. renal disease (ESRD)

end-systolic volume
end-tidal sample
end-to-end
    e.-t.-e. anastomosis
    e.-t.-e. bite
    e.-t.-e. occlusion
endurance
    muscular e.
endyma
enediol
enema
    air contrast barium e.
    analeptic e.
    barium e.
    blind e.
    cleansing e.
    contrast e.
    double contrast e.
    flatus e.
    high e.
    Hypaque e.
enemator
enemiasis
energetics
energy
    e. of activation
    e. balance equation
    binding e.
    chemical e.
    conservation of e.
    free e.
    fusion e.
    Gibbs free e.
    Helmholtz e.
    internal e.
    kinetic e.
    latent e.
    e. metabolism
    e. of position
    potential e.
    e. subtraction
energy-rich
    e.-r. bond
    e.-r. phosphate
enervation
enflurane
ENG
    electronystagmography
engagement
engastrius

NOTES

E

Engelmann
    E. basal knob
    E. disease
engine
    dental e.
    e. reamer
engineering
    biomedical e.
    dental e.
    genetic e.
Englisch sinus
English
    E. lock
    manual E.
    E. position
    E. sweating disease
englobe
englobement
engorged
engorgement
engram
engraphia
enhancement
    acoustic e.
    contrast e.
    edge e.
    immunologic e.
enhancer
enkephalinergic
enkephalins
enlargement
    cervical e.
    choroid e.
    discrete organ e.
    gingival e.
    left ventricular e.
    lumbosacral e.
enolase
    neuron-specific e.
enolization
enology
enol pyruvate
enophthalmia
enophthalmos
enorganic
enostosis
enoyl-ACP
    e.-ACP reductase
    e.-ACP reductase NADPH
enoyl-CoA
    e.-CoA hydratase
    e.-CoA reductase
enoyl hydrase
enrichment culture
ensheathing callus
ensiform
    e. appendix
    e. cartilage
    e. process

ensisternum cartilage
ensu
    equivalent normal son unit
        ensu method
ENT
    ears, nose, and throat
entactin
entad
ental
entamebiasis
Entamoeba
    E. buccalis
    E. chattoni
    E. coli
    E. dispar
    E. gingivalis
    E. hartmanni
    E. histolytica
    E. moshkovskii
    E. polecki
enteralgia
enteral hyperalimentation
enteramine
enterdynia
enterectasis
enterectomy
enterelcosis
enteric
    e. coated tablet
    e. cytopathogenic human orphan virus
    e. cytopathogenic monkey orphan virus
    e. cytopathogenic swine orphan virus
    e. fever
    e. nervous plexus
    e. tuberculosis
entericoid fever
entericus
    liquor e.
enteritidis
    Salmonella enterica e.
enteritis
    e. anaphylactica
    bacterial e.
    chronic cicatrizing e.
    diphtheritic e.
    granulomatous e.
    human eosinophilic e.
    mucomembranous e.
    e. necroticans
    e. polyposa
    pseudomembranous e.
    regional e.
    tuberculous e.
enteroanastomosis
enteroanthelone

Enterobacter
    E. aerogenes
    E. cloacae
    E. sakazakii
enterobacterium
enterobiasis
Enterobius granuloma
enterocele
enterocentesis
enterocholecystostomy
enterocholecystotomy
enterochromaffin cell
enterocidal
enterocleisis
enteroclysis
    radiologic e.
enterococcemia
Enterococcus
    E. faecalis
    E. faecium
enterocolic fistula
enterocolitis
    antibiotic e.
    hemorrhagic e.
    necrotizing e.
    pseudomembranous e.
    regional e.
enterocolostomy
enterocutaneous fistula
enterocyst
enterocystocele
enterocystoma
enterocyte cobalamin malabsorption
Enterocytozoon bieneusi
enterodynia
enteroendocrine cell
enteroenterostomy
enterogastric reflex
enterogastritis
enterogastrone
enterogenous
    e. cyanosis
    e. cyst
    e. methemoglobinemia
enterograph
enterography
enterohemorrhagic *Escherichia coli*
enterohepatic circulation
enterohepatitis
enterohepatocele
enteroidea
enteroinvasive *Escherichia coli*

enterokinase
enterokinesis
enterokinetic agent
enterolith
enterolithiasis
cnterology
enterolysis
enteromegaly, enteromegalia
enteromenia
enteromerocele
enterometer
enteromycosis
enteroparesis
enteropathica
    acrodermatitis e.
enteropathic arthritis
enteropathogen
enteropathogenic
enteropathy
    gluten e.
    protein-losing e.
enteropeptidase
enteropexy
enteroplegia
enteroproctia
enteroptosia
enteroptosis
enteroptotic
enterorenal
enterorrhagia
enterorrhaphy
enterorrhexis
enteroscope
enterosepsis
enterospasm
enterostasis
enterostenosis
enterostomy
    double e.
enterotome
enterotomy
enterotoxemia
enterotoxication
enterotoxigenic
enterotoxin
    cytotonic e.
    Escherichia coli e.
enterotoxism
enterotropic
enterovaginal fistula
enterovesical fistula
Enterovirus

E

NOTES

enterozoic
enterozoon
entgegen
enthalpy
enthesitis
enthesopathic
enthesopathy
enthlasis
Entner-Douderoff pathway
entoblast
entocele
entochoroidea
entocone
entoconid
entocornea
entocranial
entocranium
entoderm
entodermal cell
entoectad
entomion
entomology
entomophobia
Entomophthora coronata
entomophthoramycosis
entopic pregnancy
entoplasm
entoptic pulse
entoretina
entorhinal area
entosarc
entozoal
entozoon
entrails
entrainment mask
entrance block
entrapment neuropathy
entropion
    atonic e.
    cicatricial e.
entropionize
entropium
entropy
entry zone
entypy
enucleate
enucleation
enuresis
    diurnal e.
    nocturnal e.
envelope
    e. conformation
    corneocyte e.
    e. flap
    nuclear e.
    viral e.
envenomation
environment

environmental
    e. illness
    e. psychology
enzootic
    e. encephalomyelitis virus
    e. stability
enzygotic twin
enzymatic synthesis
enzyme
    acetyl-activating e.
    acyl-activating e.
    adaptive e.
    allosteric e.
    e. analog
    angiotensin-converting e. (ACE)
    e. antagonist
    antitumor e.
    autolytic e.
    branching e.
    citrate-cleavage e.
    cold-sensitive e.
    condensing e.
    constitutive e.
    cooperative e.
    D e.
    deamidizing e.
    deaminating e.
    debranching e.
    digestive e.
    disproportionating e.
    extracellular e.
    heat-stable e.
    hydrolyzing e.
    immobilized e.
    e. immunoassay
    induced e.
    inducible e.
    e. interconversion
    intracellular e.
    e. isomerization
    e. kinetics
    Kornberg e.
    malate-condensing e.
    malic e.
    marker e.
    membrane e.
    methionine-activating e.
    e. parameter
    e. regulation
    repressible e.
    e. repression
    respiratory e.
    restriction e.
enzyme-catalyzed ligation
enzyme-linked immunosorbent assay (ELISA)
enzyme-multiplied immunoassay technique (EMIT)
enzyme-substrate complex

enzymic
enzymologist
enzymology
enzymolysis
enzymopathy
EOG
electrooculography
eosin
e. B
e. I bluish
e. y, e. Y
e. yellowish
eosin-methylene blue agar
eosinocyte
eosinopenia
eosinopenic reaction
eosinophil, eosinophile
e. adenoma
e. cationic protein
e. chemotactic factor
e. granule
eosinophilia
pulmonary e.
tropical e.
eosinophilia-myalgia (E-M)
e.-m. syndrome
eosinophilic
e. cellulitis
e. cystitis
e. endomyocardial disease
e. fasciitis
e. gastritis
e. gastroenteritis
e. granuloma
e. leukemia
e. leukocyte
e. leukocytosis
e. leukopenia
e. meningitis
e. meningoencephalitis
e. pneumonia
e. pneumonopathy
e. pustular folliculitis
eosinophilocytic leukemia
eosinophiluria
eosinotactic
eosinotaxis
eosophobia
epactal
e. bone
e. ossicle

epamniotic cavity
eparterial bronchus
epaxial
ependyma
ependymal
e. cell
e. cyst
e. layer
e. zone
ependymitis
ependymoblast
ependymoblastoma
ependymocyte
ependymoma
myxopapillary e.
ephapse
ephaptic
ephebic
ephebology
ephedra
ephedrine
ephelis
ephemeral
e. fever
e. fever virus
epiandrosterone
epibatidine
epiblast
epiblastic
epiblepharon
epiboly, epibole
epibranchial placode
epibulbar
epicanthal fold
epicanthus
e. inversus
e. palpebralis
e. supraciliaris
e. tarsalis
epicardia
epicardial
epicardium
epichordal
epicillin
epicomus
epicondylalgia externa
epicondyle
lateral e.
medial e.
epicondylian
epicondylic

NOTES

317

epicondylitis
    lateral humeral e.
    medial e.
epicoracoid
epicranial
    e. aponeurosis
    e. muscle
epicranialis
    aponeurosis e.
epicranium
epicranius muscle
epicrisis
epicritic sensibility
epicystitis
epicyte
epidemic
    behavioral e.
    e. benign dry pleurisy
    e. cerebrospinal meningitis
    e. curve
    e. diaphragmatic pleurisy
    e. disease
    e. dropsy
    e. encephalitis
    e. exanthema
    e. gangrenous proctitis
    e. gastroenteritis virus
    e. hemoglobinuria
    e. hemorrhagic fever
    e. hepatitis
    e. hiccup
    e. hysteria
    e. keratoconjunctivitis
    e. keratoconjunctivitis virus
    e. myalgia
    e. myalgia virus
    e. myalgic encephalomyelitis
    e. myalgic encephalomyelopathy
    e. myositis
    e. nausea
    e. neuromyasthenia
    e. nonbacterial gastroenteritis
    e. parotiditis
    e. parotitis virus
    e. pleurodynia
    e. pleurodynia virus
    point e.
    e. polyarthritis
    e. roseola
    e. stomatitis
    e. transient diaphragmatic spasm
    e. typhus
    e. vertigo
    e. vomiting
epidemica
    neuropathia e.
    urticaria e.
epidemicity
epidemiography

epidemiological
    e. distribution
    e. genetics
epidemiologic genetics
epidemiologist
epidemiology
    clinical e.
    genetic e.
    molecular e.
epiderm, epiderma
epidermal
    e. cyst
    e. growth factor (EGF)
    e. growth factor receptor (EGFR)
    e. ridge
    e. ridge count
epidermalization
epidermal-melanin unit
epidermatic
epidermic cell
epidermidis
    stratum basale e.
    stratum corneum e.
    stratum spinosum e.
epidermidosis
epidermis
epidermitis
epidermodysplasia
epidermoid
    e. cancer
    e. carcinoma
    e. cyst
    e. tumor
epidermolysis bullosa
epidermolytic hyperkeratosis
Epidermophyton
epidermosis
epidermotropism
epidiascope
epididymal
epididymectomy
epididymidis
    cauda e.
    corpus e.
epididymis
epididymitis
epididymoorchitis
epididymoplasty
epididymotomy
epididymovasectomy
epididymovasostomy
epidural
    e. anesthesia
    e. block
    e. cavity
    e. hematoma
    e. hemorrhage
    e. meningitis
    e. space

epidurography
epiestriol
epifascial
epifascicular epineurium
epigastralgia
epigastric
    e. angle
    e. fold
    e. fossa
    e. hernia
    e. reflex
    e. region
    e. vein
    e. voice
    e. zone
epigastrica
    vena e.
epigastrium
epigastrius
epigenesis
epigenetic
epiglottic
    e. cartilage
    e. fold
    e. tubercle
    e. vallecula
epiglottidean
epiglottidectomy
epiglottiditis
epiglottis
    bifid e.
epiglottitis
epignathus
epihyal
    e. bone
    e. ligament
epihyoid
epikeratophakia
epikeratophakic keratoplasty
epikeratoprosthesis
epilamellar
epilate
epilation dose
epilatory
epilemma
epilemmal ending
epilepidoma
epilepsy
    anosognosic e.
    automatic e.
    autonomic e.
    benign childhood e.

    centrencephalic e.
    childhood absence e.
    complex precipitated e.
    cortical e.
    cryptogenic e.
    diencephalic e.
    early posttraumatic e.
    eating e.
    focal e.
    frontal lobe e.
    generalized tonic-clonic e.
    grand mal e.
    idiopathic e.
    intractable e.
    jacksonian e.
    juvenile absence e.
    juvenile myoclonic e.
    Kojewnikoff e.
    laryngeal e.
    local e.
    localization-related e.
    major e.
    masked e.
    matutinal e.
    myoclonic astatic e.
    myoclonus e.
    occipital lobe e.
    pattern-sensitive e.
    photogenic e.
    physic e.
    posttraumatic e.
    procursive e.
    psychomotor e.
    reflex e.
    rolandic e.
    sensory e.
    startle e.
    temporal lobe e.
    tonic e.
epileptic
    e. automatism
    e. dementia
    e. myoclonus
    e. seizure
    e. spasm
    e. stupor
epilepticus
    furor e.
    ictus e.
    status e.
epileptiform neuralgia
epileptogenic zone

NOTES

E

epileptogenous
epileptoid
epiloia
epiluminescence microscopy
epimandibular
epimastical fever
epimastigote
epimenorrhagia
epimenorrhea
epimer
epimerase deficiency galactosemia
epimere
epimerite
epimicroscope
epimorphosis
epimyoepithelial island
epimysiotomy
epimysium
epinephrine reversal
epinephros
epineural suture
epineurial
epineurium
    epifascicular e.
epionychium
epiotic center
epipapillary membrane
epipastic
epipericardial ridge
epipharynx
epiphenomenon
epiphora
    atonic e.
epiphrenal
epiphrenic diverticulum
epiphysial, epiphyseal
    e. arrest
    e. aseptic necrosis
    e. cartilage
    e. eye
    e. fracture
    e. line
    e. plate
epiphysiodesis
epiphysiolysis
epiphysiopathy
epiphysis
    atavistic e.
    capital e.
    e. cerebri
    pressure e.
    slipped capital femoral e. (SCFE)
    traction e.
epiphysitis
epipial
epiplocele
epiploic
    e. appendage
    e. appendix

    e. branch
    e. foramen
    e. tag
epiploica
    appendix e.
epiploon
epipodophyllotoxin
epipteric bone
epipygus
epiretinal membrane
episclera
episcleral
    e. artery
    e. lamina
    e. layer
    e. space
    e. vein
episcleritis
episioperineorrhaphy
episioplasty
episiorrhaphy
episiostenosis
episiotomy
episode
    acute schizophrenic e.
    e. of care
    manic e.
    transient cerebral ischemic e.
episodic
    e. dyscontrol syndrome
    e. hypertension
episome
epispadias
    balanitic e.
    coronal e.
epispinal
episplenitis
epistasis
epistasy
epistatic
epistaxis
epistemology
epistemophilia
epistenocardiac pericarditis
episternal bone
episternum
epistropheus
epitarsus
epitaxy
epitendineum
epitenon
epithalamus
epithalaxia
epithelial
    e. attachment
    e. body
    e. cancer
    e. cast
    e. choroid layer

e. cyst
e. downgrowth
e. dysplasia
e. dystrophy
e. ectoderm
e. inlay
e. lamina
e. membrane antigen (EMA)
e. migration
e. myoepithelial carcinoma
e. nest
e. pearl
e. plug
e. reticular cell
e. tissue
epithelialization
epitheliochorial placenta
epitheliocyte
epitheliofibril
epithelioglandular
epithelioid
e. cell
e. cell nevus
epitheliolysis
epitheliolytic
epithelioma
e. adenoides cysticum
basal cell e.
chorionic e.
e. cuniculatum
Malherbe calcifying e.
malignant ciliary e.
sebaceous e.
epitheliomatous
epitheliopathy
acute multifocal placoid pigment e.
epitheliosis
epitheliotropic
epithelium
Barrett e.
ciliated e.
columnar e.
crevicular e.
cuboidal e.
cylindrical e.
enamel e.
external dental e.
external enamel e.
germinal e.
gingival e.
glandular e.
inner dental e.

inner enamel e.
junctional e.
laminated e.
mesenchymal e.
olfactory e.
pseudostratified e.
seminiferous e.
simple squamous e.
squamous e.
stratified e.
surface e.
transitional e.
epithelization
epithem
epithermal
e. chemistry
e. neutron
epithet
epithiazide
epitope
shared e.
epitoxoid
epitrichial layer
epitrichium
epitrochlea
epitrochlear
epituberculosis
epituberculous infiltration
epitympanic
e. recess
e. space
epitympanum
epityphlitis
epizoic commensalism
epizoology
epizoon
epizootic
epizootiology
épluchage
epoetin alfa
eponychia
eponychium
eponym
eponymic
epoophoron
epoprostenol sodium
epornitic
epoxy resin
EPR
electron paramagnetic resonance
epsilon wave
Epsom salt

NOTES

E

321

EPSP
 excitatory postsynaptic potential
Epstein
 E. disease
 E. pearl
 E. sign
 E. symptom
Epstein-Barr (EB)
 E.-B. virus (EBV)
epulis
 giant cell e.
epuloid
equal
 e. bilateral breath sounds
 e. cleavage
 round, regular, and e. (RR&E)
equation
 alveolar air e.
 alveolar gas e.
 Arrhenius e.
 Bohr e.
 chemical e.
 constant field e.
 Einthoven e.
 energy balance e.
 Gay-Lussac e.
 GHK e.
 Gibbs-Helmholtz e.
 Goldman e.
 Goldman-Hodgkin-Katz e.
 Henderson-Hasselbalch e.
 Henri-Michaelis-Menten e.
 Hill e.
 Hüfner e.
 Lineweaver-Burk e.
 Michaelis-Menten e.
 e. of motion
 Nernst e.
 personal e.
 van't Hoff e.
equator
 e. bulbi oculi
 e. lentis
equatorial
 e. cleavage
 e. division
 e. plane
 e. plate
 e. staphyloma
equi
 Corynebacterium e.
 Ehrlichia e.
equianalgesic dose
equiaxial
equicaloric
equilenin
equilibration
 occlusal e.

equilibrium
 acid-base e.
 e. constant
 e. dialysis
 Donnan e.
 dynamic e.
 genetic e.
 Gibbs-Donnan e.
 Hardy-Weinberg e.
 homeostatic e.
 nutritive e.
 sense of e.
equilin
equimolar
equimolecular
equina
 cauda e.
equine
 e. encephalitis
 e. encephalomyelitis
 e. gait
 e. gonadotropin unit
 e. infectious anemia
 e. *Morbillivirus*
 e. rhinovirus
equinovalgus
 talipes e.
equinovarus
 talipes e.
equinus
 talipes e.
equiphasic complex
equitoxic
equivalence
 e. point
 e. zone
equivalency
equivalent
 combustion e.
 e. dose
 e. extract
 e. form reliability
 gold e.
 gram e.
 joule e.
 lethal e.
 metabolic e. (MET)
 nitrogen e.
 e. normal child unit (encu)
 e. normal son unit (ensu)
 e. power
 e. temperature
 e. weight
equivocal symptom
eradication
Eranko fluorescence stain
Erb
 E. disease

E. palsy
E. paralysis
Erb-Charcot disease
ERBF
    effective renal blood flow
erbium
Erb-Westphal sign
ercalcidiol
ercalciol
ercalcitriol
ERCP
    endoscopic retrograde
    cholangiopancreatography
Erdheim
    E. disease
    E. tumor
Erdmann reagent
erecta
    luxatio e.
erectile
    e. nevus
    e. tissue
erect illumination
erection
erector spinae muscle
erector-spinal reflex
eremophobia
erethism
erethismic
erethistic
erethitic
ereuthophobia
ERG
    electroretinogram
ergasia
ergasiophobia
ergasthenia
ergastoplasm
ergine
ergobasine
ergocalciferol
ergocornine
ergocristine
ergocryptine
ergodynamograph
ergoesthesiograph
ergogenic aid
ergograph
    Mosso e.
ergographic
ergoline
ergolytic

ergometer
ergometrine maleate
ergonomics
ergonovine maleate
ergosine
ergosterin
ergosterol
ergostetrine
ergot
    e. alkaloid
    e. alkaloid-associated heart disease
    corn e.
    e. poisoning
ergotamine
ergotaminine
ergothioneine
ergotism
ergotoxine
ergotropic
eriodictyon
erisophake
Erlenmeyer
    E. flask
    E. flask deformity
erode
erogenous zone
eros
erose
E-rosette test
erosion
    Dieulafoy e.
erosive
    e. adenomatosis
    e. aneurysm
    e. arthritis
    e. chancre
    e. osteoarthritis
eroticism
erotic zoophilism
erotism
    anal e.
erotization
erotogenesis
erotogenic zone
erotomania
erotomanic disorder
erotopathic
erotopathy
erotophobia
ERP
    early receptor potential

E

NOTES

ERPF
    effective renal plasma flow
erratic
erratica
    mamma e.
erroneous projection
error
    alpha e.
    beta e.
    experimental e.
    e. of the first kind
    interobserver e.
    intraobserver e.
    e. of the second kind
error-prone
    e.-p. polymerase chain reaction
    e.-p. repair
ertacalciol
erubescence
erucic acid
eructation
eruption
    accelerated e.
    butterfly e.
    clinical e.
    continuous e.
    creeping e.
    e. cyst
    delayed e.
    drug e.
    erythematous e.
    feigned e.
    fixed drug e.
    iodine e.
    Kaposi varicelliform e.
    medicinal e.
    polymorphous light e.
    pustular e.
    seabather's e.
    e. sequestrum
    serum e.
    tubercular e.
    vesicular e.
eruptive
    e. fever
    e. gingivitis
    e. phase
    e. stage
    e. xanthoma
ERV
    expiratory reserve volume
Erwinia **L-asparaginase**
erysipelas
    ambulant e.
    gangrenous e.
erysipelatous
erysipeloid

Erysipelothrix
    E. insidiosa
    E. rhusiopathiae
erysipelotoxin
erythema
    acrodynic e.
    e. anulare
    e. caloricum
    e. chronicum migrans
    cold e.
    e. dose
    e. induratum
    e. infectiosum
    e. iris
    macular e.
    e. marginatum
    e. multiforme
    e. nodosum
    e. nuchae
    e. pernio
    e. toxicum
    e. toxicum neonatorum
erythematosa
    acne e.
erythematosum
    eczema e.
erythematosus
    chilblain lupus e.
    chronic discoid lupus e.
    cutaneous lupus e.
    discoid lupus e.
    disseminated lupus e.
    lupus e. (LE)
    pemphigus e.
    systemic lupus e. (SLE)
erythematous eruption
erythematovesicular
erythermalgia
erythralgia
erythrasma
erythredema
erythremia
    altitude e.
erythremic myelosis
erythrism
erythristic
erythrite
erythritol
erythrityl tetranitrate
erythroblast
erythroblastemia
erythroblastic anemia
erythroblastopenia
erythroblastosis
    fetal e.
    e. fetalis
erythroblastotic
erythrocatalysis
erythrochromia

erythroclasis
erythroclastic
erythrocuprein
erythrocyanosis
erythrocyte
    e. adherence phenomenon
    e. adherence test
    e. fragility test
    e. index
    e. maturation factor
    reticulated e.
    e. sedimentation rate (ESR)
erythrocythemia
    induced e.
erythrocytic
    e. cycle
    e. series
erythrocytoblast
erythrocytolysin
erythrocytolysis
erythrocytometer
erythrocytometry
erythrocytopenia
erythrocytophagy
erythrocytopoiesis
erythrocytorrhexis
erythrocytoschisis
erythrocytosis
    leukemic e.
erythrocyturia
erythrodegenerative
erythroderma
    bullous congenital ichthyosiform e.
    congenital ichthyosiform e.
    e. desquamativum
    ichthyosiform e.
    e. psoriaticum
erythrodermatitis
erythrodextrin
erythrodontia
erythrodysesthesia syndrome
erythroedema
erythrogenesis imperfecta
erythrogenic toxin
erythrogonium
erythroid cell
erythroidin
erythrokeratodermia variabilis
erythrokinetics
erythroleukemia
erythroleukosis
erythrol tetranitrate

erythrolysin
erythrolysis
erythromelalgia
erythromelia
erythromycin
    e. estolate
    e. glucoheptonate
    e. propionate
    e. stearate
erythron
erythroneocytosis
erythronormoblastic anemia
erythropenia
erythrophagia
erythrophagocytosis
erythrophil
erythrophilic
erythrophore
erythroplakia
erythroplasia of Queyrat
erythropoiesis
erythropoietic
    e. hormone
    e. porphyria
    e. protoporphyria
erythropoietin
erythroprosopalgia
erythropsia
erythropyknosis
erythrorrhexis
erythrose
erythrulose
erythruria
Esbach reagent
escape
    e. beat
    e. conditioning
    e. contraction
    e. impulse
    e. interval
    junctional e.
    nasal e.
    e. phenomenon
    e. rhythm
    e. training
    ventricular e.
    e. ventricular contraction
escape-capture bigeminy
escaped beat
eschar
escharectomy
escharotic

E

NOTES

escharotomy
Escherichia
    E. coli
    E. coli enterotoxin
    E. coli RNase I
    E. freundii
escorcin
escorcinol
esculapian
esculent
esculenta
    Gyromitra e.
    Helvella e.
esculin
eseridine
eserine
    e. aminoxide
    e. oxide
    e. salicylate
Esmarch
    E. bandage
    E. tourniquet
esodeviation
esodic nerve
esophagalgia
esophageal
    e. achalasia
    e. artery
    e. atresia
    e. branch
    e. cardiogram
    e. constriction
    e. dilator
    e. dysrhythmia
    e. gland
    e. hiatus
    e. impression on liver
    e. lead
    e. manometry
    e. mucosa
    e. nervous plexus
    e. obturator airway
    e. opening
    e. reflux
    e. smear
    e. spasm
    e. speculum
    e. speech
    e. tube
    e. tuberculosis
    e. varix
    e. vein
    e. web
esophagectasia
esophagectasis
esophagectomy
    3-incision e.
    Ivor Lewis e.

    transhiatal e.
    transthoracic e.
esophagism
esophagitis
    peptic e.
    reflux e.
    thrush e.
esophagocardioplasty
esophagocele
esophagoduodenostomy
esophagodynia
esophagoenterostomy
esophagogastrectomy
esophagogastric
    e. junction
    e. orifice
    e. vestibule
esophagogastroanastomosis
esophagogastroduodenoscopy (EGD)
esophagogastromyotomy
esophagogastroplasty
esophagogastrostomy
esophagogram
esophagography
esophagology
esophagomalacia
esophagomyotomy
esophagoplasty
esophagoplication
esophagoptosia
esophagoptosis
esophagosalivary reflex
esophagoscope
    fiberoptic e.
    full-lumen e.
    optical e.
    oval e.
esophagoscopy
esophagospasm
esophagostenosis
esophagostomiasis
esophagostomy
esophagotomy
esophagram
esophagus
    adenocarcinoma in Barrett e.
    Barrett e.
esophoria
esophoric
esotropia
    A-pattern e.
    basic e.
    consecutive e.
    mixed e.
    V-pattern e.
    X-pattern e.
esotropic
ESP
    extrasensory perception

espundia
esquinancea
ESR
    erythrocyte sedimentation rate
ESRD
    end-stage renal disease
essence of rose
essential
    e. albuminuria
    e. amino acid
    e. anemia
    e. anisocoria
    e. bradycardia
    e. dysmenorrhea
    e. fatty acid
    e. fever
    e. food factor
    e. fructosuria
    e. hypertension
    e. nutrient
    e. oil
    e. pentosuria
    e. progressive atrophy
    e. pruritus
    e. tachycardia
    e. telangiectasia
    e. thrombocytopenia
    e. tremor
    e. vertigo
Esser graft
Essick cell band
Essig splint
established cell line
estazolam
ester
    Cori e.
    Embden e.
    Harden-Young e.
esterase
    butyrylcholine e.
    C1 e.
    chlorophyll e.
    choline e. I, II
esterification
esterified estrogen
Estes operation
esthematology
esthesia
esthesic
esthesiodic system
esthesiogenesis
esthesiogenic

esthesiography
esthesiology
esthesiometer
esthesiometry
esthesioneuroblastoma
esthesioneurocytoma
esthesiophysiology
esthesioscopy
esthesodic
esthetic
    e. dentistry
    denture e.'s
    e. surgery
estimate
    Kaplan-Meier e.
estimated date of confinement (EDC)
estimation
estimator
    least squares e.
    maximum likelihood e.
estival
estivation
estivoautumnal
Estlander
    E. flap
    E. operation
estolate
    erythromycin e.
estradiol
    e. benzoate
    e. benzoate unit
    e. cypionate
    e. dipropionate
    ethinyl e.
    e. undecylate
    e. valerate
estragon oil
estramustine phosphate sodium
estrane
estratriene
estrin
estriol
estrodienol
estrogen
    conjugated e.
    e. effect
    esterified e.
    e. receptor
    e. replacement therapy
estrogenic hormone
estrone unit
estrous cycle

E

NOTES

estrual
estruation
estrus
ESWL
    extracorporeal shock wave lithotripsy
esylate
etafenone
etamsylate
état
    é. criblé
    é. mamelonné
ethacridine lactate
ethacrynate sodium
ethacrynic acid
ethadione
ethamivan
ethane
ethanediamine
ethanoic acid
ethanol abuse
ethanolamine
ethchlorvynol
ethenyl
ethenylbenzene
ethenylene
ether
    anesthetic e.
    diethyl e.
    glycol e.
    guaiacol glyceryl e.
    methyl-tert-butyl e.
ethereal
    e. oil
    e. solution
    e. tincture
etherification
etherization
ethiazide
ethical
ethics
    medical e.
ethidene
ethidium bromide
ethindrone
ethinyl
    e. estradiol
    e. trichloride
ethinylestrenol
ethiodized oil
ethionamide
ethionine
ethisterone
ethmocranial
ethmofrontal
ethmoid
    e. air cell
    e. angle
    e. antrum
    e. bone

    e. infundibulum
    e. sinus mucocele
ethmoidal
    e. bulla
    e. cell
    e. crest
    e. foramen
    e. groove
    e. infundibulum
    e. labyrinth
    e. notch
    e. process
    e. sinus
    e. vein
ethmoidale
    infundibulum e.
ethmoidalia
    antra e.
ethmoidalis
    bulla e.
    hiatus e.
ethmoidal-lacrimal fistula
ethmoidectomy
ethmoiditis
ethmoidolacrimal suture
ethmoidomaxillary suture
ethmolacrimal
ethmomaxillary
ethmonasal
ethmopalatal
ethmosphenoid
ethmoturbinal
ethmovomerine plate
ethnic group
ethnocentrism
ethnology
ethnopharmacology
ethoheptazine citrate
ethohexadiol
ethologist
ethology
ethomoxane
ethopharmacology
ethyl alcohol
ethylate
ethyldichloroarsine
ethylene glycol
ethylidyne
etiocholanolone
etiogenic
etiolated
etiolation
etiologic
etiological
etiology
etiopathic
etiopathology
etioporphyrin
etiotropic

E-to-A changes
etofamide
etomidate
etoposide
etorphine
etozolin
ETP
    electron transport particle
etretinate
etymemazine
euallele
Eubacterium
    E. aerofaciens
    E. combesi
    E. contortum
    E. crispatum
    E. filamentosum
    E. lentum
    E. limosum
    E. minutum
    E. moniliforme
    E. parvum
    E. poeciloides
    E. pseudotortuosum
    E. quartum
    E. quintum
    E. rectale
    E. tenue
    E. tortuosum
eubiotics
eucaine
eucalyptol
eucalyptus
    e. gum
    e. oil
eucapnia
eucaryote
eucaryotic
eucasin
euchlorhydria
eucholia
euchromatic
euchromatin
euchromosome
eucorticalism
eucrasia
eucupine
eudiaphoresis
eudipsia
eugenic acid
eugenics
eugenism

eugenol
Euglena
    E. gracilis
    E. viridis
euglobulin clot lysis time
euglycemla
euglycemic
eugnathia
eugnathic anomaly
eugnosia
eugonic
euhydration
eukaryote
eukaryotic
eukeratin
eukinesia
Eulenburg disease
eumelanin
eumelanosome
eumetria
eumorphism
eumycetes
eumycetoma
eunuch
eunuchism
eunuchoid
    e. gigantism
    e. state
    e. voice
eunuchoidism
    hypergonadotropic e.
    hypogonadotropic e.
euosmia
eupancreatism
euparal
eupaverin
eupepsia
eupeptic
eupeptide bond
euphenics
euphoretic
euphoria
euphoriant
euphoric affect
euplasia
euplastic lymph
euploid
euploidy
eupnea
eupraxia
eurhythmia

E

NOTES

European
    E. snakeroot
    E. tarantula
    E. typhus
europium
euroxenous parasite
euryblepharon
eurycephalic
eurycephalous
eurygnathic
eurygnathism
eurygnathous
euryon
euryopic
eurysomatic
euscope
eustachian
    e. catheter
    e. cushion
    e. tonsil
    e. tube
    e. tuber
    e. valve
eustachitis
eusthenia
eustrongyloides
eusystole
eusystolic
eutectic
    e. alloy
    e. temperature
euthanasia
euthenics
eutherapeutic
euthermic
euthymia
euthymic
euthyroid
    e. hypometabolism
    e. sick syndrome
euthyroidism
euthyscope
euthyscopy
eutonic
eutrichosis
eutrophia
eutrophic
eutrophy
euvolia
evacuant
evacuate
evacuation
    dilatation and e. (D&E)
    dilation and e. (D&E)
evacuator
    Ellik e.
evagination

evaluation
    drug use e.
    physical e. (PE)
evanescent
Evans
    E. blue
    E. syndrome
evaporate
evaporation
evasion
    macular e.
event
    adverse drug e.
    life e.'s
    sentinel e.
eventration of diaphragm
eversion
evert
evidence
    dearth of e.
evidence-based
    e.-b. medicine
    e.-b. practice
evil
    king's e.
eviration
evisceration
evisceroneurotomy
evocation
evocator
evoked
    e. electromyography
    e. otoacoustic emission
    e. potential
    e. response
evolution
    biologic e.
    chemical e.
    coincidental e.
    concerted e.
    convergent e.
    darwinian e.
    divergent e.
    emergent e.
    organic e.
    saltatory e.
evolutionary fitness
evulsion
Ewart
    E. procedure
    E. sign
Ewing
    E. sarcoma
    E. sign
    E. tumor
exacerbation
    abrupt e.
    sudden e.
exaltation

examination
- bimanual e.
- cytologic e.
- detailed physical e.
- direct wet mount e.
- EMG e.
- fecal e.
- fiberoptic endoscopic e.
- ova and parasite e.
- permanent stained smear e.
- physical e. (PE)

examiner
- medical e.

examining table
exanthem
exanthema, exanthem
- Boston e.
- epidemic e.
- keratoid e.
- e. subitum

exanthematous
- e. disease
- e. fever
- e. typhus

exanthesis arthrosia
exanthrope
exanthropic
exarteritis
exarticulation
excalation
excavation
- atrophic e.
- glaucomatous e.
- ischiorectal e.
- rectoischiadic e.
- rectouterine e.
- rectovesical e.
- vesicouterine e.

excavatio papilla
excavator
- hatchet e.
- hoe e.

excavatum
- pectus e.

excementosis
excentric amputation
excess
- antibody e.
- antigen e.
- base e.
- convergence e.

- e. lactate
- negative base e.

exchange
- anion e.
- cation e.
- ion e.
- e. transfusion

exchanger
- anion e.
- cation e.
- countercurrent e.
- ion e.

excimer laser
excipient
excise
excision
- e. biopsy
- loop e.
- e. repair

excitability
- supranormal e.

excitable
- e. area
- e. gap

excitant
excitation
- anomalous atrioventricular e.
- e. spectrum
- e. wave

excitatory
- e. junction potential (EJP)
- e. postsynaptic potential (EPSP)

excited
- e. atom
- e. catatonia
- e. state

excitement
- catatonic e.
- manic e.

exciting
- e. cause
- e. electrode
- e. eye

excitoglandular
excitometabolic
excitomotor
excitomuscular
excitoreflex nerve
excitor nerve
excitosecretory
excitotoxic
excitotoxin

NOTES

E

exclamation point hair
exclave
exclusion
   allelic e.
   diagnosis by e.
exclusive provider organization
exconjugant
excoriate
excoriation
excrement
excrementitious
excrescence
   Lambl e.
excreta
excrete
excretion
excretory
   e. cystogram
   e. duct
   e. gland
   e. urography
excursion
   lateral e.
   protrusive e.
   retrusive e.
excycloduction
excyclophoria
excyclotorsion
excyclotropia
excyclovergence
excystation
exduction
exemia
exencephalia
exencephalic
exencephalocele
exencephalous
exencephaly
exenteration
   anterior pelvic e.
   pelvic e.
exenteritis
exercise
   e. economy
   e. imaging
   isometric e.
   isotonic e.
   Kegel e.'s
   nonweightbearing e.
   e. physiology
   e. prescription
   e. pressor reflex
   progressive-resistance e.
   e. radionuclide angiocardiography
   steady-rate e.
   steady-state e.
   e. stress test
   weight-supported e.

exercise-induced
   e.-i. amenorrhea
   e.-i. anemia
   e.-i. asthma
   e.-i. bronchospasm
   e.-i. urticaria
exeresis
exergonic
exertion
   dyspnea on e. (DOE)
exertional
   e. dyspnea
   e. headache
   e. rhabdomyolysis
exflagellation
exfoliation syndrome
exfoliativa
   keratolysis e.
exfoliative
   e. cytology
   e. dermatitis
   e. gastritis
   e. psoriasis
exhalation
exhaustion
   heat e.
exhibitionism
exhibitionist
exhilarant
existential
   e. anxiety
   e. psychiatry
   e. psychology
   e. psychotherapy
exit
   e. block
   e. dose
exitus
Exner plexus
exoamylase
exoantigen
exocardia
exoccipital bone
exocelomic membrane
exocrine
   e. gland
   e. pancreatic insufficiency
exocyclic
exocytosis
exodeviation
exodic nerve
exodontia
exodontist
exoenzyme
exoerythrocytic
   e. cycle
   e. stage
exogamy
exogastrula

exogenetic
exogenic toxicosis
exogenote
exogenous
 e. aneurysm
 e. buffer
 e. creatinine clearance
 e. cycle
 e. depression
 e. fiber
 e. hemochromatosis
 e. hyperglyceridemia
 e. ochronosis
 e. pigmentation
 e. pyrogen
exolever
exomphalos
exon shuffle
exonuclease
exopeptidase
Exophiala
 E. jeanselmei
 E. werneckii
exophoria
exophoric
exophthalmic
 e. goiter
 e. ophthalmoplegia
exophthalmometer
exophthalmos
 endocrine e.
 malignant e.
exophthalmos-producing substance
exophthalmus
exophyte
exophytic
exoplasm
exoserosis
exoskeleton
exospore
exosporium
exostectomy
exostosectomy
exostosis, pl. exostoses
 e. bursata
 e. cartilaginea
 hereditary multiple exostoses
 ivory e.
 tackler's e.
exoteric bacterium
exothermic
exotoxic

exotoxin
exotropia
 A-pattern e.
 basic e.
 divergence excess e.
 divergence insufficiency e.
 V-pattern e.
 X-pattern e.
expandable stent
expanded disability status scale
expander
 blood volume e.
 plasma e.
expansion
 e. arch
 clonal e.
 extensor digital e.
 hygroscopic e.
expansive delusion
expansiveness
expectation of life
expectorant
expectorate
expectoration
expenditure
 resting energy e.
 total daily energy e.
experience
 corrective emotional e.
experiential aura
experiment
 Carr-Purcell e.
 control e.
 delayed reaction e.
 double-blind e.
 double-masked e.
 factorial e.
 hertzian e.
 Mariotte e.
 Scheiner e.
experimental
 e. allergic encephalitis (EAE)
 e. allergic encephalomyelitis
 e. error
 e. group
 e. medicine
 e. method
 e. neurosis
 e. psychology
experimenter effects
expiration

NOTES

E

expiratory
  e. center
  e. dyspnea
  e. reserve volume (ERV)
  e. resistance
  e. rhonchi
  e. stridor
expire
expired gas
explant
explantation
exploration
exploratory
  e. drive
  e. incision
  e. operation
  e. surgery
exploring
  e. electrode
  e. needle
explosion
explosive
  e. decompression
  e. speech
  e. vomiting
exponent
  hydrogen e.
exponential
  e. distribution
  e. growth
exposed pulp
exposure
  e. dose
  e. keratitis
expressed
  e. mustard oil
  e. skull fracture
expression
  differential gene e.
  gene e.
  integrated rate e.
  e. library
  e. vector
expressive aphasia
expressivity
expulsive pain
exquisite
exsanguinate
exsanguination transfusion
exsanguine
exsect
exsection
exsiccant
exsiccate
exsiccated
  e. alum
  e. sodium sulfite
exsiccation fever
exsomatize

exsorption
exstrophy
  cloacal e.
extemporaneous mixture
extended
  e. care
  e. care facility (ECF)
  e. clasp
  e. family
  e. family therapy
  e. insulin zinc suspension
  e. mediastinoscopy
  e. pyelotomy
  e. radical mastectomy
  e. thymectomy
extension
  e. bridge
  Buck e.
  e. form
  joint e.
  skeletal e.
extensor
  e. aponeurosis
  e. carpi radialis brevis muscle
  e. carpi radialis longus muscle
  e. carpi ulnaris muscle
  e. compartment
  e. digital expansion
  e. digiti minimi muscle
  e. digitorum brevis muscle
  e. digitorum longus muscle
  e. digitorum muscle
  e. hallucis brevis muscle
  e. hallucis longus muscle
  e. indicis muscle
  e. pollicis brevis muscle
  e. pollicis longus muscle
  e. retinaculum
extensus
  hallux e.
exteriorize
extern
externa
  auris e.
  epicondylalgia e.
  hematorrhachis e.
  hepatitis e.
  ophthalmoplegia e.
  otitis e.
external
  e. absorption
  e. acoustic aperture
  e. acoustic foramen
  e. acoustic meatus
  e. acoustic pore
  e. anal sphincter
  e. arcuate fiber
  e. auditory foramen
  e. auditory meatus

e. auditory pore
e. axis
e. canthus
e. capsule
e. cardiac massage
e. carotid artery
e. carotid nerve
e. carotid nervous plexus
e. cephalic version
e. collateral ligament
e. conjugate
e. conjugate diameter
e. cuneate nucleus
e. defibrillator
e. dental epithelium
e. ear
e. enamel epithelium
e. exudative retinopathy
e. female genital organ
e. fistula
e. genitalia
e. hemorrhoid
e. hydrocephalus
e. iliac artery
e. iliac lymphatic plexus
e. iliac lymph node
e. iliac vein
e. inguinal ring
e. intercostal membrane
e. intercostal muscle
e. jugular vein
e. lip
e. male genital organ
e. malleolus
e. mammary artery
e. matrix
e. maxillary artery
e. maxillary plexus
e. medium
e. medullary lamina
e. meningitis
e. naris
e. nasal artery
e. nasal branch
e. nasal vein
e. nose
e. nuclear layer
e. oblique muscle
e. oblique reflex
e. oblique ridge
e. obturator muscle
e. occipital crest

e. occipital protuberance
e. opening
e. ophthalmopathy
e. ophthalmoplegia
e. os
e. pacemaker
e. pachymeningitis
e. palatine vein
e. pharyngotomy
e. phase
e. pillar cell
e. pin fixation
e. pin fixation, biphase
e. pterygoid muscle
e. pudendal artery
e. pudendal vein
e. pyocephalus
e. respiration
e. respiratory nerve
e. root sheath
e. rotation
e. salivary gland
e. saphenous nerve
e. secretion
e. semilunar fibrocartilage
e. sheath of optic nerve
e. spermatic artery
e. spermatic fascia
e. spermatic nerve
e. sphincter muscle
e. sphincterotomy
e. spiral sulcus
e. squint
e. stripper
e. surface
e. traction
e. urethral orifice
e. urethral sphincter
e. urethrotomy
e. urinary meatus

externum
filum terminale e.
hordeolum e.
externus
meatus acusticus e.
exteroceptive
exteroceptor
exterofective system
extinction
e. coefficient
specific e.
extinguish

E

NOTES

extirpation
Exton reagent
extorsion
extortor
extraabdominal desmoid
extraamniotic pregnancy
extraanatomic bypass
extraarticular
extraaxial
extrabuccal
extrabulbar
extracaliceal
extracapsular
    e. ankylosis
    e. fracture
    e. ligament
extracardiac murmur
extracarpal
extracellular
    e. enzyme
    e. fluid (ECF)
    e. fluid volume (ECFV)
    e. toxin
extrachorial pregnancy
extrachromosomal
    e. DNA
    e. element
    e. gene
    e. genetic element
    e. inheritance
extracoronal retainer
extracorporeal
    e. circulation
    e. dialysis
    e. photophoresis
    e. shock wave lithotripsy (ESWL)
extracorporeal-membrane oxygenation
extracorpuscular
extracranial
    e. arteritis
    e. ganglion
    e. pneumatocele
    e. pneumocele
extracranial-intracranial bypass
extract
    alcoholic e.
    allergenic e.
    allergic e.
    belladonna e.
    Büchner e.
    equivalent e.
    fluid e.
    hydroalcoholic e.
    liquid e.
extractant
extracting forceps
extraction
    Baker pyridine e.
    breech e.

    e. coefficient
    dilation and e.
    full-mouth e.
    e. ratio
    serial e.
extractive
extractor
extracystic
extradural
    e. anesthesia
    e. hematorrhachis
    e. hemorrhage
    e. space
extraembryonic
    e. blastoderm
    e. celom
    e. ectoderm
    e. membrane
    e. mesoderm
extraepiphysial
extragenital
extraglomerular mesangium
extrahepatic
extraligamentous
extramalleolus
extramammary Paget disease
extramedullary
extramembranous pregnancy
extramitochondrial
extramural practice
extraneous
extranodal marginal zone lymphoma
extranuclear inheritance
extraocular muscle
extraoral
    e. anchorage
    e. fracture appliance
extraovular
extrapapillary
extraparenchymal
extraperineal
extraperiosteal
extraperitoneal
    e. fascia
    e. space
extraphysiologic
extrapineal pinealoma
extraplacental
extrapleural pneumothorax
extraprostatic
extrapsychic
extrapulmonary
extrapyramidal
    e. cerebral palsy
    e. dyskinesia
    e. motor system
    e. motor system disease
    e. syndrome
extrarenal pelvis

extrasaccular hernia
extrasensory
    e. perception (ESP)
    e. thought transference
extraserous
extraskeletal chondroma
extrasomatic
extrasystole, extra-systole
    atrial e.
    atrioventricular nodal e.
    auricular e.
    AV nodal e.
    infranodal e.
    interpolated e.
    junctional e.
    return e.
    ventricular e.
extratarsal
extrathoracic airway obstruction
extrathyroidal hypermetabolism
extratracheal
extratubal
extrauterine pregnancy
extravaginal torsion
extravasate
extravasation cyst
extravascular fluid
extraventricular
extraversion
extravert
extravesical reimplantation
extravisual
extravital ultraviolet
extremal quotient
extreme capsule
extremis
    in e.
extremital
extremity
    acromial e.
    inferior e.
    left upper e. (LUE)
    lower e.
    right lower e. (RLE)
    right upper e. (RUE)
    upper e.
extrinsic
    e. allergic alveolitis
    e. asthma
    e. coagulation pathway
    e. color
    e. factor

    e. incubation period
    e. motivation
    e. muscle
    e. protein
    e. sphincter
extrogastrulation
extroversion
extrovert
extrude
extruded teeth
extrusion
extubate
extubation
exuberant tumor
exudate
exudation
    e. cell
    e. corpuscle
    e. cyst
exudativa
    retinitis e.
exudative
    e. arthritis
    e. bronchiolitis
    e. choroiditis
    e. drusen
    e. glomerulonephritis
    e. inflammation
    e. retinal detachment
    e. retinitis
    e. tuberculosis
    e. vitreoretinopathy
exude
exulcerans
exumbilication
ex vivo
eye
    amaurotic cat e.
    aphakic e.
    artificial e.
    e. bank
    black e.
    blear e.
    bleary e.
    e. capsule
    compound e.
    crossed e.'s
    e. cup
    cyclopian e.
    dark-adapted e.
    dominant e.
    e. drop

NOTES

eye *(continued)*
    e., ear, nose, and throat (EENT)
    epiphysial e.
    exciting e.
    fixing e.
    hare's e.
    e. lens
    light-adapted e.
    Listing reduced e.
    master e.
    e. ointment
    phakic e.
    photopic e.
    raccoon e.'s
    e. reflex
    scotopic e.
    shipyard e.
    e. socket
    e. speculum
    e. tooth
eyeball
    e. compression reflex
    inner layer of e.
    posterior segment of e.

eyeball-heart reflex
eyebrow
eye-closure
    e.-c. pupil reaction
    e.-c. reflex
eye-ear plane
eyeglasses
eyegrounds
eyelash
    ectopic e.
    piebald e.
    e. sign
eyelid
    e. imbrication
    inferior e.
    lower e.
eyepiece
eyespot
eyestone
eyestrain
eyewash

F

F agent
F factor
F pilus
F plasmid
F thalassemia
F wave

f

f distribution
f wave

FAB

French-American-British
FAB classification

Fab

F. fragment
F. piece

fabella

Faber

F. anemia
F. syndrome

fabism

fabrication

Fabricius ship

Fabry disease

face

bird f.
cow f.
dish f.
f. form
frog f.
hippocratic f.
masklike f.
moon f.
f. peel
f. presentation
f. region
f. validity

face-bow

adjustable axis f.-b.
f.-b. fork
kinematic f.-b.
f.-b. record

face-lift

facet, facette

acromial f.
articular f.
clavicular articular f.
corneal f.
costal f.
fibular articular f.
inferior costal f.
f. joint
lateral malleolar f.
Lenoir f.
locked f.'s

medial malleolar f.
f. rhizotomy

facetectomy

facial

f. anesthesia
f. angle
f. artery
f. aspect
f. axis
f. bone
f. canal
f. cleft
f. colliculus
f. diplegia
f. eminence
f. height
f. hemiatrophy
f. hemiatrophy of Romberg
f. hemiplegia
f. hillock
f. index
f. lymph node
f. motor nucleus
f. muscle
f. myokymia
f. nerve
f. nerve area
f. neuralgia
f. palsy
f. paralysis
f. plane
f. plexus
f. profile
f. recess approach
f. reflex
f. root
f. skeleton
f. spasm
f. surface
f. tic
f. triangle
f. vein
f. vision

facialis

herpes f.
f. phenomenon

faciei

keratosis pilaris atrophicans f.
lupus miliaris disseminatus f.
seborrhea f.

facies

adenoid f.
aortic f.
cherubic f.
Corvisart f.

F

facies *(continued)*
  elfin f.
  hippocratic f.
  hound-dog f.
  Hutchinson f.
  leonine f.
  mitral f.
  myasthenic f.
  paralytic f.
  Parkinson f.
facilitated
  f. communication
  f. diffusion
  f. transport
facilitation
  proprioceptive neuromuscular f.
facility
  acute care f. (ACF)
  adult congregate living f. (ACLF)
  extended care f. (ECF)
  intermediate care f. (ICF)
  long-term care f.
  nursing f.
  skilled nursing f. (SNF)
facing
faciodigitogenital dysplasia
faciolingual
facioplasty
facioplegia
facioscapulohumeral
  f. atrophy
  f. muscular dystrophy
factitial dermatitis
factitious
  f. disorder
  f. hyperthyroidism
  f. illness by proxy
  f. melanin
  f. purpura
  f. symptom
  f. urticaria
factor
  f. 3
  ABO f.
  accelerator f.
  acetate replacement f.
  adrenal weight f.
  adrenocorticotropic releasing f.
  angiogenesis f.
  animal protein f.
  antialopecia f.
  antianemic f.
  antiangiogenesis f.
  antiberiberi f.
  anti–black-tongue f.
  anticomplementary f.
  antidermatitis f.
  antihemophilic f. A, B
  antihemorrhagic f.

antineuritic f.
antinuclear f. (ANF)
antipellagra f.
antipernicious anemia f.
antisterility f.
atrial natriuretic f. (ANF)
f. B
bacteriocin f.
B cell differentiating f.
B cell differentiation/growth f.
biotic f.
Bittner milk f.
branching f.
C f.
capillary permeability f.
cardiac risk f. (CRF)
Castle intrinsic f.
Christmas f.
citrovorum f.
clearing f.
clotting f.
coagulation f.
cobra venom f.
coenzyme f.
colony-stimulating f. (CSF)
complement chemotactic f.
corticotropin-releasing f. (CRF)
coupling f.
f. D
debranching f.
decapacitation f.
diabetogenic f.
diffusing f.
Duran-Reynals permeability f.
Duran-Reynals spreading f.
elongation f.
endothelial relaxing f.
endothelium-derived relaxing f.
eosinophil chemotactic f.
epidermal growth f. (EGF)
erythrocyte maturation f.
essential food f.
extrinsic f.
F f.
fermentation *Lactobacillus casei* f.
fertility f.
fibrin-stabilizing f.
filtrate f.
Fitzgerald f.
Flaujeac f.
Fletcher f.
follicle-stimulating hormone-
  releasing f.
G f.
glass f.
glucose tolerance f.
glycotropic f.
f. Gm
gonadotropin-releasing f.

granulocyte colony-stimulating f. (G-CSF)
granulocyte-macrophage colony-stimulating f. (GM-CSF)
growth f.
growth hormone releasing f. (GH-RF, GHRF)
f. H
Hageman f.
hematopoietic growth f.
histamine-releasing f.
human antihemophilic f.
hyperglycemic-glycogenolytic f.
f. I, II, IIa, III
impact f.
inhibition f.
initiation f. (IF)
insulin-antagonizing f.
insulinlike growth f. (IGF)
intrinsic f.
ischemia-modifying f.
labile f.
Lactobacillus bulgaricus f.
Laki-Lorand f.
lethal f.
leukemia inhibitory f.
leukocytosis-promoting f.
leukopenic f.
lipotropic f.
liver filtrate f.
L-L f.
luteinizing hormone/follicle-stimulating hormone-releasing f. (LH/FSH-RF)
luteinizing hormone-releasing f. (LH-RF, LRF)
lymph node permeability f. (LNPF)
macrophage-activating f. (MAF)
macrophage colony-stimulating f. (M-CSF)
maize f.
mammotropic f.
maturation f.
melanotropin-releasing f.
mesodermal f.
migration-inhibitory f. (MIF)
milk f.
monocyte-derived neutrophil chemotactic f. (MDNCF)
multicolony-stimulating f.
myocardial depressant f. (MDF)
neutrophil-activating f.

osteoclast activating f.
f. P
Passavoy f.
platelet-activating f.
platelet-aggregating f.
platelet tissue f.
prolactin-inhibiting f.
prolactin-releasing f.
properdin f. A, B, D, E
recognition f.
releasing f.
resistance-transfer f.
rheumatoid f.
somatotropin-releasing f.
stem cell f.
Stuart f.
Stuart-Prower f.
sun protection f.
transfer f.
transforming f.
tumor angiogenic f.
tumor necrosis f.
f. V, Va, VIa, VII, VIII, X, Xa, XI, XII, XIII
factorial experiment
facultative
f. anaerobe
f. heterochromatin
f. hyperopia
f. parasite
f. saprophyte
Faden suture
fading time
faecalis
Enterococcus f.
Streptococcus f.
faecium
Enterococcus f.
Faget sign
fagot cell
Fahraeus-Lindqvist effect
Fahr disease
Fahrenheit scale
failure
acute renal f. (ARF)
acute respiratory f. (ARF)
backward heart f.
cardiac f.
congestive heart f.
coronary f.
electrical f.
forward heart f.

F

NOTES

failure *(continued)*
    heart f.
    high output f.
    left-sided heart f.
    left ventricular f.
    low output f.
    premature ovarian f.
    pure autonomic f.
    respiratory f.
    right ventricular f.
    f. to thrive
faint rhonchi
faith healing
falcate
falces (*pl. of* falx)
falcial
falciform
    f. cartilage
    f. crest
    f. ligament
    f. lobe
    f. margin
    f. process
    f. retinal fold
falcine
falciparum
    f. fever
    f. malaria
    Plasmodium f.
falcula
falcular
fallacy
    ecological f.
fallen arch
falling
    f. palate
    f. sickness
    f. of the womb
fallopian
    f. aqueduct
    f. arch
    f. canal
    f. hiatus
    f. ligament
    f. neuritis
    f. pregnancy
    f. tube
Fallot
    F. tetrad
    tetralogy of F.
    F. triad
    trilogy of F.
false
    f. agglutination
    f. albuminuria
    f. anemia
    f. aneurysm
    f. angina
    f. ankylosis

    f. blepharoptosis
    f. branching
    f. cast
    f. chordae tendineae
    f. conjugate
    f. coxa vara
    f. cyanosis
    f. cyst
    f. dextrocardia
    f. diphtheria
    f. diverticulum
    f. dominance
    f. glottis
    f. hellebore
    f. hematuria
    f. hermaphroditism
    f. hypertrophy
    f. image
    f. joint
    f. knot
    f. labor
    f. lumen
    f. macula
    f. membrane
    f. memory syndrome
    f. negative
    f. neuroma
    f. nucleolus
    f. pain
    f. paracusis
    f. pelvis
    f. positive
    f. pregnancy
    f. projection
    f. rib
    f. suture
    f. tendinous cord
    f. thirst
    f. vertebra
    f. vocal cord
    f. waters
false-negative reaction
false-positive reaction
falsetto
falsification
    retrospective f.
falx, pl. **falces**
    f. aponeurotica
    cerebellar f.
    f. cerebelli
    cerebral f.
    f. cerebri
    inguinal f.
    f. inguinalis
    f. septi
familial
    f. adenomatous polyposis (FAP)
    f. aggregation
    f. aminoglycoside ototoxicity

f. amyloid neuropathy
f. amyloidosis
f. aortic ectasia
f. aortic ectasia syndrome
f. bipolar mood disorder
f. cancer
f. cholemia
f. chylomicronemia syndrome
f. combined hyperlipemia
f. dysautonomia
f. emphysema
f. erythrophagocytic
  lymphohistiocytosis (FEL)
f. fat-induced hyperlipemia
f. glycinuria
f. goiter
f. hemophagocytic
  lymphohistiocytosis (FHL)
f. high density lipoprotein
  deficiency
f. hyperbetalipoproteinemia
f. hypercholesteremic xanthomatosis
f. hypercholesterolemia
f. hypercholesterolemia with
  hyperlipemia
f. hyperchylomicronemia
f. hyperlipoproteinemia
f. hyperprebetalipoproteinemia
f. hypertriglyceridemia
f. hypertrophic cardiomyopathy
f. hypobetalipoproteinemia
f. hypogonadotropic hypogonadism
f. hypoparathyroidism
f. hypophosphatemic rickets
f. hypoplastic anemia
f. juvenile nephrophthisis
f. lipoprotein lipase inhibitor
f. Mediterranean fever
f. microcytic anemia
f. multiple endocrine adenomatosis
f. myoglobinuria
f. nephrosis
f. neuroviscerolipidosis
f. nonhemolytic jaundice
f. paroxysmal polyserositis
f. paroxysmal rhabdomyolysis
f. partial lipodystrophy
f. periodic paralysis
f. polyposis coli
f. pseudoinflammatory macular
  degeneration
f. pseudoinflammatory maculopathy

f. pyridoxine-responsive anemia
f. recurrent polyserositis
f. screening
f. spinal muscular atrophy
f. tremor
f. white folded dysplasia
family
cancer f.
extended f.
gene f.
f. medicine
nuclear f.
f. physician
f. practice
f. therapy
famine dropsy
famotidine
FANA
fluorescent antinuclear antibody
FANA test
Fañanás cell
Fanconi
F. anemia
F. pancytopenia
F. syndrome
fango
fan sign
fantasy
FAP
familial adenomatous polyposis
FAPA
fever, adenitis, pharyngitis, and aphthous
ulcers
FAPA syndrome
far
F. East hemorrhagic fever
F. East Russian encephalitis
f. point
f. point of convergence
f. sight
Farabeuf
F. amputation
F. triangle
farad
Faraday
F. constant
F. law
faradism
faradization
faradocontractility
faradomuscular
faradopalpation

F

NOTES

faradotherapy
far-and-near suture
Farber
    F. disease
    F. syndrome
farcinica
    Nocardia f.
farcy
fardel
farfara
farina
    f. avenae
    f. tritici
farinaceous
farmer's
    f. lung
    f. skin
farnesene alcohol
farnesol
farnesyl pyrophosphate
farnoquinone
Farnsworth-Munsell color test
Farrant mounting fluid
Farre line
Farr law
farsightedness
Fas
    F. ligand
    F. receptor
fascia
    Abernethy f.
    f. adherens
    anal f.
    antebrachial f.
    axillary f.
    bicipital f.
    brachial f.
    broad f.
    buccopharyngeal f.
    Buck f.
    Camper f.
    f. cervicalis
    clavipectoral f.
    Colles f.
    Cooper f.
    cremasteric f.
    cribriform f.
    crural f.
    f. cruris
    Cruveilhier f.
    dartos f.
    deep cervical f.
    deep perineal f.
    dentate f.
    dorsal f.
    Dupuytren f.
    endoabdominal f.
    endopelvic f.
    endothoracic f.

    external spermatic f.
    extraperitoneal f.
    Gallaudet f.
    Gerota f.
    gluteal f.
    Godman f.
    f. graft
    Hesselbach f.
    hypothenar f.
    iliac f.
    iliopectineal f.
    inferior f.
    infraspinatus f.
    infraspinous f.
    infundibuliform f.
    internal spermatic f.
    interosseous f.
    investing f.
    lacrimal f.
    f. lata
    lumbar f.
    lumbodorsal f.
    masseteric f.
    middle cervical f.
    Monakow f.
    f. nuchae
    f. pectoralis
    pelvic f.
    perineal f.
    phrenicopleural f.
    popliteal f.
    presacral f.
    renal f.
    Scarpa f.
    superficial f.
    superficial investing f.
    thoracolumbar f.
    transversalis f.
    visceral f.
fascial
    f. graft
    f. hernia
    f. sarcoma
    f. sheath
fascicle
    anterior f.
fascicular
    f. block
    f. degeneration
    f. graft
    f. keratitis
    f. lymphosarcoma
    f. ophthalmoplegia
    f. sarcoma
    f. ulcer
fasciculata
    f. cell
    zona f.
fasciculate

fasciculated
fasciculation
fasciculus
    arcuate f.
    Burdach f.
    central tegmental f.
    cuneate f.
    dorsal longitudinal f.
    dorsolateral f.
    Flechsig f.
    Foville f.
    gracile f.
    hooked f.
    inferior longitudinal f.
    inferior occipitofrontal f.
    interfascicular f.
    intersegmental f.
    lateral pyramidal f.
    lenticular f.
    Lissauer f.
    longitudinal pontine f.
    macular f.
    mammillotegmental f.
    mammillothalamic f.
    marginal f.
    medial longitudinal f.
    superior longitudinal f.
    unciform f.
    uncinate f.
fasciectomy
fasciitis, fascitis
    eosinophilic f.
    group A streptococcal
      necrotizing f.
    nodular f.
    plantar f.
    proliferative f.
fasciodesis
fasciola
fasciolar gyrus
fascioliasis
fasciolid
fasciolopsiasis
Fasciolopsis
    F. buski
    F. rathouisi
fascioplasty
fasciorrhaphy
fasciotomy
fascitis (*var. of* fasciitis)
fast
    f. component of nystagmus

    f. protein liquid chromatography
    (FPLC)
    f. smear
fastidious organism
fastigatum
fastigial nucleus
fastigiobulbar
    f. fiber
    f. tract
fastigiospinal
    f. fiber
    f. tract
fastigium
fasting hypoglycemia
fastness
fast-neutron radiation therapy
fast-wave sleep
fat
    f. body
    brown f.
    f. cast
    f. cell
    f. embolism
    f. graft
    f. hernia
    hydrous wool f.
    f. indigestion
    f. metabolism
    f. necrosis
    f. pad
    f. solvent
    f. tide
fatality rate
fate map
fat-free body mass
father complex
fatigability
fatigable
fatigue
    auditory f.
    battle f.
    f. fever
    f. fracture
    functional vocal f.
    f. strength
fat-pad, fat pad
    Bichat f.-p.
    buccal f.-p.
    Imlach f.-p.
    infrapatellar f.-p.
    ischiorectal f.-p.
fat-soluble vitamin

F

NOTES

fat-storing cell
fatty
- f. acid
- f. acid–binding protein
- f. acid oxidation cycle
- f. acid synthase complex
- f. acid thiokinase
- f. alcohol
- f. appendix
- f. ascites
- f. atrophy
- f. cast
- f. change
- f. cirrhosis
- f. degeneration
- f. diarrhea
- f. fold
- f. heart
- f. hernia
- f. infiltration
- f. kidney
- f. layer
- f. liver
- f. metamorphosis
- f. nevus
- f. oil
- f. phanerosis
- f. renal capsule
- f. series
- f. stool
- f. tissue

fauces
faucial
- f. branch
- f. diphtheria
- f. paralysis
- f. reflex
- f. tonsil

faulty union
fauna
faun tail nevus
faveolate
faveolus
favic chandeliers
favid
FA virus
favism
Favre-Durand-Nicholas disease
Favre dystrophy
Favre-Racouchot
- F.-R. disease
- F.-R. syndrome

favus
Fazio-Londe disease
FB
- foreign body

Fc
- Fc fragment

Fc piece
Fc receptor
F&D
- fixed and dilated

feather louse
febricant
febricula
febrifacient
febriferous
febrific
febrifugal
febrifuge
febrile
- f. albuminuria
- f. convulsion
- f. crisis
- f. psychosis
- f. seizure
- f. urine
- f. urticaria

febrilis
- herpes f.

fecal
- f. abscess
- f. concentration
- f. continence
- f. examination
- f. fistula
- f. impaction
- f. incontinence
- f. tumor
- f. vomiting

fecalith
fecaloid
fecaloma
fecaluria
feces
- incontinence of f.

Fechner-Weber law
feculent
fecund
fecundate
fecundation
fecundity
Federici sign
feedback
- f. activation
- auditory f.
- f. inhibition
- f. mechanism
- f. system
- tubuloglomerular f.

feed-forward activation
feeding
- f. center
- fictitious f.
- forced f.
- forcible f.
- gastric f.

f. prosthesis
f. tube
fee-for-service insurance
feeleii
    Legionella f.
feeling tone
Feer disease
feet (*pl. of* foot)
FEF
    forced expiratory flow
Fehling
    F. reagent
    F. solution
feigned eruption
Feiss line
FEL
    familial erythrophagocytic
    lymphohistiocytosis
felbamate
feline infectious anemia
fellatio
felodipine
felon
felonious assault
felt dressing
feltwork
    Kaes f.
Felty syndrome
felypressin
female
    f. athlete triad
    f. catheter
    f. circumcision
    f. external genitalia
    genetic f.
    f. gonad
    f. hermaphroditism
    f. homosexuality
    f. internal genitalia
    f. pattern alopecia
    f. prostate
    f. pseudohermaphroditism
    f. sterility
    f. urethra
femininity complex
feminization
femoral
    f. arch
    f. branch
    f. canal
    f. fossa
    f. hernia

f. muscle
f. nerve
f. nervous plexus
f. nutrient artery
f. opening
f. reflex
f. region
f. ring
f. septum
f. sheath
f. triangle
f. vein
femoralis
    anulus f.
femoris
femoroabdominal reflex
femorocele
femoropatellar joint
femoropopliteal
    f. bypass
    f. occlusive disease
femorotibial
femur
fenbufen
fencamine
fenclofenac
fenclonine
fenestra, pl. **fenestrae**
    f. cochleae
    f. vestibuli
fenestram
    fissula ante f.
    fossula post f.
fenestrata
    placenta f.
fenestrated
    f. capillary
    f. clamp
    f. membrane
    f. sheath
    f. tenotomy
fenestration operation
Fenn effect
fennelliae
    Helicobacter f.
fenoprofen calcium
fenoterol
fentanyl citrate
fenticlor
Fenton reaction
fenugreek
Fenwick-Hunner ulcer

NOTES

F

feral
Ferguson reflex
Fergusson incision
ferment
fermentable
fermentation
    acetic f.
    acetous f.
    alcoholic f.
    amylic f.
    lactic acid f.
    f. *Lactobacillus casei* factor
fermentative dyspepsia
fermenter
fermentum
    Lactobacillus *f.*
fermium
Fernandez reaction
Fernbach flask
ferning
fern test
Ferrata cell
ferredoxin
Ferrein
    F. canal
    F. cord
    F. foramen
    F. ligament
    F. pyramid
    F. tube
    F. vasa aberrantia
ferric
    f. alum
    f. ammonium citrate
    f. ammonium sulfate
    f. chloride
    f. chloride reaction
    f. chloride test
    f. fructose
    f. glycerophosphate
    f. hydroxide
    f. oxide
    f. phosphate
ferricyanide
ferricytochrome
ferriheme chloride
ferrihemoglobin
ferriporphyrin chloride
ferriprotoporphyrin
ferritin
ferrokinetics
ferroporphyrin
ferroprotein
ferroprotoporphyrin
ferrosoferric
ferrotherapy
ferrous
    f. citrate
    f. fumarate

    f. gluconate
    f. lactate
    f. succinate
    f. sulfate
ferrugination
ferrugineum
    Microsporum *f.*
ferrugineus
    locus f.
ferruginous body
ferrule
Ferry line
Ferry-Porter law
fertile period
fertility
    f. agent
    f. factor
    f. ratio
    f. vitamin
fertilization
    f. age
    f. membrane
    in vitro f. (IVF)
    in vivo f.
fertilized ovum
fertilizin
fervescence
FESS
    functional endoscopic sinus surgery
fester
festinant
festinating gait
festination
festoon
    gingival f.
festooning
FET
    forced expiratory time
fetal
    f. adrenal cortex
    f. alcohol syndrome
    f. aspiration syndrome
    f. attitude
    biometry f.
    f. bradycardia
    f. circulation
    f. cotyledon
    f. death
    f. death rate
    f. distress
    f. dystocia
    f. electrocardiography
    f. erythroblastosis
    f. face syndrome
    f. fracture
    f. gigantism
    f. growth restriction
    f. habitus
    f. heart rate

f. heart sound
f. heart tone
f. hemoglobin
f. hydantoin syndrome
f. hydrops
f. inclusion
f. medicine
f. membrane
f. movement
f. ovoid
f. placenta
f. position
f. reticularis
f. scalp stimulation
f. souffle
f. tachycardia
f. trimethadione syndrome
f. warfarin syndrome
f. wastage
f. zone

fetalis
erythroblastosis f.
hydrops f.
ichthyosis f.
placenta f.

fetalism
fetation
feticide
fetid
fetish
fetishism
fetoglobulin
fetography
fetology
fetomaternal transfusion
fetometry
fetopathy
diabetic f.

fetoplacental anasarca
fetoprotein
fetor
f. hepaticus
f. oris

fetoscope
fetoscopy
fetotoxic
fetu
fetus in f.

fetuin
fetus
Campylobacter f.
f. in fetu

harlequin f.
impacted f.
macerated f.
mummified f.
f. papyraceus
parasitic f.
f. sanguinolentis
Vibrio f.

Feulgen
F. cytometry
F. reaction
F. stain

FEV
forced expiratory volume

fever
absorption f.
acclimating f.
Aden f.
f., adenitis, pharyngitis, and aphthous ulcers (FAPA)
aestivoautumnal f.
African hemorrhagic f.
African tick f.
African tick-bite f.
algid pernicious f.
ardent f.
Argentinean hemorrhagic f.
artificial f.
aseptic f.
Assam f.
Australian Q f.
autumn f.
benign tertian f.
bilious remittent f.
black f.
blackwater f.
f. blister
blue f.
Bolivian hemorrhagic f.
bouquet f.
boutonneuse f.
brass founder's f.
Brazilian hemorrhagic f.
Brazilian purpuric f.
Brazilian spotted f.
breakbone f.
Bunyamwera f.
Burdwan f.
Bwamba f.
cachectic f.
camp f.
canicola f.

NOTES

fever *(continued)*

catarrhal f.
cat-bite f.
catheter f.
catscratch f.
Central European tick-borne f.
cerebrospinal f.
Charcot intermittent f.
childbed f.
Colorado tick f.
Congolian red f.
continued f.
cotton-mill f.
Crimean f.
Crimean-Congo hemorrhagic f.
dandy f.
date f.
5-day f.
deer-fly f.
dehydration f.
dengue hemorrhagic f.
desert f.
digestive f.
diphasic milk f.
double quotidian f.
drug f.
Dumdum f.
Dutton relapsing f.
Ebola hemorrhagic f.
eczema, asthma, hay f. (EAHF)
elephantoid f.
enteric f.
entericoid f.
ephemeral f.
epidemic hemorrhagic f.
epimastical f.
eruptive f.
essential f.
exanthematous f.
exsiccation f.
falciparum f.
familial Mediterranean f.
Far East hemorrhagic f.
fatigue f.
field f.
Flinders Island spotted f.
flood f.
food f.
Fort Bragg f.
foundryman's f.
Gambian f.
glandular f.
Haverhill f.
hay f.
hematuric bilious f.
hemoglobinuric f.
hemorrhagic f.
hepatic intermittent f.
herpetic f.

hospital f.
icterohemorrhagic f.
Ilhéus f.
inanition f.
induced f.
intermittent malarial f.
inundation f.
island f.
jail f.
Japanese river f.
Japanese spotted f.
jungle yellow f.
Katayama f.
kedani f.
Kenya f.
Kew Gardens f.
Kinkiang f.
Korean hemorrhagic f.
Lassa hemorrhagic f.
laurel f.
malarial f.
malignant tertian f.
Malta f.
Manchurian hemorrhagic f.
Marseilles f.
marsh f.
Mediterranean erythematous f.
Mediterranean exanthematous f.
Mediterranean spotted f.
meningotyphoid f.
metal fume f.
Mexican spotted f.
miliary f.
milk f.
mill f.
miniature scarlet f.
mud f.
Oropouche f.
Oroya f.
paratyphoid f.
parenteric f.
parrot f.
Pel-Ebstein f.
pharyngoconjunctival f.
pretibial f.
puerperal f.
Q f.
quotidian f.
rat-bite f.
relapsing f.
rheumatic f.
Rocky Mountain spotted f.
scarlet f.
septic f.
Sindbis f.
South African tick-bite f.
spotted f.
swamp f.
f. therapy

tick f.
trench f.
typhoid f.
undifferentiated type f.
undulant f.
f. of unknown origin (FUO)
uveoparotid f.
Venezuelan hemorrhagic f.
yellow f.
feverish urine
few rhonchi
FF
  filtration fraction
FFA
  free fatty acid
FFP
  fresh frozen plasma
FHL
  familial hemophagocytic
  lymphohistiocytosis
fiber, fibre
  A f.
  accelerator f.
  adrenergic f.
  afferent f.
  alpha f.
  anastomosing f.
  anastomotic f.
  anterior external arcuate f.
  arcuate f.
  argyrophilic f.
  association f.
  astral f.
  augmentor f.
  autonomic nerve f.
  B f.
  Bergmann f.
  beta f.
  bulbar corticonuclear f.
  C f.
  cerebellohypothalamic f.
  cerebelloolivary f.
  cerebellospinal f.
  cholinergic f.
  chromatic f.
  circular f.
  climbing f.
  collagen f.
  collagenous f.
  commissural f.
  cone f.
  corticobulbar f.

corticomesencephalic f.
corticonuclear f.
corticopontine f.
corticoreticular f.
corticorubral f.
corticospinal f.
corticothalamic f.
cuneocerebellar f.
cuneospinal f.
delta f.
dental f.
dentatorubral f.
dentatothalamic f.
dentinal f.
depressor f.
dietary f.
efferent f.
elastic f.
enamel f.
endogenous f.
exogenous f.
external arcuate f.
fastigiobulbar f.
fastigiospinal f.
frontopontine f.
gamma f.
Gerdy f.
gracilespinal f.
Gratiolet f.
gray f.
hypothalamocerebellar f.
hypothalamospinal f.
inhibitory f.
intercolumnar f.
intercrural f.
internal arcuate f.
intrafusal f.
intrathalamic f.
intrinsic f.
James f.
kinetochore f.
Korff f.
Kühne f.
long association f.
longitudinal pontine f.
Mahaim f.
medullated nerve f.
meridional f.
mesencephalic corticonuclear f.
motor f.
muscle f.
nonmedullated f.

NOTES

fiber *(continued)*
    oblique f.
    osteogenetic f.
    perforating f.
    pontocerebellar f.
    precollagenous f.
    pressor f.
    projection f.
    Purkinje f.
    Remak f.
    reticular f.
    spinocuneate f.
    spinogracile f.
    tautomeric f.
    temporopontine f.
    unmyelinated f.
    white f.
    yellow f.
fiberoptic
    f. endoscopic examination
    f. esophagoscope
    f. gastroscope
    f. laryngoscopy
fiberoptics
fiberscope
fibrate
fibre *(var. of* fiber)
fibremia
fibrescope
fibric acid
fibril
    Alzheimer f.
    anchoring f.
    collagen f.
fibrilla
fibrillar basket
fibrillary
    f. astrocyte
    f. astrocytoma
    f. chorea
    f. contraction
    f. myoclonia
    f. neuroma
    f. wave
fibrillate
fibrillated
fibrillation
    atrial f.
    auricular f.
    f. threshold
    ventricular f.
fibrillatory wave
fibrillin
fibrilloflutter
fibrillogenesis
fibrin
    f. calculus
    split products of f.
    f. thrombus
    Weigert stain for f.
fibrinase
fibrin/fibrinogen degradation product
fibrinocellular
fibrinogen
    human f.
fibrinogenase
fibrinogenemia
fibrinogenesis
fibrinogen-fibrin conversion syndrome
fibrinogenic
fibrinogenolysis
fibrinogenopenia
fibrinogenous
fibrinoid
    f. degeneration
    f. necrosis
fibrinokinase
fibrinolysin
fibrinolysis
fibrinolysokinase
fibrinolytic purpura
fibrinopeptide
fibrinopurulent inflammation
fibrinoscopy
fibrinous
    f. adhesion
    f. bronchitis
    f. cast
    f. cataract
    f. degeneration
    f. inflammation
    f. iritis
    f. lymph
    f. pericarditis
    f. pleurisy
    f. polyp
    f. rhinitis
fibrin-stabilizing factor
fibrinuria
fibroadenoma
    giant f.
    intracanalicular f.
fibroadipose
fibroareolar
fibroblastic
fibroblast interferon
fibrocarcinoma
fibrocartilage
    basilar f.
    circumferential f.
    external semilunar f.
    interarticular f.
    internal semilunar f.
    interpubic f.
    semilunar f.
fibrocartilaginous ring
fibrocartilago

fibrocaseous peritonitis
fibrocellular
fibrochondritis
fibrochondroma
fibrocongestive
fibrocyst
fibrocystic
    f. condition
    f. disease
fibrocystoma
fibrocyte
fibrodysplasia ossificans progressiva
fibroelastic membrane of larynx
fibroelastosis
    endocardial f.
    endomyocardial f.
fibroepithelial polyp
fibroepithelioma
fibrofatty
fibrofolliculoma
fibrogenesis
fibrogliosis
fibrohyaline tissue
fibroid
    f. adenoma
    f. cataract
    f. inflammation
    f. lung
    f. tumor
fibroidectomy
fibroin
fibrolamellar liver cell carcinoma
fibroleiomyoma
fibrolipoma
fibroma
    ameloblastic f.
    aponeurotic f.
    cementoossifying f.
    central ossifying f.
    chondromyxoid f.
    concentric f.
    desmoplastic f.
    giant cell f.
    irritation f.
    lung f.
    f. molle
    f. molle gravidarum
    f. myxomatodes
    nonossifying f.
    nonosteogenic f.
    peripheral ossifying f.

    recurring digital f.
    telangiectatic f.
fibromatogenic
fibromatoid
fibromatosis
    abdominal f.
    aggressive infantile f.
    f. colli
    congenital generalized f.
    digital f.
    gingival f.
    infantile digital f.
    juvenile hyalin f.
    juvenile palmoplantar f.
    plantar f.
fibromatous
fibromectomy
fibrometer
fibromuscular
    f. disease
    f. dysplasia
    f. hyperplasia
fibromusculocartilagenous layer
fibromyalgia syndrome
fibromyectomy
fibromyoma
fibromyositis
fibromyxoma
fibronectin
    plasma f.
fibroneuroma
fibroosteoma
fibropapilloma
fibroplasia
fibroplastic
fibroplate
fibropolypus
fibroreticulate
fibrosa
    localized osteitis f.
    meninx f.
    myositis f.
fibrosarcoma
    ameloblastic f.
    Earle L f.
    infantile f.
fibrose
fibroserous
fibrosing
    f. adenomatosis
    f. adenosis
    f. alveolitis

NOTES

F

fibrosing *(continued)*
    f. colonopathy
    f. mediastinitis
fibrosis
    African endomyocardial f.
    congenital f.
    cystic f.
    endocardial f.
    endomyocardial f.
    idiopathic interstitial f.
    idiopathic pulmonary f. (IPF)
    interstitial pulmonary f.
    leptomeningeal f.
    mediastinal f.
    pulmonary f.
    radiation f.
    retroperitoneal f.
fibrositic headache
fibrositis
    cervical f.
fibrosum
    adenoma f.
fibrosus
    anulus f.
fibrothorax
fibrotic ophthalmoplegia
fibrous
    f. adhesion
    f. ankylosis
    f. appendix
    f. articular capsule
    f. astrocyte
    f. bacterial virus
    f. cavernitis
    f. cortical defect
    f. degeneration
    f. digital sheath
    f. dysplasia
    f. goiter
    f. hamartoma of infancy
    f. histiocytoma
    f. joint
    f. layer
    f. mediastinitis
    f. membrane
    f. meningioma
    f. pericarditis
    f. pericardium
    f. pneumonia
    f. polyp
    f. protein
    f. ring
    f. skeleton
    f. tendon sheath
    f. tissue
    f. trigone
    f. tubercle
    f. tunic

    f. union
    f. xanthoma
fibroxanthoma
    atypical f.
fibula
fibular
    f. articular facet
    f. articular surface
    f. collateral ligament
    f. compartment
    f. lymph node
    f. margin
    f. notch
    f. nutrient artery
    f. peroneal border
    f. tarsal tendinous sheath
    f. trochlea
    f. vein
fibularis
    f. brevis muscle
    f. longus muscle
    f. tertius muscle
fibulocalcaneal
ficin, ficain
Fick
    axes of F.
    F. laws of diffusion
    F. method
    F. principle
Ficoll-Hypaque technique
fictitious feeding
FID
    free induction decay
Fiedler myocarditis
field
    auditory f.
    f. block
    f. block anesthesia
    Broca f.
    f. carcinogenesis
    Cohnheim f.
    f. of consciousness
    f. emission tube
    f. fever
    f. of fixation
    f.'s of Forel
    free f.
    f. gradient
    H f.
    hysterical f.
    individuation f.
    involved f.
    f. lens
    magnetic f.
    microscopic f.
    F. rapid stain
    sound f.
    f. survey
    visual f.

Fielding membrane
field-vole
Fiessinger-Leroy-Reiter syndrome
fièvre boutonneuse
fifth
    f. cranial nerve
    f. digit syndrome
    f. disease
    f. finger
    f. ventricle
fight or flight reaction
figuratus
figure
    achromatic f.
    authority f.
    chromatic f.
    flame f.
    fortification f.
    f. and ground
    mitotic f.
    Purkinje f.
figure-ground perception
figure-of-8
    f.-o.-8 abnormality
    f.-o.-8 bandage
    f.-o.-8 suture
fila (*pl. of* filum)
filaceous
filaggrin
filamen, filamin
filament
    actin f.
    axial f.
    cytokeratin f.
    intermediate f.
    keratin f.
    myosin f.
    f. polymorphonuclear leukocyte
    Z f.
filamenta (*pl. of* filamentum)
filamentary
    f. keratitis
    f. keratopathy
filament-nonfilament count
filamentosa
    keratitis f.
filamentosum
    Eubacterium f.
filamentous
    f. bacterial virus
    f. bacteriophage
    f. colony
filamentum, pl. filamenta
filamin (*var. of* filamen)
filar
    f. mass
    f. micrometer
    f. substance
filarial
    f. arthritis
    f. funiculitis
    f. hydrocele
    f. periodicity
    f. synovitis
filariasis
    bancroftian f.
    Brug f.
filaricidal
filaricide
filariform larva
Filatov
    F. disease
    F. flap
Filatov-Dukes disease
Filatov-Gillies flap
file
    Hedström f.
filial generation
filiform
    f. adnatum
    f. bougie
    f. catheter
    f. and follower
    f. nucleus
    f. papilla
    f. pulse
    f. wart
filings
    iron f.
filioparental
fillet
    lateral f.
    f. layer
    medial f.
filling
    capillary f.
    f. defect
    f. internal urethral orifice
film
    absorbable gelatin f.
    f. badge
    bitewing f.

F

NOTES

355

film *(continued)*
    f. changer
    decubitus f.
    horizontal beam f.
    latitude f.
    occlusal f.
    panoramic x-ray f.
    periapical f.
    plain f.
    scout f.
    f. speed
filmless radiography
filopodium
filopressure
filovaricosis
filter
    bandpass f.
    Berkefeld f.
    bird's nest f.
    f. bleeding time
    Greenfield f.
    high-pass f.
    low-pass f.
    f. paper
filterable
filtering
    f. bleb
    f. cicatrix
    f. operation
filtrable virus
filtrate
    f. factor
    f. nitrogen
filtration
    f. angle
    f. coefficient
    f. fraction (FF)
    gel f.
    f. slit
    f. space
filtrum ventriculi
filum, pl. **fila**
    fila olfactoria
    radicular fila
    fila radicularia
    terminal f.
    f. terminale
    f. terminale externum
    f. terminale internum
fimbria, pl. **fimbriae**
fimbrial
fimbriate
fimbriated fold
fimbriation
fimbriatum
    corpus f.
fimbriectomy
fimbrin
fimbriocele

fimbriodentate sulcus
fimbrioplasty
final
    f. host
    f. impression
finasteride
Finckh test
findings
    dearth of f.
    salient f.
fine
    f. mesh dressing
    f. structure
    f. tremor
fine-needle
    f.-n. aspiration (FNA)
    f.-n. biopsy
fineness
finger
    f. agnosia
    baseball f.
    blubber f.
    clubbed f.
    dead f.
    drop f.
    drumstick f.
    fifth f.
    first f.
    fourth f.
    hammer f.
    hippocratic f.
    index f.
    jerk f.
    jersey f.
    lock f.
    mallet f.
    middle f.
    f. oximetry
    f. percussion
    f. phenomenon
    ring f.
    f. spelling
    trigger f.
    webbed f.
fingerbreadth
finger-in-glove appearance
fingernail
finger-nose test
fingerprint
    f. dystrophy
    genetic f.
fingerprinting
    DNA f.
fingerspelling
finger-thumb reflex
finger-to-finger test
finishing bur
Finkelstein test
Fink-Heimer stain

Finney
    F. operation
    F. pyloroplasty
fire
    f. ant
    Saint Anthony f.
firedamp
first
    f. aid
    f. arch syndrome
    f. cervical vertebra
    f. cranial nerve
    f. cuneiform bone
    f. dentition
    f. duodenal sphincter
    f. finger
    f. heart sound
    f. intention
    f. messenger
    f. molar
    f. parallel pelvic plane
    f. permanent molar
    f. rank symptoms (FRS)
    f. responder
    f. rib
    f. temporal convolution
    f. visceral cleft
first-degree
    f.-d. AV block
    f.-d. burn
    f.-d. prolapse
first-order reaction
first-pass
    f.-p. effect
    f.-p. metabolism
first-set rejection
Fischer
    F. projection
    F. projection formula
    F. sign
    F. symptom
fish
    f. berry
    f. eye disease
    f. poison
    f. skin
    f. tapeworm anemia
Fishberg concentration test
Fisher
    F. exact test
    F. syndrome
Fishman-Lerner unit

fishmouth
    f. incision
    f. meatus
    f. mitral stenosis
fishtank granuloma
fission
    binary f.
    bud f.
    multiple f.
    f. product
    simple f.
fissiparity
fissiparous
fissula ante fenestram
fissura, pl. **fissurae**
fissural cyst
fissurata
    lingua f.
fissuration
fissure
    abdominal f.
    Ammon f.
    anal f.
    ansoparamedian f.
    anterior median f.
    antitragohelicine f.
    ape f.
    auricular f.
    azygos f.
    Bichat f.
    branchial f.
    Broca f.
    f. bur
    calcarine f.
    callosomarginal f.
    f. caries
    caudal transverse f.
    cerebellar f.
    cerebral f.
    choroid f.
    choroidal f.
    Clevenger f.
    collateral f.
    corneal f.
    decidual f.
    dentate f.
    Duverney f.
    Ecker f.
    enamel f.
    glaserian f.
    great horizontal f.
    great longitudinal f.

NOTES

F

fissure *(continued)*
  Henle f.
  hippocampal f.
  horizontal f.
  inferior accessory f.
  inferior orbital f.
  intersemilunar f.
  intraculminate f.
  lateral cerebral f.
  left sagittal f.
  linguogingival f.
  longitudinal cerebral f.
  lunate f.
  major f.
  minor f.
  palpebral f.
  paracentral f.
  petrooccipital f.
  petrotympanic f.
  portal f.
  primary f.
  f. of Rolando
  f. sealant
  f. sign
  superior orbital f.
  f. of Sylvius
  transverse f.
  tympanomastoid f.
fissured
  f. fracture
  f. tongue
fistula
  abdominal f.
  amphibolic f.
  amphibolous f.
  anal f.
  arteriovenous f.
  biliary f.
  blind f.
  BP f.
  branchial f.
  Brescia-Cimino f.
  bronchobiliary f.
  bronchocavitary f.
  bronchoesophageal f.
  bronchopleural f.
  bronchopleural-cutaneous f.
  caroticocavernous f.
  carotid-cavernous f.
  cassia f.
  cholecystoduodenal f.
  chyle f.
  coccygeal f.
  colocutaneous f.
  coloileal f.
  colonic f.
  colovaginal f.
  colovesical f.
  complete f.

  congenital pulmonary
    arteriovenous f.
  dental f.
  duodenal f.
  dural cavernous sinus f.
  Eck f.
  enterocolic f.
  enterocutaneous f.
  enterovaginal f.
  enterovesical f.
  ethmoidal-lacrimal f.
  external f.
  fecal f.
  gastric f.
  gastrocolic f.
  gastrocutaneous f.
  gastroduodenal f.
  gastrointestinal f.
  genitourinary f.
  gingival f.
  hepatic f.
  hepatopleural f.
  horseshoe f.
  H-type tracheoesophageal f.
  incomplete f.
  internal lacrimal f.
  intestinal f.
  f. knife
  labyrinthine f.
  lacrimal f.
  lacteal f.
  lymphatic f.
  mammary f.
  Mann-Bollman f.
  metroperitoneal f.
  oronasal f.
  parietal f.
  perilymphatic f.
  perirectal f.
  rectolabial f.
  reverse Eck f.
  salivary f.
  f. test
  Thiry f.
  tracheoesophageal f.
  urethrocutaneous f.
  urethrovaginal f.
  urinary f.
  vesicocolonic f.
  vesicointestinal f.
  vesicorectal f.
  vesicoumbilical f.
  vesicouterine f.
  vesicovaginal f.
fistulation
fistulatome
fistulectomy
fistulization
fistuloenterostomy

fistulotomy
fistulous
FIT
  fusion-inferred threshold
  FIT test
fit
  goodness of f.
  induced f.
fitness
  clinical f.
  evolutionary f.
  genetic f.
  health-related physical f.
  physical f.
Fitzgerald factor
Fitz-Hugh and Curtis syndrome
fixa
  punctum f.
fixation
  ammonia f.
  arch bar f.
  f. bandage
  bifoveal f.
  binocular f.
  circumalveolar f.
  circummandibular f.
  circumzygomatic f.
  complement f.
  craniofacial f.
  crossed f.
  f. disparity
  eccentric f.
  elastic band f.
  external pin f.
  field of f.
  freudian f.
  genetic f.
  f. hook
  f. hysteria
  intermaxillary f.
  internal f.
  intraosseous f.
  line of f.
  mandibulomaxillary f.
  maxillomandibular f.
  f. nystagmus
  f. reaction
  f. suppression
fixational ocular movement
fixative
  acetone f.
  alcohol-glycerin f.

Altmann f.
Bouin f.
Carnoy f.
Champy f.
Flemming f.
formaldehyde f.
formol-calcium f.
formol-Müller f.
formol-saline f.
formol-Zenker f.
glutaraldehyde f.
Golgi osmiobichromate f.
Helly f.
Hermann f.
Kaiserling f.
Luft potassium permanganate f.
Marchi f.
methanol f.
Müller f.
Newcomer f.
Orth f.
Regaud f.
SAF f.
Schaudinn f.
single vial f.
Thoma f.
Zenker f.
fixator muscle
fixe
  idée f.
fixed
  f. alkali
  f. alkaloid
  f. bridge
  f. contracture
  f. coupling
  f. and dilated (F&D)
  f. dressing
  f. drug eruption
  f. end
  f. idea
  f. macrophage
  f. oil
  f. partial denture
  f. pupil
  f. rate pulse generator
  f. torticollis
  f. virus
fixed-rate pacemaker
fixer
fixing eye

NOTES

F

flaccid
    f. dysarthria
    f. ectropion
    f. membrane
    f. paralysis
    f. paraplegia
    f. part
flaccidity
Flack node
flagellar
    f. agglutinin
    f. antigen
Flagellata
flagellate
    collared f.
    f. diarrhea
flagellated
flagellation
flagellin
flagellosis
flagellum
flag sign
flail
    f. chest
    f. joint
    f. mitral valve
flame
    f. arc
    f. cell
    f. emission spectrophotometry
    f. figure
    f. nevus
    f. photometer
    f. spot
flammable anesthetic
flammeus
    nevus f.
flange
    buccal f.
    f. contour
    denture f.
    labial f.
    lingual f.
flank
    f. bone
    f. incision
    f. position
flap
    Abbe f.
    advancement f.
    f. amputation
    arterial f.
    axial pattern f.
    bipedicle f.
    bone f.
    buried f.
    Byars f.
    caterpillar f.
    composite f.

    compound f.
    cross f.
    delayed f.
    deltopectoral f.
    direct f.
    distant f.
    double pedicle f.
    Eloesser f.
    envelope f.
    Estlander f.
    Filatov f.
    Filatov-Gillies f.
    flat f.
    free bone f.
    full-thickness f.
    gingival f.
    hinged f.
    immediate f.
    Indian f.
    interpolated f.
    island f.
    island leg f.
    Italian f.
    jump f.
    lined f.
    liver f.
    local f.
    omental f.
    open f.
    f. operation
    osteoplastic bone f.
    partial-thickness f.
    pedicle f.
    pharyngeal f.
    random pattern f.
    rotation f.
    sliding f.
    split-thickness f.
    subcutaneous f.
    tubed f.
    waltzed f.
flapless amputation
flapping
    f. sound
    f. tremor
flare
    aqueous f.
flaring
    nasal f.
flash
    f. blindness
    f. burn
    f. dispersal
    hot f.
    f. keratoconjunctivitis
    f. method
    f. point
flashback
flashing pain syndrome

flash-lag effect
flask
    casting f.
    f. closure
    crown f.
    dcnture f.
    Dewar f.
    Erlenmeyer f.
    Fernbach f.
    Florence f.
    hatching f.
    injection f.
flasking
flat
    f. affect
    f. bone
    f. chest
    f. condyloma
    f. electroencephalogram
    f. flap
    f. muscle
    f. pelvis
    f. plate
    f. top wave
    f. wart
flat-and-rise phenomenon
Flatau law
flatfoot
flatulence
flatulent dyspepsia
flatus
    f. enema
    f. vaginalis
flatworm
Flaujeac factor
flava
    macula f.
flavedo
flavianic acid
flavin
    f. adenine dinucleotide
    electron transfer f.
    f. mononucleotide
    f. nucleotide
flavine
Flavobacterium
    F. *aquatile*
    F. *breve*
    F. *meningisepticum*
    F. *piscicida*
flavoenzyme
flavokinase

flavone
flavonoid
flavonol
flavoprotein
flavus
    Aspergillus f.
flax-dresser's disease
flaxseed oil
flea-bitten kidney
flea-borne typhus
flecainide acetate
Flechsig
    F. area
    F. fasciculus
    F. ground bundle
    F. tract
fleck
    f. dystrophy
    f. retina
flecked
    f. retina
    f. retina syndrome
Flegel disease
Fleischer
    F. ring
    F. vortex
Fleischer-Strümpell ring
Fleischmann bursa
Fleischner line
Fleisch pneumotachograph
Fleitmann test
Flemming
    F. fixative
    F. triple stain
Flesch formula
flesh
    f. fly
    goose f.
    proud f.
fleshy
    f. mole
    f. polyp
Fletcher factor
flexibilitas
    cerea f.
    f. cerea
flexibility
flexible
    f. collodion
    f. endoscope
    f. endoscopy
    f. hysteroscope

F

NOTES

fleximeter
flexion crease
flexion-extension injury
Flexner bacillus
flexneri
    Shigella f.
flexometer
flexor
    f. accessorius muscle
    f. carpi radialis muscle
    f. carpi ulnaris muscle
    f. compartment
    f. digiti minimi brevis muscle
    f. digitorum brevis muscle
    f. digitorum longus muscle
    f. digitorum profundus muscle
    f. digitorum superficialis muscle
    f. hallucis brevis muscle
    f. hallucis longus muscle
    f. pollicis brevis muscle
    f. pollicis longus muscle
    f. reflex
    f. retinaculum
flexural
    f. eczema
    f. psoriasis
flexure
    anorectal f.
    basicranial f.
    caudal f.
    cephalic f.
    cerebral f.
    cervical f.
    cranial f.
    dorsal f.
    duodenojejunal f.
    hepatic f.
    iliac f.
    inferior duodenal f.
    left colic f.
    lumbar f.
    mesencephalic f.
    pontine f.
    right colic f.
    sacral f.
    sigmoid f.
    splenic f.
    telencephalic f.
    transverse rhombencephalic f.
flexus
    hallux f.
flicker
    f. fusion
    f. fusion frequency technique
    f. perimetry
    f. photometer
flick movement
Flieringa ring

flight
    f. blindness
    f. or fight response
    f. of ideas
    f. into disease
    f. into health
    f. nurse
Flinders Island spotted fever
flint
    F. arcade
    Austin F.
    f. disease
    f. glass
    F. murmur
flip angle
flitter
flittering scotoma
floater
floating
    f. cartilage
    f. kidney
    f. organ
    f. patella
    f. rib
    f. spleen
    f. tooth sign
    f. villus
floccillation
floccose
flocculable
floccular fossa
flocculate
flocculation
    f. reaction
    f. test
floccule
flocculence
flocculent
flocculonodular lobe
flocculus, pl. flocculi
    accessory f.
flood
    f. fever
    F. ligament
flooding
floor
    f. of orbit
    f. plate
floppy valve syndrome
flora
florantyrone
Florence
    F. crystal
    F. flask
Florey unit
florid
    f. oral papillomatosis
    f. osseous dysplasia
floriform cataract

Florschütz formula
floss
    dental f.
    f. silk
flotation
    f. constant
    f. method
    Svedberg of f.
Flourens theory
floury cornea
flow
    Bingham f.
    cerebral blood f. (CBF)
    coronary blood f.
    f. cytometry
    f. cytophotometry
    f. diagram
    Doppler color f.
    effective renal blood f. (ERBF)
    effective renal plasma f. (ERPF)
    forced expiratory f. (FEF)
    gene f.
    laminar f.
    peak expiratory f.
    turbulent f.
    f. void
flow-controlled ventilator
flower
    f. basket of Bochdalek
    F. bone
    F. dental index
    elder f.
flower-spray ending
flowing hyperostosis
flowmeter
    electromagnetic f.
    peak f.
flow-over vaporizer
flow-volume
    f.-v. curve
    f.-v. loop study
floxacillin
floxuridine
flu
fluanisone
flucrylate
fluctuance
fluctuate
fluctuation
flucytosine
fludrocortisone acetate
fluence

fluency
fluent aphasia
flufenamic acid
fluffy compression dressing
fluid
    allantoic f.
    amnionic f.
    amniotic f.
    Brodie f.
    bronchoalveolar f.
    Callison f.
    cerebrospinal f. (CSF)
    crevicular f.
    Dakin f.
    dentinal f.
    extracellular f. (ECF)
    f. extract
    extravascular f.
    Farrant mounting f.
    gingival f.
    infranatant f.
    interstitial f.
    intracellular f. (ICF)
    intraocular f.
    f. mosaic model
    pleural f.
    prostatic f.
    f. retinopexy
    seminal f.
    synovial f.
    transcellular f.
    f. wave
fluidextract
fluidglycerate
fluidism
fluidity
fluidounce
fluidrachm
fluidram
fluke
    blood f.
flumazenil
flumen
flumethasone
flumethiazide
flumina pilorum
flunarizine
flunisolide
flunitrazepam
fluocinolone acetonide
fluocinonide
fluocortolone

F

NOTES

fluorapatite
fluorescamine
fluoresce
fluorescein
    f. angiography
    f. instillation test
    f. isothiocyanate
    f. sodium
    f. string test
fluorescence
    f. microscope
    f. microscopy
    f. plus Giemsa stain
    f. quenching
    f. in situ hybridization
    f. spectrum
fluorescence-activated cell sorter
fluorescent
    f. antibody
    f. antibody technique
    f. antinuclear antibody (FANA)
    f. antinuclear antibody test
    f. screen
    f. in situ hybridization
    f. stain
    f. treponemal antibody absorption (FTA-ABS)
    f. treponemal antibody-absorption test
fluoridated tooth
fluoridation
fluoride number
fluoridization
fluorine
fluorochrome
fluorochroming
fluorocyte
fluorography
fluoroimmunoassay
fluorometer
fluorometholone
fluorometry
fluorophotometry
fluoroquinolone antibiotic
fluororoentgenography
fluoroscope
fluoroscopic
fluoroscopy
fluorosis
    chronic endemic f.
fluorouracil
fluoxymesterone
flupentixol
fluphenazine
fluprednisolone
flurbiprofen
flurothyl
fluroxene

Flury
    F. strain rabies virus
    F. strain vaccine
flush
    carcinoid f.
    hectic f.
    histamine f.
    hot f.
    malar f.
    promontory f.
    f. technique
flutamide
flutter
    atrial f.
    auricular f.
    diaphragmatic f.
    impure f.
    ocular f.
    pure f.
    ventricular f.
flutter-fibrillation wave
fluvialis
    Vibrio f.
flux
    f. density
    luminous f.
    f. ratio
fluxionary hyperemia
fly
    f. agaric
    f. blister
    flesh f.
    heel f.
    louse f.
    mangrove f.
flying spot microscope
Flynn-Aird syndrome
Flynn phenomenon
FMD
    foot-and-mouth disease
    FMD virus
FNA
    fine-needle aspiration
foam
    f. cell
    human fibrin f.
    f. rubber dressing
    f. stability test
foamy
    f. agent
    f. virus
focal
    f. acrohyperkeratosis
    f. amyloidosis
    f. appendicitis
    f. condensing osteitis
    f. depth
    f. dermal hypoplasia
    f. distance

f. embolic glomerulonephritis
f. epilepsy
f. epithelial hyperplasia
f. illumination
f. infection
f. injury
f. interval
f. lesion
f. lymphocytic thyroiditis
f. metastatic disease
f. motor seizure
f. necrosis
f. nephritis
f. point
f. reaction
f. sclerosing glomerulopathy
f. sclerosis
f. segmental glomerulosclerosis
f. spot
f. spot size
focal-film distance
focimeter
focus, pl. **foci**
conjugate foci
depth of f.
Ghon f.
focused
f. grid
f. medical assessment
f. trauma assessment
focusing
isoelectric f.
fodrin
Fogarty
F. clamp
F. embolectomy catheter
fogging retinoscopy
foil
gold f.
Foix-Alajouanine
F.-A. myelitis
F.-A. syndrome
Foix-Cavany-Marie syndrome
folate
fold
adipose f.
alar f.
amnionic f.
ampullary f.
anterior axillary f.
aryepiglottic f.
arytenoepiglottidean f.

axillary f.
caval f.
cecal f.
ciliary f.
circular f.
Dennie-Morgan f.
dinucleotide f.
Douglas f.
Duncan f.
duodenojejunal f.
duodenomesocolic f.
epicanthal f.
epigastric f.
epiglottic f.
falciform retinal f.
fatty f.
fimbriated f.
gastric f.
gastropancreatic f.
genital f.
giant gastric f.
glossopalatine f.
gluteal f.
Guérin f.
Hasner f.
head f.
Houston f.
ileocecal f.
incudal f.
inferior duodenal f.
infrapatellar synovial f.
inguinal aponeurotic f.
interarytenoid f.
interdigital f.
interureteric f.
Kerckring f.
Kohlrausch f.
labioscrotal f.
lacrimal f.
lateral glossoepiglottic f.
lateral nasal f.
lateral umbilical f.
longitudinal f.
malar f.
mallear f.
mammary f.
Marshall vestigial f.
medial canthic f.
medial nasal f.
medial umbilical f.
median glossoepiglottic f.
median umbilical f.

NOTES

F

365

fold (*continued*)
    medullary f.
    mesonephric f.
    middle glossoepiglottic f.
    middle transverse rectal f.
    middle umbilical f.
    nail f.
    neural f.
    palmate f.
    rectouterine f.
    retroauricular f.
    sacrouterine f.
    semilunar conjunctival f.
    spiral f.
    tail f.
    transverse rectal f.
    ventricular f.
    vesicouterine f.
    vestibular f.
    vocal f.
foldable intraocular lens
fold-back element
folded-lung syndrome
folding fracture
Foley
    F. catheter
    F. Y-plasty pyeloplasty
folia
    f. of cerebellum
    f. linguae
foliaceous
foliaceus
    pemphigus f.
foliar
foliate
    f. papilla
    f. papillitis
folic
    f. acid
    f. acid antagonist
    f. acid conjugate
    f. acid deficiency anemia
folie
    f. à deux
    f. du doute
    f. du pourquoi
    f. gémellaire
Folin
    F. reaction
    F. reagent
    F. test
folinate
folinic acid
Folin-Looney test
folium of vermis, folium vermis
folk medicine
follian process
folliberin

follicle
    aggregated lymphatic f.
    anovular ovarian f.
    antral f.
    atretic ovarian f.
    dental f.
    gastric f.
    graafian f.
    growing ovarian f.
    hair f.
    intestinal f.
    Lieberkühn f.
    lingual f.
    luteinized unruptured f.
    lymph f.
    lymphatic f.
    mature ovarian f.
    Montgomery f.
    nabothian f.
    ovarian f.
    primary ovarian f.
    primordial ovarian f.
    sebaceous f.
    secondary f.
    solitary lymphatic f.
    splenic lymph f.
    thyroid f.
    vesicular ovarian f.
follicle-stimulating
    f.-s. hormone (FSH)
    f.-s. hormone-releasing factor
    f.-s. hormone-releasing hormone
    f.-s. principle
follicular
    f. abscess
    f. adenoma
    f. ameloblastoma
    f. antrum
    f. atrophoderma
    f. carcinoma
    f. conjunctivitis
    f. cyst
    f. cystitis
    f. epithelial cell
    f. gland
    f. goiter
    f. hormone
    f. hyperplasia
    f. impetigo
    f. iritis
    f. mucinosis
    f. ovarian cell
    f. papule
    f. predominantly large cell lymphoma
    f. predominantly small cleaved cell lymphoma
    f. stigma
    f. trachoma

f. ulcer
f. urethritis
f. vulvitis
follicularis
isolated dyskeratosis f.
keratosis f.
lichen planus f.
folliculi (*pl. of* folliculus)
folliculin hydrate
folliculitis
f. barbae
f. decalvans
eosinophilic pustular f.
f. keloidalis
f. ulerythematosa reticulata
folliculoma
folliculorum
Acarus f.
Demodex f.
folliculosis
folliculus, pl. **folliculi**
liquor folliculi
f. lymphaticus
f. pili
theca folliculi
Folling disease
Folli process
follistatin
follitropin
follitropin-releasing hormone (FRH)
follower
filiform and f.
following bougie
followup study
Foltz valvule
fomentation
fomes, pl. **fomites**
fonazine mesylate
Fonio solution
Fontan
F. operation
F. procedure
Fontana
F. canal
F. space
F. stain
Fontana-Masson silver stain
fontanelle
anterior f.
anterolateral f.
bregmatic f.
Casser f.

cranial f.
frontal f.
Gerdy f.
mastoid f.
sagittal f.
fonticulus
food
f. asthma
f. ball
f. fever
functional f.
f. impaction
f. poisoning
foot, pl. **feet**
athlete's f.
bifid f.
f. bone
cleft f.
club f., clubfoot
contracted f.
dangle f.
forced f.
immersion f.
Madura f.
f. plate
f. plugger
f. presentation
f. process
F. reticulin impregnation stain
splay f.
f. yaw
foot-and-mouth
f.-a.-m. disease (FMD)
f.-a.-m. disease virus
f.-a.-m. disease virus vaccine
footcandle
footdrop
footling presentation
footplate, foot-plate
foot-pound
foot-poundal
foot-pound-second (FPS, fps)
f.-p.-s. system
f.-p.-s. unit
footprinting
forage
foramen, pl. **foramina**
alveolar f.
anterior condyloid f.
anterior palatine f.
aortic f.
apical dental f.

F

NOTES

367

foramen *(continued)*
- arachnoid f.
- f. of Arnold
- Bichat f.
- blind f.
- Bochdalek f.
- f. of Bochdalek hernia
- Botallo f.
- carotid f.
- cecal f.
- conjugate f.
- costotransverse f.
- cribriform f.
- emissary f.
- epiploic f.
- ethmoidal f.
- external acoustic f.
- external auditory f.
- Ferrein f.
- frontal f.
- f. frontale
- great f.
- greater palatine f.
- Huschke f.
- Hyrtl f.
- incisive f.
- incisor f.
- inferior dental f.
- infraorbital f.
- internal acoustic f.
- internal auditory f.
- interventricular f.
- intervertebral f.
- f. intervertebrale
- jugular f.
- f. jugulare
- f. of Key-Retzius
- lacerated f.
- Lannelongue f.
- lesser palatine f.
- f. of Luschka
- f. of Magendie
- malar f.
- mandibular f.
- mastoid f.
- mental f.
- neural f.
- nutrient f.
- obturator f.
- olfactory f.
- omental f.
- optic f.
- oval f.
- f. ovale
- parietal f.
- f. of Retzius
- sciatic f.
- sphenopalatine f.
- stylomastoid f.

- supraorbital f.
- transverse f.
- vertebral f.
- vertebroarterial f.
- f. of Winslow
- zygomaticofacial f.
- zygomaticoorbital f.
- zygomaticotemporal f.

foraminal
- f. hernia
- f. herniation
- f. lymph node

foraminiferous

foraminotomy

foraminulum

Forbes-Albright syndrome

Forbes disease

force
- animal f.
- chewing f.
- dynamic f.
- electromotive f.
- G f.
- f. of mastication
- masticatory f.
- occlusal f.
- f. platform
- reciprocal f.
- reserve f.
- van der Waals f.

forcé
- accouchement f.
- brisement f.

forced
- f. alimentation
- f. beat
- f. cycle
- f. duction
- f. expiratory flow (FEF)
- f. expiratory time (FET)
- f. expiratory volume (FEV)
- f. feeding
- f. foot
- f. grasping reflex
- f. respiration
- f. spirometry
- f. vital capacity (FVC)

forceps
- Adson f.
- alligator f.
- Allis f.
- f. anterior
- Arruga f.
- arterial f.
- axis-traction f.
- Barton f.
- bayonet f.
- bone f.
- Brown-Adson f.

bulldog f.
bullet f.
capsule f.
cartilage f.
chalazion f.
Chamberlen f.
clamp f.
clip f.
cup biopsy f.
cutting f.
DeBakey f.
f. delivery
dental f.
dissecting f.
dressing f.
dural f.
extracting f.
frontal f.
f. frontalis
Graefe f.
hemostatic f.
inlet f.
insertion f.
jeweller f.
Kjelland f.
Lahey f.
Laplace f.
Levret f.
lion-jaw bone-holding f.
Löwenberg f.
magic f.
Magill f.
f. major
major f.
minor f.
f. minor
mosquito f.
mouse-tooth f.
needle f.
nonfenestrated f.
obstetrical f.
f. occipitalis
outlet f.
Piper f.
f. posterior
rubber dam clamp f.
speculum f.
Tarnier f.
tenaculum f.
thumb f.
tubular f.

tying f.
vulsella f., vulsellum f.
force-velocity curve
Forchheimer sign
forcible feeding
forcipate
forcipressure
Fordyce
    F. angiokeratoma
    F. disease
    F. granule
    F. spot
fore-and-aft suture
forearm
    intermediate vein of f.
forebrain
    f. eminence
    f. prominence
    f. vesicle
foreconscious
forefinger
foregut
forehead
foreign
    f. body (FB)
    f. body appendicitis
    f. body giant cell
    f. body granuloma
    f. body reaction
    f. body salpingitis
    f. body tumorigenesis
    f. protein
    f. protein therapy
    f. serum
forekidney
Forel
    F. decussation
    fields of F.
forelock
foremilk
forensic
    f. dentistry
    f. medicine
    f. odontology
    f. psychiatry
    f. psychology
foreplay
forepleasure
forequarter amputation
foreshortening
foreskin of penis
Forestier disease

F

NOTES

forestomach
forewaters
fork
    bite f.
    face-bow f.
    tuning f.
form
    appliqué f.
    arch f.
    boat f.
    chair f.
    f. constancy
    convenience f.
    extension f.
    face f.
    half-chair f.
    involution f.
    L f.
    replicative f.
Formad kidney
formaldehyde
    active f.
    f. fixative
    melamine f.
formalin-ether sedimentation concentration
formalin-ethyl acetate sedimentation concentration
formalinize
formalin pigment
formal operation
formamidase
    kynurenine f.
formant
formate
    active f.
formation
    concept f.
    personality f.
    reaction f.
    reticular f.
    rouleaux f.
formative cell
formazan
formboard
formed visual hallucination
forme fruste
formic
    f. acid
    f. aldehyde
formication
formiminoglutamic acid
formin
formocresol
formol-calcium fixative
formol-gel test
formol-Müller fixative
formol-saline fixative
formol titration

formol-Zenker fixative
formosulfathiazole
formula, pl. **formulas, formulae**
    Arneth f.
    Bazett f.
    Bernhardt f.
    Black f.
    Broca f.
    chemical f.
    Christison f.
    constitutional f.
    Demoivre f.
    dental f.
    Dreyer f.
    DuBois f.
    electrical f.
    empirical f.
    Fischer projection f.
    Flesch f.
    Florschütz f.
    Gorlin f.
    graphic f.
    Hamilton-Stewart f.
    Häser f.
    Jellinek f.
    Ledermann f.
    Long f.
    Mall f.
    Meeh f.
    Meeh-Dubois f.
    molecular f.
    official f.
    rational f.
    stereochemical f.
    structural f.
    vertebral f.
formulary
    hospital f.
formyl
    active f.
formylase
fornicate gyrus
fornication
fornicatus
    gyrus f.
fornicis
    delta f.
fornix, pl. **fornices**
    column of f.
    conjunctival f.
Forsius-Eriksson albinism
forskolin
Forssman
    F. antibody
    F. antigen
    F. antigen-antibody reaction
    F. hapten
Förster uveitis
Fort Bragg fever

fortification
    f. figure
    f. spectrum
fortified vitamin D milk
forward
    f. conduction
    f. heart failure
foscarnet
Fosdick-Hansen-Epple test
Foshay test
fossa, pl. **fossae**
    acetabular f.
    adipose f.
    amygdaloid f.
    anconal f.
    anterior cranial f.
    axillary f.
    Bichat f.
    Biesiadecki f.
    Broesike f.
    canine f.
    cerebellar f.
    Claudius f.
    condylar f.
    coronoid f.
    crural f.
    Cruveilhier f.
    cubital f.
    digastric f.
    digital f.
    duodenal f.
    duodenojejunal f.
    epigastric f.
    femoral f.
    floccular f.
    gallbladder f.
    Gerdy hyoid f.
    glenoid f.
    greater supraclavicular f.
    Gruber-Landzert f.
    hyaloid f.
    hypophysial f.
    iliac f.
    iliacosubfascial f.
    iliopectineal f.
    incisive f.
    incudal f.
    inferior duodenal f.
    infraclavicular f.
    infraduodenal f.
    infraspinous f.
    infratemporal f.

    inguinal f.
    innominate f.
    intercondylar f.
    intercondylic f.
    intercondyloid f.
    interpeduncular f.
    intrabulbar f.
    ischioanal f.
    ischiorectal f.
    Jobert de Lamballe f.
    Jonnesco f.
    jugular f.
    lacrimal f.
    Landzert f.
    lateral cerebral f.
    lateral inguinal f.
    lenticular f.
    lesser supraclavicular f.
    Malgaigne f.
    mandibular f.
    mastoid f.
    medial inguinal f.
    Merkel f.
    mesentericoparietal f.
    middle cranial f.
    Mohrenheim f.
    navicular f.
    f. olecrani
    f. ovalis
    ovarian f.
    paravesical f.
    popliteal f.
    rectocolic f.
    rhomboid f.
    subarcuate f.
    sublingual f.
    submandibular f.
    suborbital f.
    subsigmoid f.
    f. of Sylvius
    temporal f.
    f. temporalis
    tonsillar f.
    f. of vestibule of vagina
fossette
fossula post fenestram
fossulate
Foster
    F. frame
    F. Kennedy syndrome
Fothergill
    F. disease

NOTES

F

Fothergill (*continued*)
    F. neuralgia
    F. operation
    F. sign
Fouchet
    F. reagent
    F. stain
foulage
foundation
    denture f.
founder
    f. effect
    f. principle
foundryman's fever
fountain
    f. decussation
    f. syringe
fourchette
Four Corners virus
Fourier
    F. analysis
    F. transfer
    F. transform
Fournier
    F. disease
    F. gangrene
fourth
    f. cranial nerve
    f. disease
    f. finger
    f. heart sound
    f. lumbar nerve
    f. parallel pelvic plane
    f. toe
    f. turbinated bone
    f. ventricle
fourth-degree burn
fovea
    anterior f.
    central retinal f.
    inferior f.
foveate
foveated chest
foveation
foveola, pl. **foveolae**
    coccygeal f.
    granular foveolae
foveolar cell
foveolate
Foville
    F. fasciculus
    F. syndrome
Fowler position
fowl typhoid
Fox-Fordyce disease
foxglove
FPLC
    fast protein liquid chromatography

FPS, fps
    foot-pound-second
    FPS unit
fractal
fraction
    blood plasma f.
    f. collector
    dried human plasma protein f.
    ejection f.
    filtration f. (FF)
    human antihemophilic f.
    human plasma protein f.
    left ventricular ejection f.
    mole f.
    radionuclide ejection f.
fractional
    f. dilatation and curettage
    f. distillation
    f. dose
    f. epidural anesthesia
    f. spinal anesthesia
    f. sterilization
fractionation
fracture
    agenetic f.
    apophysial f.
    articular f.
    avulsion f.
    Barton f.
    basal skull f. (BSF)
    f. bed
    bending f.
    Bennett f.
    bimalleolar f.
    birth f.
    f. blister
    blowout f.
    boxer's f.
    capillary f.
    Chance f.
    chondral f.
    clay shoveler's f.
    closed skull f.
    Colles f.
    comminuted skull f.
    complex f.
    compound skull f.
    compression f.
    f. by contrecoup
    cortical f.
    cough f.
    craniofacial dysjunction f.
    dentate f.
    depressed skull f.
    derby hat f.
    diastatic skull f.
    direct f.
    dishpan f.
    dislocation f.

f. dislocation
displaced f.
double f.
Dupuytren f.
epiphysial f.
expressed skull f.
extracapsular f.
fatigue f.
fetal f.
fissured f.
folding f.
freeze f.
Galeazzi f.
Gosselin f.
greenstick f.
growing f.
Guérin f.
gutter f.
hairline f.
hangman's f.
horizontal maxillary f.
impacted f.
incomplete f.
indirect f.
intertrochanteric f.
intraarticular f.
intracapsular f.
intrauterine f.
Jones f.
Le Fort I, II, III f.
linear skull f.
longitudinal f.
Maisonneuve f.
malar f.
march f.
Monteggia f.
multiple f.
nasal f.
nasomaxillary f.
nightstick f.
oblique f.
occult f.
open f.
osteochondral f.
pathologic f.
pilon f.
Pott f.
pyramidal f.
segmental f.
Shepherd f.
silver-fork f.
simple f.

Smith f.
spiral f.
sprain f.
stellate f.
strain f.
stress f.
subcapital f.
torsion f.
torus f.
transverse f.
tripod f.
wedge f.
Fraenkel pneumococcus
fragile
    f. site
    f. X chromosome
    f. X syndrome
fragilis
    Bacteroides f.
    Dientamoeba f.
fragilitas
    f. crinium
    f. sanguinis
fragility
    capillary f.
    osmotic f.
    f. test
fragilocyte
fragilocytosis
fragment
    acentric f.
    Brimacombe f.
    butterfly f.
    1-carbon f.
    2-carbon f.
    Fab f.
    Fc f.
    Klenow f.
    f. length polymorphism
    f. reaction
fragmentation
fragmentography
fraise
Fraley syndrome
frambesia tropica
frambesiform
frambesioma
frame
    Balkan f.
    blocked reading f.
    Bradford f.
    closed reading f.

F

NOTES

frame *(continued)*
    Deiters terminal f.
    Foster f.
    Stryker f.
    trial f.
    Whitman f.
frameshift
    f. mutagen
    f. mutation
framework region
Franceschetti-Jadassohn syndrome
Franceschetti syndrome
Francisella tularensis
francium
Francke needle
frangula
frangulic acid
frangulin
frank breech presentation
Frankenhäuser ganglion
Frankfort horizontal plane
Frankfort-mandibular incisor angle
frankincense
Franklin
    F. disease
    F. spectacles
franklinic taste
Frank-Starling curve
Fräntzel murmur
Fraser-Lendrum stain
Fraser syndrome
fraternal twin
Fraunhofer line
Frazier needle
Frazier-Spiller operation
FRC
    functional residual capacity
freckle
    Hutchinson f.
    iris f.
    melanotic f.
Fredet-Ramstedt operation
free
    f. association
    f. bone flap
    f. border
    f. electrophoresis
    f. energy
    f. fatty acid (FFA)
    f. field
    f. gingiva
    f. graft
    f. induction decay (FID)
    f. ligature suture
    f. macrophage
    f. mandibular movement
    f. margin
    f. nerve ending
    f. radical

    f. tenia
    f. thyroxine index (FTI)
    f. villus
    f. water
    f. water clearance
freedom
    degrees of f.
free-floating anxiety
free-hand knife
Freeman-Sheldon syndrome
freeway space
freeze-drying
freeze fracture
freezing
    gastric f.
    f. microtome
    f. point
Freiberg
    F. disease
    F. infarction
Frei-Hoffmann reaction
Frei test
Frejka pillow splint
frémissement cattaire
fremitus
    bronchial f.
    hydatid f.
    f. pectoralis
    pericardial f.
    pleural f.
    rhonchal f.
    tactile f.
    tussive f.
    vocal f.
frena (*pl. of* frenum)
frenal
frenata
    lingua f.
French
    F. chalk
    F. scale
French-American-British (FAB)
    F.-A.-B. classification
    F.-A.-B. classification system
frenectomy
frenoplasty
frenotomy
frenulum, pl. **frenula**
    cerebellar f.
    lingual f.
frenum, pl. **frena**
frenzy
frequency
    best f.
    characteristic f.
    critical flicker fusion f.
    f. curve
    f. distribution
    f. domain

dominant f.
f. encoding
fundamental f.
gene f.
Larmor f.
modal f.
resonant f.
respiratory f.
f. spectrum
speech f.
Frerichs theory
fresh frozen plasma (FFP)
Fresnel
F. lens
F. prism
fressreflex
fretting
fretum
freudian
f. fixation
f. psychoanalysis
f. slip
Freud theory
Freund
F. anomaly
F. complete adjuvant
F. incomplete adjuvant
F. operation
freundii
Citrobacter f.
Escherichia f.
Frey
F. hair
F. syndrome
FRH
follitropin-releasing hormone
friable
fricative
friction
dynamic f.
f. murmur
pericardial f.
f. rub
f. sound
frictional attachment
Friderichsen-Waterhouse syndrome
Friedländer
F. bacillus
F. bacillus pneumonia
F. stain
Friedman curve

Friedreich
F. ataxia
F. phenomenon
F. sign
Friend
F. disease
F. leukemia virus
fright
f. neurosis
f. reaction
frigid
frigidity
frigorific
frigorism
frill
iris f.
fringe
costal f.
Froehde reagent
frog face
frog-leg
f.-l. lateral projection
f.-l. position
Fröhlich
F. dwarfism
F. syndrome
Frohn reagent
Froin syndrome
frôlement
Froment sign
frons
frontad
frontal
f. angle
f. area
f. artery
f. aspect
f. belly
f. bone
f. border
f. cortex
f. crest
f. eminence
f. fontanelle
f. foramen
f. forceps
f. groove
f. horn
f. lobe
f. lobe epilepsy
f. margin
f. nerve

F

NOTES

frontal (*continued*)
  f. notch
  f. plane
  f. plate
  f. pole
  f. process
  f. region
  f. section
  f. sinus
  f. sinus aperture
  f. sinus mucocele
  f. squama
  f. suture
  f. triangle
  f. tuber
  f. vein
frontale
  foramen f.
frontalis
  alopecia liminaris f.
  forceps f.
  incisura f.
  f. muscle
frontoanterior
  f. fetal position
  left f. (LFA)
frontoethmoidal suture
frontolacrimal suture
frontomalar suture
frontomaxillary suture
frontonasal
  f. duct
  f. process
  f. prominence
  f. suture
frontooccipital
frontoorbital area
frontoparietal
frontopolar artery
frontopontine
  f. fiber
  f. tract
frontoposterior
  f. fetal position
  left f. (LFP)
frontosphenoidal process
frontotemporal tract
frontotransverse
  f. fetal position
  left f. (LFT)
frontozygomatic suture
front-tap
  f.-t. contraction
  f.-t. reflex
Froriep ganglion
frost
  f. itch
  F. suture

  urea f.
  uremic f.
frostbite
frosted
  f. branch angiitis
  f. heart
  f. liver
frottage
frotteur
frozen
  f. pelvis
  f. section
  f. shoulder
FRS
  first rank symptoms
fructan
fructofuranose
fructokinase deficiency
fructolysis
fructosan
fructose
  ferric f.
  f. malabsorption
fructosemia
fructoside
fructosuria
  benign f.
  essential f.
fruiting body
fruit sugar
frusemide
fruste
  forme f.
frustration-aggression hypothesis
frustration tolerance
fry
  glottal f.
  vocal f.
FSH
  follicle-stimulating hormone
FTA-ABS
  fluorescent treponemal antibody
  absorption
  FTA-ABS test
FTI
  free thyroxine index
Fuchs
  F. adenoma
  angle of F.
  F. black spot
  F. coloboma
  F. endothelial dystrophy
  F. epithelial dystrophy
  F. heterochromic cyclitis
  F. position
  F. spur
  F. stoma
  F. syndrome
  F. uveitis

fuchsin
    acid f.
    aniline f.
    basic f.
    f. body
    carbol f.
    diamond f.
fuchsinophil
    f. cell
    f. granule
    f. reaction
fuchsinophilia
fuchsinophilic
fucose
fucosidosis
fugacity
fugax
    amaurosis f.
fugitive
    f. swelling
    f. wart
fugue
fugu poison
fugutoxin
fulcrum line
fulgurant
fulgurating migraine
fulguration
full
    f. denture
    f. liquid diet
fuller's earth
full-lumen esophagoscope
full-mouth
    f.-m. extraction
    f.-m. series
full-thickness
    f.-t. burn
    f.-t. flap
    f.-t. graft
fulminans
    acne f.
    glaucoma f.
    purpura f.
fulminant
    f. hepatitis
    f. hyperpyrexia
fulminating
    f. apoplexy
    f. appendicitis
    f. dysentery
    f. smallpox

fulvum
    Microsporum f.
fumarase
fumarate
    ferrous f.
    f. hydratase
    f. reductase NADH
fumaric
    f. acid
    f. acidemia
    f. aminase
    f. hydrogenase
fumarylacetoacetate hydrolase
fumigant
fumigate
fumigation
fumigatus
    Aspergillus f.
fuming
    f. nitric acid
    f. sulfuric acid
functio laesa
function
    allomeric f.
    arousal f.
    atrial transport f.
    f. corrector
    discriminant f.
    isomeric f.
    line spread f.
    liver f.
    mapping f.
    modulation transfer f.
functional
    f. activity
    f. albuminuria
    f. anatomy
    f. aphasia
    f. apoplexy
    f. appendix
    f. asplenia
    f. autonomy
    f. blindness
    f. cardiovascular disease
    f. castration
    f. chew-in record
    f. congestion
    f. contracture
    f. deafness
    f. disorder
    f. dysmenorrhea
    f. dyspepsia

F

NOTES

functional *(continued)*
f. dyspnea
f. endoscopic sinus surgery (FESS)
f. food
f. genomics
f. group
f. hearing impairment
f. hyperinsulinism
f. hypertrophy
f. illness
f. jaw orthopedics
f. mandibular movement
f. murmur
f. neck dissection
f. neurosurgery
f. occlusal harmony
f. occlusion
f. orthodontic therapy
f. paralysis
f. pathology
f. pleiotropy
f. prepubertal castration syndrome
f. psychosis
f. refractory period
f. residual air
f. residual capacity (FRC)
f. sphincter
f. splint
f. stricture
f. terminal innervation ratio
f. test
f. visual loss
f. vocal fatigue
functionale
stratum f.
functionalism
fundament
fundamental
f. frequency
f. symptom
f. tone
fundectomy
fundi *(pl. of* fundus)
fundic gland
fundiform ligament
fundoplication
Belsey f.
Collis-Belsey f.
Collis-Nissen f.
Dor f.
Nissen f.
Toupet f.
fundus, pl. **fundi**
leopard f.
f. oculi
f. reflex
tessellated f.
f. ventriculi
f. vesicae urinariae

funduscope
funduscopy
fundusectomy
fungal endocarditis
fungate
fungating chancre
fungemia
fungicidal
fungicide
fungicidin
fungiform papilla
fungilliform
fungistat
fungistatic
fungitoxic
fungitoxicity
fungoid
fungoides
mycosis f.
fungosity
fungous
fungus
f. ball
f. cerebri
dematiaceous f.
imperfect f.
perfect f.
funicle
funic souffle
funicular
f. graft
f. hernia
f. hydrocele
f. myelitis
f. myelosis
f. process
f. souffle
funiculi *(pl. of* funiculus)
funiculitis
endemic f.
filarial f.
funiculopexy
funiculus, pl. **funiculi**
anterior f.
f. anterior
cuneate f.
dorsal f.
f. dorsalis
f. gracilis
lateral f.
f. lateralis
funiculi medullae spinalis
posterior f.
f. posterior
funiform
funipuncture
funis
funisitis

funnel
> f. breast
> Büchner f.
> f. chest
> Martegiani f.
> f. plot

funnel-shaped pelvis
funny bone
FUO
> fever of unknown origin

furaltadone
furanose
furcal nerve
furcation
furcosus
> Bacteroides f.

furcula
furfur
> Malassezia f.

furfuracea
> seborrhea f.

furfuraceous
furfuryl alcohol
furious rabies
furnace
> dental f.

furnacemen's cataract
Furniss anastomosis
furnissii
> Vibrio f.

furoate
> diloxanide f.

furor epilepticus
furosemide
furred tongue
furrow
> digital f.
> genital f.
> gluteal f.
> mentolabial f.

furuncle
furuncular
furunculi (*pl. of* furunculus)
furunculoid
furunculosa
> Leishmania f.

furunculosis
furunculous
furunculus, pl. **furunculi**
fusca
> lamina f.

fuseau
fused
> f. kidney
> f. silver nitrate
> f. teeth

fusel oil
fusible metal
fusidate sodium
fusidic acid
fusiform
> f. aneurysm
> f. cataract
> f. cell
> f. gyrus
> f. layer
> f. muscle

fusimotor
fusing point
fusion
> anterior cervical discectomy and f. (ACDF)
> f. area
> f. beat
> bone block f.
> cell f.
> centric f.
> f. energy
> flicker f.
> peripheral f.
> spinal f.
> spine f.
> f. temperature wire method

fusional movement
fusion-inferred
> f.-i. threshold (FIT)
> f.-i. threshold test

fusocellular
fusospirochetal
> f. disease
> f. gingivitis
> f. stomatitis

fustic
fustigation
Futcher line
futile cycle
FVC
> forced vital capacity

Fy
> Fy antigen
> Fy blood group

F

NOTES

γ (*var. of* gamma)

G

gauss

G acid
G antigen
G cell
G factor
G force
G protein
G protein disease
G syndrome
G unit

Gaboon ulcer
G-actin
Gaddum and Schild test
gadfly
gadodiamide
gadoleic acid
gadolinium
gadopentetate
gadoteridol
Gaenslen sign
Gaffky

G. scale
G. table

gag

Crowe-Davis mouth g.
g. reflex

gagging reflex
gain

primary g.
secondary g.

Gairdner disease
Gaisböck syndrome
gait

antalgic g.
g. apraxia
ataxic g.
calcaneal g.
cerebellar g.
Charcot g.
circumduction g.
cogwheel g.
equine g.
festinating g.
gluteus maximus g.
gluteus medius g.
helicopod g.
hemiplegic g.
high-steppage g.
hysterical g.
listing g.
2-point g.
scissors g.
skater's g.

spastic g.
stamping g.
steppage g.
swing-to g.
tandem g.
Trendelenburg g.
waddling g.

GAL

gallus adenolike
GAL virus

galactacrasia
galactagogue
galactans
galactic
galactidrosis
galactitol
galactoblast
galactocele
galactogen
galactokinase

g. deficiency
g. deficiency galactosemia

galactometer
galactophagous
galactophlebitis
galactophore
galactophoritis
galactophorous

g. canal
g. duct

galactopoiesis
galactopoietic hormone
galactopyranose
galactorrhea
galactosamine
galactosaminoglycan
galactosans
galactoscope
galactose

g. cataract
g. diabetes
g. tolerance test

galactosemia

epimerase deficiency g.
galactokinase deficiency g.

galactose-1-phosphate
galactoside
galactosis
galactosuria
galactosyl
galactosylceramide lipoidosis
galactotherapy
galacturonan
galanga
galangal

G

galanthamine
Galant reflex
Galassi pupillary phenomenon
galea
Galeati gland
galeatomy
Galeazzi fracture
Galen
    G. anastomosis
    great vein of G.
    G. nerve
galena
galenic
galenical
gall
    g. bladder
    g. duct
galla
gallamine triethiodide
gallate
    dodecyl g.
Gallaudet fascia
Gallavardin phenomenon
gallbladder
    Courvoisier g.
    g. fossa
Gallego differentiating solution
gallein
gallic acid
Gallie transplant
gallinacea
    Echidnophaga g.
gallinaceous
gallinae
    Acarus g.
    Dermanyssus g.
    Microsporum g.
gallium
gallium-67, -68
gallocyanin
gallocyanine
gallon
gallop
    atrial g.
    presystolic g.
    protodiastolic g.
    g. rhythm
    g. sound
    summation g.
gallstone
    g. colic
    g. ileus
gallus
    g. adenolike (GAL)
    g. adenolike virus
GALT
    gut-associated lymphoid tissue
Galton
    G. delta

    G. law
    G. system
    G. whistle
galtonian
    g. genetics
    g. inheritance
    g. trait
Galtonian-Fisher genetics
galvanic
    g. current
    g. nystagmus
    g. skin reaction
    g. skin reflex
    g. skin response (GSR)
    g. threshold
galvanism
galvanization
galvanocaustic snare
galvanocautery
galvanocontractility
galvanofaradization
galvanometer
    d'Arsonval g.
    Einthoven string g.
galvanomuscular
galvanopalpation
galvanoscope
galvanosurgery
galvanotaxis
galvanotherapy
galvanotonus
galvanotropism
gamabufagin
gamabufogenin
gamabufotalin
Gambian
    G. fever
    G. trypanosomiasis
game
    language g.
    model g.
    g. theory
gamekeeper's thumb
gametangium
gamete
    g. intrafallopian transfer (GIFT)
    joint g.
gametic nucleus
gametocide
gametocyst
gametocyte
gametogenesis
gametogonia
gametogony
gametoid
gametokinetic hormone
gametophagia
Gamgee tissue
gamic

gamma, γ
    g. angle
    g. benzene hexachloride
    g. camera
    g. cell
    g. crystallin
    g. efferent
    g. encephalography
    g. fiber
    interferon g.
    g. knife
    g. loop
    g. motor neuron
    g. motor system
    g. radiation
    g. ray
gammacism
gammagram
gammopathy
    benign monoclonal g.
    biclonal g.
    monoclonal g.
    polyclonal g.
Gamna disease
Gamna-Favre body
Gamna-Gandy
    G.-G. body
    G.-G. nodule
gamogenesis
gamogony
gamont
gamophagia
gamophobia
ganciclovir
Gandy-Gamna
    G.-G. body
    G.-G. nodule
    G.-G. spleen
Gandy-Nanta disease
ganga
ganglia (*pl. of* ganglion)
ganglial
gangliate
gangliated nerve
gangliectomy
gangliform
gangliitis
ganglioblast
gangliocyte
gangliocytoma
ganglioform
ganglioglioma

gangliolysis
ganglioma
ganglion, pl. **ganglia**
    aberrant g.
    acoustic g.
    acousticofacial g.
    Acrel g.
    Andersch g.
    aorticorenal g.
    Arnold g.
    auditory g.
    Auerbach g.
    auricular g.
    autonomic g.
    basal ganglia
    Bezold g.
    Bochdalek g.
    Bock g.
    Böttcher g.
    cardiac g.
    carotid g.
    celiac g.
    g. cell
    cervicothoracic g.
    chain g.
    ciliary g.
    coccygeal g.
    cochlear g.
    Corti g.
    craniospinal sensory g.
    g. cyst
    diffuse g.
    dorsal root g.
    Ehrenritter g.
    extracranial g.
    Frankenhäuser g.
    Froriep g.
    gasserian g.
    geniculate g.
    Gudden g.
    hypogastric g.
    g. impar
    inferior cervical g.
    inferior mesenteric g.
    intercrural g.
    intermediate g.
    interpeduncular g.
    intervertebral g.
    intracranial g.
    jugular g.
    Laumonier g.
    Lee g.

G

NOTES

ganglion *(continued)*
    lenticular g.
    Lobstein g.
    long root of ciliary g.
    Ludwig g.
    lumbar g.
    Meckel g.
    middle cervical g.
    otic g.
    parasympathetic g.
    paravertebral g.
    pelvic g.
    phrenic g.
    prevertebral g.
    pterygopalatine g.
    renal g.
    g. ridge
    sensory g.
    spinal g.
    spiral g.
    splanchnic g.
    submandibular g.
    superior g.
    sympathetic g.
    trigeminal g.
    Troisier g.
    tympanic g.
    vestibular g.
    Walther g.

ganglionated
    g. cord
    g. nerve

ganglionectomy
ganglioneuroblastoma
ganglioneuroma
    central g.
    dumbbell g.

ganglioneuromatosis
ganglionic
    g. blockade
    g. blocking agent
    g. branch
    g. cell layer
    g. chain
    g. crest
    g. motor neuron
    g. saliva

ganglionitis
ganglionostomy
ganglionte
ganglioplegic
gangliosialidosis
ganglioside lipidosis
gangliosidosis
    generalized g.

gangosa
gangrene
    arteriosclerotic g.
    cold g.

    cutaneous g.
    decubital g.
    diabetic g.
    disseminated cutaneous g.
    dry g.
    embolic g.
    emphysematous g.
    Fournier g.
    gas g.
    gaseous g.
    hemorrhagic g.
    hospital g.
    hot g.
    Meleney g.
    moist g.
    spontaneous g.
    symmetrical g.
    wet g.
    white g.

gangrenosum
    ecthyma g.
    pyoderma g.

gangrenosus
    pemphigus g.

gangrenous
    g. appendicitis
    g. bowel
    g. cellulitis
    g. cystitis
    g. emphysema
    g. erysipelas
    g. necrosis
    g. pharyngitis
    g. pneumonia
    g. rhinitis
    g. stomatitis

ganoblast
Ganser
    G. commissure
    G. syndrome

Gant clamp
gantry
Gantzer
    G. accessory bundle
    G. muscle

Ganzfeld stimulation
gap
    air-bone g.
    anion g.
    g. arthroplasty
    auscultatory g.
    Bochdalek g.
    chromosomal g.
    DNA g.
    excitable g.
    interocclusal g.
    g. junction
    g. phenomenon

gap0
> g. period
> g. phase

gap1
> g. period
> g. phase

gap2
> g. period
> g. phase

garapata disease
Gardner-Diamond syndrome
Gardnerella
> *G. vaginalis*
> *G.* vaginitis

Gardner syndrome
gargantuan mastitis
gargle
Gariel pessary
garinii
> *Borrelia g.*

Garland triangle
garlic oil
garment
> antishock g.
> pneumatic antishock g.

Garré
> G. disease
> G. osteomyelitis

Gartner
> G. canal
> G. cyst
> G. duct

Gärtner
> G. method
> G. tonometer
> G. vein phenomenon

GAS
> group A streptococcus

gas
> g. abscess
> alveolar g.
> anesthetic g.
> arterial blood g. (ABG)
> g. bacillus
> blood g.
> carbonic acid g.
> g. cautery
> g. chromatography
> g. constant
> g. cyst
> g. embolism
> expired g.

> g. gangrene
> g. gangrene antitoxin
> hemolytic g.
> ideal alveolar g.
> inert g.
> inspircd g.
> laughing g.
> marsh g.
> mixed expired g.
> noble g.
> g. peritonitis
> g. retinopexy
> tear g.
> g. thermometer

gaseous
> g. gangrene
> g. mediastinography
> g. pulse

Gaskell
> G. bridge
> G. clamp

gas-liquid chromatography (GLC)
gasometer
gasometric
gasometry
gasserian ganglion
gassing
gaster
gastradenitis
gastralgia
gastral mesoderm
gastrea theory
gastrectasis, gastrectasia
gastrectomy
> Hofmeister g.
> physiologic g.
> Pólya g.

gastric
> g. acid inhibitor
> g. algid malaria
> g. analysis
> g. anoxia
> g. area
> g. artery
> g. branch
> g. bypass
> g. calculus
> g. canal
> g. cardia
> g. chromoscopy
> g. colic
> g. crisis

NOTES

G

gastric *(continued)*
    g. diastole
    g. digestion
    g. feeding
    g. fistula
    g. fold
    g. follicle
    g. freezing
    g. gland
    g. hemorrhage
    g. hypersecretion
    g. impression on liver
    g. impression on spleen
    g. indigestion
    g. inhibitory peptide
    g. inhibitory polypeptide (GIP)
    g. juice
    g. lymphoid nodule
    g. mucin
    g. mucosa
    g. nervous plexus
    g. neurasthenia
    g. neurectomy
    g. neurosis
    g. pit
    g. ruga
    g. smear
    g. stapling
    g. surface
    g. tetany
    g. ulcer
    g. vein
    g. vertigo
    g. volvulus
gastrica
    achylia g.
gastricsin
gastricus
gastrin
gastrinoma
gastritis
    alkaline reflux g.
    atrophic g.
    bile g.
    catarrhal g.
    eosinophilic g.
    exfoliative g.
    hypertrophic g.
    interstitial g.
    pseudomembranous g.
gastroacephalus
gastroalbumorrhea
gastroamorphus
gastroanastomosis
gastroatonia
gastroblennorrhea
gastrocardiac syndrome
gastrocele
gastrochronorrhea

gastrocnemius muscle
gastrocolic
    g. fistula
    g. ligament
    g. omentum
    g. reflex
gastrocolitis
gastrocoloptosis
gastrocolostomy
gastrocutaneous fistula
gastrocystoplasty
gastrodialysis
gastrodiaphragmatic ligament
gastroduodenal
    g. artery
    g. fistula
    g. lymph node
    g. orifice
    g. ulcer
gastroduodenitis
gastroduodenoscopy
gastroduodenostomy
gastrodynia
gastroenteric
gastroenteritis
        acute infectious nonbacterial g.
        endemic nonbacterial infantile g.
        eosinophilic g.
        epidemic nonbacterial g.
        infantile g.
        g. virus type A, B
gastroenteroanastomosis
gastroenterocolitis
gastroenterocolostomy
gastroenterologist
gastroenterology
gastroenteropathy
gastroenteroplasty
gastroenteroptosis
gastroenterostomy
gastroenterotomy
gastroepiploic
    g. artery
    g. vein
gastroesophageal
    g. hernia
    g. reflux
    g. reflux disease (GERD)
    g. vestibule
gastroesophagitis
gastroesophagostomy
gastrogastrostomy
gastrogavage
gastrogenic
gastrogenous diarrhea
Gastrografin swallow
gastrograph
gastrohepatic omentum
gastrohydrorrhea

gastroileac reflex
gastroileitis
gastroileostomy
gastrointestinal (GI)
    g. autonomic nerve tumor
    g. fistula
    g. hormone
    g. smooth muscle
    g. stromal tumor
    g. tract
gastrojejunal
    g. loop obstruction syndrome
    g. ulcer
gastrojejunocolic
gastrojejunostomy
gastrokinesograph
gastrolavage
gastrolienal ligament
gastrolith
gastrolithiasis
gastrologist
gastrology
gastrolysis
gastromalacia
gastromegaly
gastromelus
gastromyxorrhea
gastronesteostomy
gastroomental artery
gastropagus
gastropancreatic fold
gastroparalysis
gastroparasitus
gastroparesis diabeticorum
gastropathic
gastropathy
    hypertrophic hypersecretory g.
gastropexy
gastrophrenic ligament
gastroplasty
    Collis g.
    vertical banded g.
gastroplication
gastropneumonic
gastropod
gastroptosia
gastroptosis
gastroptyxis
gastropulmonary
gastropylorectomy
gastropyloric
gastrorrhagia

gastrorrhaphy
gastrorrhea
gastrorrhexis
gastroschisis
gastroscope
    fiberoptic g.
gastroscopic
gastroscopy
gastrospasm
gastrosplenic
    g. ligament
    g. omentum
gastrostaxis
gastrostenosis
gastrostogavage
gastrostolavage
gastrostomy
gastrothoracopagus
gastrotome
gastrotomy
gastrotonometer
gastrotonometry
gastrotoxic
gastrotoxin
gastrotropic
gastroxia
gastroxynsis
gastrula
gastrulation
Gatch bed
gate-control
    g.-c. hypothesis
    g.-c. theory
gated
    g. radionuclide angiocardiography
    g. system
gatekeeper
gating
    cardiac g.
    g. mechanism
    respiratory g.
Gaucher
    G. cell
    G. disease
gauge
    bite g.
    Boley g.
    Bourdon g.
    catheter g.
    g. pressure
gaultheria oil
gaultherin

G

NOTES

gauntlet bandage
gauss (G)
    g. sign
gaussian
    g. curve
    g. distribution
gauze bandage
gavage
Gavard muscle
gay
    g. bowel syndrome
    G. gland
Gay-Lussac
    G.-L. equation
    G.-L. law
gaze
    conjugate g.
    dysconjugate g.
    horizontal g.
    g. palsy
    g. paretic nystagmus
G-banding stain
GBG
    gonadal steroid-binding globulin
GB virus
G-CSF
    granulocyte colony-stimulating factor
Ge antigen
gedoelstiosis
Geigel reflex
Geiger-Müller
    G.-M. counter
    G.-M. tube
gel
    aluminum hydroxide g.
    aluminum phosphate g.
    colloidal g.
    g. diffusion
    g. diffusion precipitin test
    g. diffusion reaction
    g. electrophoresis
    g. filtration
    g. filtration chromatography
    g. structure
gelastic seizure
gelate
gelatin
    glycerinated g.
    Irish moss g.
    g. sugar
gelatinase
gelatiniferous
gelatinization
gelatinize
gelatinoid
gelatinous
    g. ascites
    g. bone marrow
    g. droplike corneal dystrophy

    g. infiltration
    g. nucleus
    g. polyp
    g. scleritis
    g. substance
    g. tissue
    g. varix
gelation
gelatum
Gélineau syndrome
Gell
    G. and Coombs Classification
    G. and Coombs reaction
Gellé test
gelosis
gelsemine
gelsolin
Gély suture
gémellaire
    folie g.
Gemella morbillorum
gemellology
gemellus
gemfibrozil
geminate
geminated teeth
gemination
geminous
gemistocyte
gemistocytic
    g. astrocyte
    g. astrocytoma
    g. cell
    g. reaction
gemistocytoma
gemma
gemmation
gemmule
    Hoboken g.
gena
genal gland
gender
    g. crisis
    g. dysphoria syndrome
    g. identity
    g. identity disorder
    g. role
gene
    g. activation
    allelic g.
    autosomal g.
    BCR/ABL g.
    BRCA1 g.
    BRCA2 g.
    C g.
    codominant g.
    control g.
    g. deletion
    dominant g.

g. dosage compensation
g. dosage effect
g. duplication
g. expression
extrachromosomal g.
g. family
g. flow
g. frequency
H g.
histocompatibility g.
holandric g.
homeotic g.
housekeeping g.
immune response g.
jumping g.
lethal g.
g. library
g. mapping
mimic g.
mitochondrial g.
modifier g.
g. mosaicism
mutant g.
operator g.
pleiotropic g.
polyphenic g.
g. pool
reciprocal g.
g. regulation
regulator g.
repressor g.
silent g.
g. splicing
structural g.
suicide g.
supplementary g.
g. therapy
tumor suppressor g.
X-linked g.
Y-linked g.
genealogy
general
g. adaptation reaction
g. adaptation syndrome
g. anatomy
g. anesthesia
g. anesthetic
g. bloodletting
g. duty nurse
g. fertility rate
g. hospital
g. immunity

g. paresis
g. peritonitis
g. physiology
g. practice
g. sensation
g. sensorium
g. somatic afferent column
g. somatic efferent column
g. stimulant
g. surgery
g. symptom
g. transduction
g. visceral afferent column
g. visceral efferent column
generalis
acne g.
generalist
generalization
generalized
g. anaphylaxis
g. anxiety disorder
g. chondromalacia
g. cortical hyperostosis
g. elastolysis
g. emphysema
g. epidermolytic hyperkeratosis
g. eruptive histiocytoma
g. gangliosidosis
g. glycogenosis
g. lentiginosis
g. myokymia
g. paralysis
g. plane xanthomatosis
g. pustular psoriasis
g. Shwartzman phenomenon
g. tetanus
g. tonic-clonic epilepsy
g. tonic-clonic seizure
g. tuberculosis
g. vaccinia
g. xanthelasma
generate
generated occlusal path
generation
asexual g.
g. effect
filial g.
nonsexual g.
parental g.
sexual g.
spontaneous g.
generational

G

NOTES

generative empathy
generator
    aerosol g.
    asynchronous pulse g.
    atrial synchronous pulse g.
    atrial triggered pulse g.
    demand pulse g.
    fixed rate pulse g.
    g. potential
    pulse g.
    radionuclide g.
generic
    g. name
    g. substitution
genesial
genesiology
genesis
genetic
    g. amplification
    g. association
    g. burden
    g. carrier
    g. code
    g. colonization
    g. compound
    g. counseling
    g. deafness
    g. death
    g. determinant
    g. disequilibrium
    g. dominance
    g. drift
    g. engineering
    g. epidemiology
    g. equilibrium
    g. female
    g. fingerprint
    g. fitness
    g. fixation
    g. heterogeneity
    g. homeostasis
    g. human male
    g. isolate
    g. lethal
    g. linkage
    g. load
    g. locus
    g. map
    g. marker
    g. material
    g. model
    g. penetrance
    g. polymorphism
    g. psychology
    g. recombination
    g. testing
geneticist
genetics
    behavioral g.

    biochemical g.
    classical g.
    clinical g.
    epidemiologic g.
    epidemiological g.
    galtonian g.
    Galtonian-Fisher g.
    human g.
    mathematical g.
    medical g.
    mendelian g.
    microbial g.
    modern g.
    molecular g.
    population g.
genetotrophic
Geneva lens measure
Gengou phenomenon
genial tubercle
genian
genicular
    g. anastomosis
    g. artery
    g. vein
geniculate
    g. body
    g. ganglion
    g. neuralgia
    g. otalgia
    g. zoster
geniculated
geniculocalcarine
    g. radiation
    g. tract
geniculum
genioglossal muscle
genioglossus muscle
geniohyoid muscle
genion
genioplasty
genital
    g. ambiguity
    g. area
    g. branch
    g. cord
    g. corpuscle
    g. duct
    g. eminence
    g. fold
    g. furrow
    g. gland
    g. herpes
    g. ligament
    g. organ
    g. phase
    g. primacy
    g. primordium
    g. ridge
    g. stage

g. swelling
g. system
g. tract
g. tubercle
g. tuberculosis
g. wart
genitalia
ambiguous external g.
external g.
female external g.
female internal g.
indifferent g.
male external g.
male internal g.
genitalis
herpes g.
genitality
genitocrural nerve
genitofemoral nerve
genitoinguinal ligament
genitourinary (GU)
g. apparatus
g. fistula
g. region
g. surgeon
g. system
genius
Gennari
G. band
line of G.
G. stria
genoblast
genocopy
genodermatology
genodermatosis
genome
genomic
g. clone
g. DNA
g. imprinting
g. library
genomics
functional g.
genospecies
genote
genotoxic
genotype
genotypic
genotypical
gentamicin
gentian
g. aniline water

g. root
g. violet
gentianophil
gentianophile
gentianophilous
gcntianophobic
gentiobiase
gentiobiose
gentisic acid
genu
g. recurvatum
g. valgum
g. varum
genual
genucubital position
genufacial position
genupectoral position
genus
genyantrum
geode
geographic
g. choroidopathy
g. information system
g. keratitis
g. retinal atrophy
g. stippling
g. tongue
geographica
lingua g.
geomedicine
geometric
g. isomer
g. isomerism
g. mean
g. sense
g. unsharpness
geopathology
geophagia
geophagism
geophagy
geophilic
geotaxis
geotrichosis
geotropism
gephyrin
gephyrophobia
gepirone
geraniol
geranylgeranyl pyrophosphate
geranyl pyrophosphate
geratology
Gerbich antigen

NOTES

Gerbode defect
GERD
    gastroesophageal reflux disease
Gerdy
    G. fiber
    G. fontanelle
    G. hyoid fossa
    G. interatrial loop
    G. ligament
    G. tubercle
Gerhardt
    G. reaction
    G. test
Gerhardt-Mitchell disease
geriatric
    dental g.'s
    g. medicine
    g. therapy
Gerlach
    G. annular tendon
    G. tonsil
    G. valve
    G. valvula
Gerlier disease
germ
    g. cell
    dental g.
    g. disc
    enamel g.
    g. layer
    g. layer theory
    g. line
    g. membrane
    g. nucleus
    tooth g.
    g. tube
    g. tube test
German
    G. measles
    G. measles virus
germanium
germicidal
germicide
germinal
    g. aplasia
    g. area
    g. cell
    g. cord
    g. disc
    g. epithelium
    g. localization
    g. membrane
    g. mosaicism
    g. pole
    g. rod
    g. streak
    g. vesicle
germinativa
    area g.

germinative layer
germine
germinoma
Germiston virus
geroderma
gerodontics
gerodontology
geromarasmus
gerontal
gerontine
gerontologist
gerontology
gerontophilia
gerontophobia
gerontotherapeutics
gerontotherapy
gerontoxon
Gerota
    G. capsule
    G. fascia
    G. method
Gerstmann-Sträussler-Scheinker syndrome
Gerstmann syndrome
gestagen
gestagenic
gestalt
    g. phenomenon
    g. psychology
    g. theory
    g. therapy
gestaltism
gestation
    abdominal g.
gestational
    g. age
    g. diabetes
    g. edema
    g. hypertension
    g. proteinuria
    g. ring
    g. sac
    g. trophoblastic disease
gestationis
    herpes g.
gestin
gestosis
Gey solution
GFR
    glomerular filtration rate
GH
    growth hormone
ghatti gum
GHK equation
Ghon
    G. complex
    G. focus
    G. primary lesion
    G. tubercle

ghost
  g. cell
  g. cell glaucoma
  g. corpuscle
  g. tooth
ghoul hand
GH-RF, GHRF
  growth hormone-releasing factor
GH-RH, GHRH
  growth hormone-releasing hormone
GHz
  gigahertz
GI
  gastrointestinal
  GI tract
Giacomini
  band of G.
Giannuzzi crescent
Gianotti-Crosti syndrome
giant
  g. axonal neuropathy
  g. cell
  g. cell aortitis
  g. cell arteritis
  g. cell carcinoma
  g. cell epulis
  g. cell fibroma
  g. cell glioblastoma multiforme
  g. cell granuloma
  g. cell hepatitis
  g. cell hyaline angiopathy
  g. cell monstrocellular sarcoma of Zülch
  g. cell myeloma
  g. cell myocarditis
  g. cell pneumonia
  g. cell sarcoma
  g. cell thyroiditis
  g. cell tumor
  g. chromosome
  g. colon
  g. condyloma
  g. fibroadenoma
  g. follicular lymphoblastoma
  g. follicular thyroiditis
  g. gastric fold
  g. hives
  g. hypertrophy
  g. melanosome
  g. nevus
  g. osteoid osteoma
  g. papillary conjunctivitis
  g. pigmented nevus
  g. urticaria
giantism
Giardia
  G. intestinalis
  G. lamblia
giardiasis
gibberellic acid
gibberellins
gibbous
Gibb phase rule
Gibbs
  G. energy of activation
  G. free energy
  G. theorem
Gibbs-Donnan equilibrium
Gibbs-Helmholtz equation
gibbus
Gibney
  G. boot
  G. fixation bandage
Gibson
  G. bandage
  G. murmur
Giemsa chromosome banding stain
Gierke
  G. cell
  G. disease
  G. respiratory bundle
Gifford reflex
GIFT
  gamete intrafallopian transfer
gigahertz (GHz)
gigantiform cementoma
gigantism
  acromegalic g.
  cerebral g.
  eunuchoid g.
  fetal g.
  pituitary g.
gigantocellular
  g. glioma
  g. nucleus
gigantomastia
Gigli saw
GIH
  growth hormone-inhibiting hormone
Gila monster
Gilbert
  G. disease
  G. syndrome
gilbert

NOTES

Gilchrist disease
Gilead
>   balm of G.

gill
>   g. arch skeleton
>   g. cleft

Gilles
>   G. de la Tourette disease
>   G. de la Tourette syndrome

Gillespie syndrome
Gillette suspensory ligament
Gilliam operation
Gillies operation
Gillmore needle
Gilmer wiring
Gil-Vernet operation
Gimbernat ligament
ginger
>   Chinese g.
>   Indian g.
>   g. oleoresin
>   g. paralysis

gingili oil
gingiva, pl. **gingivae**
>   alveolar g.
>   attached g.
>   buccal g.
>   free g.
>   labial g.
>   lingual g.

gingival
>   g. abrasion
>   g. abscess
>   g. atrophy
>   g. clamp
>   g. cleft
>   g. contour
>   g. crest
>   g. crevice
>   g. curvature
>   g. cyst
>   g. elephantiasis
>   g. embrasure
>   g. enlargement
>   g. epithelium
>   g. festoon
>   g. fibromatosis
>   g. fistula
>   g. flap
>   g. fluid
>   g. groove
>   g. hyperplasia
>   G. Index
>   g. line
>   g. margin
>   g. massage
>   g. mucosa
>   g. papilla
>   g. pocket

>   g. proliferation
>   g. recession
>   g. repositioning
>   g. resorption
>   g. retraction
>   g. septum
>   g. space
>   g. sulcus
>   g. tissue
>   g. trough
>   g. zone

gingivalis
>   *Entamoeba g.*

gingivectomy
gingivitis
>   acute necrotizing ulcerative g.
>   (ANUG)
>   atypical g.
>   chronic desquamative g.
>   diabetic g.
>   Dilantin g.
>   diphenylhydantoin g.
>   eruptive g.
>   fusospirochetal g.
>   herpetic g.
>   hormonal g.
>   hyperplastic g.
>   leukemic hyperplastic g.
>   marginal g.
>   necrotizing ulcerative g.
>   pregnancy g.
>   suppurative g.
>   ulceromembranous g.

gingivoaxial
gingivobuccal
>   g. groove
>   g. sulcus

gingivodental ligament
gingivoglossitis
gingivolabial
>   g. groove
>   g. sulcus

gingivolingual
>   g. groove
>   g. sulcus

gingivolinguoaxial
gingivo-osseous
gingivoplasty
gingivosis
gingivostomatitis
>   primary herpetic g.

ginglyform
ginglymoarthrodial
ginglymoid joint
ginglymus
>   helicoid g.
>   lateral g.

Ginkgo biloba
ginseng

Giordano-Giovannetti diet
Giovannetti diet
GIP
    gastric inhibitory polypeptide
Girard reagent
girdle
    g. anesthesia
    Hitzig g.
    Neptune g.
    g. pain
    pectoral g.
    pelvic g.
    g. sensation
    shoulder g.
    white limbal g.
Girdlestone procedure
gitalin
Gitelman syndrome
githagism
gitogenin
gitonin
gitoxigenin
gitoxin
gitter cell
gitterzelle
glabella
glabellad
glabellar
    g. frown line
    g. wrinkle
glabrata
    Candida g.
glabrate
glabrous skin
glacial
    g. acetic acid
    g. phosphoric acid
gladiate
gladiatorum
    herpes g.
gladiolus
glairy mucus
glancing wound
gland
    accessory lacrimal g.
    accessory parotid g.
    accessory suprarenal g.
    accessory thyroid g.
    acid g.
    acinotubular g.
    acinous g.
    admaxillary g.

adrenal g.
aggregate g.
agminate g.
agminated g.
Albarran g.
albuminous g.
alveolar g.
anal g.
anterior lingual g.
apical g.
apocrine sweat g.
areolar g.
arteriococcygeal g.
arytenoid g.
Aselli g.
axillary sweat g.
Bartholin g.
basal g.
Bauhin g.
Baumgarten g.
biliary g.
Blandin g.
Bowman g.
brachial g.
bronchial g.
Bruch g.
Brunner g.
buccal g.
bulbourethral g.
cardiac g.
ceruminous g.
cervical g.
Ciaccio g.
ciliary g.
circumanal g.
coccygeal g.
coil g.
compound g.
conjunctival g.
convoluted g.
Cowper g.
cutaneous g.
ductless g.
duct of Skene g.
duodenal g.
Duverney g.
Ebner g.
eccrine g.
ecdysial g.
Eglis g.
endocrine g.
endometrial g.

G

NOTES

gland (*continued*)
 esophageal g.
 excretory g.
 exocrine g.
 external salivary g.
 follicular g.
 fundic g.
 Galeati g.
 gastric g.
 Gay g.
 genal g.
 genital g.
 Gley g.
 glomiform g.
 greater vestibular g.
 Guérin g.
 hemal g.
 hematopoietic g.
 hemolymph g.
 Henle g.
 hibernating g.
 holocrine g.
 internal salivary g.
 interscapular g.
 interstitial g.
 intestinal g.
 intraepithelial g.
 isthmus of thyroid g.
 jugular g.
 Knoll g.
 Krause g.
 labial g.
 lacrimal g.
 lactiferous g.
 laryngeal g.
 lesser vestibular g.
 Lieberkühn g.
 lingual g.
 Littré g.
 Luschka cystic g.
 lymph g.
 major salivary g.
 malpighian g.
 mammary g.
 marrow-lymph g.
 master g.
 maxillary g.
 meibomian g.
 merocrine g.
 Méry g.
 mesenteric g.
 milk g.
 minor salivary g.
 mixed g.
 molar g.
 Moll g.
 mucous g.
 olfactory g.
 palatine g.

 parathyroid g.
 parotid g.
 pileous g.
 pineal g.
 pituitary g.
 preputial g.
 prostate g.
 pyloric g.
 racemose g.
 Rosenmüller g.
 saccular g.
 salivary g.
 sebaceous g.
 seminal g.
 sentinel g.
 seromucous g.
 serous g.
 sublingual g.
 submandibular g.
 suprarenal g.
 sweat g.
 target g.
 tarsal g.
 thymus g.
 thyroid g.
 tubular g.
 tubuloacinar g.
 unicellular g.
 urethral g.
 uterine g.
 vaginal g.
 Zeis g.
glanders
glandilemma
glandula, pl. **glandulae**
glandular
 g. abscess
 g. branch
 g. cancer
 g. carcinoma
 g. epithelium
 g. fever
 g. lobe
 g. mastitis
 g. plague
 g. substance
 g. system
 g. tularemia
glandularis
 cheilitis g.
 cystitis g.
glandule
glandulopreputial lamella
glandulous
glans
 g. clitoridis
 g. penis
glanular hypospadias

Glanzmann
  G. disease
  G. thrombasthenia
glaphenine
glare
  blinding g.
  dazzling g.
  g. of light
glarometer
glaserian
  g. artery
  g. fissure
Glasgow
  G. coma scale
  G. sign
glass
  g. bead sterilizer
  g. body
  cover g.
  Crookes g.
  crown g.
  cupping g.
  g. electrode
  g. factor
  flint g.
  g. ionomer cement
  g. ray
  3-g. test
  Wood g.
2-glass test
glassworker's cataract
glassy membrane
Glauber salt
glaucine
glaucoma
  absolute g.
  acute g.
  air block g.
  angle-closure g.
  aphakic g.
  auricular g.
  capsular g.
  chronic g.
  closed-angle g.
  combined g.
  compensated g.
  congenital g.
  corticosteroid-induced g.
  g. fulminans
  ghost cell g.
  hemorrhagic g.
  hypersecretion g.

  low-tension g.
  malignant g.
  narrow-angle g.
  normal-tension g.
  open-angle g.
  phacogenic g.
  phacomorphic g.
  pseudoexfoliative g.
  secondary g.
  simple g.
  g. simplex
  traumatic g.
  wide-angle g.
glaucomatocyclitic crisis
glaucomatous
  g. cataract
  g. cup
  g. excavation
  g. halo
  g. nerve-fiber bundle scotoma
  g. ring
glaucosuria
GLC
  gas-liquid chromatography
Gleason
  G. score
  G. tumor grade
Glenn
  G. operation
  G. shunt
Glenner-Lillie stain
glenohumeral
  g. articulation
  g. joint
  g. ligament
glenoid
  g. cavity
  g. fossa
  g. labrum
  g. ligament
  g. surface
glenoidal lip
Gley gland
glia cell
gliacyte
gliadin
glial
  g. fibrillary acidic protein
  g. limiting membrane
gliclazide
glide
  mandibular g.

G

NOTES

397

glidewire
gliding
    g. joint
    g. occlusion
glioblast
glioblastoma multiforme
glioblastosis cerebri
glioma
    brainstem g.
    gigantocellular g.
    mixed g.
gliomatosis
gliomatous
gliomyxoma
glioneuroma
gliosarcoma
gliosis
    hemispheric g.
    isomorphous g.
    spinal g.
    g. uteri
glipizide
Glisson
    G. capsule
    G. cirrhosis
    G. sphincter
glissonitis
glitter cell
global
    g. aphasia
    g. burden of disease
    g. paralysis
    g. warming
globi (*pl. of* globus)
globin zinc insulin
Globocephalus
globoid
    g. cell
    g. cell leukodystrophy
globoside
globosus nucleus
globotriaosylceramide
globular
    g. heart
    g. leukocyte
    g. process
    g. protein
    g. sputum
    g. thrombus
globule
    dentin g.
    Morgagni g.
globuliferous
globulin
    accelerator g.
    antihemophilic g. A, B
    antihuman g.
    antilymphocyte g.
    corticosteroid-binding g.

    1E g.
    1F g.
    gonadal steroid-binding g. (GBG)
    hepatitis B immune g.
    human gamma g.
    immune serum g.
    plasma accelerator g.
    Rh-immune g.
    serum accelerator g.
globulinuria
globulomaxillary cyst
globulus
globus, pl. **globi**
    g. hystericus
    g. major
    g. minor
    g. pallidus
glomal
glomangioma
glomangiosis
glome
glomectomy
glomera (*pl. of* glomus)
glomerular
    g. capsule
    g. crescent
    g. cyst
    g. filtration rate (GFR)
    g. insufficiency
    g. layer
    g. necrosis
    g. nephritis
    g. sclerosis
glomeruli (*pl. of* glomerulus)
glomerulitis
glomerulonephritis
    acute crescentic g.
    acute hemorrhagic g.
    acute poststreptococcal g.
    antibasement membrane g.
    Berger focal g.
    chronic g.
    diffuse g.
    exudative g.
    focal embolic g.
    hypocomplementemic g.
    immune complex g.
    lobular g.
    local g.
    membranoproliferative g.
    membranous g.
    mesangial proliferative g.
    mesangiocapillary g.
glomerulopathy
    focal sclerosing g.
glomerulosa
    g. cell
    zona g.

glomerulosclerosis
    diabetic g.
    focal segmental g.
    intercapillary g.
glomerulose
glomerulus, pl. **glomeruli**
    juxtamedullary g.
    malpighian g.
glomiform gland
glomus, pl. **glomera**
    aortic glomera
    glomera aortica
    g. body
    choroid g.
    intravagal g.
    jugular g.
    g. jugulare tumor
    g. tympanicum tumor
glossa
glossagra
glossal
glossalgia
glossectomy
glossitis
    atrophic g.
    benign migratory g.
    g. desiccans
    Hunter g.
    median rhomboid g.
    Moeller g.
    parenchymatous g.
glossocele
glossocinesthetic
glossodontotropism
glossodynamometer
glossodynia
glossodyniotropism
glossoepiglottic ligament
glossoepiglottidean
glossograph
glossohyal
glossokinesthetic
glossolabiolaryngeal paralysis
glossolabiopharyngeal paralysis
glossolalia
glossology
glossoncus
glossopalatine
    g. arch
    g. fold
glossopalatinus
glossopalatolabial paralysis

glossopathy
glossopharyngeal
    g. breathing
    g. nerve
    g. neuralgia
    g. tic
glossopharyngeolabial paralysis
glossopharyngeus
glossoplasty
glossoplegia
glossoptosia
glossoptosis
glossopyrosis
glossorrhaphy
glossospasm
glossosteresis
glossotomy
glossotrichia
glossy skin
glottal
    g. attack
    g. fry
glottalization
glotte
    coup de g.
glottic
glottidis
    atrium g.
    edema g.
glottidospasm
glottis
    false g.
    g. vocalis
glottitis
glottology
glove anesthesia
gloved-finger sign
glover
    G. phenomenon
    g. suture
glucagon
    gut g.
glucagonlike
    g. insulinotropic peptide
    g. peptide
glucagonoma syndrome
glucal
glucan
gluceptate
gluciphore
glucoamylase
glucoascorbic acid

NOTES

399

glucocerebroside
glucocorticoid
glucocorticotrophic
glucocyamine
glucofuranose
glucogenesis
glucogenic
glucoheptonate
    erythromycin g.
glucoinvertase
glucokinase
glucokinetic
glucolipid
glucolysis
gluconate
    calcium g.
    ferrous g.
gluconeogenesis
gluconic acid
gluconolactonase
glucopenia
glucoplastic
glucoprotein
glucopyranose
glucosamine
glucosaminoglycan
glucosan
glucose
    activated g.
    g. dehydrogenase
    liquid g.
    g. oxidase
    g. oxidase method
    g. oxidase paper strip test
    g. oxyhydrase
    g. 6-phosphate
    g. tolerance factor
    g. tolerance test
    g. transport maximum
glucose-dependent insulinotropic polypeptide
glucosidase inhibitor
glucosidases
glucoside
glucosinolate
glucosone
glucosulfone sodium
glucosuria
glucosyl
glucosylceramide
glucosyltransferase
glucuronate
glucurone
glucuronic acid
glucuronide
glucuronolyticum
    Corynebacterium g.
glucuronoside

glucuronosyltransferase
    bilirubin-glucuronoside g.
glue ear
glue-sniffing
Gluge corpuscle
glusulase
glutaconic acid
glutamate
    arginine g.
    monosodium g.
    g. synthase
glutamic acid
glutamic-oxaloacetic transaminase
glutamic-pyruvic transaminase
glutaminase
glutamine
glutaminyl
glutamoyl
glutamyl
glutaraldehyde fixative
glutaric acid
glutathione
glutathionuria
gluteal
    g. cleft
    g. crest
    g. fascia
    g. fold
    g. furrow
    g. hernia
    g. line
    g. lymph node
    g. reflex
    g. region
    g. ridge
    g. surface
    g. tuberosity
    g. vein
glutelins
gluten
    g. ataxia
    g. casein
    g. enteropathy
gluten-free diet
glutenin
gluteofemoral bursa
gluteoinguinal
glutethimide
gluteus
    g. maximus gait
    g. maximus muscle
    g. medius bursae
    g. medius gait
    g. medius muscle
    g. minimus bursa
    g. minimus muscle
glutinoid
glutinous
glutitis

glyburide
glycal
glycan
glycanohydrolase
glycate
glycated hemoglobin
glycation
glycemia
glycemic index
glyceraldehyde
glyceric
    g. acid
    g. aldehyde
glyceridase
glyceride
    mixed g.'s
glycerin
    g. jelly
    g. suppository
glycerinated
    g. gelatin
    g. tincture
glycerite
glycerogelatin
glycerokinase
glycerol
    g. dehydration test
    iodopropylidene g.
    g. kinase
    g. phosphate
glycerone
glycerophosphate
    ferric g.
    g. shuttle
glycerophosphocholine
glycerophosphoric acid
glycerophosphorylcholine
glycerulose
glyceryl
    g. alcohol
    g. iodide
glycinate
glycine
    g. acyltransferase
    g. amidinotransferase
    g. betaine
    g. cleavage complex
    g. dehydrogenase
    g. synthase
    g. transamidinase
glycineamide ribonucleotide
glycine-succinate cycle

glycinin
glycinium
glycinuria
    familial g.
glycoaldehyde
    active g.
glycobiarsol
glycocalyx
glycocholate sodium
glycocholic acid
glycoconjugate
glycocorticoid
glycocyamine
glycogelatin
glycogen
    g. cardiomegaly
    g. granule
    g. loading
    g. phosphorylase
    g. starch synthase
    g. supercompensation
    g. synthase
glycogenase
glycogenesis
glycogenetic
glycogenic
    g. acanthosis
    g. cardiomegaly
glycogenolysis
glycogenosis
    brancher deficiency g.
    generalized g.
    hepatophosphorylase deficiency g.
    type 1–6 g.
glycogen-storage disease
glycogeusia
glycoglycinuria
glycohemoglobin
glycohistochemistry
    lectin g.
glycol
    g. ether
    ethylene g.
glycolaldehyde
glycolate
glycoleucine
glycolic
    g. acid
    g. aciduria
glycolipid lipidosis
glycolyl
glycolylurea

G

NOTES

glycolysis
glycolytic
glyconeogenesis
glyconic acid
glycopenia
glycopeptide antibiotic
Glycophagus
glycophilia
glycophorins
glycoprotein
glycoptyalism
glycopyrrolate
glycorrhachia
glycorrhea
glycosaminoglycan
glycosecretory
glycosialia
glycosialorrhea
glycosidase
glycoside
    cardiac g.
    cyanogenic g.
glycosidic
glycosphingolipid
glycostatic
glycosuria
    alimentary g.
    benign g.
    digestive g.
    phloridzin g.
    phlorizin g.
    renal g.
glycosylated hemoglobin
glycosylation
glycosyl compound
glycosyltransferase
glycotropic, glycotrophic
    g. factor
glycuresis
glycuronate
glycuronic acid
glycuronidase
glycuronide
glycuronuria
glycyclamide
glycyl
glycyrrhiza
glyoxal
glyoxalase
glyoxylate transacetylase
glyoxyldiureide
glyoxylic
    g. acid
    g. acid cycle
Gm
    G. allotype
    G. antigen
    factor G.

GM-CSF
    granulocyte-macrophage colony-
      stimulating factor
Gmelin test
gnashing
gnat
gnathic index
gnathion
gnathocephalus
gnathodynamics
gnathodynamometer
gnathography
gnathological
gnathology
gnathoplasty
gnathoschisis
gnathostatics
gnathostomiasis
gnoscopine
gnosia
gnotobiology
gnotobiota
gnotobiote
gnotobiotic
GnRH
    gonadotropin-releasing hormone
goatpox virus
goat's milk anemia
goblet cell
Godélier law
Godman fascia
Godwin tumor
Goeckerman treatment
Goethe bone
Gofman test
Goggia sign
goiter
    aberrant g.
    acute g.
    adenomatous g.
    Basedow g.
    cabbage g.
    colloid g.
    cystic g.
    diffuse g.
    diving g.
    endemic g.
    exophthalmic g.
    familial g.
    fibrous g.
    follicular g.
    intrathoracic g.
    lingual g.
    microfollicular g.
    multinodular g.
    nontoxic g.
    parenchymatous g.
    simple g.
    substernal g.

suffocative g.
toxic g.
wandering g.
goitrogen
goitrogenic
goitrous
gold
g. alloy
g. casting
cohesive g.
colloidal radioactive g.
g. equivalent
g. foil
g. inlay
mat g.
g. number
g. standard
g. thioglucose
Goldblatt
G. hypertension
G. kidney
golden
g. hour
g. seal
Goldenhar syndrome
Goldflam disease
Goldie-Coldman hypothesis
Goldman equation
Goldman-Fox knife
Goldman-Hodgkin-Katz equation
Goldmann
G. applanation tonometer
G. perimeter
Goldmann-Favre syndrome
gold-myokymia syndrome
Goldscheider test
Goldstein toe sign
golfer's skin
golf-hole ureteral orifice
Golgi
G. apparatus
G. body
G. complex
G. corpuscle
G. epithelial cell
G. internal reticulum
G. osmiobichromate fixative
G. stain
G. tendon organ
G. type I, II neuron
G. zone
Golgi-Mazzoni corpuscle

golgiokinesis
Goll column
Goltz syndrome
Gombault triangle
gomitoli
Gomori aldehyde fuchsin stain
Gomori-Jones periodic acid-methenamine-silver stain
Gompertz
G. hypothesis
G. law
gompholic joint
gomphosis
gonad
g. dose
female g.
indifferent g.
male g.
g. nucleus
gonadal
g. agenesis
g. aplasia
g. cord
g. dose
g. dysgenesis
g. hormone
g. mosaicism
g. ridge
g. steroid-binding globulin (GBG)
g. streak
gonadectomy
gonadoblastoma
gonadocrin
gonadoliberin
gonadopathy
gonadorelin hydrochloride
gonadotroph
gonadotrophic cycle
gonadotropic hormone
gonadotropin, gonadotrophin
anterior pituitary g.
chorionic g. (CG)
human chorionic g. (HCG, hCG)
human menopausal g. (HMG, hMG)
gonadotropin-producing adenoma
gonadotropin-releasing
g.-r. factor
g.-r. hormone (GnRH, GRH)
gonaduct
gonalgia
gonane

G

NOTES

gonangiectomy
gonarthritis
gonarthrotomy
gonecyst
gonecystis
gongylonemiasis
goniocraniometry
goniodysgenesis
goniometer
gonion
goniopuncture
gonioscope
gonioscopy
goniosynechia
goniotomy
gonocele
gonochorism
gonochorismus
gonocide
gonococcal
  g. arthritis
  g. conjunctivitis
  g. endocarditis
  g. stomatitis
gonococcemia
gonococcic
gonococcicide
gonococcus
gonocyte
gonohemia
gono-opsonin
gonophage
gonophore
gonophorus
gonorrhea
  oropharyngeal g.
  pharyngeal g.
gonorrheal
  g. arthritis
  g. conjunctivitis
  g. ophthalmia
  g. rheumatism
  g. salpingitis
  g. urethritis
gonorrhoeae
  Neisseria g.
gonosome
gonotoxemia
gonotoxin
gonotyl
gonycampsis
good
  G. antigen
  g. object
Goodell sign
Goodenough draw-a-man test
goodness
  g. of fit
  g. of fit test

Goodpasture
  G. stain
  G. syndrome
Goormaghtigh cell
gooseflesh
goose flesh
gooseneck deformity
Gopalan syndrome
Gordon
  G. reflex
  G. sign
  G. and Sweet stain
  G. symptom
gorget
Gorham
  G. disease
  G. syndrome
Goriaew rule
Gorlin
  G. cyst
  G. formula
  G. sign
  G. syndrome
Gorlin-Chaudhry-Moss syndrome
gormanii
  Legionella g.
goserelin
Gosselin fracture
Gothic
  G. arch
  G. arch tracing
  G. palate
Göthlin test
Gougerot and Blum disease
Gougerot-Carteaud syndrome
Gougerot-Sjögren disease
Gould suture
Gouley catheter
goundou
gout
  abarticular g.
  articular g.
  calcium g.
  g. diet
  idiopathic g.
  interval g.
  latent g.
  lead g.
  masked g.
  secondary g.
  tophaceous g.
gouty
  g. arthritis
  g. diathesis
  g. pearl
  g. tophus
  g. urine
government hospital

Gower-1
  hemoglobin G.-1
Gower-2
  hemoglobin G.-2
Gowers
  G. column
  G. contraction
  G. disease
  G. syndrome
  G. tract
Gower sign
Goyrand hernia
G-protein
graafian follicle
gracile
  g. fasciculus
  g. habitus
  g. lobule
  g. nucleus
  g. tubercle
gracilespinal fiber
gracilis
  Euglena g.
  funiculus g.
  g. muscle
  g. syndrome
grade
  Gleason tumor g.
  g. I–IV astrocytoma
graded exercise test
Gradenigo syndrome
gradient
  atrioventricular g.
  concentration g.
  density g.
  electrochemical g.
  g. elution
  g. encoding
  field g.
  magnetic field g.
  mitral g.
gradient-recalled
  g.-r. acquisition
  g.-r. acquisition in the steady state
    (GRASS)
grading
  activity g.
graduated
  g. compress
  g. pipette
  g. tenotomy
graduate nurse

Graefe
  G. forceps
  G. knife
  G. operation
  G. sign
Graefenberg ring
Graffi virus
graft
  accordion g.
  allogeneic g.
  animal g.
  autodermic g.
  autogeneic g.
  autogenous g.
  autologous fat g.
  autoplastic g.
  Blair-Brown g.
  bolus g.
  bone g.
  cable g.
  chip g.
  chorioallantoic g.
  composite g.
  corneal g.
  Davis g.
  delayed g.
  dermal g.
  dermal-fat g.
  dowel g.
  Esser g.
  fascia g.
  fascial g.
  fascicular g.
  fat g.
  free g.
  full-thickness g.
  funicular g.
  H g.
  heterogenous g.
  heterologous g.
  heteroplastic g.
  heterotopic g.
  homogenous g.
  homologous g.
  homoplastic g.
  inlay g.
  isogeneic g.
  isologous g.
  isoplastic g.
  Krause g.
  Krause-Wolfe g.
  mesh g.

NOTES

G

graft *(continued)*
  Ollier g.
  Ollier-Thiersch g.
  omental g.
  partial-thickness g.
  penetrating corneal g.
  periosteal g.
  Phemister g.
  pinch g.
  punch g.
  split-thickness g.
  vascularized g.
  g. versus host (GVH)
  g. versus host disease
  g. versus host reaction (GVHR)
  white g.
  Wolfe g.
grafting
Graham
  G. law
  G. Steell murmur
Graham-Cole test
grain
  g. alcohol
  g. itch
gram
  g. calorie
  g. equivalent
  G. iodine
  G. stain
gram-atomic weight
gram-centimeter
Gram-chromotrope stain
gram-ion
gram-meter
gram-molecular weight
gram-molecule
Gram-negative
Gram-positive
grana *(pl. of* granum)
granatum
grand
  g. mal
  g. mal epilepsy
  g. mal seizure
  g. multipara
granddaughter cyst
grandeur
  delusion of g.
grandiose delusion
Granger
  G. line
  G. projection
Granit loop
granny knot
Gr antigen
granular
  g. cast
  g. cell myoblastoma

g. cell tumor
g. conjunctivitis
g. corneal dystrophy
g. cortex
g. degeneration
g. endoplasmic reticulum
g. foveolae
g. kidney
g. layer
g. leukocyte
g. lid
g. ophthalmia
g. pharyngitis
g. pit
g. pneumonocyte
g. trachoma
g. urethritis
granulated opium
granulation
  arachnoid g.
  arachnoidal g.
  g. tissue
granulationes arachnoideae
granule
  acidophil g.
  acrosomal g.
  alpha g.
  Altmann g.
  amphophil g.
  argentaffin g.
  azurophil g.
  basal g.
  basophil g.
  Bensley specific g.
  beta g.
  Birbeck g.
  Bollinger g.
  g. cell
  chromatic g.
  chromophil g.
  chromophobe g.
  cone g.
  Crooke g.
  delta g.
  diazo stain for argentaffin g.
  elementary g.
  eosinophil g.
  Fordyce g.
  fuchsinophil g.
  glycogen g.
  iodophil g.
  juxtaglomerular g.
  kappa g.
  keratohyalin g.
  lamellar g.
  Langerhans g.
  Langley g.
  membrane-coating g.
  metachromatic g.

Neusser g.
Nissl g.
proacrosomal g.
rod g.
seminal g.
granuloblast
granulocyte
g. colony-stimulating factor (G-CSF)
immature g.
granulocyte-macrophage colony-stimulating factor (GM-CSF)
granulocytic
g. leukemia
g. sarcoma
g. series
granulocytopenia
granulocytopoiesis
granulocytopoietic
granulocytosis
granuloma
actinic g.
amebic g.
apical g.
beryllium g.
bilharzial g.
Capillaria g.
cholesterol g.
coccidioidal g.
cutaneous leishmaniasis g.
dental g.
Enterobius g.
eosinophilic g.
fishtank g.
foreign body g.
giant cell g.
infectious g.
g. inguinale
laryngeal g.
lethal midline g.
lipoid g.
lipophagic g.
lymphatic filariasis g.
Majocchi g.
malignant g.
midline lethal g.
midline malignant reticulosis g.
Miescher g.
g. multiforme
ocular larva migrans g.
paracoccidioidal g.
Paragonimus g.

periapical g.
pyogenic g.
g. pyogenicum
reparative g.
sarcoidal g.
telangiectatic g.
trichinosis g.
g. tropicum
ulcerating g.
g. venereum
granulomatosa
cheilitis g.
granulomatosis
allergic g.
bronchocentric g.
lipid g.
lipoid g.
lymphomatoid g.
Wegener g.
granulomatous
g. arteritis
g. colitis
g. disease
g. encephalomyelitis
g. endophthalmitis
g. enteritis
g. inflammation
g. mastitis
g. nocardiosis
g. rosacea
g. vasculitis
granulomere
granulopenia
granuloplasm
granuloplastic
granulopoiesis
granulopoietic
granulosa
g. cell tumor
g. lutein cell
pars g.
granulosis rubra nasi
granulosus
Echinococcus g.
granulovacuolar degeneration
granum, pl. **grana**
granzyme
grape
g. ending
g. sugar
graphanesthesia
graphesthesia

NOTES

G

graphic
> g. aphasia
> g. formula

graphite
graphology
graphomania
graphomotor aphasia
graphopathology
graphophobia
graphorrhea
graphospasm
grappe
> en g.

grasping reflex
grasp reflex
GRASS
> gradient-recalled acquisition in the steady
> state

grass bacillus
Grasset
> G. law
> G. phenomenon
> G. sign

Grasset-Gaussel phenomenon
grating
> diffraction g.

Gratiolet
> G. fiber
> G. radiation

grattage
gratuitous inducer
gravel
> coarse g.
> g. voice

Graves
> G. disease
> G. ophthalmopathy
> G. optic neuropathy
> G. orbitopathy

grave wax
gravida
gravidae
> hydrorrhea g.

gravidarum
> chorea g.
> fibroma molle g.
> hydrorrhea g.
> hyperemesis g.
> melasma g.
> nausea g.
> pruritus g.

gravidic
gravidism
gravidity
gravid uterus
gravimeter
gravimetric
gravireceptor

gravis
> anemia g.
> icterus g.
> myasthenia g.

gravitation
> g. abscess
> newtonian constant of g.

gravitational
> g. insecurity
> g. ulcer
> g. unit

gravity
> center of g.
> g. concentration
> g. cystogram
> specific g.

Grawitz
> G. basophilia
> G. tumor

gray
> g. baby syndrome
> g. cataract
> g. column
> g. commissure
> g. degeneration
> g. fiber
> g. hepatization
> g. induration
> g. infiltration
> g. literature
> g. matter
> g. ramus communicantes
> g. scale
> g. substance
> g. tuber
> g. tubercle
> g. wing

grayi
> *Listeria g.*

gray-scale ultrasonography
greaseless cream
great
> g. adductor muscle
> g. alveolar cell
> g. anastomotic artery
> g. auricular nerve
> g. cardiac vein
> g. cerebral vein
> g. foramen
> g. horizontal fissure
> g. longitudinal fissure
> g. radicular artery
> g. saphenous vein
> g. sciatic nerve
> g. segmental medullary artery
> g. superior pancreatic artery
> g. toe
> g. vein of Galen

greater
  g. alar cartilage
  g. arterial circle
  g. circulation
  g. cul-de-sac
  g. curvature
  g. horn of hyoid bone
  g. multangular bone
  g. occipital nerve
  g. omentum
  g. palatine artery
  g. palatine canal
  g. palatine foramen
  g. palatine groove
  g. palatine nerve
  g. pancreatic artery
  g. pectoral muscle
  g. pelvis
  g. peritoneal cavity
  g. posterior rectus muscle
  g. psoas muscle
  g. rhomboid muscle
  g. ring
  g. sciatic notch
  g. splanchnic nerve
  g. superficial petrosal nerve
  g. supraclavicular fossa
  g. trochanter
  g. tubercle
  g. tuberosity
  g. tympanic spine
  g. vestibular gland
  g. wing
  g. zygomatic muscle
greatest length
great-toe reflex
greedy bowel
green
  bromcresol g.
  bromocresol g.
  g. hemoglobin
  indocyanine g.
  malachite g.
  methyl g.
  g. monkey virus
  g. pus
  g. soap
  g. soap tincture
  g. sputum
  g. stain
  g. tobacco sickness

  g. tooth
  g. vision
Greenfield filter
greenstick fracture
gregaloid
gregarine
gregarinosis
Greig cephalopolysyndactyly syndrome
grenz
  g. ray
  g. zone
gression
Greville bath
Grey Turner sign
GRH
  gonadotropin-releasing hormone
grid
  Amsler g.
  focused g.
  g. ratio
gridiron suture
Gridley stain
Griesinger
  bilious typhoid of G.
  G. disease
  G. sign
grin
  sardonic g.
grindelia
grinder's phthisis
grinding-in
grinding surface
grip
  devil g.
grippe
gripping reflex
griseofulvin
griseum
  indusium g.
griseus
Grisonella ratellina
gristle
Gritti operation
Gritti-Stokes amputation
Grocco
  G. sign
  G. triangle
grocer itch
Grocott-Gomori methenamine-silver stain
Groenouw corneal dystrophy
groin
Grönblad-Strandberg syndrome

NOTES

Grondahl-Finney operation
groove
   alveolobuccal g.
   alveololabial g.
   alveololingual g.
   ampullary g.
   anterior auricular g.
   anterior intermediate g.
   anterior interventricular g.
   anterolateral g.
   anteromedian g.
   arterial g.
   atrioventricular g.
   auriculoventricular g.
   bicipital g.
   branchial g.
   carotid g.
   carpal g.
   cavernous g.
   chiasmatic g.
   coronary g.
   costal g.
   dental g.
   developmental g.
   digastric g.
   ethmoidal g.
   frontal g.
   gingival g.
   gingivobuccal g.
   gingivolabial g.
   gingivolingual g.
   greater palatine g.
   Harrison g.
   inferior petrosal g.
   infraorbital g.
   interosseous g.
   intertubercular g.
   interventricular g.
   lacrimal g.
   laryngotracheal g.
   lateral bicipital g.
   linguogingival g.
   Lucas g.
   major g.
   malleolar g.
   mastoid g.
   medial bicipital g.
   median g.
   medullary g.
   middle meningeal artery g.
   minor g.
   neural g.
   pharyngeal g.
   pontomedullary g.
   popliteal g.
   primitive g.
   g. sign
   supplemental g.

   g. suture
   urethral g.
grooved tongue
gross
   g. anatomy
   g. hematuria
   g. lesion
   G. leukemia virus
   g. reproduction rate
ground
   g. bundle
   figure and g.
   g. itch
   g. itch anemia
   g. lamella
   g. state
   g. substance
ground-glass
   g.-g. appearance
   g.-g. cytoplasm
   g.-g. pattern
group
   ABO blood g.
   activity g.
   g. agglutination
   g. agglutinin
   aluminum g.
   ambulatory patient g.
   g. antigen
   g. A streptococcal necrotizing
      fasciitis
   g. A streptococcus (GAS)
   Auberger blood g.
   Au blood g.
   Bethesda-Ballerup g.
   blood g.
   g. B streptococcus
   calcium g.
   characterizing g.
   chlorine g.
   connective tissue g.
   control g.
   cytophil g.
   determinant g.
   diagnosis-related g. (DRG)
   Di blood g.
   Diego blood g.
   difarnesyl g.
   Dombrock blood g.
   Duffy blood g.
   g. dynamics
   encounter g.
   ethnic g.
   experimental g.
   functional g.
   Fy blood g.
   HACEK g.
   g. hospital
   g. immunity

Jk blood g.
K blood g., k blood g.
Kell blood g.
ketole g.
Kidd blood g.
Le blood g.
Lewis blood g.
linkage g.
Lu blood g.
matched g.'s
MNSs blood g.
g. model HMO
nitrogen g.
g. practice
prosthetic g.
g. psychotherapy
g. reaction
g. test
training g.
g. transfer
g. translocation
vanadium g.
grouping
blood g.
Grover disease
growing
g. fracture
g. ovarian follicle
g. pain
growth
accretionary g.
appositional g.
g. arrest line
auxetic g.
bacterial g.
g. curve
differential g.
exponential g.
g. factor
g. hormone (GH)
g. hormone-inhibiting hormone (GIH)
g. hormone-producing adenoma
g. hormone-releasing factor (GH-RF, GHRF)
g. hormone-releasing hormone (GH-RH, GHRH)
interstitial g.
intussusceptive g.
g. medium
g. plate
g. rate

g. rate of population
g. regulator
growth-onset diabetes
Gruber
G. cul-de-sac
G. hernia
G. method
G. reaction
Gruber-Landzert fossa
Gruber-Widal reaction
gruel
grumous
Grunert spur
Grunstein-Hogness assay
Grynfeltt
G. hernia
G. triangle
gryochrome
gryposis penis
GSR
galvanic skin response
gt.
gutta
GU
genitourinary
guaiac
g. gum
g. test
guaiacin
guaiacol
g. glyceryl ether
g. phosphate
guaifenesin
Guama virus
guanabenz acetate
guanacline sulfate
guanadrel sulfate
Guanarito virus
guanase
guanfacine
guanidine
guanidinium
guanidinoacetate N-methyltransferase
guanine
g. aminase
g. cell
g. deaminase
g. deoxyribonucleotide
g. ribonucleotide
guanochlor sulfate
guanosine
guanylic acid

NOTES

G

guarana
guaranine
guardian ad litem
guarding
    abdominal g.
    involuntary g.
guar gum
Guarnieri body
Guaroa virus
gubernacular
    g. canal
    g. cord
gubernaculum
    g. dentis
    Hunter g.
Gubler
    G. line
    G. paralysis
    G. sign
    G. syndrome
Gudden
    G. commissure
    G. ganglion
    G. tegmental nucleus
Guedel airway
Guéneau
    G. de Mussy
    G. de Mussy point
Guérin
    G. fold
    G. fracture
    G. gland
    G. sinus
    G. valve
guidance
    condylar g.
    incisal g.
guide
    anterior g.
    catheter g.
    condylar g.
    incisal g.
    mold g.
    g. plane
    g. wire
guided tissue regeneration
guideline
    clasp g.
    clinical practice g.
    Cummer g.
    practice g.
guidewire
guiding symptom
Guillain-Barré
    G.-B. reflex
    G.-B. syndrome
guillotine amputation

guinea
    g. green B
    g. pig
Guldberg-Waage law
Gulf War syndrome
gullet
Gullstrand slitlamp
gulose
gum
    g. arabic
    Bassora g.
    g. benjamin
    g. benzoin
    British g.
    g. contour
    eucalyptus g.
    ghatti g.
    guaiac g.
    guar g.
    Indian g.
    karaya g.
    g. lancet
    g. line
    locust g.
    g. opium
    g. resection
    g. resin
gumboil
gumma, pl. gummata, gummas
gummatous
    g. abscess
    g. ulcer
Gumprecht shadow
Gunn
    G. crossing sign
    G. dot
    G. phenomenon
    G. pupil
    G. syndrome
Günning reaction
Gunning splint
gunshot wound
gunstock deformity
Günzberg
    G. reagent
    G. test
Günz ligament
gurgling rale
gurney
gusher
    perilymphatic g.
Gussenbauer
    G. operation
    G. suture
gustation
gustatory
    g. agnosia
    g. anesthesia
    g. aura

g. bud
g. cell
g. hallucination
g. hyperesthesia
g. hyperhidrosis
g. lemniscus
g. nucleus
g. organ
g. pore
g. receptor
g. rhinorrhea
g. sweating syndrome
gustatory-sudorific reflex
gustducin
gut
blind g.
g. glucagon
primitive g.
primordial g.
gut-associated lymphoid tissue (GALT)
Guthrie
G. muscle
G. test
gutta (gt.)
g. serena
gutta-percha
g.-p. cone
g.-p. point
g.-p. spreader
guttata
keratopathia g.
guttate psoriasis
gutter
g. dystrophy
g. fracture
g. wound
Guttman scale
guttural
g. duct
g. pulse
g. rale
gutturotetany
Gutzeit test
guyanensis
Leishmania braziliensis g.
Guyon
G. amputation
canal of G.
G. canal
G. isthmus
G. sign
G. tunnel syndrome

GVH
graft versus host
GVH disease
GVHR
graft versus host reaction
gymnastics
gymnophobia
gymnothecium
GYN
gynecology
gynandrism
gynandroblastoma
gynandroid
gynandromorphism
gynandromorphous
gynatresia
gynecic
gynecogenic
gynecoid
g. obesity
g. pelvis
gynecologic
gynecological
gynecologist
gynecology (GYN)
gynecomania
gynecomastia
gynecomasty
gynecophoric canal
gynephobia
gyniatrics
gyniatry
gynocardia oil
gynogenesis
gynopathy
gynoplastics
gynoplasty
gypseum
Microsporum g.
gypsum
gyrase
gyrate atrophy
gyration
gyrectomy
gyrencephalic
gyri (*pl. of* gyrus)
gyrochrome cell
gyromagnetic ratio
Gyromitra esculenta
gyrorum
impressiones g.
gyrose

G

NOTES

gyrospasm
gyrus, pl. **gyri**
    angular g.
    annectent g.
    anterior central g.
    anterior paracentral g.
    anterior piriform g.
    anterior transverse temporal g.
    ascending frontal g.
    ascending parietal g.
    callosal g.
    central g.
    cerebral g.
    cingulate g.
    deep transitional g.
    dentate g.
    fasciolar g.
    fornicate g.
    g. fornicatus
    fusiform g.
    Heschl g.
    hippocampal g.
    inferior frontal g.
    inferior occipital g.
    inferior parietal g.
    inferior temporal g.
    insular g.
    interlocking gyri
    lateral occipitotemporal g.
    lateral olfactory g.
    lingual g.
    long g.
    marginal g.
    medial frontal g.
    medial occipitotemporal g.
    medial olfactory g.
    middle frontal g.
    middle temporal g.
    orbital g.
    parahippocampal g.
    postcentral g.
    precentral g.
    short g.
    straight g.
    subcallosal g.
    superior frontal g.
    supramarginal g.
    transitional g.
    transverse temporal g.
    uncinate g.

H

H agglutinin
H antigen
H band
H chain
H colony
H and D curve
H disc
H field
H gene
H graft
H ray
H reflex
H shunt
H substance

H-2

H-2 antigen
H-2 complex

HA1 virus
HA2 virus
HAA

hepatitis-associated antigen

Haase rule
habena, pl. **habenae**
habenal
habenar
habenula, pl. **habenulae**

Haller h.

habenular

h. commissure
h. nucleus
h. sulcus
h. trigone

habenulointerpeduncular tract
habenulopeduncular tract
Haber syndrome
Haber-Weiss reaction
habit

h. chorea
h. cough
h. scoliosis
h. spasm
h. tic

habitual

h. abortion
h. centric
h. pitch

habituation
habitus

fetal h.
gracile h.

HACEK group
Haeckel

H. gastrea theory
H. law

haematobium

Schistosoma h.
schistosomiasis h.

haemolyticum

Corynebacterium h.

haemolyticus

Haemophilus h.

Haemophilus

H. actinomycetemcomitans
H. aegyptius
H. aphrophilus
H. ducreyi
H. haemolyticus
H. influenzae
H. influenzae type b
H. influenzae type B vaccine
H. parahaemolyticus
H. parainfluenzae
H. paratropicalis
H. segnis

Haff disease
Haffkine vaccine
hafnium
hafussi bath
Hagedorn needle
Hageman factor
hagiotherapy
Haglund

H. deformity
H. disease

Hahn

H. operation
H. oxine reagent

hahnemannian
hahnium
Haidinger brush
Haight anastomosis
Hailey-Hailey disease
hair

auditory h.
axillary h.
h. ball
bamboo h.
bayonet h.
beaded h.
h. bulb
burrowing h.
h. cast
h. cell
club h.
h. cycle
h. disc
downy h.
exclamation point h.
h. follicle

H

hair *(continued)*
    Frey h.
    ingrown h.
    kinky h.
    lanugo h.
    moniliform h.
    h. papilla
    h. root
    scalp h.
    h. shaft
    spun glass h.
    stellate h.
    h. stream
    taste h.
    terminal h.
    h. transplant
    twisted h.'s
    h. whorl
hairline fracture
hairpin
    h. loop
    h. vessel
hairworm
hairy
    h. cell
    h. cell leukemia
    h. heart
    h. leukoplakia
    h. mole
    h. nevus
    h. tongue
halation
halazone
Halberstaedter-Prowazek body
Haldane
    H. apparatus
    H. effect
    H. relationship
    H. transformation
    H. tube
Haldane-Priestley sample
Hale colloidal iron stain
Hales piesimeter
half
    h. amplitude pulse duration
    h. axial view
    h. cystine
    h. and half nail
    h. hapten
half-axial projection
half-chair form
half-glass spectacles
half-hapten
half-life
    biologic h.-l.
    effective h.-l.
half-moon

half-time
half-value (HV)
    h.-v. layer (HVL)
halfway house
halibut liver oil
halide
haliphagia
halisteresis
halisteretic
halitosis
halitus
hallachrome
Hallé point
Haller
    H. ansa
    H. anulus
    H. arch
    H. cell
    H. circle
    H. cone
    H. habenula
    H. insula
    H. line
    H. plexus
    H. rete
    H. tripod
    H. vascular tissue
Hallermann-Streiff-François syndrome
Hallermann-Streiff syndrome
Hallervorden-Spatz
    H.-S. disease
    H.-S. syndrome
Hallervorden syndrome
hallex, pl. **hallices**
Hallgren syndrome
Hallopeau disease
hallucal
halluces (*pl. of* hallux)
hallucination
    auditory h.
    blank h.
    command h.
    formed visual h.
    gustatory h.
    haptic h.
    hypnagogic h.
    hypnopompic h.
    kinesthesia h.
    mood-congruent h.
    mood-incongruent h.
    olfactory h.
    stump h.
    tactile h.
    visual h.
hallucinatory neuralgia
hallucinogen
hallucinogenesis
hallucinogenic
hallucinosis

hallus
hallux, pl. **halluces**
   h. dolorosus
   h. extensus
   h. flexus
   h. malleus
   h. rigidus
   h. valgus
   h. varus
halo
   anemic h.
   h. cast
   h. effect
   glaucomatous h.
   h. nevus
   h. sign
   h. traction
   h. vision
haloalkylamine
halogen acne
halogenation
halogenoderma
Halogeton
halometer
halophil
halophile
halophilic
halosteresis
halothane-ether azeotrope
halothane hepatitis
Halstead-Reitan battery
Halsted
   H. law
   H. operation
   H. suture
halter traction
halzoun
hamamelis
hamartia
hamartoblastoma
hamartochondromatosis
hamartoma
   pulmonary h.
hamartomatous
hamartophobia
hamate
   h. bone
   hook of h.
hamatum
Hamburger
   H. law
   H. phenomenon

Hamilton
   H. anxiety rating scale
   H. depression rating scale
Hamilton-Stewart
   H.-S. formula
   H.-S. method
Hamman
   H. disease
   H. murmur
   H. sign
   H. syndrome
Hamman-Rich
   H.-R. disease
   H.-R. syndrome
Hammarsten reagent
hammer
   h. finger
   h. nose
   h. palsy
   h. toe
Hammerschlag method
hammock
   h. bandage
   h. ligament
Hammond disease
Hampton
   H. hump
   H. line
   H. maneuver
   H. technique
hamstring
   h. muscle
   h. tendon
Ham test
hamular
   h. notch
   h. process
hamulus, pl. **hamuli**
   lacrimal h.
Hancock amputation
hand
   accoucheur h.
   ape h.
   cleft h.
   club h., clubhand
   crab h.
   drop h.
   h. eczema
   ghoul h.
   Marinesco succulent h.
   obstetric h.
   obstetrical h.

NOTES

H

hand *(continued)*
    h. ratio
    split h.
    writing h.
hand-and-foot syndrome
handedness
hand-foot-and-mouth
    h.-f.-a.-m. disease
    h.-f.-a.-m. disease virus
hand-foot syndrome
handicap
Handley operation
handpiece
Hand-Schüller-Christian disease
handshapes
HANE
    hereditary angioneurotic edema
Hanes plot
hanging
    h. drop
    h. septum
hanging-block culture
hangman's fracture
hangnail
Hanhart syndrome
Hanks
    H. dilator
    H. solution
Hannover canal
Hanot cirrhosis
Hansemann macrophage
Hansen
    H. bacillus
    H. disease
Hantaan virus
Hantavirus
hantavirus pulmonary syndrome
hapalonychia
haphalgesia
haphazard sampling
haphephobia
haplodont
haploid set
haplology
haploprotein
haploscope
    mirror h.
haploscopic vision
Haplosporidia
haplotype
happy puppet syndrome
Hapsburg
    H. jaw
    H. lip
hapten
    conjugated h.
    Forssman h.
    half h.
haptic hallucination

haptics
haptodysphoria
haptoglobin
haptometer
Harada
    H. disease
    H. syndrome
Harada-Ito procedure
Harada-Mori filter paper strip culture
hard
    h. cataract
    h. chancre
    h. corn
    h. drusen
    h. nevus
    h. palate
    h. papilloma
    h. paraffin
    h. pulse
    h. ray
    h. soap
    h. sore
    h. tissue
    h. tubercle
    h. ulcer
    h. water
hardened pelvis
hardening
Harden-Young ester
hardiness
Harding-Passey melanoma
hardness
    indentation h.
    h. scale
hardware
Hardy-Rand-Ritter test
Hardy-Weinberg
    H.-W. equilibrium
    H.-W. law
harelip
hare's eye
harlequin
    h. fetus
    h. ichthyosis
    h. reaction
harmaline
harmidine
harmine
harmonia
harmonic
    h. mean
    h. suture
harmonious retinal correspondence
harmony
    functional occlusal h.
harpaxophobia
harpoon
Harrington-Flocks test

Harris
    H. hematoxylin
    H. line
    H. migraine
    H. and Ray test
    H. syndrome
Harrison groove
harsh rhonchi
Hartel technique
Hartmann
    H. curette
    H. operation
    H. pouch
    H. solution
Hartmannella
hartmanni
    Entamoeba h.
Hartman solution
Hartnup
    H. disease
    H. syndrome
hartshorn
harvest bug
harvester
    h. ant
    h. lung
hasamiyami
Häser formula
Hashimoto
    H. disease
    H. struma
    H. thyroiditis
hashish
Hasner fold
Hassall
    H. body
    H. concentric corpuscle
Hassall-Henle body
Hasson
    H. cannula
    H. trocar
hat band migraine
hatchet excavator
hatching flask
Hauch
    ohne H.
Haudek niche
haustorium
haustra coli
haustral
haustration
haustrum

haustus
HAV
    hepatitis A virus
Haverhill fever
Haverhillia multiformis
haversian
    h. canal
    h. lamella
    h. space
    h. system
Hawkins impingement sign
Hawley
    H. appliance
    H. retainer
Haworth projection
Hawthorne effect
hay
    h. asthma
    h. bacillus
    h. fever
Hayem
    H. hematoblast
    H. solution
Hayem-Widal syndrome
Hayflick limit
Haygarth node
hazard rate
hazelwort
Hb
    hemoglobin
HBcAb
    antibody to the hepatitis B core antigen
HBcAg
    hepatitis B core antigen
HbChesapeake
    hemoglobin Chesapeake
HBE
    His bundle electrogram
HBe, HBeAg
    hepatitis B e antigen
HBeAb
    antibody to the hepatitis B e antigen
Hb S
    sickle cell hemoglobin
HBsAb
    antibody to the hepatitis B surface antigen
HBsAg
    hepatitis B surface antigen
HBV
    hepatitis B virus

NOTES

H

419

HCG, hCG
  human chorionic gonadotropin
HCS
  human chorionic somatomammotropin
Hct
  hematocrit
HCV
  hepatitis C virus
Hcy
  homocysteine
HDCV
  human diploid cell vaccine
HDL
  high-density lipoprotein
HDV
  hepatitis delta virus
head
  absorber h.
  H. area
  h. botflies
  bulldog h.
  h. cap
  h. cavity
  clavicular h.
  h. cold
  h. dependent position
  h. fold
  hourglass h.
  humeral h.
  humeroulnar h.
  h. kidney
  lateral h.
  H. line
  long h.
  medial h.
  Medusa h.
  h. mirror
  h. nurse
  h. presentation
  h. process
  saddle h.
  h. tremor
  H. zone
headache
  benign exertional h.
  bilious h.
  blind h.
  cluster h.
  coital h.
  exertional h.
  fibrositic h.
  histaminic h.
  Horton h.
  ice pick h.
  idiopathic stabbing h.
  jolt h.
  meningeal h.
  migraine without h.
  muscle contraction h.

  neuralgic h.
  paraplegic h.
  postconcussional h.
  posttraumatic h.
  sick h.
  spinal h.
  tension h.
  tension-type h.
  thunderclap h.
  traumatic h.
  vascular h.
head-bobbing doll syndrome
head-dropping test
4-headed muscle
headgear
headgut
head-nodding
head-tilt
healed
  h. tuberculosis
  h. ulcer
healer
healing
  faith h.
  h. by first intention
  h. by second intention
  h. by third intention
health
  h. behavior
  behavioral h.
  h. care
  h. center
  dental public h.
  h. education
  flight into h.
  h. indicator
  h. information system
  H. Level-7 (HL-7)
  h. maintenance organization (HMO)
  mental h.
  h. promotion
  h. psychology
  h. risk appraisal
  h. risk assessment
  h. status index
health-related physical fitness
healthy worker effect
Heaney operation
He antigen
hearing
  h. aid
  color h.
  h. impairment
  h. instrument
  h. level
  h. loss
  h. protector
  Weber test for h.

heart
- h. antigen
- armor h.
- armored h.
- h. arrest
- artificial h.
- athlete's h.
- athletic h.
- h. attack
- h. beat
- beer h.
- beriberi h.
- h. block
- bony h.
- h. chamber remodeling
- chaotic h.
- crisscross h.
- dextroposition of h.
- dextroversion of h.
- h. disease
- drop h.
- h. failure
- h. failure cell
- fatty h.
- frosted h.
- globular h.
- hairy h.
- Holmes h.
- horizontal h.
- h. hormone
- hyperthyroid h.
- hypoplastic h.
- icing h.
- intermediate h.
- Jarvik artificial h.
- left h.
- h. massage
- mechanical h.
- ox h.
- h. position
- h. rate
- h. rate reserve
- h. rate turbulence
- right h.
- round h.
- h. sac
- semihorizontal h.
- semivertical h.
- h. sounds
- stone h.
- h. stroke
- h. tamponade
- tobacco h.
- h. tones
- h. transplantation
- h. valve prosthesis
- vertical h.

heartbeat

heartburn

heart-lung
- h.-l. machine
- h.-l. preparation
- h.-l. transplantation

heart-shaped
- h.-s. pelvis
- h.-s. uterus

heartworm

heat
- h. apoplexy
- atomic h.
- h. capacity
- h. coagulation test
- conductive h.
- convective h.
- conversive h.
- h. cramps
- h. edema
- h. exhaustion
- h. hyperpyrexia
- initial h.
- innate h.
- h. instability test
- h. lamp
- latent h.
- molecular h.
- prickly h.
- h. prostration
- h. rash
- h. rigor
- h. shock protein
- h. stress index
- h. stroke
- h. treatment
- h. urticaria

heat-curing resin

heat-labile

Heaton operation

heat-rigor point

heat-stable enzyme

heatstroke

heavy
- h. chain
- h. chain disease
- h. hydrogen

NOTES

H

heavy *(continued)*
    h. liquid petrolatum
    h. metal
    h. metal neuropathy
    h. nitrogen
    h. oxygen
    h. water
heavy-meromyosin
hebephrenia
hebephrenic
    h. dementia
    h. schizophrenia
Heberden
    H. angina
    H. asthma
    H. node
hebetic
hebetude
hebiatrics
hebraeum
    Amblyomma h.
Hebra prurigo
hecateromeric
hecatomeral
hecatomeric
Hecht pneumonia
Heck disease
hectic flush
hectogram
hectoliter
hectometer
hedeoma
hederiform ending
hedonophobia
Hedström file
heel
    black h.
    h. bone
    cracked h.
    h. fly
    h. jar
    h. pad
    painful h.
    prominent h.
    h. region
    h. spur
    h. tap
    h. tendon
heel-tap
    h.-t. reaction
    h.-t. test
heel-to-knee-to-toe test
heel-to-shin test
Heerfordt disease
Hegar
    H. dilator
    H. sign

Hegglin
    H. anomaly
    H. syndrome
Hehner
    H. number
    H. value
Heidelberger curve
Heidenhain
    H. azan stain
    H. crescent
    H. demilune
    H. iron hematoxylin stain
    H. law
    H. pouch
height
    anterior facial h. (AFH)
    h. of contour
    cusp h.
    facial h.
    h. vertigo
height-length index
Heilbronner thigh
heilmannii
    Helicobacter h.
Heim-Kreysig sign
Heimlich maneuver
Heineke-Mikulicz pyloroplasty
Heinz
    H. body
    H. body anemia
    H. body test
Heinz-Ehrlich body
Heister
    H. diverticulum
    H. valve
HeLa cell
helcomenia
Held
    H. bundle
    H. decussation
helianthine
helical
    h. computed tomography
    h. CT
    h. suture
helices (*pl. of* helix)
helicine artery
helicis
    h. major muscle
    h. minor muscle
Helicobacter
    H. cinaedi
    H. fennelliae
    H. heilmannii
    H. pylori
helicoid
    h. choroidopathy
    h. ginglymus
helicopod gait

helicopodia
helicotrema
Helie bundle
heliencephalitis
helioaerotherapy
hcliopathy
heliophobia
heliosis
heliotaxis
heliotropism
helium
    h. speech
    h. therapy
helium-3, -4
helix, pl. helices
    collagen h.
    DNA h.
    double h.
    Watson-Crick h.
hellebore
    false h.
helleborin
helleborism
helleborus
hellem
    Encephalitozoon h.
Heller
    H. myotomy
    H. operation
    H. plexus
Hellin law
HELLP
    hemolysis, elevated liver function, and
    low platelets
    HELLP syndrome
Helly fixative
helmet cell
Helmholtz
    H. axis ligament
    H. energy
Helmholtz-Gibbs theory
helminth
helminthagogue
helminthemesis
helminthiasis
helminthic, helmintic
    h. abscess
    h. dysentery
helminthism
helminthoid
helminthology
helminthoma

helminthophobia
Helminthosporium
helmintic (*var. of* helminthic)
heloma
    h. durum
    h. molle
helotomy
help
    cry for h.
helper
    h. cell
    h. virus
helplessness
    learned h.
Helvella esculenta
Helweg bundle
Helweg-Larssen syndrome
Helwig bundle
hemachrome
hemacyte
hemacytometer
hemacytozoon
hemadostenosis
hemadsorption
    h. virus test
    h. virus type 1, 2
hemafacient
hemagglutinating cold autoantibody
hemagglutination
    h. inhibition
    passive h.
    reverse passive h.
    h. test
    viral h.
hemagglutinin
hemagglutinin-protease
hemagogic
hemal
    h. arch
    h. gland
    h. node
    h. spine
hemalum
hemamebiasis
hemanalysis
hemangiectasia
hemangiectasis
hemangiectatic hypertrophy
hemangioblast
hemangioblastoma
hemangioendothelioblastoma
hemangioendothelioma

NOTES

H

hemangiofibroma
    juvenile h.
hemangioma
    capillary h.
    cavernous h.
    dyschondroplasia with h.
    lobular capillary h.
    sclerosing h.
    scrotal h.
    senile h.
    strawberry h.
    verrucous h.
hemangiomatosis
hemangiopericytoma
hemangiosarcoma
hemapheic
hemaphein
hemapheism
hemapophysis
hemarthrosis
hemastrontium
hematachometer
hematapostema
hematein
    Baker acid h.
hematemesis
hematencephalon
hematherapy
hematherm
hemathermal
hemathermous
hemathorax
hematic
hematid
hematidrosis
hematimeter
hematin
    h. chloride
    reduced h.
hematinemia
hematinic principle
hematobilia
hematobium
hematoblast
    Hayem h.
hematocele
hematocephaly
hematochezia
hematochlorin
hematochyluria
hematocolpometra
hematocolpos
hematocrit (Hct)
hematocryal
hematocyst
hematocystis
hematocyte
hematocytoblast
hematocytolysis

hematocytometer
hematocytozoon
hematodyscrasia
hematodystrophy
hematogenesis
hematogenetic calculus
hematogenic
hematogenous
    h. abscess
    h. embolism
    h. jaundice
    h. metastasis
    h. osteitis
    h. pigment
hematohistioblast
hematohiston
hematoid
hematoidin crystal
hematologist
hematology
hematolymphangioma
hematolysis
hematolytic
hematoma
    auricle h.
    communicating h.
    epidural h.
    intracranial h.
    intramural h.
    retroperitoneal h.
    subdural h.
    subungual h.
hematometra
hematometry
hematomphalocele
hematomyelia
hematomyelopore
hematonic
hematopathology
hematopathy
hematopenia
hematophagia
hematophagous
hematophagus
hematoplast
hematoplastic
hematopoiesis
hematopoietic
    h. gland
    h. growth factor
    h. system
hematopoietin
hematoporphyria
hematoporphyrin
hematoporphyrinemia
hematoporphyrinuria
hematopsia
hematorrhachis
    h. externa

extradural h.
h. interna
hematosalpinx
hematosepsis
hematosin
hematosis
hematospectroscope
hematospectroscopy
hematospermatocele
hematospermia
hematostatic
hematostaxis
hematosteon
hematothermal
hematotoxic
hematotoxin
hematotropic
hematotympanum
hematoxic
hematoxin
hematoxylin
h. body
Boehmer h.
Delafield h.
h. and eosin stain
Harris h.
iron h.
hematoxyphil body
hematozoic
hematozoon
hematuria
Egyptian h.
endemic h.
false h.
gross h.
initial h.
microscopic h.
profound h.
renal h.
urethral h.
vesical h.
hematuric bilious fever
heme protein
hemeralopia
hemeranopia
hemerythrin
hemerythrins
hemiacardius
hemiacetal
hemiacrosomia
hemiageusia, hemiageustia
hemialgia

hemianalgesia
hemianencephaly
hemianesthesia
alternate h.
crossed h.
hemianopia
absolute h.
altitudinal h.
binasal h.
bitemporal h.
complete h.
congruous h.
crossed h.
heteronymous h.
homonymous h.
incomplete h.
incongruous h.
temporal h.
unilateral h.
hemianopic
h. scotoma
h. spectacles
hemianopsia
hemianosmia
hemiaplasia
hemiapraxia
hemiarthroplasty
hemiasynergia
hemiataxia
hemiathetosis
hemiatrophy
facial h.
lingual h.
hemiazygos vein
hemiballism
hemiballismus
hemiblock
hemibody radiation
hemic
h. calculus
h. distomiasis
h. murmur
hemicardia
h. dextra
h. sinistra
hemicellulose
hemicentrum
hemicephalalgia
hemicephalia
hemicerebrum
hemicholinium
Hemichordata, Hemichorda

NOTES

H

425

hemichorea
hemicolectomy
hemicorporectomy
hemicrania
hemicraniectomy
hemicraniosis
hemicraniotomy
hemidesmosomes
hemidiaphoresis
hemidrosis
hemidysesthesia
hemidystrophy
hemiectromelia
hemifacial spasm
hemigastrectomy
hemigeusia
hemiglossal
hemiglossectomy
hemiglossitis
hemignathia
hemihepatectomy
hemihidrosis
hemihydranencephaly
hemihypalgesia
hemihyperesthesia
hemihyperhidrosis
hemihypertonia
hemihypertrophy
hemihypesthesia
hemihypoesthesia
hemihypotonia
hemikaryon
hemiketal
hemilaminectomy
hemilaryngectomy
hemilateral chorea
hemilesion
hemilingual
hemimacroglossia
hemimandibulectomy
hemimelia
    dysplasia epiphysialis h.
hemimetabolous
hemin
hemiopalgia
hemipagus
hemipancreatectomy
hemiparesis
hemipelvectomy
hemiplegia
    alternating h.
    contralateral h.
    crossed h.
    double h.
    facial h.
    infantile h.
    spastic h.
hemiplegic
    h. amyotrophy

    h. gait
    h. migraine
hemisection
hemisensory
hemiseptum
hemispasm
hemisphere
    cerebellar h.
    cerebral h.
    dominant h.
hemispherectomy
hemispheric gliosis
hemisphericum
hemispherium
hemistrumectomy
hemisubstance
hemisulfur mustard
hemisyndrome
hemisystole
hemiterpene
hemithermoanesthesia
hemithoracic duct
hemithorax
hemithyroidectomy
hemitransfixion incision
hemitremor
hemitruncus
hemivertebra
hemizona assay
hemizygosity
hemizygote
hemizygotic
hemizygous
hemlock
hemoagglutination
hemoagglutinin
hemoantitoxin
hemobilia
hemoblast
    lymphoid h.
hemoblastosis
hemocatharsis
hemocatheresis
hemocatheretic
Hemoccult test
hemocele
hemocholecystitis
hemochorial placenta
hemochromatosis
    exogenous h.
    primary h.
    secondary h.
hemochrome
hemochromogen
hemoclasia
hemoclasis
hemoclastic reaction
hemoconcentration
hemoconia

hemoconiosis
hemocryoscopy
hemocuprein
hemocyanin
hemocyte
hemocytoblast
hemocytocatheresis
hemocytolysis
hemocytoma
hemocytometer
hemocytometry
hemocytotripsis
hemocytozoon
hemodiafiltration
hemodiagnosis
hemodialysis
hemodialyzer
hemodiastase
hemodilution
hemodynamic
hemodynamics
hemodyscrasia
hemodystrophy
hemoendothelial placenta
hemofiltration
hemoflagellate
hemofuscin
hemogenesis
hemogenic
hemoglobin (Hb)
    h. A2
    h. A, A2
    aberrant h.
    h. AIc
    h. anti-Lepore
    h. Bart
    bile pigment h.
    h. C
    carbon monoxide h.
    h. C disease
    h. Chesapeake (HbChesapeake)
    h. Constant Spring
    h. E
    embryonic h.
    h. F
    fetal h.
    glycated h.
    glycosylated h.
    h. Gower-1
    h. Gower-2
    green h.
    h. H

    h. H disease
    h. I
    h. $J_{Capetown}$
    h. Kansas
    h. Lepore
    h. M
    mean corpuscular h. (MCH)
    muscle h.
    h. Portland
    h. Rainier
    reduced h.
    h. S
    sickle cell h. (Hb S)
    h. Yakima
hemoglobinemia
    paroxysmal nocturnal h.
hemoglobinocholia
hemoglobinolysis
hemoglobinometry
hemoglobinopathy
hemoglobinopepsia
hemoglobinophilic
hemoglobinuria
    epidemic h.
    intermittent h.
    malarial h.
    march h.
    paroxysmal cold h.
    paroxysmal nocturnal h.
    toxic h.
hemoglobinuric
    h. fever
    h. nephrosis
hemogram
hemohistioblast
hemolamella
hemolipase
hemolith
hemology
hemolymph
    h. gland
    h. node
hemolysate
hemolysin
    bacterial h.
    cold h.
    heterophil h.
    immune h.
    h. unit
hemolysinogen
hemolysis
    biologic h.

NOTES

H

hemolysis *(continued)*
  conditioned h.
  h., elevated liver function, and low
    platelets (HELLP)
  immune h.
  phenylhydrazine h.
hemolytic
  h. anemia
  h. crisis
  h. disease
  h. gas
  h. jaundice
  h. plaque assay
  h. splenomegaly
  h. streptococcus
  h. unit
  h. uremic syndrome
hemolyzation
hemolyze
hemomediastinum
hemometra
hemometry
hemonectin
hemoparasite
hemopathology
hemopathy
hemoperfusion
hemopericardium
hemoperitoneum
hemopexin
hemophagia
hemophagocyte
hemophagocytosis
hemophil, hemophile
hemophilia
  h. A, B, C
  classic h.
hemophiliac
hemophilic
  h. arthritis
  h. joint
hemophilioid
hemophilosis
hemophobia
hemophoresis
hemophthalmia
hemophthalmus
hemophthisis
hemoplastic
hemoplasty
hemopneumopericardium
hemopneumothorax
hemopoiesis
hemopoietic tissue
hemopoietin
hemoporphyrin
hemoprecipitin
hemoprotein

hemoptysis
  endemic h.
  paracytic h.
hemopyelectasia
hemopyelectasis
hemorepellant
hemorheology
hemorrhachis
hemorrhage
  brainstem h.
  cerebral h.
  concealed h.
  Duret h.
  epidural h.
  extradural h.
  gastric h.
  intermediate h.
  internal h.
  intracerebral h.
  intracranial h.
  intrapartum h.
  intraventricular h. (IVH)
  parenchymatous h.
  petechial h.
  postpartum h.
  primary h.
  punctate h.
  recalcitrant h.
  secondary h.
  splinter h.
  subarachnoid h.
  subdural h.
hemorrhagic
  h. abscess
  h. anemia
  h. ascites
  h. bronchitis
  h. colitis
  h. cyst
  h. cystitis
  h. dengue
  h. disease
  h. endovasculitis
  h. enterocolitis
  h. fever
  h. gangrene
  h. glaucoma
  h. infarct
  h. iritis
  h. measles
  h. nephritis
  h. pachymeningitis
  h. pericarditis
  h. plague
  h. pleurisy
  h. rickets
  h. scurvy
  h. shock

h. smallpox
h. urticaria
hemorrhagica
metropathia h.
purpura h.
scarlatina h.
hemorrhagicum
corpus h.
hemorrhagin
hemorrhoid
combined h.
cutaneous h.
external h.
internal h.
lingual h.
mixed h.
mucocutaneous h.
prolapsed h.
strangulated h.
thrombosed h.
hemorrhoidal
h. cushion
h. nerve
h. plexus
h. vein
h. zone
hemorrhoidalis
anulus h.
hemorrhoidectomy
hemosalpinx
hemosialemesis
hemosiderin
hemosiderosis
idiopathic pulmonary h.
hemospermia
h. spuria
h. vera
hemosporidium
hemosporine
hemostasia
hemostasis
hemostat
hemostatic
h. clamp
h. collodion
h. forceps
hemostyptic
hemosuccus pancreaticus
hemotachogram
hemotachometer
hemotachometry
hemotherapeutics

hemotherapy
hemothorax
hemotoxic
hemotoxin
cobra h.
hemotroph, hemotrophe
hemotropic
hemotympanum
hemoximeter
hemoximetry
hemozoic
hemozoon
HEMPAS
hereditary erythroblastic multinuclearity
associated with positive acidified serum
HEMPAS cell
henbane
hen-cluck stertor
Henderson-Hasselbalch equation
Hendersonula toruloidea
Hendra virus
Henke space
Henle
H. ampulla
H. ansa
H. fenestrated elastic membrane
H. fiber layer
H. fissure
H. gland
H. loop
H. nervous layer
H. reaction
H. sheath
H. spine
H. tubule
H. wart
henna
Hennebert sign
Henoch
H. chorea
H. purpura
Henoch-Schönlein
H.-S. purpura
H.-S. syndrome
henpuye
Henri-Michaelis-Menten equation
henry
Henry-Gauer response
Henry law
henselae
Bartonella h.

NOTES

H

429

Hensen
- H. canal
- H. cell
- H. disc
- H. duct
- H. knot
- H. line
- H. node
- H. stripe

Hensing ligament

heparan
- h. N-sulfatase
- h. sulfate

heparin
- h. complement
- h. eliminase
- h. lock
- h. lyase
- h. sodium
- h. unit

heparinase

heparinemia

heparinic acid

heparinize

heparinolytica
- *Prevotella h.*

heparitin sulfate

hepar lobatum

hepatatrophia

hepatatrophy

hepatectomize

hepatectomy

hepatic
- h. adenoma
- h. amebiasis
- h. artery
- h. artery proper
- h. branch
- h. capsulitis
- h. colic
- h. coma
- h. cord
- h. cyst
- h. diverticulum
- h. duct
- h. encephalopathy
- h. fistula
- h. flexure
- h. infantilism
- h. insufficiency
- h. intermittent fever
- h. laminae
- h. lobule
- h. lymph node
- h. nervous plexus
- h. porphyria
- h. portal system
- h. portal vein
- h. prominence

- h. segment
- h. steatosis
- h. triad
- h. vein catheterization

hepaticodochotomy

hepaticoduodenostomy

hepaticoenterostomy

hepaticogastrostomy

hepaticolithotomy

hepaticolithotripsy

hepaticopulmonary

hepaticostomy

hepaticotomy

hepaticus
- fetor h.

hepatin

hepatis
- peliosis h.

hepatitic

hepatitis
- h. A, B, C, D, E, F, G
- active chronic h.
- acute parenchymatous h.
- anicteric viral h.
- anicteric virus h.
- h. A virus (HAV)
- h. B core antigen (HBcAg)
- h. B e antigen (HBe, HBeAg)
- h. B immune globulin
- h. B surface antigen (HBsAg)
- h. B vaccine
- h. B virus (HBV)
- cholangiolitic h.
- cholestatic h.
- chronic active h.
- chronic interstitial h.
- chronic persistent h.
- chronic persisting h.
- h. C virus (HCV)
- delta h.
- h. delta virus (HDV)
- drug-induced h.
- h. D virus
- epidemic h.
- h. E virus (HEV)
- h. externa
- fulminant h.
- giant cell h.
- h. G virus (HGV)
- halothane h.
- infectious h. (IH)
- long incubation h.
- lupoid h.
- neonatal h.
- non–A-E h.
- persistent chronic h.
- viral h.
- viral h. type A, B, D

hepatitis-associated antigen (HAA)

hepatization
  gray h.
  red h.
  yellow h.
hepatoblastoma
hepatocarcinoma
hepatocele
hepatocellular
  h. adenoma
  h. carcinoma
  h. jaundice
hepatocholangioenterostomy
hepatocholangiojejunostomy
hepatocholangiostomy
hepatocholangitis
hepatocolic ligament
hepatocuprein
hepatocystic duct
hepatocyte
hepatoduodenal ligament
hepatoduodenostomy
hepatodysentery
hepatoenteric recess
hepatoerythropoietic porphyria
hepatoesophageal ligament
hepatofugal
hepatogastric ligament
hepatogenic
hepatogenous
  h. jaundice
  h. pigment
hepatography
hepatohemia
hepatoid
hepatojugular
  h. reflex
  h. reflux
hepatojugularometer
hepatolenticular degeneration
hepatolienography
hepatolienomegaly
hepatolith
hepatolithectomy
hepatolithiasis
hepatologist
hepatology
hepatolysin
hepatoma
  malignant h.
hepatomalacia
hepatomegalia
hepatomegaly

hepatomelanosis
hepatomphalocele
hepatomphalos
hepatonecrosis
hepatonephoric syndrome
hepatonephric syndrome
hepatonephromegaly
hepatopancreatic
  h. ampulla
  h. sphincter
hepatopathic
hepatopathy
hepatoperitonitis
hepatopetal
hepatopexy
hepatophosphorylase deficiency
  glycogenosis
hepatophyma
hepatopleural fistula
hepatopneumonic
hepatoportal
hepatoptosis
hepatopulmonary
hepatorenal
  h. ligament
  h. pouch
  h. recess
  h. syndrome
hepatorrhagia
hepatorrhaphy
hepatorrhexis
hepatoscopy
hepatosplenitis
hepatosplenography
hepatosplenomegaly
hepatosplenopathy
hepatostomy
hepatotherapy
hepatotomy
hepatotoxemia
hepatotoxic
hepatotoxicity
hepatotoxin
heptachlor
heptad
heptanal
heptapeptide
heptose
heptulose
herald
  h. patch
  h. plaque

NOTES

H

431

herbivorous
Hercules
    infant H.
herd
    h. immunity
    h. instinct
hereditaria
    adynamia episodica h.
    alopecia h.
hereditary
    h. alopecia
    h. amyloidosis
    h. angioedema
    h. angioneurotic edema (HANE)
    autosomal h.
    h. benign telangiectasia
    h. cerebellar ataxia
    h. chorea
    h. clubbing
    h. coproporphyria
    h. deafness
    h. deforming chondrodystrophy
    dominant h.
    h. epithelial dystrophy
    h. erythroblastic multinuclearity
    associated with positive acidified
    serum (HEMPAS)
    h. folate malabsorption
    h. fructose intolerance
    h. hearing impairment
    h. hemorrhagic telangiectasia
    h. hemorrhagic thrombasthenia
    h. hypersegmentation
    h. hyperthyroidism
    h. hypertrophic neuropathy
    h. hypophosphatemic rickets
    h. lymphedema
    h. methemoglobinemia
    h. methemoglobinemic cyanosis
    h. multiple exostoses
    h. multiple trichoepithelioma
    h. myokymia
    h. nephritis
    h. nonpolyposis colorectal cancer
    h. opalescent dentin
    h. photomyoclonus
    h. progressive arthroophthalmopathy
    h. pyropoikilocytosis
    h. renal hypouricuria
    h. sensory radicular neuropathy
    h. spherocytosis
    h. spinal ataxia
    h. syphilis
heredity
heredofamilial tremor
heredopathia atactica polyneuritiformis
heredotaxia
Hering
    canal of H.

    H. sinus nerve
    H. test
    H. theory
Hering-Breuer reflex
heritability
Herlitz syndrome
Hermann fixative
Hermansky-Pudlak syndrome
hermaphrodite
hermaphroditism, hermaphrodism
    adrenal h.
    bilateral h.
    dimidiate h.
    false h.
    female h.
    lateral h.
    male h.
    transverse h.
    unilateral h.
hermetic
hernia
    abdominal h.
    acquired h.
    amniotic h.
    Barth h.
    Béclard h.
    bilocular femoral h.
    Birkett h.
    Bochdalek h.
    cecal h.
    cerebral h.
    Cloquet h.
    complete h.
    concealed h.
    congenital diaphragmatic h.
    Cooper h.
    crural h.
    diaphragmatic h.
    direct inguinal h.
    diverticular h.
    double loop h.
    dry h.
    duodenojejunal h.
    h. en bissac
    encysted h.
    epigastric h.
    extrasaccular h.
    fascial h.
    fat h.
    fatty h.
    femoral h.
    foramen of Bochdalek h.
    foraminal h.
    funicular h.
    gastroesophageal h.
    gluteal h.
    Goyrand h.
    Gruber h.
    Grynfeltt h.

Hesselbach h.
Hey h.
hiatal h.
Holthouse h.
iliacosubfascial h.
incarcerated h.
incisional h.
indirect inguinal h.
infantile h.
inguinal h.
inguinocrural h.
inguinofemoral h.
inguinolabial h.
inguinoproperitoneal h.
inguinoscrotal h.
inguinosuperficial h.
intermuscular h.
internal h.
interparietal h.
intersigmoid h.
interstitial h.
intraepiploic h.
intrailiac h.
intrapelvic h.
irreducible h.
ischiatic h.
ischiorectal h.
h. knife
Krönlein h.
labial h.
lateral ventral h.
Laugier h.
levator h.
linea alba h.
Littré h.
Littré-Richard h.
lumbar h.
Malgaigne h.
Maydl h.
meningeal h.
mesenteric h.
mesocolic h.
Morgagni foramen h.
mucosal h.
oblique h.
obturator h.
omental h.
ovarian h.
pannicular h.
pantaloon h.
paraesophageal h.
paraperitoneal h.

parasaccular h.
parasternal h.
paraumbilical h.
parietal h.
pectineal h.
perineal h.
Petit h.
properitoneal h.
pudendal h.
pulsion h.
rectal h.
reducible h.
retrograde h.
retroperitoneal h.
Richter h.
Rokitansky h.
sciatic h.
scrotal h.
sliding h.
slipped h.
strangulated h.
subpubic h.
synovial h.
thyroidal h.
tonsillar h.
Treitz h.
tunicary h.
umbilical h.
uterine h.
vaginal h.
vaginolabial h.
Velpeau h.
ventral h.
vesicle h.
vitreous h.
voluminous h.
Von Bergman h.
hernial
    h. aneurysm
    h. sac
herniated disc
herniation
    caudal transtentorial h.
    cingulate h.
    contained disc h.
    disc h.
    foraminal h.
    noncontained disc h.
    uncal h.
hernioappendectomy
hernioenterotomy
herniography

NOTES

H

hernioid
herniolaparotomy
hernioplasty
herniopuncture
herniorrhaphy
    Bassini h.
herniotome
    Cooper h.
herniotomy
    Petit h.
heroic
heroin overdose syndrome
herpangina
herpes
    h. B encephalomyelitis
    buccal h.
    h. catarrhalis
    h. corneae
    h. digitalis
    h. facialis
    h. febrilis
    genital h.
    h. genitalis
    h. gestationis
    h. gladiatorum
    h. iris
    h. labialis
    lingual h.
    nasal h.
    neonatal h.
    pharyngeal h.
    h. simplex
    h. simplex encephalitis
    h. simplex virus (HSV)
    h. whitlow
    h. zoster
    h. zoster ophthalmicus
    h. zoster oticus
    h. zoster varicellosus
    h. zoster virus
herpesvirus
    cercopithecrine h.
    Herpesvirus saimiri
    human h. 1–8 (HHV)
herpetic
    h. fever
    h. gingivitis
    h. keratitis
    h. keratoconjunctivitis
    h. meningoencephalitis
    h. ulcer
    h. whitlow
herpeticum
    eczema h.
herpetiform aphthae
herpetiformis
    dermatitis h.
    impetigo h.
herpetologist

herpetology
Herpetomonas
Herpetoviridae
herpetovirus
Herring
    H. body
    H. law
herring-worm disease
Herrmann syndrome
hersage
Hers disease
Hershberg test
Hertwig sheath
hertz (Hz)
hertzian experiment
Herxheimer reaction
herz hormone
herzstoss
Heschl gyrus
hesitancy
hesitant
hesperidin
Hess
    H. law
    H. screen
Hesselbach
    H. fascia
    H. hernia
    H. ligament
    H. triangle
hetastarch
heteradelphus
heteralius
heteraxial
heterecious
heterecism
heteresthesia
heteroagglutinin
heteroallele
heteroantibody
heteroantiserum
heteroatom
heteroautoplasty
heteroblastic
heterocellular
heterocentric
heterocephalus
heterocheiral, heterochiral
heterochromatic
heterochromatin
    constitutive h.
    facultative h.
heterochromia
    atrophic h.
    binocular h.
heterochromic
    h. cyclitis
    h. uveitis
heterochromosome

heterochromous
heterochron
heterochronia
heterochronic
heterochronous
heterocladic
heterocrine
heterocrisis
heterocyclic compound
heterocytotropic antibody
heterodetic peptide
heterodisperse
heterodont
heterodromous
heteroduplex
heterodymus
heteroerotic
heteroeroticism
heteroerotism
heterogametic embryo
heterogamous
heterogamy
heterogeneic antigen
heterogeneity
    genetic h.
heterogeneous
    h. nuclear RNA
    h. nucleation
    h. radiation
    h. system
heterogenesis
heterogenetic
    h. antibody
    h. antigen
    h. parasite
heterogenic enterobacterial antigen
heterogenote
heterogenous
    h. graft
    h. keratoplasty
    h. vaccine
heteroglycan
heterogonic life cycle
heterograft
heterokaryon
heterokaryotic
heterokeratoplasty
heterokinesia
heterokinesis
heterolalia
heterolateral
heterolipid

heteroliteral
heterologous
    h. antiserum
    h. desensitization
    h. graft
    h. insemination
    h. protein
    h. serotype
    h. stimulus
    h. tumor
    h. twin
heterology
heterolysin
heterolysis
heterolytic
heteromastigote
heteromeral
heteromeric
    h. cell
    h. peptide
heteromerous
heterometabolous metamorphosis
heterometaplasia
heterometric autoregulation
heterometropia
heteromorphism
heteromorphosis
heteromorphous
heteronomous psychotherapy
heteronomy
heteronuclear
heteronymous
    h. diplopia
    h. hemianopia
    h. image
    h. parallax
heteropagus
heteropathy
heterophagy
heterophemia
heterophemy
heterophil, heterophile
    h. antibody
    h. antigen
    h. hemolysin
heterophonia
heterophoria
heterophthalmus
heterophthongia
heterophyiasis
heterophyid
heterophyidiasis

NOTES

H

heteroplasia
heteroplastic graft
heteroplastid
heteroploid
heteroploidy
heteropolar bond
heteropolysaccharide
heteroproteose
heteropyknosis
heteropyknotic chromatin
heteroreceptor
heterosaccharide
heteroscedasticity
heteroscope
heterosexual
heterosexuality
heteroside
heterosis
heterosmia
heterosomal aberration
heterosome
heterospecific
heterosuggestion
heterotaxia
    cardiac h.
heterotaxic
heterotaxis
heterotaxy
heterothallic
heterotherm
heterothermic
heterotic
heterotonia
heterotopia maculae
heterotopic
    h. bone
    h. graft
    h. pregnancy
    h. stimulus
heterotopous
heterotransplantation
heterotrichosis
heterotroph
heterotrophic oral gastrointestinal cyst
heterotrophy
heterotropia
heterotropy
heterotype mitosis
heterotypical chromosome
heterotypic cortex
heterovaccine therapy
heteroxanthine
heteroxenous parasite
heterozoic
heterozygosis
heterozygosity
heterozygote
    compound h.
    manifesting h.

heterozygous
    doubly h.
Heubner
    H. arteritis
    H. artery
Heuser membrane
HEV
    hepatitis E virus
hexacanth embryo
hexachloride
    gamma benzene h.
hexachlorocyclohexane
hexachlorophane
hexachlorophene
hexacosanoic acid
hexacosanol
hexacosyl
hexad
hexadactylism
hexadactyly
hexadecanoic acid
hexafluorenium bromide
hexamer
hexameric
hexametazime
hexamethylpropyleneamine oxime
hexamidine isethionate
hexamine
hexane
hexanoate
hexanoyl
hexapeptide
hexaploidy
hexaxial reference system
hexazonium salt
hexestrol
hexitol
hexokinase method
hexon antigen
hexone base
hexonic acid
hexosamine
hexosaminidase A, B
hexosan
hexose
    h. monophosphate pathway
    h. monophosphate shunt
    h. phosphatase
hexosebisphosphatase,
    hexosediphosphatase
hexosephosphate isomerase
hexulose
hexuronic acid
hexyl
Hey
    H. amputation
    H. Groves operation
    H. hernia
    H. ligament

Heyer-Pudenz valve
HGE
    human granulocytic ehrlichiosis
HGH
    human growth hormone
HGSIL
    high-grade squamous intraepithelial
      lesion
HGV
    hepatitis G virus
HHV
    human herpesvirus
    human herpesvirus 1–8
hians
    Diphyllobothrium h.
hiatal hernia
hiatopexy
hiatus
    adductor h.
    aortic h.
    Breschet h.
    esophageal h.
    h. ethmoidalis
    fallopian h.
    h. maxillaris
    maxillary h.
    h. sacralis
    semilunar h.
hibernating
    h. gland
    h. myocardium
hibernation
    myocardial h.
hibernoma
    interscapular h.
Hib vaccine
hiccup, hiccough
    epidemic h.
Hickman catheter
HIDA
    dimethyl iminodiacetic acid
    HIDA scan
hidden
    h. border
    h. nail skin
    h. part
hidradenitis suppurativa
hidradenoma
    clear cell h.
    papillary h.
    h. papilliferum
hidroa

hidrocystoma
    apocrine h.
hidromeiosis
hidropoiesis
hidroschesis
hidrosis
hidrotic ectodermal dysplasia
hierarchy
    dominance h.
    Maslow h.
    h. of terms
hierophobia
hierotherapy
high
    h. altitude chamber
    h. convex
    h. dose tolerance
    h. endothelial postcapillary venule
    h. enema
    h. forceps delivery
    h. lip line
    h. lithotomy
    h. molecular weight kininogen
    h. osmolar contrast agent (HOCA)
    h. osmolar contrast medium
      (HOCM)
    h. output failure
    h. pressure oxygen
    h. risk register
    h. spinal anesthesia
    h. wine
high-calorie diet
high-density lipoprotein (HDL)
high-dose-rate brachytherapy
high-egg-passage vaccine
high-energy
    h.-e. compound
    h.-e. phosphate
    h.-e. phosphate bond
higher
    h. order conditioning
    h. order pregnancy
highest
    h. concha
    h. intercostal artery
    h. intercostal vein
    h. nuchal line
    h. thoracic artery
    h. turbinated bone
high-fat diet
high-fiber diet

NOTES

H

high-frequency
    h.-f. current
    h.-f. hearing impairment
    h.-f. transduction
    h.-f. ventilation
high-grade squamous intraepithelial lesion (HGSIL, HSIL)
high-kV technique
Highmore body
high-pass filter
high-performance liquid chromatography
high-pitched rhonchi
high-pressure liquid chromatography (HPLC)
high-quality filter paper
high-resolution
    h.-r. banding
    h.-r. computed tomography (HRCT)
high-steppage gait
high-tension burn
Higoumenakia sign
Hikojima antigen
hila (*pl. of* hilum)
hilar
    h. carcinoma
    h. cell tumor
    h. dance
    h. lymph node
    h. shadow
hilitis
Hill
    H. coefficient
    H. constant
    H. criteria
    H. equation
    H. operation
    H. phenomenon
    H. plot
    H. reaction
    H. sign
Hillis-Müller maneuver
hillock
    axon h.
    facial h.
Hill-Sachs lesion
Hilton
    H. law
    H. method
    H. sac
    H. white line
hilum, pl. **hila**
hilus cell
himantosis
hindbrain vesicle
hindfoot
    h. valgus
    h. varus
hindgut
hind kidney

hindquarter amputation
hindwater
Hines-Brown test
hinge
    h. axis
    h. joint
    h. movement
    h. position
    h. region
hinge-bow
hinged flap
Hinman syndrome
Hinton test
hinzii
    Bordetella h.
hip
    h. bone
    h. joint
    h. phenomenon
    h. pointer
hipberries
hip-flexion phenomenon
hippocampal
    h. commissure
    h. convolution
    h. fissure
    h. gyrus
    h. sclerosis
    h. sulcus
hippocampus
    major h.
    h. major
    minor h.
    h. minor
Hippocrates of Cos
hippocratic
    h. face
    h. facies
    h. finger
    h. nail
    H. Oath
    h. school
    h. succussion
    h. succussion sound
hippocratism
hippurate
    calcium h.
    methenamine h.
hippuria
hippuric acid
hippuricase
hippus
hircismus
hircus, pl. **hirci**
    barbula hirci
Hirschberg
    H. method
    H. test
Hirschfeld canal

Hirsch-Peiffer stain
Hirschsprung disease
hirsute
hirsutism, hirsuties
 constitutional h.
 idiopathic h.
hirtellous
hirudicide
hirudin
hirudiniasis
hirudinization
His
 H. band
 H. bundle
 H. bundle deflection
 H. bundle electrogram (HBE)
 H. copula
 isthmus of H.
 H. line
 H. perivascular space
 H. spindle
Hiss stain
Histalog test
histaminase
histamine
 h. flush
 h. liberator
 h. phosphate
 h. shock
 h. test
histamine-fast
histaminemia
histamine-releasing factor
histaminic
 h. cephalalgia
 h. headache
histaminuria
histangic
His-Tawara system
histidase
histidinal
histidinase
histidine decarboxylase
histidinemia
histidino
histidinuria
histidyl
histioblast
histiocyte
 cardiac h.

histiocytic
 h. leukopenia
 h. lymphoma
histiocytoma
 fibrous h.
 generalized eruptive h.
 malignant fibrous h.
histiocytosis
 Langerhans cell h.
 lipid h.
 malignant h.
 h. X, Y
histiogenic
histioid
histioma
histionic
histoangic
histoblast
histochemistry
histocompatibility
 h. antigen
 h. complex
 h. gene
 h. testing
histocyte
histocytosis
histodifferentiation
histofluorescence
histogenesis
histogenetic
histogenous
histogeny
histogram
histoid
 h. leprosy
 h. neoplasm
 h. tumor
histoincompatibility
histologic
 h. accommodation
 h. lesion
histological internal os
histologist
histology
histolysis
histolytica
 Entamoeba h.
histolyticum
 Clostridium h.
histoma
histometaplastic
histomoniasis

NOTES

H

histomorphometry
histone base
histonectomy
histoneurology
histonomy
histonuria
histopathogenesis
histopathology
histophysiology
Histoplasma capsulatum
histoplasmin
histoplasmin-latex test
histoplasmoma
histoplasmosis
    acute h.
    African h.
    chronic mediastinal h.
    disseminated h.
    presumed ocular h.
historadiography
historrhexis
history
    incongruous h.
    nursing h.
    past medical h. (PMH)
    past surgical h. (PSH)
    h. and physical (H&P)
    h. of present illness (HPI)
    social h.
histotome
histotomy
histotope
histotoxic anoxia
histotroph
histotrophic
histotropic
histozoic
histozyme
histrionic personality disorder
hitchhiker thumb
hitting the wall
Hitzig girdle
HIV
    human immunodeficiency virus
    HIV encephalopathy
    HIV wasting syndrome
HIV-1
    human immunodeficiency virus-1
HIV-2
    human immunodeficiency virus-2
hive
    giant h.'s
HL-7
    Health Level-7
HLA
    human leukocyte antigen
    HLA complex
    HLA typing

HME
    human monocytic ehrlichiosis
H-meromyosin
HMG, hMG
    human menopausal gonadotropin
    HMG CoA-reductase inhibitor
HMO
    health maintenance organization
    group model HMO
    independent practice association
     HMO
    staff model HMO
Hoagland sign
Ho antigen
hoarhound
hoarseness
hobnail
    h. cell
    h. liver
    h. tongue
Hoboken
    H. gemmule
    H. nodule
    H. valve
HOCA
    high osmolar contrast agent
Hoche
    H. bundle
    H. tract
Hochenegg operation
hockey-stick incision
HOCM
    high osmolar contrast medium
    hypertrophic obstructive cardiomyopathy
Hodge pessary
Hodgkin
    H. disease
    H. lymphoma
Hodgkin-Key murmur
Hodgson disease
hodoneuromere
hodophobia
hoe
    h. excavator
    h. scaler
HOECHST 33258
Hofbauer cell
Hoffa operation
Hoffmann
    H. duct
    H. muscular atrophy
    H. phenomenon
    H. reflex
    H. sign
Hoffman violet
Hofmann bacillus
hofmannii
    Corynebacterium h.

Hofmeister
- H. gastrectomy
- H. operation
- H. series

Hofmeister-Pólya anastomosis

hog
- h. cholera vaccine
- h. cholera virus

Hogben number
Hogness box
holandric
- h. gene
- h. inheritance

holarthritic
holarthritis
Holden line
hole
- h. in retina
- h. saw

holiday
- drug h.
- h. heart syndrome

holism
holistic
- h. medicine
- h. psychology

Hollander test
Hollenhorst plaque
Holliday
- H. junction
- H. structure

Holl ligament
hollow
- h. back
- h. bone

hollow-cathode lamp
Holmes
- H. heart
- H. stain

Holmes-Adie
- H.-A. pupil
- H.-A. syndrome

Holmes-Rahe questionnaire
Holmgrén-Golgi canal
Holmgren wool test
holmium
holo-ACP synthase
holoacrania
holoanencephaly
holoblastic cleavage
holocarboxylase synthetase
holocephalic

holocord
holocrine gland
holodiastolic
holoendemic disease
holoenzyme
hologastroschisis
hologram
holography
hologynic inheritance
holomastigote
holometabolous metamorphosis
holomiantic infection
holomorphosis
holophytic
holoprosencephaly
holoprotein
holorachischisis
holoside
holosystolic murmur
holotelencephaly
holothurins
holotrichous
holozoic
Holter monitor
Holthouse hernia
Holt-Oram syndrome
Holzknecht unit
homalocephalous
homaluria
Homans sign
homatropine
homaxial
home
- h. health care
- h. health nurse
- H. lobe
- h. monitor
- nursing h.

homeobox
homeodomain
homeometric autoregulation
homeomorphous
homeopath
homeopathic
homeopathist
homeopathy
homeoplasia
homeoplastic
homeorrhesis
homeosis
homeostasis
- Bernard-Cannon h.

NOTES

homeostasis *(continued)*
    genetic h.
    Lerner h.
    physiologic h.
homeostatic
    h. equilibrium
    h. lag
homeotherapeutic
homeotherapeutics
homeotherapy
homeotherm
homeothermal
homeothermic
homeotic gene
homeotypical
homergy
Homer-Wright rosettes
homidium bromide
homigrade scale
hominal physiology
homing value
hominis
    Blastocystis h.
    Dermatobia h.
    Mycoplasma h.
    poliovirus h.
homoarginine
homobiotin
homoblastic
homocarnosine
homocarnosinosis
homocentric
homochronous
homocitrullinuria
homocladic
homocyclic compound
homocysteine (Hcy)
homocystine
homocystinemia
homocystinuria
homocytotropic antibody
homodetic peptide
homodont
homodromous
homoeroticism
homoerotism
homogametic embryo
homogamy
homogenate
homogeneous
    h. immersion
    h. nucleation
    h. radiation
    h. system
homogenesis
homogenization
homogenize

homogenous
    h. graft
    h. keratoplasty
homogentisic
    h. acid
    h. acid oxidase
homogeny
homoglycan
homogonic life cycle
homograft reaction
homoioplasia
homoiothermal
homokaryon
homokaryotic
homokeratoplasty
homolateral
homolecithal egg
homolipid
homolog, homologue
homologous
    h. antigen
    h. antiserum
    h. chromosome
    h. desensitization
    h. graft
    h. insemination
    h. protein
    h. recombination
    h. series
    h. serotype
    h. serum jaundice
    h. stimulus
    h. tumor
homology
    DNA h.
homolysin
homolysis
homomeric peptide
homomorphic
homonomous
homonomy
homonuclear
homonymous
    h. diplopia
    h. hemianopia
    h. image
    h. parallax
homophene
homophil
homophobia
    internalized h.
homoplastic graft
homoplasty
homopolymer
homoproline
homoprotocatechuic acid
homorganic
homosalate
Homo sapiens

homoscedasticity
homoserine
    h. deaminase
    h. dehydratase
    h. lactone
homosexuality
    ego-dystonic h.
    female h.
    latent h.
    male h.
    overt h.
homosexual panic
homosteroid
homothallic
homothermal
homotonic
homotopic
homotransplantation
homotropic
homotype
homotypical
homotypic cortex
homovanillic
    h. acid
    h. acid test
homozoic
homozygosis
homozygosity
homozygote
homozygous
    h. achondroplasia
    h. by descent
homunculus
honeycomb
    h. lung
    h. macula
    h. pattern
    h. ringworm
honey urine
Hong Kong influenza
hood
    dorsal h.
    H. and Kirklin incision
hooded prepuce
hook
    calvarial h.
    dural h.
    fixation h.
    h. of hamate
    h. of spiral lamina
hookean behavior

hooked
    h. bone
    h. bundle of Russell
    h. fasciculus
Hooke law
hooklet
hook-shaped cataract
hookworm
    h. anemia
    h. disease
Hoover sign
Hopkins rod-lens telescope
Hoplopsyllus anomalus
Hopmann
    H. papilloma
    H. polyp
hordei
    Acarus h.
hordenine
hordeolum
    h. externum
    h. internum
    h. meibomianum
horehound
horizon
    Streeter developmental h.
horizontal
    h. atrophy
    h. beam film
    h. cell
    h. fissure
    h. gaze
    h. growth phase
    h. heart
    h. laryngectomy
    h. mattress suture
    h. maxillary fracture
    h. osteotomy
    h. overlap
    h. plane
    h. plate
    h. resorption
    h. tear
    h. transmission
    h. vertigo
horizontalis
hormesis
hormion
hormogonal
hormonal gingivitis
hormone
    adipokinetic h.

NOTES

H

hormone *(continued)*
    adrenal androgen-stimulating h. (AASH)
    adrenocortical h.
    adrenocorticotropic h. (ACTH)
    adrenomedullary h.
    adrenotropic h.
    androgenic h.
    anterior pituitary-like h.
    antidiuretic h. (ADH)
    anti-müllerian h.
    cardiac h.
    chorionic gonadotrophic h.
    chorionic gonadotropic h.
    corpus luteum h.
    cortical h.
    corticotropic h.
    corticotropin-releasing h. (CRH)
    ectopic h.
    endocrine h.
    erythropoietic h.
    estrogenic h.
    follicle-stimulating h. (FSH)
    follicle-stimulating hormone-releasing h.
    follicular h.
    follitropin-releasing h. (FRH)
    galactopoietic h.
    gametokinetic h.
    gastrointestinal h.
    gonadal h.
    gonadotropic h.
    gonadotropin-releasing h. (GnRH, GRH)
    growth h. (GH)
    growth hormone-inhibiting h. (GIH)
    growth hormone-releasing h. (GH-RH, GHRH)
    heart h.
    herz h.
    human chorionic somatomammotropic h.
    human growth h. (HGH)
    hypophysiotropic h.
    inappropriate h.
    interstitial cell-stimulating h. (ICSH)
    lactation h.
    lactogenic h.
    lipid-mobilizing h.
    lipotropic pituitary h.
    local h.
    luteinizing h. (LH)
    luteinizing hormone-releasing h. (LH-RH, LRH)
    luteotropic h.
    mammotropic h.
    melanocyte-stimulating h.
    melanotropin release-inhibiting h. (MIH)
    melanotropin-releasing h.
    parathyroid h.
    pituitary gonadotropic h.
    pituitary growth h.
    placental growth h.
    progestational h.
    prolactin-inhibiting h.
    prolactin-releasing h.
    proparathyroid h.
    releasing h.
    h. replacement therapy (HRT)
    sex h.
    somatotropic h.
    somatotropin release-inhibiting h.
    somatotropin-releasing h.
    steroid h.
    thyroid-stimulating h.
    thyrotropin-releasing h. (TRH)
hormone-prolactin
    chorionic growth h.-p.
hormonogenesis
hormonogenic
hormonopoiesis
hormonopoietic
hormonoprivia
hormonotherapy
horn
    Ammon h.
    anterior h.
    cicatricial h.
    coccygeal h.
    cutaneous h.
    frontal h.
    iliac h.
    inferior h.
    lateral h.
    posterior h.
    pulp h.
    H. sign
    h. of uterus
    ventral h.
Horner
    H. muscle
    H. pupil
    H. syndrome
    H. teeth
Horner-Trantas dot
horny
    h. cell
    h. layer
horopter
    empirical h.
horripilation
horse
    charley h.
horsefly
horsepower
horsepox virus
horseradish peroxidase

horseshoe
  h. fistula
  h. kidney
  h. placenta
Horsley bone wax
Hortega
  H. cell
  H. neuroglia stain
Horton
  H. arteritis
  H. cephalalgia
  H. headache
hose
  TED h.
hospice
hospital
  acute care h.
  base h.
  camp h.
  closed h.
  day h.
  h. fever
  h. formulary
  h. gangrene
  general h.
  government h.
  group h.
  maternity h.
  mental h.
  h. nurse
  open h.
  h. record
  h. sore throat
  teaching h.
hospital-acquired pneumonia
hospital-based physician
hospitalist
hospitalization
host
  accidental h.
  amplifier h.
  h. cell
  dead-end h.
  definitive h.
  final h.
  graft versus h. (GVH)
  intermediary h.
  intermediate h.
  reservoir h.
hostile behavior
hot
  h. abscess

  h. flash
  h. flush
  h. gangrene
  h. nodule
  h. pack
  h. salt sterilizer
  h. snare
  h. spot
Hottentot tea
hot-wire flow-measuring device
houghtoni
  Diphyllobothrium h.
hound-dog facies
Hounsfield
  H. number
  H. unit
hour
  golden h.
hourglass
  h. chest
  h. contraction
  h. head
  h. murmur
  h. pattern
  h. stomach
  h. vertebra
house
  halfway h.
  h. officer
  h. staff
housefly
housekeeping gene
housemaid's knee
Houssay
  H. animal
  H. phenomenon
  H. syndrome
Houston
  H. fold
  H. muscle
Houston-Harris syndrome
Hovius
  canal of H.
Howard test
Howell-Jolly body
Howell unit
Howship lacunae
Hoyer
  H. anastomosis
  H. canal
H&P
  history and physical

NOTES

H

HPI
> history of present illness

HPL
> human placental lactogen

HPLC
> high-pressure liquid chromatography

HPV
> human papillomavirus

HR conduction time

HRCT
> high-resolution computed tomography

HRT
> hormone replacement therapy

Hruby lens

H-shape vertebra

HSIL
> high-grade squamous intraepithelial lesion

HSV
> herpes simplex virus

HTLV
> human T-cell lymphoma/leukemia virus

HTLV-I
> human T-cell lymphotropic virus, type 1

HTLV-II
> human T-cell lymphotropic virus, type 2

HTLV-III
> human T-cell lymphotropic virus, type 3

H-type tracheoesophageal fistula

Hu antigen

Hubbard tank

Hubrecht protochordal knot

Hückel rule

Hucker-Conn stain

Hudson-Stähli line

Hueck ligament

Hueter maneuver

Hüfner equation

Hughes-Stovin syndrome

Huguier
> H. canal
> H. circle
> H. sinus

Huhner test

Hull triad

hum
> venous h.

human
> h. antihemophilic factor
> h. antihemophilic fraction
> h. antimouse antibody
> h. babesiosis
> h. botfly
> h. botfly myiasis
> h. calorimeter
> chickenpox immune globulin h.
> h. chorionic gonadotropin (HCG, hCG)

> h. chorionic somatomammotropic hormone
> h. chorionic somatomammotropin (HCS)
> h. communication
> h. companionship
> h. diploid cell rabies vaccine
> h. diploid cell vaccine (HDCV)
> h. ecology
> h. ehrlichiosis
> h. eosinophilic enteritis
> h. fibrin foam
> h. fibrinogen
> h. gamma globulin
> h. genetics
> h. glandular kallikrein 3
> h. granulocytic ehrlichiosis (HGE)
> h. growth hormone (HGH)
> h. herpesvirus (HHV)
> h. herpesvirus 1–8 (HHV)
> h. immunodeficiency virus (HIV)
> h. immunodeficiency virus-1 (HIV-1)
> h. immunodeficiency virus-2 (HIV-2)
> h. insulin
> h. interleukin-11
> h. leukocyte antigen (HLA)
> measles immune globulin h.
> h. measles immune serum
> h. menopausal gonadotropin (HMG, hMG)
> h. monocytic ehrlichiosis (HME)
> h. normal immunoglobulin
> h. papilloma virus
> h. papillomavirus (HPV)
> h. pertussis immune serum
> h. placental lactogen (HPL)
> h. plasma protein fraction
> h. scarlet fever immune serum
> h. serum jaundice
> h. T-cell lymphoma/leukemia virus (HTLV)
> h. T-cell lymphotropic virus
> h. T-cell lymphotropic virus, type 1 (HTLV-I)
> h. T-cell lymphotropic virus, type 2 (HTLV-II)
> h. T-cell lymphotropic virus, type 3 (HTLV-III)
> h. thrombin
> h. T lymphotrophic virus

humanistic psychology

humectant

humectation

humeral
> h. articulation
> h. axillary lymph node
> h. head

446

h. joint
h. nutrient artery
humeri (*pl. of* humerus)
humeroradial
h. articulation
h. joint
humeroscapular
humeroulnar
h. head
h. joint
humerus, pl. **humeri**
humidifier
bubble-through h.
hygroscopic condenser h.
humidity
absolute h.
relative h.
humin
Hummelsheim
H. operation
H. procedure
humming rhonchi
humor
aqueous h.
h. aquosus
ocular h.
vitreous h.
h. vitreus
humoral
h. doctrine
h. hypercalcemia
h. immunity
h. pathology
h. regulator
h. theory
humoralism
humoris
humorism
hump
buffalo h.
dowager h.
Hampton h.
humpback
Humphry ligament
humulus
hunchback
hunger
affect h.
air h.
h. contraction
h. pain
h. swelling

Hung method
Hunner ulcer
Hunt
H. neuralgia
H. paradoxic phenomenon
H. syndrome
Hunter
H. canal
H. and Driffield curve
H. glossitis
H. gubernaculum
H. ligament
H. line
H. membrane
H. operation
H. syndrome
Hunter-Schreger
H.-S. band
H.-S. line
Hunter-Thompson dwarfism
hunting
h. reaction
h. response
Huntington
H. chorea
H. disease
Hurler
H. disease
H. syndrome
Hurler-Scheie syndrome
Hurst
H. bougie
H. disease
Hürthle
H. cell
H. cell adenoma
H. cell carcinoma
H. cell tumor
Huschke
H. auditory teeth
H. cartilage
H. foramen
H. valve
Hutchinson
H. crescentic notch
H. facies
H. freckle
H. incisor
H. mask
H. patch
H. pupil

NOTES

H

Hutchinson *(continued)*
    H. teeth
    H. triad
Hutchinson-Gilford
    H.-G. disease
    H.-G. syndrome
Hutchison syndrome
Huxley
    H. layer
    H. membrane
    H. sheath
Huygens
    H. ocular
    H. principle
HV
  half-value
    HV conduction time
    HV interval
HVL
  half-value layer
hyalin
    alcoholic h.
hyaline
    h. body
    h. cartilage
    h. cast
    h. degeneration
    h. leukocyte
    h. membrane
    h. membrane disease
    h. membrane syndrome
    h. necrosis
    h. thrombus
    h. tubercle
hyalinization
hyalinosis
hyalinuria
hyalitis
    suppurative h.
hyalobiuronic acid
hyalocapsular ligament
hyalocyte
hyalogen
hyalohyphomycosis
hyaloid
    h. artery
    h. body
    h. canal
    h. fossa
    h. membrane
hyaloideoretinal degeneration
hyalomere
hyalophagia
hyalophagy
hyalophobia
hyaloplasm
hyaloplasma
hyaloserositis

hyalosis
    asteroid h.
    punctate h.
hyalosome
hyalurate
hyaluronate lyase
hyaluronic
    h. acid
    h. lyase
hyaluronidase
hyaluronoglucosaminidase
hyaluronoglucuronidase
H-Y antigen
hybaroxia
hybenzate
hybrid
    DNA-RNA h.
    h. prosthesis
hybridism
hybridization
    cell h.
    cross h.
    DNA h.
    fluorescence in situ h.
    fluorescent in situ h.
    in situ h.
hybridoma
hyclate
hydantoin
hydantoinate
hydatid
    h. cyst
    h. disease
    h. fremitus
    h. mole
    h. polyp
    h. pregnancy
    h. rash
    h. resonance
    h. sand
    h. thrill
hydatidiform mole
hydatidocele
hydatidoma
hydatidosis
hydatidostomy
hydatoid
hydnocarpus oil
hydracetin
hydradenitis
hydradenoma
hydragogue
hydralazine syndrome
hydrallostane
hydramnion
hydramnios
hydranencephaly
hydrargyria
hydrargyrism

hydrargyrum
hydrarthrodial
hydrarthrosis
  intermittent h.
hydrase
  enoyl h.
hydrastine
hydrastinine
hydrastis
hydratase
  aconitate h.
  enoyl-CoA h.
  fumarate h.
  urocanate h.
hydrate
  aluminum h.
  amyl h.
  amylene h.
  benzoyl h.
  caffeine h.
  h. crystal
  folliculin h.
  h. microcrystal theory
hydrated
  h. alumina
  h. pyelogram
hydration
  absolute h.
hydraulic conductivity
hydrazide
hydrazine yellow
hydrazinolysis
hydrazone
hydremia
hydremic edema
hydrencephalocele
hydrencephalomeningocele
hydrencephalus
hydriatic
hydriatric
hydric
hydride ion
hydrindantin
hydroalcoholic
  h. extract
  h. tincture
hydroappendix
hydrobilirubin
hydrobromate
hydrobromic acid

hydrobromide
  dextromethorphan h.
  hyoscine h.
hydrocalycosis
hydrocarbon
  Diels h.
hydrocele
  cervical h.
  communicating h.
  congenital h.
  cord h.
  Dupuytren h.
  encysted h.
  filarial h.
  funicular h.
  noncommunicating h.
  scrotal h.
hydrocelectomy
hydrocephalic
hydrocephalocele
hydrocephaloid
hydrocephalus
  communicating h.
  congenital h.
  double compartment h.
  external h.
  h. ex vacuo
  internal h.
  noncommunicating h.
  normal pressure h.
  obstructive h.
hydrocephaly
hydrochloric acid
hydrochloride
  cocaine h.
  gonadorelin h.
  tocainide h.
hydrochlorothiazide
hydrocholecystis
hydrocholeresis
hydrocholeretic
hydrocodone
hydrocolloid
  irreversible h.
hydrocolpocele
hydrocolpos
hydrocortisone
hydrocotarnine
hydrocyanism
hydrocyst
hydrocystoma
hydrodiascope

NOTES

H

hydrodipsia
hydrodipsomania
hydrodiuresis
hydrodynamics
hydroelectric bath
hydroencephalocele
hydrogel
hydrogen
    h. acceptor
    activated h.
    arseniureted h.
    h. bond
    h. bromide
    h. carrier
    h. chloride
    h. cyanide
    h. dehydrogenase
    h. dioxide
    h. donor
    h. electrode
    h. exponent
    heavy h.
    h. ion
    h. number
    h. peroxide
    h. phosphide
    h. pump
    h. sulfide
    h. transport
hydrogen-1, -2, -3
hydrogenase
    cytochrome c3 h.
    fumaric h.
hydrogenation
hydrogenlyase
hydrokinetic
hydrokinetics
hydrolabile
hydrolability
hydrolase
    fumarylacetoacetate h.
hydrolyase
hydrolymph
hydrolysate
hydrolysis
hydrolytic cleavage
hydrolyze
hydrolyzing enzyme
hydroma
hydromassage
hydromeningocele
hydrometer
hydrometra
hydrometric
hydrometrocolpos
hydrometry
hydromicrocephaly
hydromphalus
hydromyelia

hydromyelocele
hydromyoma
hydronephrosis
hydronephrotic
hydronium ion
hydroparasalpinx
hydropathic
hydropathy
hydropenia
hydropenic
hydropericarditis
hydropericardium
hydroperitoneum
hydroperitonia
hydroperoxidase
hydroperoxide
hydrophil, hydrophile
    h. colloid
hydrophila
    Aeromonas h.
hydrophilia
hydrophilic
    h. colloid
    h. lens
    h. ointment
    h. petrolatum
hydrophilous
hydrophobia
hydrophobic
    h. bond
    h. colloid
    h. interaction
hydrophthalmia
hydrophthalmos
hydrophthalmus
hydropic degeneration
hydropneumatosis
hydropneumogony
hydropneumopericardium
hydropneumoperitoneum
hydropneumothorax
hydroposia
hydrops
    endolymphatic h.
    fetal h.
    h. fetalis
    immune fetal h.
hydropyonephrosis
hydroquinol
hydroquinone
hydrorchis
hydrorheostat
hydrorrhea
    h. gravidae
    h. gravidarum
hydrosalpinx
    intermittent h.
hydrosarca
hydrosarcocele

hydrosol
hydrosphygmograph
hydrostat
hydrostatic
    h. dilator
    h. pressure
    h. weighing
hydrosudopathy
hydrosudotherapy
hydrosyringomyelia
hydrotaxis
hydrotherapeutic
hydrotherapeutics
hydrotherapy
hydrothermal
hydrothionemia
hydrothionuria
hydrothorax
    chylous h.
hydrotomy
hydrotropism
hydrotubation
hydroureter
hydroureteronephrosis
hydrous wool fat
hydrovarium
hydroxamic acid
hydroxide
    aluminum h.
    barium h.
    bismuth h.
    calcium h.
    corticotropin-zinc h.
    ferric h.
    magnesium h.
hydroxocobalamin
hydroxocobemine
hydroxyacetic acid
hydroxy acid
hydroxyanisole
    butylated h.
hydroxyapatite
    amorphous h.
hydroxybenzoate
    methyl h.
hydroxycarbamide
hydroxychloroquine sulfate
hydroxychroman
hydroxychromene
hydroxyephedrine
hydroxyfatty acid
hydroxyhemin

hydroxykynureninuria
hydroxyl
hydroxylapatite
hydroxylase
hydroxylation
hydroxynervone
hydroxynervonic acid
hydroxyphenyluria
hydroxyprolinemia
hydroxystilbamidine isethionate
hydroxytoluene
    butylated h.
hydroxytoluic acid
hydroxytryptophan decarboxylase
hydroxyurea
hydroxyzine
hygieiology
hygiene
    bronchial h.
    criminal h.
    industrial h.
    mental h.
    oral h.
hygienic laboratory coefficient
hygienist
    dental h.
hygric acid
hygroma
    cervical h.
    cystic h.
hygrometer
hygrometry
hygrophobia
hygroscopic
    h. condenser humidifier
    h. expansion
hygrostomia
hyla
hylephobia
hymen
    h. bifenestratus
    h. biforis
    cribriform h.
    denticulate h.
    imperforate h.
    infundibuliform h.
    h. sculptatus
    h. subseptus
hymenal
    h. caruncula
    h. cyst

NOTES

H

hymenal *(continued)*
    h. membrane
    h. orifice
hymenectomy
hymenitis
hymenoid
hymenolepiasis
hymenolepidid
hymenology
hymenorrhaphy
hymenotomy
hyobranchial cleft
hyoepiglottic ligament
hyoepiglottidean
hyoglossal
    h. membrane
    h. muscle
hyoglossus muscle
hyoid
    h. apparatus
    h. arch
    h. bone
    lesser horn of h.
hyointestinalis
    Campylobacter h.
hyomandibular cleft
hyoscine hydrobromide
hyoscyamine sulfate
hyoscyamus
hyothyroid
hypacusis, hypacusia
hypalbuminemia
hypalgesia
hypalgesic
hypalgetic
hypamnion
hypamnios
hypanakinesia, hypanakinesis
Hypaque
    H. enema
    H. swallow
hyparterial bronchus
hypaxial
hypazoturia
hypencephalon
hypengyophobia
hyperabduction syndrome
hyperacidity
hyperactive child syndrome
hyperactivity
hyperacusia
hyperacusis
hyperacute
    h. purulent conjunctivitis
    h. rejection
hyperadenosis
hyperadiposis
hyperadiposity
hyperadrenalcorticalism

hyperadrenocorticalism
hyperalaninemia
hyperaldosteronism
hyperalgesia
hyperalgesic
hyperalgetic
hyperalimentation
    enteral h.
    total parenteral h.
hyperallantoinuria
hyperalphalipoproteinemia
hyperaminoaciduria
hyperammonemia
hyperamylasemia
hyperanakinesia, hyperanacinesia
hyperanakinesis, hyperanacinesis
hyperaphia
hyperaphic
hyperargininemia
hyperbaric
    h. chamber
    h. medicine
    h. oxygen
    h. oxygenation
    h. oxygen therapy
    h. spinal anesthesia
hyperbarism
hyperbasic aminoaciduria
hyperbetalipoproteinemia
    familial h.
hyperbilirubinemia
    constitutional h.
    neonatal h.
hyperbrachycephaly
hypercalcemia
    humoral h.
    idiopathic h.
hypercalcemic
    h. sarcoidosis
    h. uremia
hypercalciuria, hypercalcinuria
hypercalcuria
hypercapnia
hypercapnic acidosis
hypercarbia
hypercardia
hypercatabolic
hypercatabolism
hypercatharsis
hypercathexis
hypercementosis
hyperchloremia
hyperchloremic acidosis
hyperchlorhydria
hyperchloruria
hypercholesteremia
hypercholesterinemia
hypercholesterolemia
    familial h.

hypercholesterolia
hypercholia
hyperchromaffinism
hyperchromasia
hyperchromatic
  h. anemia
  h. macrocythemia
hyperchromatism
hyperchromia
  macrocytic h.
hyperchromic
  h. anemia
  h. effect
hyperchylia
hyperchylomicronemia
  familial h.
hypercinesia (var. of hyperkinesia)
hypercinesis (var. of hyperkinesis)
hypercoagulability
hypercoagulable
hypercorticoidism
hypercortisolism
hypercryalgesia
hypercryesthesia
hypercupremia
hypercyanotic angina
hypercyesis, hypercyesia
hypercythemia
hypercytochromia
hypercytosis
hyperdicrotic
hyperdicrotism
hyperdiploid
hyperdipsia
hyperdistention
hyperechoic
hyperekplexia
hyperemesis
  h. gravidarum
  h. lactentium
hyperemetic
hyperemia
  active h.
  arterial h.
  Bier h.
  collateral h.
  constriction h.
  fluxionary h.
  passive h.
  reactive h.
  venous h.
hyperemic

hyperencephaly
hyperendemic disease
hypereosinophilia
hypereosinophilic syndrome
hyperergasia
hyperergia
hyperergic encephalitis
hypererythrocythemia
hyperesophoria
hyperesthesia
  auditory h.
  cervical h.
  gustatory h.
  h. olfactoria
  h. optica
hyperesthetic
hypereuryprosopic
hyperexophoria
hyperextension
hyperextension-hyperflexion injury
hyperferremia
hyperfibrinogenemia
hyperfibrinolysis
hyperflexion
hyperfractionated radiation
hyperfructosemia
hyperfunction
hyperfunctional occlusion
hypergalactosis
hypergammaglobulinemia
hyperganglionosis
hypergenesis
hypergenetic
hypergenic teratosis
hypergenitalism
hypergeusia
hypergia
hypergic
hyperglandular
hyperglobulia
hyperglobulinemia
hyperglobulinemic purpura
hyperglobulism
hyperglycemia
  ketotic h.
hyperglycemic-glycogenolytic factor
hyperglyceridemia
  endogenous h.
  exogenous h.
hyperglycerolemia
  infantile-type h.
  juvenile-type h.

NOTES

H

453

hyperglycinemia
   ketotic h.
hyperglycinuria
hyperglycogenolysis
hyperglycorrhachia
hyperglycosemia
hyperglycosuria
hyperglyoxylemia
hypergnosis
hypergonadism
hypergonadotropic
   h. eunuchoidism
   h. hypogonadism
hypergranulosis
hyperguanidinemia
hypergynecosmia
hyperhedonia
hyperhedonism
hyperhemoglobinemia
hyperheparinemia
hyperhidrosis
   gustatory h.
hyperhydration
hyperhydrochloria
hyperhydrochloridia
hyperhydropexis
hyperhydropexy
hyperhydroxyprolinemia
hyperidrosis
hyper-IgM syndrome
hyperimidodipeptiduria
hyperimmune serum
hyperimmunity
hyperimmunization
hyperimmunoglobulin E syndrome
hyperindicanemia
hyperinfection
hyperinflation
hyperinosemia
hyperinosis
hyperinsulinemia
hyperinsulinism
   alimentary h.
   functional h.
   iatrogenic h.
hyperinvolution
hyperisotonic
hyperkalemia, hyperkaliemia
hyperkalemic periodic paralysis
hyperkaluresis
hyperkeratinization
hyperkeratosis
   h. congenita
   diffuse h.
   epidermolytic h.
   generalized epidermolytic h.
hyperketonemia
hyperketonuria
hyperkinemia

hyperkinesia, hypercinesia
hyperkinesis, hypercinesis
hyperkinetic
   h. dysarthria
   h. heart syndrome
hyperlactation
hyperleukocytosis
hyperlexia
hyperlipemia
   carbohydrate-induced h.
   familial combined h.
   familial fat-induced h.
   familial hypercholesterolemia
     with h.
   idiopathic h.
   mixed h.
hyperlipidemia
   mixed h.
hyperlipoidemia
hyperlipoproteinemia
   acquired h.
   familial h.
   type I–V familial h.
hyperliposis
hyperlithuria
hyperlogia
hyperlordosis
hyperlucent lung
hyperlysinemia
hyperlysinuria
hypermagnesemia
hypermastia
hypermature cataract
hypermenorrhea
hypermetabolism
   extrathyroidal h.
hypermetamorphosis
hypermethioninemia
hypermetria
hypermetrope
hypermetropia
   index h.
hypermnesia
hypermobility
hypermorph
hypermotor seizure
hypermyotonia
hypermyotrophy
hypernasality
hypernatremia
hypernatremic encephalopathy
hyperneocytosis
hypernephroid
hypernoia
hypernomic
hypernormal
hypernutrition
hyperoncotic
hyperonychia

hyperope
hyperopia
    absolute h.
    axial h.
    curvature h.
    facultative h.
    latent h.
    manifest h.
    total h.
hyperopic astigmatism
hyperorality
hyperorchidism
hyperorexia
hyperornithinemia
hyperorthocytosis
hyperosmia
hyperosmolality
hyperosmolarity
hyperosmolar nonketotic coma
hyperosmotic
hyperosteoidosis
hyperostosis
    ankylosing h.
    diffuse idiopathic skeletal h.
    (DISH)
    flowing h.
    generalized cortical h.
    infantile cortical h.
hyperostotic spondylosis
hyperovarianism
hyperoxaluria
hyperoxia
hyperoxidation
hyperpancreatism
hyperparasite
hyperparasitism
hyperparathyroidism
hyperparotidism
hyperpathia
hyperpepsia
hyperpepsinia
hyperperistalsis
hyperphagia
hyperphalangism
hyperphenylalaninemia
    malignant h.
hyperphonesis
hyperphonia
hyperphoria
hyperphosphatasemia
hyperphosphatasia
hyperphosphatemia

hyperphosphaturia
hyperphrenia
hyperpiesis, hyperpiesia
hyperpietic
hyperpigmentation
hyperpipecolatemia
hyperpipecolic acidemia
hyperpituitarism
hyperplasia
    adenomatous h.
    angiofollicular mediastinal lymph
     node h.
    angiolymphoid h.
    atypical endometrial h.
    atypical melanocytic h.
    basal cell h.
    benign giant lymph node h.
    benign prostatic h. (BPH)
    cementum h.
    complex endometrial h.
    congenital virilizing adrenal h.
    cystic prostatic h.
    denture h.
    ductal h.
    endometrial h.
    fibromuscular h.
    focal epithelial h.
    follicular h.
    gingival h.
    inflammatory fibrous h.
    inflammatory papillary h.
    intravascular papillary endothelial h.
    polypoid h.
    simple endometrial h.
    Swiss-cheese h.
hyperplastic
    h. arteriosclerosis
    h. gingivitis
    h. inflammation
    h. osteoarthritis
    h. polyp
    h. pulpitis
hyperpnea
hyperpolarization
hyperponesis
hyperpotassemia
hyperprebetalipoproteinemia
    familial h.
hyperprochoresis
hyperproinsulinemia
hyperprolactinemia
hyperprolactinemic amenorrhea

NOTES

H

hyperprolinemia
hyperproteinemia
hyperproteosis
hyperpyretic
hyperpyrexia
    fulminant h.
    heat h.
    malignant h.
hyperpyrexial
hyperreactive malarious splenomegaly
hyperreflexia
    autonomic h.
    detrusor h.
hyperreflexic bladder
hyperresonance
hyperresonant
hyperrhinophonia
hypersalemia
hypersaline
hypersalivation
hypersarcosinemia
hypersecretion
    gastric h.
    h. glaucoma
    mucous h.
hypersegmentation
    hereditary h.
hypersegmented neutrophil
hypersensibility
hypersensitive
    h. dentin
    h. xiphoid syndrome
hypersensitivity
    h. angiitis
    contact h.
    delayed h.
    delayed-type h. (DTH)
    immediate h.
    h. pneumonitis
    h. reaction
    h. vasculitis
hypersensitization
hyperserotonemia
hyperskeocytosis
hypersomatotropism
hypersomnia
    paroxysmal h.
    periodic h.
hypersonic
hypersphyxia
hypersplenism
hypersteatosis
hypersthenia
hypersthenic
hypersthenuria
hypersusceptibility
hypersystole
hypersystolic

hypertelorism
    Bixler type h.
    canthal h.
    ocular h.
hypertensinogen
hypertension
    accelerated h.
    adrenal h.
    benign h.
    borderline h.
    episodic h.
    essential h.
    gestational h.
    Goldblatt h.
    idiopathic h.
    labile h.
    malignant h.
    paroxysmal h.
    portal h.
    pregnancy-induced h.
    pulmonary h.
    renal h.
    renovascular h.
    secondary h.
hypertensive
    h. arteriopathy
    h. arteriosclerosis
    h. crisis
    h. encephalopathy
    h. renal disease
    h. retinopathy
    h. upper esophageal sphincter
    h. vascular disease
hypertensor
hypertestoidism
hyperthecosis
hyperthelia
hyperthermalgesia
hyperthermia
    malignant h.
hyperthermoesthesia
hyperthrombinemia
hyperthymia
hyperthymic
hyperthymism
hyperthymization
hyperthyrea
hyperthyroid heart
hyperthyroidism
    apathetic h.
    factitious h.
    hereditary h.
    iodine-induced h.
    masked h.
hyperthyroxinemia
hypertonia polycythemica
hypertonica
    polycythemia h.
hypertonic bladder

hypertonicity
hypertoxic
hypertrichiasis
hypertrichophrydia
hypertrichosis
hypertriglyceridemia
    familial h.
hypertroph
hypertrophia
hypertrophic
    h. arthritis
    h. cervical pachymeningitis
    h. dystrophy
    h. gastritis
    h. hypersecretory gastropathy
    h. interstitial neuropathy
    h. obstructive cardiomyopathy
    (HOCM)
    h. pulmonary osteoarthropathy
    h. pulpitis
    h. pyloric stenosis
    h. rhinitis
    h. rosacea
    h. scar
hypertrophica
    acne h.
hypertrophicus
    lichen planus h.
hypertrophy
    adaptive h.
    adenoid h.
    benign prostatic h. (BPH)
    compensatory h.
    complementary h.
    concentric h.
    eccentric h.
    endemic h.
    false h.
    functional h.
    giant h.
    hemangiectatic h.
    lipomatous h.
    myocardial h.
    physiologic h.
    ventricular h.
    vicarious h.
hypertropia
hypertyrosinemia
hyperuracil thyminuria
hyperuricemia
hyperuricemic
hyperuricuria

hypervaccination
hypervalinemia
hypervariable region
hypervascular
hyperventilation
    h. syndrome
    h. test
    h. tetany
hyperviscosity syndrome
hypervitaminosis
hypervolemia
hypervolemic
hypervolia
hypesthesia
hypha
hyphedonia
hyphema
hyphemia
    intertropical h.
hypnagogic
    h. hallucination
    h. image
hypnagogue
hypnapagogic
hypnoanalysis
hypnoanalytic
hypnocatharsis
hypnocyst
hypnogenesis
hypnogenetic spot
hypnogenic spot
hypnogenous
hypnoidal
hypnoid state
hypnophobia
hypnopompic
    h. hallucination
    h. image
hypnosis
    lethargic h.
    major h.
    minor h.
hypnotherapy
hypnotic
    h. psychotherapy
    h. relationship
    h. sleep
    h. state
    h. suggestion
hypnotism
hypnotist
hypnotize

NOTES

H

hypnozoite
hypoacidity
hypoacusis
hypoadenia
hypoadrenalism
hypoalbuminemia
hypoaldosteronism
    hyporeninemic h.
    isolated h.
hypoaldosteronuria
hypoalgesia
hypoalimentation
hypoazoturia
hypobaria
hypobaric spinal anesthesia
hypobarism
hypobaropathy
hypobetalipoproteinemia
    familial h.
hypoblast
hypoblastic
hypobranchial eminence
hypobromite
hypobromous acid
hypocalcemia
    neonatal h. (NHC)
hypocalcemic cataract
hypocalcification
    enamel h.
hypocapnia
hypocarbia
hypocelom
hypochloremia
hypochloremic
hypochlorhydria
hypochlorite
hypochlorous acid
hypochloruria
hypocholesteremia
hypocholesterolemia, hypocholesterinemia
hypocholia
hypochondria
hypochondriacal
    h. melancholia
    h. neurosis
hypochondriac region
hypochondrial reflex
hypochondriasis
hypochondrium
hypochondroplasia
hypochordal
hypochromasia
hypochromatic
hypochromatism
hypochromia
hypochromic
    h. effect
    h. microcytic anemia
hypochrosis

hypochylia
hypocinesia
hypocinesis
hypocitraturia
hypocomplementemia
hypocomplementemic
    h. glomerulonephritis
    h. vasculitis
hypocone
hypoconid
hypoconule
hypoconulid
hypocorticoidism
hypocupremia
hypocycloidal tomography
hypocystotomy
hypocythemia
hypocytosis
hypodactylia
hypodactylism
hypodactyly
hypoderm
hypodermatoclysis
hypodermatomy
hypodermatosis
hypodermic
    h. injection
    h. needle
    h. syringe
    h. tablet
hypodermis
hypodermoclysis
hypodiploid
hypodipsia
hypodontia
hypodynamia cordis
hypodynamic
hypoeccrisis
hypoeccritic
hypoechoic
hypoeosinophilia
hypoesophoria
hypoesthesia
    acoustic h.
    olfactory h.
    tactile h.
hypoexophoria
hypoferremia
hypoferric anemia
hypofibrinogenemia
hypofractionated radiation
hypofrontality
hypofunction
hypogalactia
hypogalactous
hypogammaglobinemia
hypogammaglobulinemia
    acquired h.

transient h.
X-linked infantile h.
hypoganglionosis
hypogastric
    h. artery
    h. ganglion
    h. nerve
    h. reflex
    h. region
    h. vein
hypogastrium
hypogastrocele
hypogastropagus
hypogastroschisis
hypogenesis
hypogenetic
hypogenitalism
hypogeusia
hypoglobulia
hypoglossal
    h. canal
    h. eminence
    h. nerve
    h. nucleus
    h. trigone
hypoglottis
hypoglycemia
    fasting h.
    ketotic h.
    leucine-induced h.
    leucine-sensitive h.
    mixed h.
hypoglycemic coma
hypoglycogenolysis
hypoglycorrhachia
hypognathous
hypognathus
hypogonadism
    familial hypogonadotropic h.
    hypergonadotropic h.
    hypogonadotropic h.
    hypothalamic obesity with h.
    male h.
    h. with anosmia
hypogonadotropic
    h. eunuchoidism
    h. hypogonadism
hypogranulocytosis
hypohepatia
hypohidrosis
hypohidrotic ectodermal dysplasia
hypohydration

hypohydremia
hypohydrochloria
hypoisotonic
hypokalemia
hypokalemic
    h. alkalosis
    h. nephropathy
    h. periodic paralysis
hypokinemia
hypokinesis, hypokinesia
hypokinetic dysarthria
hypoleukemia
hypoleydigism
hypolipoproteinemia
hypoliposis
hypologia
hypolymphemia
hypomagnesemia
hypomania
hypomastia
hypomelancholia
hypomelanosis of Ito
hypomelia
hypomenorrhea
hypomere
hypometabolic
    h. state
    h. syndrome
hypometabolism
    euthyroid h.
hypometria
hypomnesia
hypomorph
hypomotility
hypomotor seizure
hypomyelination
hypomyelinogenesis
hypomyotonia
hypomyxia
hyponasality
hyponatremia
    depletional h.
    dilutional h.
hyponeocytosis
hyponoia
hyponychial
hyponychium
hyponychon
hypooncotic
hypoorthocytosis
hypoovarianism
hypopancreatism

NOTES

H

hypopancreorrhea
hypoparathyroidism
    familial h.
    immunodeficiency with h.
    h. syndrome
hypoparathyroid tetany
hypopepsia
hypoperistalsis
hypophalangism
hypopharyngeal diverticulum
hypopharyngoscope
hypopharynx
hypophonesis
hypophonia
hypophoria
hypophosphatasemia
hypophosphatasia
    adult h.
    childhood h.
    congenital h.
hypophosphatemia
hypophosphaturia
hypophosphite
    calcium h.
hypophosphorous acid
hypophrasia
hypophyseal (*var. of* hypophysial)
hypophysectomize
hypophysectomy
hypophyseoportal system
hypophyseopriva
    cachexia h.
hypophyseoprivic
hypophyseotropic
hypophysial, hypophyseal
    h. amenorrhea
    h. cachexia
    h. duct
    h. dwarf
    h. fossa
    h. infantilism
    h. portal circulation
    h. portal system
    h. pouch
    h. syndrome
hypophysin
hypophysioportal system
hypophysioprivic
hypophysiosphenoidal syndrome
hypophysiotropic hormone
hypophysis
    h. cerebri
    h. sicca
hypophysitis
    lymphocytic h.
    lymphoid h.
hypopiesis
hypopigmentation
hypopituitarism

hypoplasia
    adrenal h.
    cartilage-hair h.
    congenital generalized muscular h.
    craniofacial h.
    enamel h.
    focal dermal h.
    renal h.
hypoplastic
    h. anemia
    h. fetal chondrodystrophy
    h. heart
    h. left heart syndrome
hypopnea
hypoposia
hypopotassemia
hypopraxia
hypoproaccelerinemia
hypoproconvertinemia
hypoproteinemia
hypoproteinosis
hypoprothrombinemia
hypoptyalism
hypopyon ulcer
hyporeflexia
hyporeninemia
hyporeninemic hypoaldosteronism
hyporhinophonia
hyporiboflavinosis
hyposalivation
hyposcheotomy
hyposcleral
hyposensitivity
hyposensitization
hyposkeocytosis
hyposmia
hyposmosis
hyposmotic
hyposomatotropism
hyposomia
hyposomniac
hypospadiac
hypospadias
    balanic h.
    coronal h.
    glanular h.
    penile h.
    perineal h.
    scrotal h.
hyposphygmia
hyposplenism
hypostasis
hypostatic
    h. abscess
    h. congestion
    h. ectasia
    h. pneumonia
hyposthenia
hyposthenic

hyposthenuria
hypostome
hypostomia
hypostosis
hyposupradrenalism
hyposystole
hypotelorism
hypotension
    arterial h.
    controlled h.
    idiopathic orthostatic h.
    induced h.
    intracranial h.
    orthostatic h.
hypotensive anesthesia
hypotensor
hypothalamic
    h. amenorrhea
    h. infundibulum
    h. obesity
    h. obesity with hypogonadism
    h. sulcus
hypothalamocerebellar fiber
hypothalamohypophysial
    h. portal circulation
    h. portal system
    h. tract
hypothalamospinal fiber
hypothalamus
hypothenar
    h. eminence
    h. fascia
    h. prominence
hypothermal
hypothermia
    accidental h.
    moderate h.
    regional h.
    total body h.
hypothermic anesthesia
hypothesis
    adaptor h.
    alternative h.
    autocrine h.
    Avogadro h.
    Bayesian h.
    frustration-aggression h.
    gate-control h.
    Goldie-Coldman h.
    Gompertz h.
    insular h.
    Knudsen h.

    Lyon h.
    Makeham h.
    Michaelis-Menten h.
    mnemic h.
    monoamine h.
    null h.
    Starling h.
    upregulation/downregulation h.
    zwitter h.
hypothetical
    h. mean organism
    h. mean strain
hypothrombinemia
hypothromboplastinemia
hypothymia
hypothymic
hypothymism
hypothyroid
    h. dwarf
    h. dwarfism
    h. infantilism
    h. obesity
hypothyroidism
    congenital h.
    infantile h.
hypothyroxinemia
hypotonia
    benign congenital h.
hypotonic
hypotonicity
hypotonus
hypotony
    ocular h.
hypotoxicity
hypotrichiasis
hypotrichosis
hypotrophy
hypotropia
hypotympanotomy
hypotympanum
hypouresis
hypouricemia
hypouricuria
    hereditary renal h.
hypovarianism
hypoventilation coma
hypovitaminosis
hypovolemia
hypovolemic shock
hypovolia
hypoxanthine
hypoxemia test

NOTES

H

hypoxemic
hypoxia
  anemic h.
  diffusion h.
  hypoxic h.
  ischemic h.
  oxygen affinity h.
  h. warning system
hypoxic
  h. hypoxia
  h. ischemic encephalopathy
  h. nephrosis
hypoxic-hypercarbic encephalopathy
hypsarhythmia
hypsarrhythmia
hypsibrachycephalic
hypsicephaly
hypsiconchous
hypsiloid
  h. angle
  h. cartilage
  h. ligament
hypsistaphylia
hypsistenocephalic
hypsocephaly
hypsochromic
hypsodont
hypurgia
Hyrtl
  H. anastomosis
  H. epitympanic recess
  H. foramen
  H. loop
  H. sphincter
hysteralgia
hysteratresia
hysterectomy
  abdominal h.
  abdominovaginal h.
  cesarean h.
  chemical h.
  laparoscopic-assisted vaginal h.
  modified radical h.
  paravaginal h.
  partial h.
  radical h.
  supracervical h.
  supravaginal h.
  vaginal h.
hysteresis
hystereurysis
hysteria
  anxiety h.
  conversion h.
  degenerative h.
  dissociative h.
  epidemic h.
  fixation h.
  masked h.

  mass h.
  minor h.
hysterical, hysteric
  h. amblyopia
  h. anesthesia
  h. aphonia
  h. ataxia
  h. blindness
  h. chorea
  h. convulsion
  h. field
  h. gait
  h. hearing impairment
  h. joint
  h. neurosis
  h. paralysis
  h. personality
  h. personality disorder
  h. polydipsia
  h. pregnancy
  h. psychosis
  h. rigidity
  h. syncope
  h. torticollis
  h. tremor
  h. vertigo
  h. vomiting
hysterics
hystericus
  globus h.
hysterocatalepsy
hysterocele
hysterocleisis
hysterocolposcope
hysterocystopexy
hysterodynia
hysteroepilepsy
hysterogenic
hysterogenous
hysterogram
hysterograph
hysterography
hysteroid convulsion
hysterolysis
hysterometer
hysteromyoma
hysteromyomectomy
hysteromyotomy
hystero-oophorectomy
hysteropathy
hysteropexy
  abdominal h.
hysteroplasty
hysterorrhaphy
hysterorrhexis
hysterosalpingectomy
hysterosalpingography
hysterosalpingo-oophorectomy
hysterosalpingostomy

hysteroscope
    contact h.
    flexible h.
hysteroscopy
hysterospasm
hysterostat
hysterosystole
hysterothermometry
hysterotome

hysterotomy
    abdominal h.
hysterotrachelectomy
hysterotracheloplasty
hysterotrachelorrhaphy
hysterotrachelotomy
hysterotubography
Hz
    hertz

NOTES

H

463

I
- I antigen
- I band
- I cell
- I disc
- I region

IAHS
- infection-associated hemophagocytic syndrome

IAP
- intermittent acute porphyria

iatraliptic
iatric
iatrochemical
iatrochemist
iatrochemistry
iatrogenic
- i. hyperinsulinism
- i. pneumothorax
- i. transmission

iatrology
iatromathematical school
iatromechanical
iatrophysical
iatrophysicist
iatrophysics
iatrotechnique
IBC
- iron-binding capacity

ibogaine
ibotenic acid
ibuprofen
iccosomes
ice
- dry i.
- i. pack
- i. pick headache

Iceland
- I. disease
- I. moss

I-cell disease
ICF
- intermediate care facility
- intracellular fluid

ichor
ichoremia
ichoroid
ichorous pus
ichorrhea
ichorrhemia
ichthammol
ichthyism
ichthyohemotoxin
ichthyohemotoxism
ichthyoid

ichthyootoxin
ichthyophagous
ichthyophobia
ichthyosarcotoxin
ichthyosarcotoxism
ichthyosiform erythroderma
ichthyosis
- acquired i.
- i. congenita
- i. fetalis
- harlequin i.
- lamellar i.
- i. simplex
- i. vulgaris

ichthyotic
ichthyotoxicology
ichthyotoxicon
ichthyotoxin
ichthyotoxism
icing heart
ICM
- intercostal margin

iconic sign
icosahedral
ICP
- intracranial pressure

ICSH
- interstitial cell-stimulating hormone

ictal
icteric
icteroanemia
icterogenic
icterohematuric
icterohemoglobinuria
icterohemorrhagic fever
icterohepatitis
icteroid
icterus
- acquired hemolytic i.
- benign familial i.
- chronic familial i.
- congenital hemolytic i.
- cythemolytic i.
- i. gravis
- infectious i.
- i. melas
- i. neonatorum
- physiologic i.
- i. praecox
- scleral i.

ictometer
ictus
- i. cordis
- i. epilepticus

ictus *(continued)*
  i. paralyticus
  i. solis
ICU
  intensive care unit
  ICU psychosis
IDDM
  insulin-dependent diabetes mellitus
idea
  autochthonous i.
  compulsive i.
  dominant i.
  fixed i.
  flight of i.'s
  i. of reference
ideal
  i. alveolar gas
  ego i.
ideation
ideational
idée fixe
identical twin
identification
  projective i.
  synthetic sentence i.
identity
  i. crisis
  i. disorder
  ego i.
  gender i.
  i. matrix
ideokinetic apraxia
ideology
ideomotion
ideomotor apraxia
ideophobia
idioagglutinin
idiodynamic control
idiogenesis
idioglossia
idioglottic
idiogram
idiographic approach
idioheteroagglutinin
idioheterolysin
idiohypnotism
idioisoagglutinin
idioisolysin
idiojunctional rhythm
idiolalia
idiolysin
idiomuscular contraction
idionodal rhythm
idiopathetic
idiopathic
  i. abscess
  i. aldosteronism
  i. bilateral vestibulopathy
  i. bone cavity

  i. bradycardia
  i. cardiomyopathy
  i. disease
  i. epilepsy
  i. fibrous mediastinitis
  i. fibrous retroperitonitis
  i. gout
  i. hirsutism
  i. hypercalcemia
  i. hypercalcemic sclerosis
  i. hyperlipemia
  i. hypertension
  i. hypertrophic osteoarthropathy
  i. hypertrophic subaortic stenosis
  i. infantilism
  i. interstitial fibrosis
  i. megacolon
  i. myocarditis
  i. myoglobinuria
  i. neuralgia
  i. neutropenia
  i. orthostatic hypotension
  i. paroxysmal rhabdomyolysis
  i. proctitis
  i. pulmonary fibrosis (IPF)
  i. pulmonary hemosiderosis
  i. roseola
  i. stabbing headache
  i. subglottic stenosis
  i. thrombocytopenic purpura (ITP)
idiopathy
idiophrenic
idiopsychologic
idioreflex
idiosome
idiosyncrasy
idiosyncratic sensitivity
idiotope
idiot-prodigy
idiotrophic
idiotropic
idiot-savant
idiotype autoantibody
idiotypic
  i. antibody
  i. antigenic determinant
idioventricular
  i. kick
  i. rhythm
iditol
IDL
  intermediate density lipoprotein
idose
idoxuridine
id reaction
iduronate sulfatase
iduronic acid
IEP
  isoelectric point

IF
  initiation factor
Ig
  immunoglobulin
IgA
  immunoglobulin A
    IgA nephropathy
IgD
  immunoglobulin D
IgE
  immunoglobulin E
IGF
  insulinlike growth factor
IgG
  immunoglobulin G
IgM
  immunoglobulin M
    immunodeficiency with elevated
      IgM
    IgM nephropathy
ignatia
ignipedites
ignipuncture
ignotine
IH
  infectious hepatitis
IJP
  inhibitory junction potential
ikota
IL-1
  interleukin-1
IL-2
  interleukin-2
IL-3
  interleukin-3
IL-4
  interleukin-4
IL-5
  interleukin-5
IL-6
  interleukin-6
IL-7
  interleukin-7
IL-8
  interleukin-8
IL-9
  interleukin-9
IL-10
  interleukin-10
IL-11
  interleukin-11

IL-12
  interleukin-12
IL-13
  interleukin-13
IL-14
  interleukin-14
IL-15
  interleukin-15
IL-16
  interleukin-16
IL-17
  interleukin-17
IL-18
  interleukin-18
ILA
  insulinlike activity
ileac
ileal
    i. artery
    i. atresia
    i. bladder
    i. conduit
    i. intussusception
    i. orifice
    i. papilla
    i. sphincter
    i. ureter
    i. vein
ileale
    ostium i.
ileectomy
ileitis
    backwash i.
    distal i.
    regional i.
    terminal i.
ileoanal pouch
ileocecal
    i. eminence
    i. fold
    i. intussusception
    i. junction
    i. opening
    i. orifice
    i. tuberculosis
    i. valve
ileocecocolic sphincter
ileocecocystoplasty
ileocecostomy
ileocecum
ileocolic
    i. artery

NOTES

ileocolic *(continued)*
    i. intussusception
    i. lymph node
    i. valve
    i. vein
ileocolitis
ileocolonic
ileocolostomy
ileocystoplasty
ileoentectropy
ileoileal intussusception
ileoileostomy
ileojejunitis
ileopexy
ileoproctostomy
ileorectostomy
ileorrhaphy
ileosigmoidostomy
ileostomy
    Brooke i.
    Kock i.
ileotomy
ileotransverse colostomy
ileotransversostomy
ileum duplex
ileus
    adynamic i.
    duodenal i.
    dynamic i.
    gallstone i.
    mechanical i.
    meconium i.
    occlusive i.
    paralytic i.
    spastic i.
    i. subparta
Ilhéus
    I. encephalitis
    I. fever
    I. virus
iliac
    i. artery
    i. bone
    i. branch
    i. bursa
    i. colon
    i. crest
    i. fascia
    i. flexure
    i. fossa
    i. horn
    i. muscle
    i. nervous plexus
    i. region
    i. roll
    i. spine
    i. steal
    i. tubercle

    i. tuberosity
    i. vein
iliacosubfascial
    i. fossa
    i. hernia
iliacus
    i. branch
    i. minor muscle
iliadelphus
iliococcygeal
    i. muscle
    i. raphe
iliococcygeus muscle
iliocolotomy
iliocostalis
    i. cervicis muscle
    i. lumborum muscle
    i. thoracis muscle
iliocostal muscle
iliofemoral
    i. ligament
    i. triangle
iliofemoroplasty
iliohypogastric nerve
ilioinguinal nerve
iliolumbar
    i. artery
    i. ligament
    i. vein
iliopagus
iliopectineal
    i. arch
    i. bursa
    i. eminence
    i. fascia
    i. fossa
    i. ligament
    i. line
iliopelvic sphincter
iliopsoas muscle
iliopubic
    i. eminence
    i. tract
iliosacral
iliosciatic notch
iliospinal
iliothoracopagus
iliotibial
    i. band
    i. band friction syndrome
    i. tract
iliotrochanteric ligament
ilioxiphopagus
ilium
Ilizarov technique
illegal abortion
illicium
illinition

illness
  debilitating i.
  environmental i.
  functional i.
  history of present i. (HPI)
  manic-depressive i.
  mass sociogenic i.
  mental i.
  nonspecific building-related i.'s
  refractory i.
  severity of i.
  specific building-related i.'s
illumination
  axial i.
  central i.
  contact i.
  critical i.
  dark-field i.
  dark-ground i.
  direct i.
  erect i.
  focal i.
  Köhler i.
  lateral i.
illuminism
illusion
  i. of doubles
  i. of movement
illusional
ilocanum
  Echinostoma i.
Ilosvay reagent
IM
  intramuscular
image
  accidental i.
  i. amplifier
  amplitude i.
  body i.
  catatropic i.
  i. cytometer
  direct i.
  double i.
  eidetic i.
  false i.
  heteronymous i.
  homonymous i.
  hypnagogic i.
  hypnopompic i.
  i. intensifier
  inverted i.
  latent i.

  magnitude i.
  mental i.
  mirror i.
  motor i.
  optical i.
  phase i.
  i. point
  Purkinje-Sanson i.
  Sanson i.
  sensory i.
  tactile i.
imagery
imaginal
imaging
  blood pool i.
  i. department
  exercise i.
  magnetic resonance i.
imago
imbalance
  autonomic i.
  occlusal i.
  vasomotor i.
imbecile
imbed
imbibition
imbricata
  tinea i.
imbricate
imbricated suture
imbrication
  eyelid i.
Imerslünd-Grasbeck syndrome
imidazole alkaloid
imidazolyl
imide
imidodipeptidase
imidodipeptiduria
imidole
iminazolyl
imino acid
iminocarbonyl
iminodipeptidase
iminoglycinuria
iminohydrolase
iminopeptidase
  proline i.
iminostilbene
imipenem
imiquimod
Imlach fat-pad

NOTES

immature
 i. birth
 i. cataract
 i. granulocyte
 i. neutrophil
 i. teratoma
immediate
 i. allergy
 i. amputation
 i. auscultation
 i. energy system
 i. flap
 i. hypersensitivity
 i. hypersensitivity reaction
 i. insertion denture
 i. percussion
 i. posttraumatic automatism
 i. posttraumatic convulsion
 i. transfusion
immedicable
immersion
 i. bath
 i. burn
 i. foot
 homogeneous i.
 i. lens
 i. microscopy
 i. objective
imminent abortion
immiscible
immission
immitis
 Dirofilaria i.
immittance
 acoustic i.
immobility
immobilization
immobilize
immobilized enzyme
immobilizing
 i. antibody
 i. bandage
immortalization
immotile cilia syndrome
immovable
 i. bandage
 i. joint
immune
 i. adherence
 i. adherence phenomenon
 i. adhesion test
 i. adsorption
 i. agglutination
 i. agglutinin
 i. complex
 i. complex disease
 i. complex disorder
 i. complex glomerulonephritis
 i. complex nephritis

 i. deficiency
 i. deviation
 i. dysfunction syndrome
 i. electron microscopy
 i. elimination
 i. fetal hydrops
 i. hemolysin
 i. hemolysis
 i. inflammation
 i. interferon
 i. opsonin
 i. paralysis
 i. precipitation
 i. protein
 i. reaction
 i. response
 i. response gene
 i. serum
 i. serum globulin
 i. suppression
 i. surveillance
 i. system
 i. thrombocytopenia
 i. thrombocytopenic purpura
immunifacient
immunity
 acquired i.
 active i.
 adoptive i.
 antiviral i.
 artificial active i.
 artificial passive i.
 bacteriophage i.
 cell-mediated i. (CMI)
 cellular i.
 concomitant i.
 i. deficiency
 general i.
 group i.
 herd i.
 humoral i.
 infection i.
 innate i.
 local i.
 maternal i.
 natural i.
 nonspecific i.
 passive i.
 specific i.
immunization
 active i.
immunize
immunoadjuvant
immunoagglutination
immunoassay
 chemiluminescence i.
 double antibody i.
 enzyme i.
immunobiology

immunoblast
immunoblastic
>   i. lymphadenopathy
>   i. lymphoma
>   i. sarcoma

immunoblot
immunoblotting
immunochemical assay
immunochemistry
immunocompetence
immunocompetent
immunocomplex
immunocompromised
immunoconglutinin
immunocyte
immunocytoadherence
immunocytochemistry
immunodeficiency
>   cellular i.
>   combined i.
>   common variable i.
>   i. syndrome
>   i. with elevated IgM
>   i. with hypoparathyroidism

immunodeficient
immunodepressant
immunodepressor
immunodiagnosis
immunodiffusion
>   double i.

immunoelectrophoresis
>   crossed i.

immunoenhancement
immunoenhancer
immunoferritin
immunofluorescence
>   direct i.
>   indirect i.
>   i. method
>   i. microscopy

immunofluorescent stain
immunogen
>   behavioral i.

immunogenetics
immunogenic
immunogenicity
immunoglobulin (Ig)
>   i. A (IgA)
>   anti-D i.
>   chickenpox i.
>   i. D (IgD)
>   i. domain

>   i. E (IgE)
>   i. G (IgG)
>   i. G subclass deficiency
>   human normal i.
>   i. M (IgM)
>   measles i.
>   monoclonal i.
>   thyroid-stimulating i.

immunohematology
immunohistochemistry
immunolocalization
immunologic
>   i. competence
>   i. deficiency
>   i. enhancement
>   i. high dose tolerance
>   i. mechanism
>   i. paralysis
>   i. pregnancy test

immunological
>   i. mechanism
>   i. paralysis
>   i. surveillance

immunologically
>   i. activated cell
>   i. competent cell
>   i. privileged sites

immunologist
immunology
immunomodulatory
immunopathology
immunoperoxidase technique
immunophilin
immunopotentiation
immunopotentiator
immunoprecipitation
immunoproliferative
>   i. disorder
>   i. small intestinal disease

immunoradiometric assay
immunoreaction
immunoreactive insulin
immunoselection
immunosorbent
immunosuppressant
immunosuppression
immunosuppressive
immunosurveillance
immunosympathectomy
immunotherapy
>   adoptive i.
>   biologic i.

NOTES

471

immunotolerance
immunotransfusion
impact
    i. factor
    i. resistance
impacted
    i. fetus
    i. fracture
    i. tooth
impaction
    dental i.
    fecal i.
    food i.
impaired
    i. affect
    i. glucose tolerance
impairment
    Alexander hearing i.
    conductive hearing i.
    functional hearing i.
    hearing i.
    hereditary hearing i.
    high-frequency hearing i.
    hysterical hearing i.
    mental i.
    Mondini hearing i.
    organic hearing i.
    perceptive hearing i.
    psychogenic hearing i.
    Scheibe hearing i.
    sensory hearing i.
impar
    ganglion i.
impatent
impedance
    acoustic i.
    i. angle
    i. matching
    i. method
    i. plethysmography
imperative conception
imperception
imperfect
    i. fungus
    i. stage
    i. state
imperfecta
    dentinogenesis i.
    enamelogenesis i.
    erythrogenesis i.
    osteogenesis i.
imperforate
    i. anus
    i. hymen
imperforation
impermeable junction
impermeant
impersistence
impervious

impetiginization
impetiginous cheilitis
impetigo
    Bockhart i.
    bullous i.
    i. circinata
    i. contagiosa
    i. contagiosa bullosa
    follicular i.
    i. herpetiformis
    i. neonatorum
    i. vulgaris
impetus
impingement
    i. sign
    i. syndrome
    i. test
implant
    carcinomatous i.
    cochlear i.
    corneal i.
    dental i.
    i. denture
    i. denture substructure
    i. denture superstructure
    endometrial i.
    endo-osseous i.
    endosteal i.
    inflatable i.
    intracorneal i.
    intraocular i.
    magnetic i.
    root-form i.
    sponge i.
    surface i.
    threaded i.
    tunneled i.
    wire mesh i.
implantation
    central i.
    circumferential i.
    collagen i.
    i. cone
    cortical i.
    i. cyst
    eccentric i.
    interstitial i.
implanted suture
implosion
implosive therapy
impotence
impotency
impregnate
impregnated dressing
impregnation
    silver i.
impression
    aortic i.
    i. area

basilar i.
colic i.
complete denture i.
i. compound
deltoid i.
digitate i.
dircct bone i.
final i.
i. material
mental i.
i. tray
impressiones
i. digitatae
i. gyrorum
impressive aphasia
imprinting
genomic i.
impromidine
impulse
apical i.
cardiac i.
i. control disorder
ectopic i.
escape i.
irresistible i.
point of maximal i. (PMI)
impulsion
impulsive
i. act
i. obsession
impure flutter
imus
IMV
intermittent mandatory ventilation
in
i. extremis
i. phase
i. situ
i. situ hybridization
i. utero
i. vacuo
i. vitro
i. vitro fertilization (IVF)
i. vivo
i. vivo fertilization
inaction
inactivate
inactivated
i. poliovirus vaccine (IPV)
i. serum
inactivation
insertional i.

inactivator
anaphylatoxin i.
inactive
i. mutant
i. repressor
i. tuberculosis
inactivity
i. atrophy
electrocerebral i.
inadequate
i. personality
i. stimulus
in-and-out surgery
inanimate
inanition fever
inapparent infection
inappetence
inappropriate
i. affect
i. hormone
i. polycythemia
inarticulate
inassimilable
inattention
inborn
i. error of metabolism
i. lysosomal disease
i. reflex
inbred
inbreeding
coefficient of i.
incarcerated
i. hernia
i. placenta
incarceration symptom
incarial bone
incarnant
incarnative
incasement theory
incendiarism
incentive spirometer
inception rate
incest barrier
incestuous
incidence
i. density
i. rate
incident
i. angle
i. command system
i. management system

NOTES

incident *(continued)*
    i. point
    i. ray
incidental
    i. learning
    i. parasite
incidentaloma
incipient
    i. caries
    i. cataract
    i. heart attack
incisal
    i. edge
    i. embrasure
    i. guidance
    i. guide
    i. guide angle
    i. margin
    i. path
    i. point
    i. rest
    i. surface
incise
incised wound
incision
    abdominal i.
    abdominothoracic i.
    Agnew-Verhoeff i.
    alar i.
    angular i.
    aortotomy i.
    arcuate i.
    areolar i.
    arteriotomy i.
    i. biopsy
    bivalved i.
    bucket-handle i.
    celiotomy i.
    cervical i.
    chevron i.
    chevron-shaped i.
    circumareolar i.
    circumcision i.
    circumferential i.
    circumlimbal i.
    circumscribing i.
    clamshell i.
    collar i.
    corneoscleral i.
    crescent i.
    cruciate i.
    Deaver i.
    dorsolateral i.
    Dührssen i.
    endaural i.
    exploratory i.
    Fergusson i.
    fishmouth i.
    flank i.

    hemitransfixion i.
    hockey-stick i.
    Hood and Kirklin i.
    inframammary i.
    infraumbilical i.
    inguinal i.
    intercartilaginous i.
    intracapsular i.
    Kocher i.
    lamellar i.
    lateral flank i.
    lateral rectus i.
    limbal i.
    linear i.
    longitudinal i.
    lumbotomy i.
    mastoid i.
    McBurney i.
    meatal i.
    median i.
    midline i.
    muscle-splitting i.
    Ollier i.
    Orr i.
    perianal i.
    periareolar i.
    perilimbal i.
    periscapular i.
    peritoneal i.
    Pfannenstiel i.
    postauricular i.
    proximal i.
    recumbent i.
    relief i.
    retroauricular i.
    rim i.
    thoracoabdominal i.
    thoracotomy i.
    transection i.
    transmeatal i.
    transrectus i.
    Whipple i.
    Z-flap i.
    zigzag i.
incisional hernia
3-incision esophagectomy
incisive
    i. bone
    i. canal
    i. canal cyst
    i. duct
    i. foramen
    i. fossa
    i. papilla
    i. suture
incisivum
    os i.
incisor
    i. canal

I

central i.
i. crest
i. foramen
Hutchinson i.
lateral i.
shovel-shaped i.
i. tooth
incisura
i. acetabuli
i. angularis
i. frontalis
i. lacrimalis
incisure
angular i.
Lanterman i.
Schmidt-Lanterman i.
inclination
condylar guidance i.
enamel rod i.
lateral condylar i.
i. of pelvis
inclinometer
inclusion
i. blennorrhea
i. body
i. body disease
i. body encephalitis
i. cell
i. cell disease
i. compound
i. conjunctivitis
i. conjunctivitis virus
i. cyst
i. dermoid
Döhle i.
fetal i.
leukocyte i.
incoherent
incomitant strabismus
incompatibility
Rh antigen i.
incompatible blood transfusion reaction
incompetence
aortic i.
cardiac valvular i.
mitral i.
incompetency
incompetent
i. cervical os
i. cervix
incomplete
i. abortion

i. achromatopsia
i. agglutinin
i. alexia
i. antibody
i. antigen
i. ascertainment
i. atrioventricular block
i. atrioventricular dissociation
i. AV dissociation
i. breech
i. cleavage
i. conjoined twins
i. disinfectant
i. fistula
i. foot presentation
i. fracture
i. hemianopia
i. metamorphosis
i. neurofibromatosis
i. tetanus
incongruent nystagmus
incongruous
i. hemianopia
i. history
inconstant
incontinence
fecal i.
i. of feces
overflow i.
paralytic i.
stress urinary i.
urge i.
urgency i.
i. of urine
incontinent
incontinentia
incoordination
incorporation
increase
absolute cell i.
base i.
increased markings emphysema
increment
incremental line
increta
placenta i.
incretin
incretion
incrustation
incrusted cystitis
incubation period
incubative stage

NOTES

incubator
incubatory carrier
incubus
incudal
    i. fold
    i. fossa
incudectomy
incudes (*pl. of* incus)
incudiform uterus
incudis
incudomalleal
incudomalleolar
    i. articulation
    i. joint
incudostapedial
    i. articulation
    i. joint
incurable
incurvation
incus, pl. incudes
    long crus of i.
incycloduction
incyclophoria
incyclotropia
indanedione derivatives
indanediones
indeciduate
indenization
indentation hardness
independence
    causal i.
independent
    i. assortment
    i. living model
    i. practice association
    i. practice association HMO
    i. variable
indeterminate
    i. cleavage
    i. leprosy
index, pl. indices, indexes
    absorbancy i.
    alveolar i.
    i. ametropia
    amnionic fluid i.
    anesthetic i.
    antitryptic i.
    apnea-hypopnea i.
    Arneth i.
    auricular i.
    Ayala i.
    basilar i.
    Bödecker i.
    body mass i.
    buffer i.
    cardiac i.
    i. case
    centromeric i.
    cephalic i.

cephaloorbital i.
cerebral i.
cerebrospinal i.
chemotherapeutic i.
chest i.
cranial i.
Dean fluorosis i.
degenerative i.
dental i. (DI)
diet quality i.
DMFS caries i.
effective temperature i.
empathic i.
endemic i.
erythrocyte i.
i. extensor muscle
facial i.
i. finger
Flower dental i.
free thyroxine i. (FTI)
Gingival I.
glycemic i.
gnathic i.
health status i.
heat stress i.
height-length i.
i. hypermetropia
international sensitivity i.
iron i.
karyopyknotic i.
length-breadth i.
length-height i.
leukopenic i.
master patient i.
maturation i.
metacarpal i.
mitotic i.
molar absorbancy i.
i. myopia
opsonic i.
palatal i.
Pearl i.
phagocytic i.
pressure-volume i.
refractive i.
reticulocyte production i.
Robinson i.
root caries i.
Russell Periodontal I.
saturation i.
short increment sensitivity i.
Simplified Oral Hygiene I. (OHI-S)
small increment sensitivity i.
stroke work i.
therapeutic i.
ultraviolet i.
vital i.
volume i.
windchill i.

indexical sign
India ink capsule stain
Indian
    I. flap
    I. ginger
    I. gum
    I. podophyllum
    I. podophyllum resin
    I. sickness
    I. tick typhus
indican
    metabolic i.
indicanidrosis
indicant
indicanuria
indication
    off label i.
indicator
    alizarin i.
    biologic i.
    clinical i.
    i. dilution method
    health i.
    i. system
    i. yellow
indicator-dilution curve
indices (*pl. of* index)
indifference
    i. to pain syndrome
    i. reaction
indifférence
    belle i.
    la belle i.
indifferent
    i. cell
    i. electrode
    i. genitalia
    i. gonad
    i. oxide
    i. tissue
    i. water
indigenous
indigestion
    acid i.
    fat i.
    gastric i.
    nervous i.
indigo
    i. blue
    i. carmine
indigotin
indigouria

indiguria
indirect
    i. agglutination
    i. assay
    i. calorimetry
    i. Coombs test
    i. diuretic
    i. fluorescent antibody test
    i. fracture
    i. hemagglutination test
    i. immunofluorescence
    i. inguinal hernia
    i. laryngoscopy
    i. lead
    i. nuclear division
    i. ophthalmoscope
    i. ophthalmoscopy
    i. oxidase
    i. pulp capping
    i. pupillary reaction
    i. ray
    i. reacting bilirubin
    i. retainer
    i. retention
    i. symptom
    i. technique
    i. transfusion
    i. vision
indiscriminate lesion
indisposition
indium
indium-111
    i.-111 chloride
    i.-111 trichloride
indium-113m
individual
    i. differences
    i. psychology
    i. therapy
    i. tolerance
    I.'s with Disabilities Education Act
individualized education program
individuation field
indocyanine
    i. green
    i. green angiography
indocybin
indolaceturia
indolamine
indolent
    i. bubo
    i. ulcer

NOTES

indole test
indolic acid
indologenes
>Kingella i.

indologenous
indoluria
indolyl
indomethacin
indophenol
>i. method
>i. oxidase

indophenolase
indoramin
indoxyl
indoxyluria
induce
induced
>i. abortion
>i. apnea
>i. enzyme
>i. erythrocythemia
>i. fever
>i. fit
>i. fit model
>i. hypotension
>i. malaria
>i. mutation
>i. phagocytosis
>i. psychosis
>i. psychotic disorder
>i. radioactivity
>i. sensitivity
>i. symptom
>i. trance

inducer
>i. cell
>embryonal i.
>gratuitous i.

inducible enzyme
inductance
induction
>i. chemotherapy
>electromagnetic i.
>lysogenic i.
>i. period

inductive resistance
inductor
inductorium
inductotherm
inductothermy
indulin
indulinophil, indulinophile
indurata
>acne i.

indurated
>i. cellulitis
>i. chancre
>i. lymphangitis

induration
>brawny i.
>brown i.
>cyanotic i.
>gray i.
>red i.

indurative myocarditis
induratum
>erythema i.

indusium griseum
industrial
>i. disease
>i. hearing loss
>i. hygiene
>i. methylated spirit
>i. psychiatry
>i. psychology

indwelling catheter
inebriant
inebriation
inebriety
inert gas
inertia
>magnetic i.
>i. time

inevitable abortion
inexorable
infancy
>fibrous hamartoma of i.

infant
>i. death
>i. Hercules
>liveborn i.
>i. mortality rate
>postmature i.
>postterm i.
>preterm i.
>stillborn i.

infanticide
infantile
>i. acropustulosis
>i. acute hemorrhagic edema
>i. autism
>i. beriberi
>i. cataract
>i. celiac disease
>i. colic
>i. convulsion
>i. cortical hyperostosis
>i. digital fibromatosis
>i. diplegia
>i. dwarfism
>i. eczema
>i. fibrosarcoma
>i. gastroenteritis
>i. gastroenteritis virus
>i. hemiplegia
>i. hernia
>i. hypothyroidism

i. leishmaniasis
i. muscular atrophy
i. myofibromatosis
i. myxedema
i. neuroaxonal dystrophy
i. neuronal degeneration
i. osteomalacia
i. pellagra
i. progressive spinal muscular
  atrophy
i. purulent conjunctivitis
i. scurvy
i. sexuality
i. spasm
i. spastic paraplegia
i. spinal muscular atrophy
i. tetany
i. torticollis
infantile-type hyperglycerolemia
infantilis
roseola i.
infantilism
Brissaud i.
dysthyroidal i.
hepatic i.
hypophysial i.
hypothyroid i.
idiopathic i.
Lorain-Lévi i.
sexual i.
infantum
dermatitis exfoliativa i.
dermatitis gangrenosa i.
osteopathia hemorrhagica i.
roseola i.
infarct
anemic i.
bland i.
bone i.
Brewer i.
embolic i.
hemorrhagic i.
Roesler-Dressler i.
septic i.
white i.
Zahn i.
infarction
acute myocardial i. (AMI)
anterior myocardial i.
anteroinferior myocardial i.
anterolateral myocardial i.
anteroseptal myocardial i.

apical i.
atrial i.
cardiac i.
diaphragmatic myocardial i.
Freiberg i.
inferior myocardial i.
inferolateral myocardial i.
lateral myocardial i.
myocardial i. (MI)
rule out myocardial i.
silent myocardial i.
watershed i.
infect
infected abortion
infection
agonal i.
airborne i.
apical i.
i. calculus
i. control nurse
cross i.
cryptogenic i.
disseminated gonococcal i.
droplet i.
endogenous i.
focal i.
holomiantic i.
i. immunity
inapparent i.
latent i.
mass i.
mixed i.
recurrent upper respiratory tract i.
reservoir of i.
terminal i.
i. transmission parameter
tunnel i.
upper respiratory i. (URI)
upper respiratory tract i. (URTI)
urinary tract i.
vector-borne i.
Vincent i.
**infection-associated hemophagocytic
syndrome (IAHS)**
infection-exhaustion psychosis
infection-immunity
infectiosity
infectiosum
erythema i.
infectious
i. anemia
i. bovine keratoconjunctivitis

NOTES

infectious (*continued*)
    i. crystalline keratopathy
    i. disease
    i. ectromelia virus
    i. eczematoid dermatitis
    i. endocarditis
    i. granuloma
    i. hepatitis (IH)
    i. hepatitis virus
    i. icterus
    i. jaundice
    i. mononucleosis
    i. myositis
    i. nucleic acid
    i. papilloma virus
    i. plasmid
    i. polyneuritis
    i. porcine encephalomyelitis virus
    i. stomatitis
    i. wart
infectiousness
infective
    i. disease
    i. embolism
    i. endocarditis
    i. jaundice
    i. thrombus
infectivity
infecundity
inference
inferential statistics
inferior
    i. aberrant ductule
    i. accessory fissure
    i. alveolar artery
    i. alveolar nerve
    i. anal nerve
    i. anastomotic vein
    arcus dentalis i.
    arcus palpebralis i.
    i. articular process
    i. basal vein
    i. border
    i. calcaneonavicular ligament
    i. cardiac vein
    i. carotid triangle
    i. cerebellar peduncle
    i. cerebral surface
    i. cerebral vein
    i. cervical cardiac branch
    i. cervical cardiac nerve
    i. cervical ganglion
    i. choroid vein
    i. clunial nerve
    i. constrictor muscle
    i. costal facet
    i. costal pit
    i. dental arch
    i. dental artery

i. dental branch
i. dental canal
i. dental foramen
i. dental nerve
i. dental nervous plexus
i. dental ramus
i. duodenal flexure
i. duodenal fold
i. duodenal fossa
i. duodenal recess
i. epigastric artery
i. epigastric lymph node
i. epigastric vein
i. esophageal constriction
i. esophageal sphincter
i. extensor retinaculum
i. extremity
i. eyelid
i. fascia
i. fibular retinaculum
i. fovea
i. frontal convolution
i. frontal gyrus
i. frontal sulcus
i. gemellus muscle
i. gingival branch
i. gluteal artery
i. gluteal nerve
i. gluteal vein
i. hemiazygos vein
i. hemorrhoidal artery
i. hemorrhoidal nerve
i. hemorrhoidal plexus
i. hemorrhoidal vein
i. horn
i. hypogastric nervous plexus
i. hypophysial artery
i. ileocecal recess
i. internal parietal artery
i. labial artery
i. labial branch
i. labial vein
i. laryngeal artery
i. laryngeal cavity
i. laryngeal nerve
i. laryngeal vein
i. laryngotomy
i. lateral brachial cutaneous nerve
i. lateral genicular artery
i. limb
i. lingual muscle
i. lingular artery
i. lingular branch
i. lingular bronchopulmonary segment
i. lingular segment
i. lobar artery
i. longitudinal fasciculus
i. longitudinal muscle

i. longitudinal sinus
i. lumbar triangle
i. macular arteriole
i. macular venule
i. margin
i. maxillary nerve
i. medial genicular artery
i. mediastinum
i. medullary velum
i. member
i. mesenteric artery
i. mesenteric ganglion
i. mesenteric lymph node
i. mesenteric nervous plexus
i. mesenteric vein
i. myocardial infarction
i. nasal arteriole of retina
i. nasal colliculus
i. nasal concha
i. nasal retinal venule
i. nasal venule of retina
i. nuchal line
i. oblique muscle
i. occipital gyrus
i. occipital triangle
i. occipitofrontal fasciculus
i. olivary complex
i. olivary nucleus
i. olive
i. omental recess
i. ophthalmic vein
i. orbital fissure
i. palpebral arterial arch
i. palpebral vein
i. pancreatic artery
i. pancreaticoduodenal artery
i. parietal gyrus
i. parietal lobule
i. pelvic aperture
i. peroneal retinaculum
i. petrosal groove
i. petrosal sinus
i. petrosal sulcus
i. phrenic artery
i. phrenic lymph node
i. phrenic vein
i. pole
i. polioencephalitis
i. posterior serratus muscle
i. pubic ligament
i. pubic ramus

i. quadrigeminal brachium
i. radioulnar joint
i. rectal artery
i. rectal nerve
i. rectal nervous plexus
i. rectal vein
i. rectus muscle
i. renal segment
i. root
i. sagittal sinus
i. salivary nucleus
i. salivatory nucleus
i. segmental artery
i. semilunar lobule
i. subtendinous bursa
i. suprarenal artery
i. tarsal muscle
i. tarsus
i. temporal convolution
i. temporal gyrus
i. temporal line
i. temporal retinal arteriole
i. temporal retinal venule
i. temporal sulcus
i. thalamic peduncle
i. thalamic radiation
i. thalamostriate vein
i. thoracic aperture
i. thyroid artery
i. thyroid notch
i. thyroid plexus
i. thyroid tubercle
i. thyroid vein
i. tibiofibular joint
i. tracheobronchial lymph node
i. transverse scapular ligament
i. triangle sign
i. trunk
i. turbinated bone
i. tympanic artery
i. ulnar collateral artery
i. vena cava (IVC)
i. vena cava pressure (IVCP)
i. venacavography
i. ventricular vein
i. vesical artery
i. vesical venous plexus
i. vestibular area
i. vestibular nucleus
i. wall
inferiority complex

NOTES

inferius
    labrale i.
    mediastinum i.
inferolateral
    i. margin
    i. myocardial infarction
    i. surface
inferomedial margin
infertile male syndrome
infertility
infest
infestation
infibulation
infiltrate
    Assmann tuberculous i.
    infraclavicular i.
infiltration
    adipose i.
    i. anesthesia
    calcareous i.
    cellular i.
    epituberculous i.
    fatty i.
    gelatinous i.
    gray i.
    inflammatory i.
    lipomatous i.
    lymphocytic i.
infinite distance
infinity
infirm
infirmary
infirmity
inflamed ulcer
inflammable
inflammation
    active i.
    acute i.
    adhesive i.
    allergic i.
    alterative i.
    atrophic i.
    catarrhal i.
    chronic active i.
    degenerative i.
    exudative i.
    fibrinopurulent i.
    fibrinous i.
    fibroid i.
    granulomatous i.
    hyperplastic i.
    immune i.
    interstitial i.
    necrotic i.
    necrotizing i.
    proliferative i.
    pseudomembranous i.
    purulent i.
    serous i.

    subacute i.
    suppurative i.
inflammatory
    i. carcinoma
    i. corpuscle
    i. edema
    i. fibrous hyperplasia
    i. infiltration
    i. linear verrucous epidermal nevus
    i. lymph
    i. macrophage
    i. papillary hyperplasia
    i. polyp
    i. pseudotumor
    i. rheumatism
inflatable
    i. implant
    i. splint
inflation
inflator
inflection
inflexion
influenza
    i. A, B, C
    Asian i.
    i. bacillus
    endemic i.
    Hong Kong i.
    i. nostras
    i. pneumonia
    Spanish i.
    i. virus
    i. virus vaccine
influenzae
    Haemophilus i.
influenzal virus pneumonia
infold
informatics
information
    i. system
    i. theory
informational RNA
informed consent
informofer
informosome
infraauricular
    i. deep parotid lymph node
    i. subfascial parotid lymph node
infraaxillary
infrabony pocket
infrabulge
infracardiac bursa
infracerebral
infraclavicular
    i. fossa
    i. infiltrate
    i. part
    i. triangle
infraclinoid aneurysm

infraclusion
infracortical
infracostal line
infracotyloid
infracristal
infraction
infradentale
infradian
infradiaphragmatic
infraduction
infraduodenal fossa
infraglenoid
   i. tubercle
   i. tuberosity
infraglottic
   i. cavity
   i. space
infragranular layer
infrahepatic
infrahyoid
   i. branch
   i. bursa
   i. muscle
inframamillary
inframammary
   i. incision
   i. region
inframandibular
inframarginal
inframaxillary
infranatant fluid
infranodal extrasystole
infraocclusion
infraorbital
   i. artery
   i. canal
   i. foramen
   i. groove
   i. margin
   i. nerve
   i. region
   i. suture
infraorbitomeatal plane
infrapalpebral sulcus
infrapatellar
   i. branch
   i. fat body
   i. fat-pad
   i. synovial fold
infrapsychic
infrared
   i. cataract

i. light
i. microscope
i. ray
i. spectroscopy
i. spectrum
i. thermography
infrascapular
   i. artery
   i. region
infrasegmental
   i. part
   i. vein
infrasonic
infraspinatus
   i. bursa
   i. fascia
   i. muscle
infraspinous
   i. fascia
   i. fossa
infrasplenic
infrasternal angle
infrasubspecific
infratemporal
   i. approach
   i. crest
   i. fossa
   i. surface
infrathoracic
infratonsillar
infratrochlear nerve
infraumbilical incision
infraversion
infriction
infundibular
   i. part
   i. recess
   i. stalk
   i. stem
   i. stenosis
infundibulectomy
infundibuliform
   i. fascia
   i. hymen
   i. sheath
infundibulin
infundibulofolliculitis
infundibuloma
infundibuloovarian ligament
infundibulopelvic ligament
infundibulum
   ethmoid i.

NOTES

infundibulum *(continued)*
    ethmoidal i.
    i. ethmoidale
    hypothalamic i.
infusible
infusion
    i. cannula
    i. pyelogram
infusion-aspiration drainage
infusorian
Ingelfinger rule
ingestion
ingestive
Ingrassia process
ingravescent
ingrowing toenail
ingrown
    i. hair
    i. nail
inguen
inguinal
    i. aponeurotic fold
    i. branch
    i. canal
    i. crest
    i. falx
    i. fossa
    i. hernia
    i. incision
    i. ligament
    i. lymphatic plexus
    i. part
    i. region
    i. triangle
    i. trigone
inguinale
    granuloma i.
    lymphogranuloma i.
inguinalis
    falx i.
inguinocrural hernia
inguinodynia
inguinofemoral hernia
inguinolabial hernia
inguinoperitoneal
inguinoproperitoneal hernia
inguinoscrotal hernia
inguinosuperficial hernia
inhalant abuse
inhalation
    i. analgesia
    i. anesthesia
    i. anesthetic
    i. therapy
inhalational bronchopneumonia
inhale
inhaler
    metered-dose i.
inherent

inheritance
    alternative i.
    blending i.
    codominant i.
    collateral i.
    cytoplasmic i.
    dominant i.
    extrachromosomal i.
    extranuclear i.
    galtonian i.
    holandric i.
    hologynic i.
    maternal i.
    mendelian i.
    mosaic i.
    multifactorial i.
    recessive i.
    sex-influenced i.
    sex-limited i.
    sex-linked i.
inherited
    i. albumin variant
    i. character
inhibin
inhibit
inhibiting antibody
inhibition
    allogeneic i.
    central i.
    competitive i.
    contact i.
    end product i.
    i. factor
    feedback i.
    hemagglutination i.
    noncompetitive i.
    reflex i.
    selective i.
inhibitor
    angiotensin-converting enzyme i.
      (ACEI)
    aromatase i.
    Bowman-Birk i.
    carbonate dehydratase i.
    carbonic anhydrase i.
    C1 esterase i.
    cholinesterase i.
    familial lipoprotein lipase i.
    gastric acid i.
    glucosidase i.
    HMG CoA-reductase i.
    lipoprotein-associated coagulation i.
      (LACI)
    mechanism-based i.
    monoamine oxidase i.
    nonnucleoside reverse
      transcriptase i. (NNRTI)
    protease i.
    proton pump i.

5-reductase i.
selective norepinephrine reuptake i.
selective serotonin reuptake i.
uncompetitive i.

inhibitory
    i. fiber
    i. junction potential (IJP)
    i. nerve
    i. obsession
    i. postsynaptic potential (IPSP)

iniac
iniad
inial
iniencephaly
inion
iniopagus
iniops
initial
    i. assessment
    i. contact
    i. dose
    i. heat
    i. hematuria
    i. rate
    i. velocity

initiating
    i. agent
    i. codon

initiation
    i. codon
    i. factor (IF)
    i. tRNA

initis
inject
injectable
injected
injection
    adrenal cortex i.
    collagen i.
    depot i.
    i. flask
    hypodermic i.
    insulin i.
    intracytoplasmic sperm i.
    intradermal i.
    intrathecal i.
    intraventricular i.
    jet i.
    lactated Ringer i.
    i. mass
    i. molding

injector
    jet i.

injury
    acceleration-deceleration i.
    blast i.
    brachial plexus i.
    closed head i. (CHI)
    contrecoup i.
    coup i.
    current of i.
    degloving i.
    diffuse i.'s
    egg-white i.
    flexion-extension i.
    focal i.
    hyperextension-hyperflexion i.
    Lisfranc i.
    open head i.
    i. potential
    whiplash i.

inkblot test
inlay
    epithelial i.
    gold i.
    i. graft
    i. wax

inlet
    i. forceps
    laryngeal i.
    pelvic i.

innate
    i. heat
    i. immunity
    i. reflex

inner
    i. border
    i. cell mass
    i. dental epithelium
    i. enamel epithelium
    i. layer of eyeball
    i. limiting layer
    i. lip
    i. malleolus
    i. membrane
    i. nuclear layer
    i. plexiform layer
    i. sheath of optic nerve
    i. spiral sulcus
    i. stripe
    i. table of skull
    i. zone

innermost intercostal muscle

NOTES

innervation apraxia
innidiation
innocens
    diabetes i.
innocent
    i. bystander cell
    i. murmur
    i. tumor
innocuous
innominatal
innominate
    i. artery
    i. bone
    i. cardiac vein
    i. fossa
    i. substance
innoxious
INO
    internuclear ophthalmoplegia
inoculability
inoculable
inoculate
inoculation
inoculum
inopectic
inoperable
inopexia
inorganic
    i. acid
    i. catalyst
    i. chemistry
    i. compound
    i. dental cement
    i. diphosphatase
    i. murmur
    i. orthophosphate
    i. phosphate
    i. pyrophosphatase
inosamine
inoscopy
inosemia
inosinate
inosine pranobex
inosinic acid
inosinicase
inosinyl
inosite
inositide
inositol
inosituria
inosuria
inotropic agent
inpatient
inquest
inquiline parasite
INR
    international normalized ratio
insalubrious
insanitary

insanity
    criminal i.
    i. defense
inscription
inscriptio tendinea
insectarium
insecticide
insectifuge
insectivorous
insect virus
insecurity
    gravitational i.
insemination
    artificial i.
    donor i.
    heterologous i.
    homologous i.
    intrauterine i. (IUI)
insenescence
insensible
    i. perspiration
    i. thirst
insertion
    i. forceps
    i. sequence
insertional
    i. inactivation
    i. mutagenesis
insheathed
insidiosa
    Erysipelothrix i.
insidious
insight
    i. and judgment
    i. learning
insipidus
    diabetes i.
    nephrogenic diabetes i.
insolation
insoluble soap
insomnia
    conditioned i.
insomniac
insorption
inspection
    visual i.
inspersion
inspiration
    crowing i.
inspiratory
    i. capacity
    i. center
    i. reserve volume (IRV)
    i. rhonchi
    i. stridor
inspire
inspired gas
inspirometer
inspissate

inspissated
>   i. bile syndrome
>   i. cerumen

inspissation

inspissator

inspissatum
>   cerumen i.

instability
>   detrusor i.
>   spinal i.

instantaneous
>   i. electrical axis
>   i. vector

instar

instep

instillation

instillator

instinct
>   aggressive i.
>   death i.
>   ego i.
>   herd i.
>   life i.

instinctive

instinctual

institutional review board

instructive theory

instrument
>   diamond cutting i.
>   hearing i.
>   purse-string i.
>   stereotactic i.

instrumental
>   i. amusia
>   i. conditioning

instrumentarium

instrumentation

insuccation

insudate

insufficiency
>   accommodative i.
>   acute adrenocortical i.
>   adrenocortical i.
>   aortic i.
>   cardiac i.
>   chronic adrenocortical i.
>   convergence i.
>   coronary i.
>   divergence i.
>   exocrine pancreatic i.
>   glomerular i.
>   hepatic i.

>   latent adrenocortical i.
>   mitral i.
>   myocardial i.
>   primary adrenocortical i.
>   pulmonary i.
>   secondary adrenocortical i.
>   tricuspid i.
>   valvular i.
>   velopharyngeal i.
>   venous i.

insufflate

insufflation
>   i. anesthesia
>   peritoneal i.

insufflator

insula, pl. **insulae**
>   Haller i.

insular
>   i. area
>   i. artery
>   i. cortex
>   i. gyrus
>   i. hypothesis
>   i. lobe
>   i. part
>   i. sclerosis
>   i. vein

insulate

insulation

insulator

insulin
>   i. antagonist
>   biphasic i.
>   i. coma therapy
>   i. coma treatment
>   globin zinc i.
>   human i.
>   i. hypoglycemia test
>   immunoreactive i.
>   i. injection
>   isophane i.
>   lente i.
>   i. lipoatrophy
>   i. lipodystrophy
>   lispro i.
>   NPH i.
>   i. receptor substrate-1
>   i. resistance
>   i. shock
>   i. shock treatment
>   i. unit
>   i. zinc suspension

NOTES

insulin-antagonizing factor
insulin-dependent diabetes mellitus (IDDM)
insulinemia
insulinlike
    i. activity (ILA)
    i. growth factor (IGF)
insulinogenesis
insulinogenic
insulinoma
insulinopenic diabetes
insulitis
insulogenic
insuloma
insurance
    fee-for-service i.
insusceptibility
intake
    caloric i.
    i. and output (I&O)
integral
    i. dose
    i. protein
integrated rate expression
integration
    sensory i.
integument
integumentary system
integumentum commune
intellectual aura
intellectualization
intelligence
    abstract i.
    artificial i.
    measured i.
    mechanical i.
    i. quotient (IQ)
    i. test
intemperance
intensification chemotherapy
intensifier
    image i.
intensifying screen
intensity
    luminous i.
    performance i.
    point of maximal i. (PMI)
    radiant i.
    i. of sound
intensive
    i. care
    i. care unit (ICU)
    i. psychotherapy
intention
    first i.
    healing by first i.
    healing by second i.
    healing by third i.
    i. myoclonus
    secondary i.
    i. spasm
    i. tremor
intentional
    i. replantation
    i. spasm
intentionem
    per primam i.
intention-to-treat analysis
interacinar
interacinous
interaction
    apolar i.
    drug i.
    hydrophobic i.
    i. process analysis
interalveolar
    i. pore
    i. septum
    i. space
interannular segment
interarch distance
interarticular
    i. fibrocartilage
    i. joint
interarticularis
    pars i.
interarytenoid
    i. fold
    i. notch
interasteric
interatrial
    i. block
    i. conduction time
    i. foramen primum
    i. foramen secundum
    i. septum
    i. sulcus
interaural attenuation
interauricular arc
interbody
intercadence
intercadent
intercalary
    i. neuron
    i. staphyloma
intercalated
    i. disc
    i. duct
    i. nucleus
intercalation
intercanalicular
intercapillary
    i. cell
    i. glomerulosclerosis
intercapitular vein
intercarotic

intercarotid
  i. body
  i. nerve
intercarpal
  i. joint
  i. ligament
intercartilaginous
  i. incision
  i. part
intercavernous sinus
intercellular
  i. bridge
  i. canaliculus
  i. cement
  i. digestion
  i. junction
  i. lymph
intercentral
interceptive occlusal contact
intercerebral
interchondral
  i. articulation
  i. joint
intercilium
interclavicular
  i. ligament
  i. notch
interclinoid ligament
intercoccygeal
intercolumnar
  i. fiber
  i. tubercle
intercondylar
  i. eminence
  i. fossa
  i. line
  i. notch
  i. tubercle
intercondylic fossa
intercondyloid
  i. eminence
  i. fossa
  i. notch
interconversion
  enzyme i.
intercornual ligament
intercostal
  i. anesthesia
  i. artery
  i. ligament
  i. lymph node
  i. margin (ICM)

  i. membrane
  i. nerve
  i. neuralgia
  i. space
  i. vein
intercostobrachial nerve
intercostohumeralis
intercostohumeral nerve
intercourse
  sexual i.
intercricothyrotomy
intercrine
intercristal
intercross
intercrural
  i. fiber
  i. ganglion
intercuneiform
  i. joint
  i. ligament
intercurrent disease
intercuspal position
intercuspation
intercusping
intercutaneomucous
interdeferential
interdental
  i. canal
  i. caries
  i. papilla
  i. septum
  i. splint
interdentium
interdigit
interdigital fold
interdigitating reticulum cell
interdigitation
interdisciplinary
interectopic interval
interest
  conflict of i.
  region of i.
interface
  crystalline i.
  dermoepidermal i.
  metal i.
interfacial
  i. canal
  i. surface tension
interfascial space
interfascicular fasciculus
interfemoral

NOTES

interference
    bacterial i.
    i. beat
    cuspal i.
    dissociation by i.
    i. dissociation
    i. microscope
interferometer
    electron i.
interferometry
    electron i.
interferon
    i. alfa 2b
    i. alpha
    antigen i.
    i. beta
    i. beta 1b
    fibroblast i.
    i. gamma
    immune i.
    leukocyte i.
    i. omega
    i. tau
    trophoblast i.
    i. type I, II
interfibrillar
interfibrillary
interfibrous
interfilamentous
interfoveolar ligament
interfrontal
interganglionic branch
intergemmal
intergenal
intergenic
    i. complementation
    i. suppression
interglobular
    i. dentin
    i. space
intergluteal cleft
intergonial
intergyral
interhemicerebral
interictal
intérieur
    milieu i.
interiliac lymph node
interim denture
interior
interischiadic
interjudge reliability
interkinesis
interlamellar
interlaminar jelly

interleukin
interleukin-1 (IL-1)
interleukin-2 (IL-2)
interleukin-3 (IL-3)
interleukin-4 (IL-4)
interleukin-5 (IL-5)
interleukin-6 (IL-6)
interleukin-7 (IL-7)
interleukin-8 (IL-8)
interleukin-9 (IL-9)
interleukin-10 (IL-10)
interleukin-11 (IL-11)
    human i.-11
    recombinant human i.-11
interleukin-12 (IL-12)
interleukin-13 (IL-13)
interleukin-14 (IL-14)
interleukin-15 (IL-15)
interleukin-16 (IL-16)
interleukin-17 (IL-17)
interleukin-18 (IL-18)
interlobar
    i. artery
    i. duct
    i. surface
    i. vein
interlobitis
interlobular
    i. artery
    i. duct
    i. ductule
    i. emphysema
    i. pleurisy
    i. septum
    i. vein
interlocal additivity
interlocking
    i. gyri
    i. suture
intermalleolar
intermammary
intermammillary
intermarriage
intermaxilla
intermaxillary
    i. anchorage
    i. bone
    i. elastic
    i. fixation
    i. relation
    i. segment
    i. suture
    i. traction
intermedia
    Prevotella i.
intermediary
    i. host
    i. metabolism
    i. movements

i. nerve
i. system
intermediate
   i. abutment
   i. acoustic stria
   i. amputation
   i. antebrachial vein
   i. atrial branch
   i. basilic vein
   i. body
   i. bronchus
   i. care facility (ICF)
   i. cephalic vein
   i. cervical septum
   i. column
   i. cubital vein
   i. cuneiform bone
   i. density lipoprotein (IDL)
   i. disc
   i. dorsal cutaneous nerve
   i. filament
   i. ganglion
   i. great muscle
   i. heart
   i. hemorrhage
   i. hepatic vein
   i. host
   i. hypothalamic area
   i. hypothalamic region
   i. junction
   i. lacunar lymph node
   i. lamella
   i. laryngeal cavity
   i. leprosy
   i. line
   i. lumbar lymph node
   i. mass
   i. mesoderm
   i. part
   i. ray
   i. sacral crest
   i. supraclavicular nerve
   i. temporal artery
   i. temporal branch
   i. trait
   i. uveitis
   i. variable
   i. vastus muscle
   i. vein of forearm
   i. white layer
   i. zone

intermediolateral
   i. cell column
   i. nucleus
intermediomedial
   i. frontal branch
   i. nucleus
intermedius
   bronchus i.
intermembrane space
intermembranous
intermeningeal
intermenstrual pain
intermesenteric
   i. arterial anastomosis
   i. nervous plexus
intermetacarpal joint
intermetameric
intermetatarsal
   i. articulation
   i. joint
intermetatarseum
   os i.
intermission
intermit
intermittence
intermittency
intermittens
   diabetes i.
   dyskinesia i.
intermittent
   i. acute porphyria (IAP)
   i. albuminuria
   i. arthralgia
   i. claudication
   i. compression
   i. cramp
   i. explosive disorder
   i. hemoglobinuria
   i. hydrarthrosis
   i. hydrosalpinx
   i. malaria
   i. malarial fever
   i. mandatory ventilation (IMV)
   i. positive pressure breathing
   (IPPB)
   i. positive pressure ventilation
   (IPPV)
   i. pulse
   i. self-obturation
   i. sterilization
   i. tetanus

NOTES

intermuscular
    i. gluteal bursa
    i. hernia
    i. septum
intern
interna
    auris i.
    hematorrhachis i.
    ophthalmoplegia i.
    otitis i.
internal
    i. acoustic canal
    i. acoustic foramen
    i. acoustic meatus
    i. acoustic opening
    i. acoustic pore
    i. adhesive pericarditis
    i. anal sphincter
    i. arcuate fiber
    i. attachment
    i. auditory artery
    i. auditory foramen
    i. auditory meatus
    i. auditory vein
    i. axis
    i. base
    i. canthus
    i. capsule
    i. capsule syndrome
    i. carotid artery
    i. carotid nerve
    i. carotid nervous plexus
    i. carotid venous plexus
    i. cephalic version
    i. cerebral vein
    i. collateral ligament
    i. conjugate
    i. conversion electron
    i. decompression
    i. ear
    i. energy
    i. female genital organ
    i. fixation
    i. hemorrhage
    i. hemorrhoid
    i. hernia
    i. hydrocephalus
    i. iliac artery
    i. iliac lymph node
    i. iliac vein
    i. inguinal ring
    i. intercostal membrane
    i. intercostal muscle
    i. jugular vein
    i. lacrimal fistula
    i. lip
    i. male genital organ
    i. malleolus
    i. mammary artery
    i. mammary plexus
    i. maxillary artery
    i. maxillary plexus
    i. medicine
    i. medullary lamina
    i. meningitis
    i. naris
    i. nasal branch
    i. nostril
    i. oblique muscle
    i. obturator muscle
    i. occipital crest
    i. occipital protuberance
    i. ophthalmopathy
    i. ophthalmoplegia
    i. phase
    i. pillar cell
    i. podalic version
    i. proctotomy
    i. pterygoid muscle
    i. pudendal artery
    i. pudendal vein
    i. pyocephalus
    i. ramus
    i. representation
    i. resorption
    i. respiration
    i. root sheath
    i. rotation
    i. salivary gland
    i. saphenous nerve
    i. semilunar fibrocartilage
    i. sheath of optic nerve
    i. spermatic artery
    i. spermatic fascia
    i. sphincter muscle
    i. sphincterotomy
    i. spiral sulcus
    i. squint
    i. stripper
    i. surface
    i. table
    i. thoracic artery
    i. thoracic lymphatic plexus
    i. thoracic vein
    i. traction
    i. urethral opening
    i. urethral orifice
    i. urethral sphincter
    i. urethrotomy
internalization
internalized homophobia
internarial
internasal suture
international
    i. normalized ratio (INR)
    i. sensitivity index
    i. unit (IU)

interne
    milieu i.
internet addiction disorder
interneuromeric cleft
interneuron
internodal segment
internode
internuclear ophthalmoplegia (INO)
internum
    filum terminale i.
    hordeolum i.
internuncial neuron
interobserver error
interocclusal
    i. clearance
    i. distance
    i. gap
    i. record
    i. rest space
interoceptive
interoceptor
interofective system
interolivary
interorbital
interosseal
interosseous
    i. border
    i. cartilage
    i. crest
    i. cubital bursa
    i. cuneocuboid ligament
    i. cuneometatarsal ligament
    i. fascia
    i. groove
    i. margin
    i. membrane
    i. metacarpal ligament
    i. metacarpal space
    i. metatarsal ligament
    i. metatarsal space
    i. muscle
    i. nerve
    i. sacroiliac ligament
    i. talocalcaneal ligament
    i. tibiofibular ligament
interosseus, pl. **interossei**
interpalatine suture
interpalpebral zone
interpapillary ridge
interparietal
    i. bone
    i. hernia

    i. sulcus
    i. suture
interparoxysmal
interpectoral lymph node
interpediculate
interpeduncular
    i. cistern
    i. fossa
    i. ganglion
    i. nucleus
interpelviabdominal amputation
interpersonal conflict
interphalangeal
    i. articulation
    distal i. (DIP)
    i. joint
    i. ostearthritis
interphase
interphyletic
interplant
interplanting
interpleural space
interpolated
    i. extrasystole
    i. flap
interposition arthroplasty
interpositospinal tract
interpositus nucleus
interpretation
interproximal
    i. papilla
    i. space
    i. surface
interpubic
    i. disc
    i. fibrocartilage
interpulmonary septum
interpupillary
interradial
interradicular
    i. alveoloplasty
    i. space
interrenal
interridge distance
interrod enamel
interrupted
    i. respiration
    i. suture
interruptus
    coitus i.
interscalene triangle

NOTES

interscapular
    i. gland
    i. hibernoma
    i. reflex
interscapulothoracic amputation
interscapulum
intersciatic
intersection
intersegmental
    i. fasciculus
    i. part
    i. vein
intersemilunar fissure
interseptal
interseptovalvular space
interseptum
intersexual
intersexuality
intersheath space
intersigmoid
    i. hernia
    i. recess
interspace
interspinal
    i. line
    i. muscle
    i. plane
interspinales
    i. cervicis muscle
    i. lumborum muscle
    i. thoracis muscle
interspinous
    i. ligament
    i. plane
intersternebral joint
interstice
interstitial
    i. absorption
    i. amygdaloid nucleus
    i. brachytherapy
    i. cell
    i. cell-stimulating hormone (ICSH)
    i. cell tumor
    i. cystitis
    i. deletion
    i. disease
    i. edema
    i. emphysema
    i. fluid
    i. gastritis
    i. gland
    i. growth
    i. hernia
    i. implantation
    i. inflammation
    i. keratitis
    i. lamella
    i. mastitis
    i. myositis

    i. nephritis
    i. neuritis
    i. pattern
    i. plasma cell pneumonia
    i. pregnancy
    i. pulmonary fibrosis
    i. radiation
    i. therapy
    i. tissue
interstitiospinal tract
interstitium
intertarsal
    i. articulation
    i. joint
intertendinous connection
interthalamica
    adhesio i.
interthalamic adhesion
intertragic notch
intertransversarii muscle
intertransverse
    i. ligament
    i. muscle
intertriginous
intertrigo
    eczema i.
intertrochanteric
    i. crest
    i. fracture
    i. line
intertropical hyphemia
intertubercular
    i. groove
    i. line
    i. plane
    i. sulcus
    i. tendon sheath
intertubular zone
interureteral
interureteric
    i. crest
    i. fold
intervaginal subarachnoid space
interval
    a-c i.
    AH i.
    AN i.
    atrioventricular i.
    auriculoventricular i.
    AV i.
    BH i.
    c-a i.
    calibration i.
    cardioarterial i.
    confidence i.
    coupling i.
    escape i.
    focal i.
    i. gout

I

HV i.
interectopic i.
isovolumic i.
lucid i.
i. operation
PA i.
PJ i.
PQ i.
PR i.
QR i.
QRB i.
QS2 i.
QT i.
i. scale
serial i.
sphygmic i.
Sturm i.
systolic time i.
i. training
intervascular
intervening
    i. sequence
    i. variable
intervenous tubercle
intervention
    crisis i.
interventional
    i. angiography
    i. radiology
interventricular
    i. foramen
    i. groove
    i. septal branch
    i. septum
intervertebral
    i. cartilage
    i. disc
    i. foramen
    i. ganglion
    i. notch
    i. symphysis
    i. vein
intervertebrale
    foramen i.
interview
    Zarit burden i.
intervillous
    i. lacuna
    i. space
interzonal mesenchyme
intestinal
    i. anastomosis

i. angina
i. anthrax
i. arterial arcade
i. artery
i. atresia
i. calculus
i. capillariasis
i. cecum
i. digestion
i. emphysema
i. fistula
i. follicle
i. gland
i. intoxication
i. juice
i. lymphangiectasis
i. lymphatic trunk
i. metaplasia
i. myiasis
i. pseudoobstruction
i. rotation
i. sand
i. schistosomiasis
i. sepsis
i. stasis
i. steatorrhea
i. surface
i. tube
i. villus
intestinale
    Encephalitozoon i.
intestinalis
    Encephalitozoon i.
    Giardia i.
    Lamblia i.
intestine
    large i.
    small i.
intestinotoxin
in-the-canal hearing aid
in-the-ear hearing aid
intima
intimal
intimitis
intoe
intolerance
    hereditary fructose i.
    lactose i.
    lysinuric protein i.
intorsion
intortor
intoxation

NOTES

intoxicant
intoxication
    acid i.
    anaphylactic i.
    intestinal i.
intraabdominal
intraacinous
intraadenoidal
intraalveolar septum
intraaortic
    i. balloon
    i. balloon counterpulsation
    i. balloon pump
intraarterial
intraarticular
    i. cartilage
    i. fracture
    i. sternocostal ligament
intraatrial
    i. block
    i. conduction
    i. conduction time
intraaural
intraauricular
intrabony pocket
intrabronchial
intrabuccal
intrabulbar fossa
intracanalicular fibroadenoma
intracapsular
    i. ankylosis
    i. fracture
    i. incision
    i. ligament
    i. rupture
    i. temporomandibular joint
       arthroplasty
intracardiac
    i. catheter
    i. lead
    i. pressure curve
    i. thrombosis
intracarpal
intracartilaginous
intracatheter
intracavernous
    i. aneurysm
    i. plexus
intracavitary
intracelial
intracellular
    i. canaliculus
    i. digestion
    i. enzyme
    i. fluid (ICF)
    i. toxin
    i. water
intracerebellar
intracerebral hemorrhage

intracerebroventricular
intracervical
intrachromosomal aberration
intracisternal
intracolic
intracordal
intracorneal implant
intracoronal retainer
intracorporeal
intracorpuscular
intracostal
intracranial
    i. aneurysm
    i. cavity
    i. ganglion
    i. granulomatous arteritis
    i. hematoma
    i. hemorrhage
    i. hypotension
    i. pneumatocele
    i. pneumocele
    i. pressure (ICP)
intracrine
intractable
    i. epilepsy
    i. pain
intraculminate fissure
intracutaneous reaction
intracystic papilloma
intracytoplasmic sperm injection
intrad
intradermal
    i. injection
    i. mattress suture
    i. nevus
    i. reaction
    i. test
intradermic
intraduct
intraductal
    i. carcinoma
    i. papilloma
intradural
intraembryonic mesoderm
intraepidermal carcinoma
intraepiphysial
intraepiploic hernia
intraepithelial
    i. carcinoma
    i. dyskeratosis
    i. gland
    i. plexus
intrafaradization
intrafascicular
intrafebrile
intrafilar
intrafusal fiber
intragalvanization
intragastric

intragemmal
intragenal
intragenic
    i. complementation
    i. suppression
intraglandular deep parotid lymph node
intraglobular
intragracile sulcus
intragyral
intrahepatic cholestasis
intrahyoid
intrailiac hernia
intrajugular process
intralaminar nucleus
intralaryngeal
intralesional therapy
intraligamentary pregnancy
intraligamentous
intralobar part
intralobular duct
intralocal additivity
intralocular
intraluminal
    i. catheter
    i. stripper
intramaxillary anchorage
intramedullary
    i. anesthesia
    i. drill
    i. reamer
    i. tractotomy
    i. transfusion
intramembranous ossification
intrameningeal
intramitochondrial
intramolecular
intramural
    i. hematoma
    i. part
    i. practice
    i. pregnancy
intramuscular (IM)
intramyocardial
intramyometrial
intranasal
    i. anesthesia
    i. antrostomy
intranatal
intraneural
in-transit metastasis
intranuclear
intraobserver error

intraocular
    i. fluid
    i. implant
    i. neuritis
    i. part
    i. pressure
intraoral
    i. anchorage
    i. anesthesia
    i. antrostomy
    i. fracture appliance
intraorbital
intraosseous
    i. anesthesia
    i. fixation
intraosteal
intraovarian
intraovular
intrapapillary drusen
intraparietal sulcus
intraparotid plexus
intrapartum
    i. hemorrhage
    i. period
intrapelvic hernia
intrapericardiac
intrapericardial
intraperitoneal
    i. catheter
    i. pregnancy
intrapersonal conflict
intrapial
intrapleural
intrapontine
intraprostatic
intraprotoplasmic
intrapsychic
intrapulmonary
    i. blood vessel
    i. lymph node
intrapyretic
intrarachidian
intrarectal
intrarenal
    i. artery
    i. reflux
intraretinal space
intrarrhachidian
intrascrotal
intrasegmental
    i. bronchus

NOTES

intrasegmental *(continued)*
    i. part
    i. vein
intraseptal alveoloplasty
intraspinal anesthesia
intrasplenic
intrastromal
intrasynovial
intratarsal
intratendinous olecranon bursa
intrathalamic fiber
intrathecal injection
intrathoracic
    i. airway obstruction
    i. goiter
intrathyroid cartilage
intratonsillar
intratracheal
    i. anesthesia
    i. intubation
    i. tube
intratubal
intratubular
intratympanic
intrauterine
    i. amputation
    i. contraceptive device (IUCD)
    i. device (IUD)
    i. fetal death
    i. fracture
    i. growth retardation (IUGR)
    i. insemination (IUI)
    i. pneumonia
    i. transfusion
intravagal glomus
intravaginal torsion
intravascular
    i. ligature
    i. lymph
    i. papillary endothelial hyperplasia
intravenous
    i. anesthesia
    i. anesthetic
    i. bolus
    i. cholangiogram (IVC)
    i. cholangiography
    i. drip
    i. narcosis
    i. pyelogram (IVP)
    i. pyelography (IVP)
    i. regional anesthesia
    i. urogram (IVU)
    i. urography
intraventricular (I-V, IV)
    i. block (IVB)
    i. conduction
    i. hemorrhage (IVH)
    i. injection
intravesical

intravital
    i. stain
    i. ultraviolet
intra vitam
intravitelline
intravitreous
intrinsic
    i. asthma
    i. coagulation pathway
    i. color
    i. deflection
    i. dysmenorrhea
    i. factor
    i. fiber
    i. motivation
    i. muscle
    i. PEEP
    i. protein
    i. proteinuria
    i. reflex
    i. sphincter
    i. sympathomimetic activity (ISA)
intrinsicoid deflection
introducer
introflection
introflexion
introgastric
introitus
introject
introjection
intromission
intromittent organ
intron
introspection
introspective method
introsusception
introversion
introvert
intubate
intubation
    altercursive i.
    aqueductal i.
    blind nasotracheal i.
    endotracheal i.
    intratracheal i.
    i. tube
intubator
intuitive stage
intumesce
intumescence
intumescent cataract
intumescentia
intussusception
    cecocolic i.
    colic i.
    colocolic i.
    double i.
    ileal i.
    ileocecal i.

ileocolic i.
ileoileal i.
jejunogastric i.
intussusceptive growth
intussusceptum
inulinase
inulin clearance
inulol
inunction
inundation fever
invaccination
invaginata
trichorrhexis i.
invaginated nipple
invaginate planula
invagination
basilar i.
invaginator
invalid
invalidism
invasin
invasion
invasive
i. carcinoma
i. mole
i. pituitary adenoma
inventory
Minnesota Multiphasic
Personality I. (MMPI)
invermination
inversa
angina i.
inverse
i. anaphylaxis
i. ocular bobbing
i. square law
i. symmetry
i. syntropy
inversed jaw-winking syndrome
inverse-ratio ventilation
inversion recovery
inversus
dextrocardia with situs i.
epicanthus i.
situs i.
invertase
invertebrate
inverted
i. cone bur
i. follicular keratosis
i. image
i. papilloma

i. pelvis
i. radial reflex
i. repeat
i. suture
invertin
invertor
invert sugar
investigatory reflex
investing
i. cartilage
i. fascia
i. layer
i. tissue
investment cast
inveterate
inviscation
invisible
i. differentiation
i. light
i. spectrum
involucra (*pl. of* involucrum)
involucre
involucrin
involucrum, pl. **involucra**
involuntary
i. activity
i. guarding
i. muscle
i. nervous system
involutional
i. depression
i. melancholia
involution form
involved field
I&O
intake and output
iobenzamic acid
iocetamic acid
iodamide
iodate
calcium i.
i. reaction
iodic acid
iodide
i. acne
bismuth i.
colloidal silver i.
dithiazanine i.
echothiophate i.
glyceryl i.
mercurous i.
metocurine i.

NOTES

iodide *(continued)*
    i. peroxidase
    i. transport defect
iodimetry
iodinase
iodinate
iodinated
    i. 131I human serum albumin
    i. 125I serum albumin
iodine
    butanol-extractable i.
    casein i.
    i. eruption
    Gram i.
    i. number
    i. reaction
    i. stain
    i. test
    i. tincture
    i. value
iodine-123, -125, -127, -131, -132
iodine-fast
iodine-induced hyperthyroidism
iodinophil
iodinophile
iodinophilous
iodipamide
iodism
iodixanol
iodize
iodized
    i. collodion
    i. oil
iodoacetamide
iodobehenate
    calcium i.
iodochlorol
iododerma
iodoform
iodoglobulin
iodogorgoic acid
iodohippurate sodium
iodomethamate sodium
iodometric
iodometry
iodopanoic acid
iodophendylate
iodophil granule
iodophilia
iodophor
iodophthalein
iodopropylidene glycerol
iodoprotein
iodopsin
iodopyracet
iodoquinol
iodotherapy
iodothyronine

iodotyrosine
    i. deiodase
    i. deiodinase defect
iodoxamate meglumine
ioduria
ioglycamic acid
iohexol
iometer
ion
    i. channel
    i. channel disorder
    dipolar i.'s
    i. exchange
    i. exchange chromatography
    i. exchanger
    hydride i.
    hydrogen i.
    hydronium i.
    i. pump
ion-exchange resin
ionic
    i. medication
    i. strength
ionium
ionization chamber
ionize
ionized atom
ionizing radiation
ionogram
ionone
ionopherogram
ionophore
ionophoresis
ionophoretic
ion-selective electrode
iontophoresis
iontophoretic
iontotherapy
iopamidol
iopanoic acid
iopentol
iophendylate
iophenoic acid
iophenoxic acid
iophobia
iopromide
iota
iotacism
iothalamic acid
iothiouracil sodium
iotrol
iotrolan
ioversol
ioxaglate
ioxilan
ioxithalamate
ipecac syrup
ipecacuanha
    deemetinized i.

IPF
idiopathic pulmonary fibrosis
ipodate
calcium i.
ipomea resin
IPPB
intermittent positive pressure breathing
IPPV
intermittent positive pressure ventilation
ipsefact
ipsilateral reflex
IPSP
inhibitory postsynaptic potential
IPV
inactivated poliovirus vaccine
IQ
intelligence quotient
irascibility
iridal
iridectomy
basal i.
buttonhole i.
laser i.
iridencleisis
irideremia
iridescent virus
iridesis
iridial part
iridian
iridic
iridin
iridium
iridoavulsion
iridocele
iridochoroiditis
iridocoloboma
iridocorneal
i. angle
i. endothelial syndrome
i. mesenchymal dysgenesis
iridocyclectomy
iridocyclitis septica
iridocyclochoroiditis
iridocystectomy
iridodiagnosis
iridodialysis
iridodilator
iridodonesis
iridokinetic
iridology
iridomalacia
iridomesodialysis

iridomotor
iridoparalysis
iridopathy
iridoplegia
complete i.
iridoptosis
iridopupillary lamina
iridorrhexis
iridoschisis
iridosclerotomy
iridotomy
laser i.
Iridoviridae
Iridovirus
irigenin
iris
i. bicolor
i. bombé
i. dehiscence
erythema i.
i. freckle
i. frill
herpes i.
i. pit
i. prolapse
i. scissors
i. spatula
umbrella i.
Irish
I. moss
I. moss gelatin
irisin
iris-nevus syndrome
iritic
iritis
diabetic i.
fibrinous i.
follicular i.
hemorrhagic i.
spongy i.
iron
i. albuminate
albuminized i.
i. alum
i. deficiency anemia
i. filings
i. hematoxylin
i. index
i. line
i. lung
i. protoporphyrin

NOTES

iron *(continued)*
    i. pyrites
    i. sulfate
iron-52, -55, -59
iron-binding capacity (IBC)
iron-dextran complex
iron-storage disease
iron-sulfur protein
irradiate
irradiated vitamin D milk
irradiation
irrational
irreducible hernia
irregular
    i. astigmatism
    i. bone
    i. dentin
    i. emphysema
    i. nystagmus
    i. pulse
irresistible impulse
irrespirable
irresponsibility
    criminal i.
irresuscitable
irreversible
    i. colloid
    i. hydrocolloid
    i. pulpitis
    i. reaction
    i. shock
irrigate
irrigation cannula
irrigator
irritability
    electric i.
    myotatic i.
irritable
    i. bowel syndrome
    i. breast
    i. colon
irritant contact dermatitis
irritation
    i. cell
    i. dentin
    i. fibroma
irritative miosis
irrumation
irruption
irruptive
IRV
    inspiratory reserve volume
Irvine-Gass syndrome
ISA
    intrinsic sympathomimetic activity
Isaac-Merton syndrome
Isaac syndrome
isauxesis

ischemia-modifying factor
ischemia retinae
ischemic
    i. contracture
    i. heart disease
    i. hypoxia
    i. lumbago
    i. mitral regurgitation
    i. muscular atrophy
    i. necrosis
    i. optic neuropathy
    i. palsy
ischesis
ischiadic
    i. plexus
    i. spine
ischial
    i. bone
    i. bursa
    i. bursitis
    i. ramus
    i. spine
    i. tuberosity
ischialgia
ischiatic
    i. hernia
    i. notch
ischioanal fossa
ischiobulbar
ischiocapsular ligament
ischiocavernosus
ischiocavernous muscle
ischiocele
ischiococcygeal
ischiococcygeus
ischiodynia
ischiofemoral ligament
ischiofibular
ischiomelus
ischionitis
ischiopagus
ischioperineal
ischiopubic ramus
ischiorectal
    i. abscess
    i. excavation
    i. fat-pad
    i. fossa
    i. hernia
ischiosacral
ischiothoracopagus
ischiotibial
ischiovaginal
ischiovertebral
ischium
ischochymia
ischuretic
ischuria

isethionate
    hexamidine i.
    hydroxystilbamidine i.
isethionic acid
Ishihara test
Isinglass
island
    blood i.
    bone i.
    i. of Calleja
    cartilage i.
    i. disease
    epimyoepithelial i.
    i. fever
    i. flap
    Langerhans i.
    i. leg flap
    i. of Reil
islet
    blood i.
    i. cell
    i. cell tumor
    i. of Langerhans
    i. tissue
isoacceptor tRNA
isoagglutination
isoagglutinin
isoagglutinogen
isoallele
isoallotypic determinant
isoalloxazine
isoaminile
isoamyl
isoamylase
isoandrosterone
isoantibody
isoantigen
isobar
isobaric spinal anesthesia
isobornyl thiocyanoacetate
isobutane
isobuteine
isobutyl nitrite
isobutyric acid
isocapnia
isocellular
isochoric
isochromatic
isochromatophil
isochromatophile
isochromic anemia
isochromosome

isochronia
isochronous
isocitrase
isocitratase
isocitrate
    i. dehydrogenase
    i. lyase
isocitric
    i. acid
    i. acid dehydrogenase
isocitritase
isocline
isoconazole
isocoria
isocortex
isocyanate
isocyanic acid
isocyanide
isocyclic compound
isocytolysin
isodactylism
isodemographic map
isodense
isodesmosine
isodiphasic complex
isodose
isodulcit
isodynamic law
isodynamogenic
isoelectric
    i. electroencephalogram
    i. focusing
    i. line
    i. period
    i. point (IEP)
    i. zone
isoenergetic
isoenzyme
    creatine kinase i.
    i. electrophoresis
isoerythrolysis
isofluorphate
isoflurane
isogamete
isogamy
isogeneic graft
isogenic strain
isogenous
    i. chondrocyte
    i. nest
isogentiobiose
isoglutamine

NOTES

isognathous
isograft
isohemagglutination
isohemagglutinin
isohemolysin
isohemolysis
isohydric
isohydruria
isoimmune neonatal thrombocytopenia
isoimmunization
isoionic point
isolate
    genetic i.
    mating i.
isolated
    i. abutment
    i. dextrocardia
    i. dyskeratosis follicularis
    i. explosive disorder
    i. hypoaldosteronism
    i. parietal endocarditis
    i. proteinuria
isolation
    body substance i.
isolé
    cerveau i.
    encéphale i.
isolecithal
    i. egg
    i. ovum
isoleucine
isoleucyl
isoleukoagglutinin
isologous graft
isolysin
isolysis
isolytic
isomaltase
isomaltose
isomastigote
isomer
    geometric i.
isomerase
    hexosephosphate i.
    retinal i.
    triosephosphate i.
isomeric
    i. function
    i. transition
isomerism
    geometric i.
    optic i.
    optical i.
    structural i.
isomerization
    enzyme i.
isomerous
isomethadone
isometheptene

isometric
    i. chart
    i. contraction
    i. contraction period
    i. exercise
    i. relaxation
    i. relaxation period
    i. ruler
    i. traction
isometropia
isomorphic response
isomorphism
isomorphous gliosis
isonaphthol
isoncotic
isoniazid
    i. neuropathy
    i. polyneuropathy
isonicotinic acid
isonitrile
isonitrosoacetone
isoosmotic
isopathy
isopentenylpyrophosphate
isopentyl
isopeptide bond
isoperistaltic anastomosis
isophagy
isophane insulin
isoplassont
isoplastic graft
isopleth
isopotential
isoprecipitin
isoprenaline sulfate
isoprene rule
isoprenoid
isoprenylation
isopropanol
isopropyl alcohol
isopropylcarbinol
isopropylthiogalactoside
isoproterenol sulfate
isopter
isopycnic zone
isopyknic
isopyrocalciferol
isoquinoline
isorhythmic dissociation
isoriboflavin
isorrhea
isosbestic point
isoschizomer
isosensitize
isoserum treatment
isosexual
isosmotic
isosorbide dinitrate
Isospora

isosporiasis
isostere
isostery
isosthenuria
isosuccinic acid
isosulfan blue
isothermal
isothiocyanate
 fluorescein i.
isothipendyl
isotone
isotonia
isotonic
 i. coefficient
 i. contraction
 i. exercise
 i. traction
isotonicity
isotope
 i. clearance
 daughter i.
 radioactive i.
 stable i.
isotopic
isotransplantation
isotretinoin
isotropic
 i. disc
 i. lipid
isotropous
isotype
isotypic
isovaleric
 i. acid
 i. acidemia
isovalthine
isovolume pressure-flow curve
isovolumetric relaxation
isovolumic
 i. interval
 i. period
 i. relaxation
isozyme
israelii
 Actinomyces i.
isthmectomy
isthmian
isthmic
isthmoparalysis
isthmoplegia
isthmus
 aortic i.

 Guyon i.
 i. of His
 Krönig i.
 i. of pharynx
 i. of prostate
 rhombencephalic i.
 i. of thyroid gland
 i. of uterus
itaconic acid
Itai-Itai disease
Italian flap
itch
 azo i.
 baker i.
 barber i.
 bath i.
 copra i.
 Cuban i.
 frost i.
 grain i.
 grocer i.
 ground i.
 jock i.
 kabure i.
 straw i.
 straw-bed i.
 swimmer's i.
 water i.
Ito
 I. cell
 hypomelanosis of I.
 I. nevus
ITO method
ITP
 idiopathic thrombocytopenic purpura
itramin tosylate
IU
 international unit
IUCD
 intrauterine contraceptive device
IUD
 intrauterine device
IUGR
 intrauterine growth retardation
IUI
 intrauterine insemination
I-V, IV
 intraventricular
  I-V block
IVB
 intraventricular block

NOTES

IVC
  inferior vena cava
  intravenous cholangiogram
IVCP
  inferior vena cava pressure
Ivemark syndrome
ivermectin
IVF
  in vitro fertilization
IVH
  intraventricular hemorrhage
Ivor Lewis esophagectomy
ivory
    i. exostosis
    i. membrane
    i. osteoma
    i. vertebra
IVP
  intravenous pyelogram
  intravenous pyelography
IVU
  intravenous urogram
Ivy
    I. bleeding time test
    I. loop wiring
ixodiasis
ixodic
ixodid
Ixodidae

J

joule
  J chain
  J point

J_{Capetown}
  hemoglobin J.

Jaboulay
  J. amputation
  J. operation
  J. pyloroplasty

Jaccoud
  J. arthritis
  J. arthropathy

jacket
  j. crown
  Minerva j.

jackscrew

Jackson
  J. law
  J. membrane
  J. rule
  J. sign
  J. veil

Jackson-Babcock operation

jacksonian
  j. epilepsy
  j. seizure

Jacobaeus operation

Jacobson
  J. anastomosis
  J. canal
  J. cartilage
  J. nerve
  J. organ
  J. plexus
  J. reflex

Jacquart facial angle
Jacquemet recess
Jacquemin test
Jacques plexus
jactitation
Jadassohn-Lewandowski syndrome
Jadassohn nevus
Jadassohn-Pellizzari anetoderma
Jaeger test type
Jaffe
  J. reaction
  J. test

Jaffe-Lichtenstein disease
Jahnke syndrome
jail fever
jake paralysis
jalap resin
Jamaican vomiting sickness

jambes
  maladie des j.

James
  J. fiber
  J. tract

Jamestown
  J. Canyon virus
  J. weed

Janet test
Janeway lesion
janiceps
  j. asymmetrus
  j. parasiticus

Jansen operation
Jansky-Bielschowsky disease
Jansky classification
Janus green B
Japanese
  J. B encephalitis
  J. B encephalitis virus
  J. river fever
  J. schistosomiasis
  J. spotted fever

Japan wax
japonica
  cutaneous schistosomiasis j.
  schistosomiasis j.

japonicum
  Schistosoma j.

jar
  heel j.

jargon aphasia
Jarisch-Herxheimer reaction
Jarman score
Jarvik artificial heart
Jatene procedure
jaundice
  acholuric j.
  anhepatic j.
  anhepatogenous j.
  choleric j.
  cholestatic j.
  chronic acholuric j.
  chronic familial j.
  chronic idiopathic j.
  congenital hemolytic j.
  constitutional j.
  familial nonhemolytic j.
  hematogenous j.
  hemolytic j.
  hepatocellular j.
  hepatogenous j.
  homologous serum j.
  human serum j.
  infectious j.

J

jaundice *(continued)*
    infective j.
    leptospiral j.
    malignant j.
    mechanical j.
    nonobstructive j.
    nuclear j.
    obstructive j.
    physiologic j.
    recurrent j.
    regurgitation j.
    retention j.
    j. root
    transfusion j.
jaw
    j. bone
    crackling j.
    Hapsburg j.
    j. jerk
    j. joint
    lower j.
    lumpy j.
    j. reflex
    j. repositioning
    j. separation
    j. skeleton
    j. winking
Jaworski body
jaw-winking
    j.-w. phenomenon
    j.-w. syndrome
jaw-working reflex
JC virus
jeanselmei
    Exophiala j.
Jeanselme nodule
Jeghers-Peutz syndrome
jeikeium
    Corynebacterium j.
jejunal artery
jejunectomy
jejuni
    Campylobacter j.
    Campylobacter fetus j.
jejunitis
jejunocolostomy
jejunogastric intussusception
jejunoileal
    j. bypass
    j. shunt
jejunoileitis
jejunoileostomy
jejunojejunostomy
jejunoplasty
jejunostomy
jejunotomy
jejunum
Jellinek formula

jelly
    box j.
    cardiac j.
    glycerin j.
    interlaminar j.
    Wharton j.
jellyfish
Jendrassik maneuver
Jenner-Kay unit
Jenner stain
Jensen
    J. disease
    J. sarcoma
jensenii
    Lactobacillus j.
Jericho boil
jerk
    ankle j.
    chin j.
    crossed adductor j.
    crossed knee j.
    elbow j.
    j. finger
    jaw j.
    knee j.
jerky
    j. nystagmus
    j. pulse
    j. respiration
Jerne
    J. plaque assay
    J. technique
jersey finger
Jervell and Lange-Nielsen syndrome
Jesuits bark
Jesuit tea
jet
    j. ejector pump
    j. injection
    j. injector
    j. lag
    j. nebulizer
Jeune syndrome
jeweller forceps
Jewett
    J. sound
    J. and Strong staging
JH virus
jigger
jimson weed
Jk
    J. antigen
    J. blood group
Jobbins antigen
Jobert
    J. de Lamballe fossa
    J. de Lamballe suture
Job syndrome
Jocasta complex

J

jock itch
Jod-Basedow phenomenon
Joffroy
    J. reflex
    J. sign
Johanson-Blizzard syndrome
Johnson method
joint
    acromioclavicular j.
    ankle j.
    anterior intraoccipital j.
    arthrodial j.
    atlantoaxial j.
    atlantooccipital j.
    ball-and-socket j.
    biaxial j.
    bicondylar j.
    bilocular j.
    j. branch
    Budin obstetrical j.
    calcaneocuboid j.
    capitular j.
    j. capsule
    carpal j.
    carpometacarpal j.
    cartilaginous j.
    j. cavity
    Charcot j.
    Chopart j.
    Clutton j.
    coccygeal j.
    cochlear j.
    complex j.
    composite j.
    compound j.
    condylar j.
    costochondral j.
    costotransverse j.
    costovertebral j.
    cotyloid j.
    cranial synovial j.
    cricoarytenoid j.
    cricothyroid j.
    Cruveilhier j.
    cubital j.
    cuboideonavicular j.
    cuneocuboid j.
    cuneometatarsal j.
    cuneonavicular j.
    cylindrical j.
    dentoalveolar j.
    diarthrodial j.

    digital j.
    DIP j.
    distal interphalangeal j.
    distal radioulnar j.
    distal tibiofibular j.
    dry j.
    j. effusion
    elbow j.
    ellipsoidal j.
    enarthrodial j.
    j. extension
    facet j.
    false j.
    femoropatellar j.
    fibrous j.
    flail j.
    j. gamete
    ginglymoid j.
    glenohumeral j.
    gliding j.
    gompholic j.
    hemophilic j.
    hinge j.
    hip j.
    humeral j.
    humeroradial j.
    humeroulnar j.
    hysterical j.
    immovable j.
    incudomalleolar j.
    incudostapedial j.
    inferior radioulnar j.
    inferior tibiofibular j.
    interarticular j.
    intercarpal j.
    interchondral j.
    intercuneiform j.
    intermetacarpal j.
    intermetatarsal j.
    interphalangeal j.
    intersternebral j.
    intertarsal j.
    jaw j.
    knee j.
    lateral atlantoaxial j.
    lateral atlantoepistrophic j.
    Lisfranc j.
    lumbosacral j.
    Luschka j.
    mandibular j.
    manubriosternal j.
    median atlantoaxial j.

NOTES

joint *(continued)*
    metacarpophalangeal j.
    metatarsophalangeal j.
    midcarpal j.
    middle atlantoepistrophic j.
    middle carpal j.
    middle radioulnar j.
    midtarsal j.
    mortise j.
    j. mouse
    movable j.
    multiaxial j.
    neuropathic j.
    j. oil
    patellofemoral j.
    pivot j.
    plane j.
    polyaxial j.
    j. probability
    radiocarpal j.
    rotary j.
    rotatory j.
    saddle j.
    scapulothoracic j.
    j. sense
    shoulder j.
    simple j.
    slip j.
    spheroid j.
    spiral j.
    sternoclavicular j.
    stress-broken j.
    subtalar j.
    synarthrodial j.
    synchondrodial j.
    synovial j.
    talocalcaneal j.
    talocalcaneonavicular j.
    talocrural j.
    tarsal j.
    tarsometatarsal j.
    temporomandibular j. (TMJ)
    transverse tarsal j.
    trochoid j.
    uniaxial j.
    unilocular j.
    wedge-and-groove j.
    wrist j.
jojoba oil
joker elevator
Jolles test
Jolly
    J. body
    J. reaction
jolt headache
Jones
    J. criteria
    J. fracture
    J. I, II test

    J. test
    J. transfer
Jonesia denitrificans
Jonnesco fossa
Joubert syndrome
joule (J)
    j. equivalent
Js antigen
J-sella deformity
Juanism
    Don J.
Judet view
judgment
    insight and j.
Judkins technique
jugal
    j. bone
    j. ligament
    j. point
jugomaxillary
jugular
    j. bulb
    j. duct
    j. foramen
    j. foramen syndrome
    j. fossa
    j. ganglion
    j. gland
    j. glomus
    j. lymphatic plexus
    j. lymphatic trunk
    j. nerve
    j. notch
    j. process
    j. pulse
    j. sinus
    j. tubercle
    j. vein
    j. venous arch
    j. venous distention (JVD)
    j. venous pressure (JVP)
    j. venous pulse (JVP)
    j. wall
jugulare
    foramen j.
jugulodigastric lymph node
juguloomohyoid lymph node
jugum
juice
    appetite j.
    cherry j.
    gastric j.
    intestinal j.
jumper disease
jump flap
jumping
    j. the bite
    j. disease
    j. gene

junction
  adhering j.
  amelodental j.
  amelodentinal j.
  amnioembryonic j.
  anorectal j.
  AV j.
  cardioesophageal j.
  cementodentinal j.
  cementoenamel j.
  choledochoduodenal j.
  communicating j.
  corneoscleral j.
  costochondral j.
  dentinocemental j.
  dentinoenamel j. (DEJ)
  duodenojejunal j.
  electrotonic j.
  esophagogastric j.
  gap j.
  Holliday j.
  ileocecal j.
  impermeable j.
  intercellular j.
  intermediate j.
  j. of lips
  manubriosternal j.
  mucocutaneous j.
  myoneural j.
  j. nevus
  tight j.
  ureteropelvic j.
  ureterovesical j. (UVJ)
junctional
  j. complex
  j. cyst
  j. epithelium
  j. escape
  j. escape rhythm
  j. extrasystole
  j. tachycardia
junctura
juncture
jungian psychoanalysis
jungle yellow fever
Jüngling disease
Jung muscle
Junin virus
juniper
  j. berry oil
  j. tar
junk DNA

jurisprudence
  dental j.
  medical j.
Jurkat cell
juvenile
  j. absence epilepsy
  j. angiofibroma
  j. arrhythmia
  j. carcinoma
  j. cataract
  j. cell
  j. cerebellar astrocytoma
  j. chorea
  j. chronic arthritis
  j. cirrhosis
  j. delinquent
  j. diabetes
  j. elastoma
  j. hemangiofibroma
  j. hyalin fibromatosis
  j. kyphosis
  j. muscular atrophy
  j. myoclonic epilepsy
  j. neutrophil
  j. osteomalacia
  j. osteoporosis
  j. palmoplantar fibromatosis
  j. papillomatosis
  j. pattern
  j. pelvis
  j. periodontitis
  j. plantar dermatosis
  j. polyp
  j. retinoschisis
  j. rheumatoid arthritis
  j. spinal muscular atrophy
  j. xanthogranuloma
juvenile-onset diabetes
juvenile-type hyperglycerolemia
juxtaarticular nodule
juxtacolic artery
juxtacortical
  j. chondroma
  j. osteogenic sarcoma
juxtacrine
juxtaepiphysial
juxtaesophageal pulmonary lymph node
juxtaglomerular
  j. apparatus
  j. body
  j. cell
  j. cell tumor

NOTES

juxtaglomerular *(continued)*
    j. complex
    j. granule
juxtaintestinal mesenteric lymph node
juxtallocortex
juxtamedullary glomerulus
juxtapapillaris
    retinochoroiditis j.
juxtaphrenic peak

juxtaposition
juxtapupillary choroiditis
juxtarestiform body
JVD
    jugular venous distention
JVP
    jugular venous pressure
    jugular venous pulse

κ (*var. of* kappa)

K
    kelvin
        K antigen
        K blood group
        K capture
        K cell
        K complex
        K region
        K shell
        K virus

K1
    vitamin K1

K2
    vitamin K2

K:A
    ketogenic-antiketogenic
    K:A ratio

kabure itch

Kader-Senn operation

Kaes
    K. feltwork
    line of K.
    K. line

Kaes-Bechterew
    band of K.-B.

Kaffir pox

kafindo

kainate receptor

kainic acid

kairomones

Kaiserling fixative

kala azar

kalemia

kaliopenia

kaliopenic

kalium

kaliuresis

kaliuretic

kallak

kallidin
    k. 9, 10
    k. I, II

kallikrein system

Kallmann syndrome

kaluresis

kaluretic

kangaroo tendon suture

kang cancer

kangri
    k. burn carcinoma
    k. cancer

Kanner syndrome

Kansas
    hemoglobin K.

kansasii
    Mycobacterium k.

kanyemba

kaodzera

kaolin clotting time

kaolinosis

Kaplan-Meier
    K.-M. analysis
    K.-M. estimate

Kaposi
    K. sarcoma
    K. varicelliform eruption

kappa, κ
    k. angle
    k. granule
    k. particle

kappacism

karaya gum

Karman cannula

Karmen unit

Karnofsky scale

Kartagener
    K. syndrome
    K. triad

karyochrome cell

karyoclasis

karyocyte

karyogamic

karyogamy

karyogenesis

karyogenic

karyogonad

karyogram

karyology

karyolymph

karyolysis

karyolytic

karyomere

karyomicrosome

karyomitome

karyomorphism

karyon

karyophage

karyoplasm

karyoplasmolysis

karyoplast

karyoplastin

karyopyknosis

karyopyknotic index

karyorrhexis

karyosome

karyostasis

karyotheca

karyotype

karyozoic

K

Kasabach-Merritt syndrome
Kasai operation
Kashin-Bek disease
Kasokero virus
Kasten
    K. fluorescent Feulgen stain
    K. fluorescent PAS stain
    K. fluorescent Schiff reagent
Kast syndrome
katal
katathermometer
Katayama
    K. disease
    K. fever
    K. syndrome
    K. test
kathexis
kava
Kawasaki
    K. disease
    K. syndrome
Kayser-Fleischer ring
Kazanjian operation
kb
    kilobase
k blood group
kc
    kilocycle
kcal
    kilocalorie
    kilogram calorie
Kearns-Sayre syndrome
Keating-Hart method
kedani fever
keel
keeled chest
Keen operation
keep vein open (KVO)
Kegel exercises
Kehr sign
Keith
    K. bundle
    K. and Flack node
kelectome
Kelev strain rabies virus
Kell
    K. antigen
    K. blood group
Keller bunionectomy
Keller-Madlener operation
Kelly
    K. clamp
    K. operation
    K. rectal speculum
keloid
    acne k.
keloidalis
    folliculitis k.
keloidosis

keloplasty
kelosomia
kelvin (K)
Kelvin scale
Kempner diet
Kendall
    K. compound
    K. substance
Kennedy
    K. classification
    K. disease
    K. syndrome
Kenny-Caffey syndrome
Kenny treatment
Kent bundle
Kent-His bundle
Kenya fever
kephalin
Kerandel sign
kerasin
keratan sulfate
keratectasia
keratectomy
    automated lamellar k.
    phototherapeutic k.
keratein
keratic precipitates
keratin
    k. filament
    k. pearl
keratinase
keratinization
keratinized cell
keratinizing odontogenic cyst
keratinocyte
keratinophilic
keratinosome
keratinous cyst
keratitis
    actinic k.
    deep punctate k.
    dendriform k.
    dendritic k.
    diffuse deep k.
    Dimmer k.
    disciform k.
    k. disciformis
    exposure k.
    fascicular k.
    filamentary k.
    k. filamentosa
    geographic k.
    herpetic k.
    interstitial k.
    lagophthalmic k.
    k. linearis migrans
    marginal k.
    metaherpetic k.
    mycotic k.

necrotizing k.
neuroparalytic k.
neurotrophic k.
k. nummularis
phlyctenular k.
k. profunda
k. punctata
sclerosing k.
k. sicca
stromal k.
trachomatous k.
vesicular k.
keratoacanthoma
keratoangioma
keratocele
keratoconjunctivitis
atopic k.
epidemic k.
flash k.
herpetic k.
infectious bovine k.
microsporidian k.
k. sicca
superior limbic k.
ultraviolet k.
virus k.
keratoconus
circumscribed posterior k.
keratocricoid
keratocyst
odontogenic k.
keratocyte
keratoderma
lymphedematous k.
mutilating k.
k. plantare sulcatum
keratodermatitis
keratoectasia
keratoelastoidosis marginalis
keratoepithelioplasty
keratogenesis
keratogenetic
keratogenous membrane
keratoglobus
keratography
keratohyal
keratohyalin granule
keratoid exanthema
keratoleptynsis
keratoleukoma
keratolysis
k. exfoliativa

pitted k.
k. plantare sulcatum
keratolytic
keratoma
k. disseminatum
k. hereditarium mutilans
k. plantare sulcatum
keratomalacia
keratome
keratometer
keratometry
keratomileusis
laser-assisted in situ k. (LASIK)
keratomycosis
keratonosis
keratopachyderma
keratopathia guttata
keratopathy
band-shaped k.
bullous k.
chronic actinic k.
climatic droplike k.
filamentary k.
infectious crystalline k.
Labrador k.
lipid k.
neuroparalytic k.
keratophakia
keratophakic keratoplasty
keratoplasia
keratoplasty
allopathic k.
autogenous k.
epikeratophakic k.
heterogenous k.
homogenous k.
keratophakic k.
lamellar k.
layered k.
optical k.
refractive k.
tectonic k.
keratoprosthesis
keratorefractive surgery
keratorhexis
keratorrhexis
keratorus
keratosa
acne k.
keratoscleritis
keratoscope
keratoscopy

K

NOTES

keratose
keratosis
    actinic k.
    arsenical k.
    k. blennorrhagica
    k. follicularis
    inverted follicular k.
    k. labialis
    lichenoid k.
    lichen planus-like k.
    k. obturans
    k. palmaris et plantaris
    k. pilaris
    k. pilaris atrophicans faciei
    k. punctata
    seborrheic k.
    k. seborrheica
    k. senilis
keratosulfate
keratotome
keratotomy
    delimiting k.
    radial k.
    refractive k.
keraunophobia
Kerckring
    K. center
    K. fold
    K. ossicle
    K. valve
kerion
    tinea k.
Kerley A, B, C line
kernicterus
Kernig sign
Kernohan notch
kern-plasma relation theory
keroid
kerosene
Kestenbaum
    K. number
    K. procedure
    K. sign
ketal
ketamine
ketanserin
ketene
ketimine
keto acid
ketoacidemia
ketoacidosis
    diabetic k. (DKA)
ketoaciduria
    branched chain k.
ketoconazole
ketogenesis

ketogenic
    k. corticoids test
    k. diet
ketogenic-antiketogenic (K:A)
    k.-a. ratio
ketoheptose
ketohexose
ketohydroxyestrin
ketol
ketole group
ketolytic
ketone
    k. alcohol
    k. body
    dimethyl k.
    methyl isobutyl k.
ketone-aldehyde mutase
ketonemia
ketonic
ketonimine dye
ketonization
ketonuria
    branched chain k.
ketopantoic acid
ketopentose
ketorolac
ketose reductase
ketosis
    bovine k.
ketosis-prone diabetes
ketosis-resistant diabetes
ketosuccinic acid
ketosuria
ketotetrose
ketotic
    k. hyperglycemia
    k. hyperglycinemia
    k. hypoglycemia
ketotriose
Kety-Schmidt method
keV
    kiloelectron volt
Kew Gardens fever
key
    k. attachment
    k. ridge
    k. vein
keyhole
    k. deformity
    k. pupil
key-in-lock maneuver
Key-Retzius
    foramen of K.-R.
keyway attachment
kg
    kilogram
khat
khellin

kick
  atrial k.
  idioventricular k.
Kidd
  K. antigen
  K. blood group
kidney
  amyloid k.
  Armanni-Ebstein k.
  arteriolosclerotic k.
  arteriosclerotic k.
  artificial k.
  Ask-Upmark k.
  atrophic k.
  k. basin
  cake k.
  k. carbuncle
  contracted k.
  cow k.
  crush k.
  cystic k.
  decapsulation of k.
  disc k.
  duplex k.
  fatty k.
  flea-bitten k.
  floating k.
  Formad k.
  fused k.
  Goldblatt k.
  granular k.
  head k.
  hind k.
  horseshoe k.
  k.'s, liver, spleen (KLS)
  k. lobe
  medullary sponge k.
  middle k.
  pancake k.
  polycystic k.
  k. scan
  k. stone
  k.'s, ureters, bladder (KUB)
  wandering k.
  waxy k.
Kiel classification
Kienböck
  K. disease
  K. dislocation
  K. unit
Kiernan space
Kiesselbach area

Kikuchi disease
Kilham rat virus
Kiliani-Fischer
  K.-F. reaction
  K.-F. synthesis
Kilian line
killer
  k. cell
  natural k. (NK)
Killian
  K. bundle
  K. operation
  K. triangle
kilobase (kb)
kilocalorie (kcal)
kilocycle (kc)
kiloelectron volt (keV)
kilogram (kg)
  k. calorie (kcal)
kilogram-meter
kilogram-metre
kilohertz
kilohm
kilojoule
kilovolt (kv)
  k.'s peak (kVp)
kilovoltmeter
Kimmelstiel-Wilson
  K.-W. disease
  K.-W. syndrome
Kimura disease
kinanesthesia
kinase
  acetate k.
  adenosine k.
  adenylate k.
  carbamate k.
  choline k.
  creatine k. (CK)
  glycerol k.
  k. II
  mevalonate k.
  pyruvate k.
kind
  error of the first k.
  error of the second k.
kindred
  degree of k.
kinematic
  k. chain
  k. face-bow
  k. viscosity

K

NOTES

kinematics
kinemometer
kineplastic amputation
kineplastics
kinesalgia
kinesia
kinesialgia
kinesiatrics
kinesics
kinesimeter
kinesin
kinesiology
kinesiometer
kinesipathist
kinesis
kinesitherapy
kinesophobia
kinesthesia hallucination
kinesthesiometer
kinesthesis
kinesthetic
>k. aura
>k. awareness
>k. sense
kinetic
>k. analyzer
>k. ataxia
>k. energy
>k. measurement
>k. perimetry
>k. strabismus
>k. system
>k. tremor
kinetics
>chemical k.
>enzyme k.
kinetocardiogram
kinetocardiograph
kinetochore fiber
kinetogenic
kinetoplasm
kinetoplast
kinetoscope
kinetosome
king
>k. evil
>K. unit
kingae
>*Kingella k.*
King-Armstrong unit
Kingella
>*K. indologenes*
>*K. kingae*
Kingsley splint
kinic acid
kinin 9
kininogen
>high molecular weight k.
>low molecular weight k.

kininogenase
kininogenin
kink
>Lane k.
kinked aorta
Kinkiang fever
kinky-hair, kinky hair
>k.-h. disease
kinocentrum
kinocilium
kinomometer
kinoplasm
kinoplasmic
kinship
>coefficient of k.
Kinyoun stain
kion
Kirk amputation
Kirkland knife
Kirschner
>K. apparatus
>K. wire
Kisch reflex
kissing
>k. puncta
>k. spines
Kitasato bacillus
Kjeldahl
>K. apparatus
>K. method
Kjelland forceps
Kjer optic atrophy
Klatskin tumor
Klebsiella
>*K. mobilis*
>*K. oxytoca*
>*K. pneumoniae*
>*K. pneumoniae ozaenae*
>*K. rhinoscleromatis*
Klebs-Loeffler bacillus
kleeblattschädel
Kleihauer-Betke technique
Kleihauer stain
Kleine-Levin syndrome
Klein-Gumprecht shadow nucleus
Klemm sign
Klenow fragment
kleptomania
kleptomaniac
kleptophobia
Klestadt cyst
Klinefelter syndrome
Klinger-Ludwig acid-thionin stain
Klippel-Feil syndrome
Klippel-Trenaunay-Weber syndrome
KLS
>kidneys, liver, spleen

Klumpke
K. palsy
K. paralysis
Klüver-Barrera Luxol fast blue stain
Klüver-Bucy syndrome
Km
K. allotype
K. antigen
Knapp
K. streak
K. stria
knee
above k. (A-K)
below the k. (B-K)
Brodie k.
k. complex
k. disarticulation amputation
housemaid's k.
k. jerk
k. joint
locked k.
k. presentation
k. reflex
runner's k.
Wilbrand k.
knee-ankle-foot orthosis
kneecap
knee-chest position
knee-elbow position
knee-jerk reflex
KNF
Koshland-Némethy-Filmer
KNF model
Kniest syndrome
knife
amputation k.
Beer k.
cartilage k.
cautery k.
chemical k.
electrode k.
fistula k.
free-hand k.
gamma k.
Goldman-Fox k.
Graefe k.
hernia k.
Kirkland k.
lenticular k.
Liston k.
Merrifield k.
k. needle

knife-rest crystal
knismogenic
knitted vascular prosthesis
knob
aortic k.
Engelmann basal k.
malarial k.
knock-knee
knock-out drop
Knoll gland
Knoop
K. hardness number
K. hardness test
K. theory
knot
false k.
granny k.
Hensen k.
Hubrecht protochordal k.
laparoscopic k.
primitive k.
square k.
surgeon's k.
syncytial k.
Knott technique
knuckle
aortic k.
cervical aortic k.
k. pad
k. sign
Knudsen hypothesis
Kobberling-Dunnigan syndrome
Kobelt tubule
Kober test
Köbner phenomenon
Koch
K. bacillus
K. law
K. node
K. old tuberculin
K. phenomenon
K. postulate
K. triangle
Kocher
K. clamp
K. incision
K. sign
K. ulcer
Kocher-Debré-Sémélaigne syndrome
Koch-Weeks bacillus

K

NOTES

519

Kock
  K. ileostomy
  K. pouch
Koenig syndrome
Koerber-Salus-Elschnig syndrome
Koerte-Ballance operation
Koettstorfer number
Köhler
  K. disease
  K. illumination
Kohlmeier-Degos syndrome
Kohlrausch
  K. fold
  K. muscle
Kohn pore
Kohnstamm phenomenon
koilocyte
koilocytosis
koilonychia
koilosternia
Kojewnikoff epilepsy
kojic acid
kokoi venom
Kokoskin stain
Kölliker
  K. layer
  K. reticulum
Kollmann dilator
Kolmer test
kolytic
Kommerell diverticulum
Kondoleon operation
koniocortex
Konno procedure
Konno-Rastan procedure
konzo
Koongol virus
Koplik spot
kopophobia
Korean
  K. hemorrhagic fever
  K. hemorrhagic fever virus
Korff fiber
Kornberg enzyme
koro
koronion
Korotkoff
  K. sound
  K. test
Korsakoff
  K. psychosis
  K. syndrome
koseri
  Citrobacter k.
Koshland-Némethy-Filmer (KNF)
  K.-N.-F. model
Kossa stain
Kostmann syndrome
Krabbe disease

K-radiation
krait
Kraske operation
kraurosis vulvae
Krause
  K. bone
  K. end bulb
  K. gland
  K. graft
  K. ligament
  K. respiratory bundle
  K. valve
Krause-Wolfe graft
krebiozen
Krebs
  K. ornithine cycle
  K. urea cycle
Krebs-Henseleit cycle
Krebs-Kornberg cycle
Krebs-Ringer solution
Kretschmann space
Kreysig sign
kriging
Krimsky test
kringle
Krogh spirometer
Kronecker stain
Krönig
  K. isthmus
  K. step
Krönlein
  K. hernia
  K. operation
Krueger instrument stop
Krukenberg
  K. amputation
  K. spindle
  K. tumor
  K. vein
Kruse brush
krypton laser
KTP laser
KUB
  kidneys, ureters, bladder
Kufs disease
Kugel anastomotic artery
Kugelberg-Welander disease
Kühne
  K. fiber
  K. methylene blue
  K. phenomenon
  K. plate
  K. spindle
Kuhnt space
Kulchitsky cell
Külz cylinder
Kunin antigen
Küntscher nail
Kupffer cell

kurchi bark
Kürsteiner canal
kurtosis
Kurtzke multiple sclerosis disability
  scale
kuru
Kurzrok-Ratner test
Kuskokwim syndrome
Kussmaul
    K. breathing
    K. coma
    K. disease
    K. respiration
    K. sign
Kussmaul-Kien respiration
kv
  kilovolt
Kveim
    K. antigen
    K. test
Kveim-Siltzbach
    K.-S. antigen
    K.-S. test
KVO
  keep vein open

kVp
  kilovolts peak
kwashiorkor
  marasmic k.
Kyasanur
    K. Forest disease
    K. Forest disease virus
kymatism
kymogram
kymograph
kymography
kymoscope
kynurenic acid
kynureninase
kynurenine formamidase
kyphos
kyphoscoliosis
kyphoscoliotic pelvis
kyphosis
    juvenile k.
    k. sacralis
    thoracic k.
    k. thoracica
kyphotic pelvis
Kyrle disease

K

NOTES

L
- L chain
- L dose
- L form
- L selectin
- L shell

la
- l. belle indifférence
- L. Crosse virus

Laband syndrome

Labbé
- L. triangle
- L. vein

labeled
- l. atom
- l. thyroxine

labia (*pl. of* labium)

labial
- l. arch
- l. bar
- l. branch
- l. commissure
- l. embrasure
- l. flange
- l. gingiva
- l. gland
- l. hernia
- l. occlusion
- l. splint
- l. sulcus
- l. swelling
- l. tubercle
- l. vein
- l. vestibule

labialis
- herpes l.
- keratosis l.

labialism

labially

labii
- modiolus l.

labile
- l. affect
- l. current
- l. element
- l. factor
- l. hypertension
- l. pulse

lability
- emotional l.

labiocervical

labiochorea

labioclination

labiodental sulcus

labiogingival lamina

labioglossolaryngeal

labioglossopharyngeal

labiograph

labiolingual
- l. appliance
- l. plane

labiomental

labionasal

labiopalatine

labioplacement

labioplasty

labioscrotal
- l. fold
- l. swelling

labioversion

labitome

labium, pl. **labia**
- l. majus
- l. minus
- labia oris
- l. urethrae
- labia uteri

labor
- active l.
- arrest of l.
- artificial l.
- l. curve
- dry l.
- false l.
- missed l.
- obstructed l.
- l. pain
- precipitate l.
- premature l.
- prodromal l.
- spurious l.
- stage of l.

laboratorian

laboratory
- l. diagnosis
- physician office l.

labored
- l. breathing
- l. respiration

labra (*pl. of* labrum)

Labrador keratopathy

labrale
- l. inferius
- l. superius

labrocyte

labrum, pl. **labra**
- acetabular l.
- articular l.
- glenoid l.

L

labyrinth
    acoustic l.
    bony l.
    cochlear l.
    ethmoidal l.
    Ludwig l.
    membranous l.
    renal l.
labyrinthectomy
    membranous l.
labyrinthine
    l. apoplexy
    l. artery
    l. deafness
    l. fistula
    l. nystagmus
    l. placenta
    l. righting reflex
    l. torticollis
    l. vein
    l. vertigo
    l. wall
labyrinthitis
labyrinthotomy
lacerable
lacerated foramen
lacerating wound (LW)
laceration
    brain l.
    zigzag l.
lacertus
Lachman test
lachrymal
LACI
    lipoprotein-associated coagulation
    inhibitor
laciniate ligament
lacis cell
Lac operon
lacquer
    l. crack
    l. stain
lacrimal
    l. apparatus
    l. artery
    l. bay
    l. bone
    l. border
    l. calculus
    l. canaliculus
    l. caruncle
    l. duct
    l. fascia
    l. fistula
    l. fold
    l. fossa
    l. gland
    l. groove
    l. hamulus

    l. lake
    l. margin
    l. mucocele
    l. nerve
    l. notch
    l. opening
    l. papilla
    l. pathway
    l. punctum
    l. reflex
    l. sac
    l. vein
lacrimalis
    incisura l.
lacrimation
lacrimator
lacrimatory
lacrimoconchal suture
lacrimogustatory reflex
lacrimomaxillary suture
lacrimotomy
lactacidemia
lactacidosis
lactacid oxygen debt
lactalbumin
lactam
lactamase
lactase
    l. persistence
    l. restriction
lactate
    amrinone l.
    calcium l.
    l. dehydrogenase
    l. dehydrogenase virus
    ethacridine l.
    excess l.
    ferrous l.
    magnesium l.
    l. paradox
    squalamine l.
    l. threshold
lactated
    l. Ringer (LR)
    l. Ringer injection
    l. Ringer solution (LRS)
lactating adenoma
lactation
    l. amenorrhea
    l. hormone
lactational mastitis
lactea
    crusta l.
lacteal
    central l.
    l. cyst
    l. fistula
    l. vessel
lactenin

lactentium
  hyperemesis l.
lactescent
lactic
  l. acid
  l. acid bacillus
  l. acid dehydrogenase
  l. acidemia
  l. acid fermentation
  l. acidosis
  l. acid oxygen debt
lactiferous
  l. ampulla
  l. duct
  l. gland
  l. sinus
lactifugal
lactifuge
lactigenous
lactigerous
lactim
lactimorbus
lactinated
lactis
lactobacillary milk
lactobacillic acid
Lactobacillus
  L. *acidophilus*
  L. *brevis*
  L. *buchneri*
  L. *bulgaricus*
  L. *bulgaricus* factor
  L. *casei*
  L. *catenaformis*
  L. *crispatus*
  L. *curvatus*
  L. *delbrueckii*
  L. *fermentum*
  L. *jensenii*
  L. *plantarum*
  L. *salivarius*
  L. *trichodes*
lactobezoar
lactobutyrometer
lactocele
lactochrome
lactocrit
lactodensimeter
lactoferrin
lactoflavin
lactogen
  human placental l. (HPL)

lactogenesis
lactogenic hormone
lactoglobulin
lactometer
lactonase
lactone
  homoserine l.
lacto-ovo-vegetarian
lactoperoxidase
lactophenol cotton blue stain
lactophosphate
  calcium l.
lactoprotein
lactorrhea
lactoscope
lactose
  l. intolerance
  l. synthase
lactosuria
lactotherapy
lactotrophic
lactotropin
lactovegetarian
lactoylglutathione lyase
lactulose
lacuna, pl. **lacunae**
  bone l.
  cartilage l.
  cerebral l.
  l. cerebri
  Howship lacunae
  intervillous l.
  lacunae laterales
  l. magna
  l. musculorum
  l. musculorum retroinguinalis
  osseous l.
  l. pharyngis
  resorption lacunae
  trophoblastic l.
  l. urethralis
  vascular l.
  l. vasorum
  l. vasorum retroinguinalis
lacunar
  l. amnesia
  l. ligament
  l. state
  l. tonsillitis
lacunar-molecular layer
lacunule
lacus seminalis

L

NOTES

LAD
    left anterior descending
Ladd
    L. band
    L. operation
ladder
    sequence l.
    l. splint
Ladd-Franklin theory
Lady Windemere's syndrome
Laelaps echidninus
Laënnec
    L. cirrhosis
    L. pearl
laesa
    functio l.
laetrile
Lafora
    L. body
    L. body disease
lag
    anaphase l.
    homeostatic l.
    jet l.
    nitrogen l.
    l. phase
lagena
lagging
lagomorph
Lagomorpha
lagophthalmia
lagophthalmic keratitis
lagophthalmos
Lahey
    L. forceps
    L. operation
Lahore sore
laidlawii
    Acholeplasma l.
Laimer-Haeckerman area
lake
    capillary l.
    lacrimal l.
    lateral l.
    seminal l.
    subchorial l.
Laki-Lorand factor
laky blood
laliatry
laliophobia
Lallemand body
lalling
Lallouette pyramid
lalochezia
lalognosis
laloplegia
lamarckian theory
Lamaze method
lambdacism

Lambda phage
lambdoid
    l. border
    l. margin
    l. suture
Lambert
    L. law
    L. syndrome
Lambert-Eaton syndrome
Lambl excrescence
lamblia
    Giardia l.
Lamblia intestinalis
Lambrinudi operation
lamella, pl. **lamellae**
    articular l.
    l. of bone
    circumferential l.
    concentric l.
    cornoid l.
    elastic l.
    enamel l.
    endosteal l.
    glandulopreputial l.
    ground l.
    haversian l.
    intermediate l.
    interstitial l.
    vitreous l.
lamellar
    l. bone
    l. cataract
    l. granule
    l. ichthyosis
    l. incision
    l. keratoplasty
lamellate
lamellated corpuscle
lamellipodium
lamina, pl. **laminae**
    alar l.
    anterior elastic l.
    anterior limiting l.
    basal l.
    basement l.
    basilar l.
    boundary l.
    capillary l.
    l. cribrosa sclerae
    cribrous l.
    deep l.
    dental l.
    dentogingival l.
    elastic l.
    episcleral l.
    epithelial l.
    external medullary l.
    l. fusca
    hepatic laminae

hook of spiral l.
internal medullary l.
iridopupillary l.
labiogingival l.
lateral medullary l.
l. limitans anterior corneae
l. limitans posterior corneae
medial medullary l.
medullary l.
membranous l.
osseous spiral l.
posterior elastic l.
l. propria
tragal l.
vascular l.

laminagram
laminagraph
laminagraphy
laminar
l. cortical necrosis
l. cortical sclerosis
l. flow
laminaria
laminarin sulfate
laminated
l. clot
l. cortex
l. epithelial plug
l. epithelium
l. thrombus
lamination
laminectomy
laminin receptor
laminitis
laminography
laminotomy
lamins
lamotrigine
lamp
annealing l.
Edridge-Green l.
heat l.
hollow-cathode l.
mercury vapor l.
mignon l.
spirit l.
Wood l.
lampbrush, lamp-brush
l. chromosome
lanae
adeps l.
Lan antigen

Lancaster red green test
lance
Lancefield classification
lancet
gum l.
lancinating pain
Lancisi sign
Landau-Kleffner syndrome
Landolfi sign
Landouzy-Dejerine dystrophy
Landouzy-Grasset law
Landry
L. paralysis
L. syndrome
Landry-Guillain-Barré syndrome
landscape ecology
Landschutz tumor
land scurvy
Landsteiner-Donath test
Landström muscle
Landzert fossa
Lane
L. band
L. disease
L. kink
L. operation
Lange
L. solution
L. test
Langenbeck triangle
Langendorff method
Lange-Nielsen
Langer
L. arch
L. line
L. muscle
Langerhans
L. cell
L. cell histiocytosis
L. granule
L. island
islet of L.
Langer-Saldino syndrome
Langhans
L. cell
L. layer
L. stria
Langhans-type giant cell
Langley granule
Langmuir trough
language
l. board

L

NOTES

language *(continued)*
  body l.
  l. game
  l. zone
laniary
lankamycin
Lannelongue
  L. foramen
  L. ligament
lanolin
  anhydrous l.
lanosterol
Lanterman
  L. incisure
  L. segment
lanthanic
lanthanides
lanthanum
lanthionine
lanuginous
lanugo hair
Lanz line
LAO
  left anterior oblique
laparocele
laparocystidotomy
laparoendoscopic
laparogastroscopy
laparogastrostomy
laparogastrotomy
laparohepatotomy
laparoileotomy
laparomyositis
laparorrhaphy
laparosalpingo-oophorectomy
laparoscope
laparoscopic
  l. cannula
  l. cholecystotomy
  l. knot
  l. nephrectomy
  l. surgery
  l. uterosacral nerve ablation
laparoscopically assisted surgery
**laparoscopic-assisted vaginal
  hysterectomy**
laparoscopy
  closed l.
laparotomy pad
Lapicque law
lapinization
lapinized
Laplace
  L. forceps
  L. law
Laquer stain
larch turpentine
lard
  benzoinated l.

lardaceous
  l. liver
  l. spleen
large
  l. bowel
  l. calorie
  l. cell carcinoma
  l. cell lymphoma
  l. interarch distance
  l. intestine
  l. loop excision of transformation
    zone (LLETZ)
  l. pelvis
  l. pudendal lip
  l. saphenous vein
lari
  Campylobacter l.
larkspur
Larmor frequency
Laron-type dwarfism
Laroyenne operation
Larrey
  L. amputation
  L. cleft
Larsen syndrome
Larson-Johansson disease
larva, pl. **larvae**
  l. currens
  filariform l.
  l. migrans
larvaceous
larval
  l. conjunctivitis
  l. plague
larvate
larvicidal
larvicide
larviparous
larviphagic
laryngeal
  l. aditus
  l. aperture
  l. atresia
  l. bursa
  l. cavity
  l. chorea
  l. crisis
  l. diphtheria
  l. epilepsy
  l. gland
  l. granuloma
  l. inlet
  l. lymphoid nodule
  l. mask
  l. mucosa
  l. papillomatosis
  l. part
  l. pharynx
  l. polyp

l. pouch
l. prominence
l. rale
l. reflex
l. saccule
l. sinus
l. stenosis
l. stridor
l. syncope
l. tonsil
l. vein
l. ventricle
l. vertigo
l. web

laryngectomy
horizontal l.
partial l.
supraglottic l.
total l.

larynges (*pl. of* larynx)
laryngis
pachyderma l.
sacculus l.
laryngismus stridulus
laryngitic
laryngitis
chronic posterior l.
chronic subglottic l.
croupous l.
membranous l.
l. sicca
l. stridulosa
syphilitic l.
tuberculous l.

laryngocele
laryngofissure
laryngograph
laryngography
laryngology
laryngomalacia
laryngoparalysis
laryngopharyngeal branch
laryngopharyngectomy
laryngopharyngeus
laryngopharyngitis
laryngopharynx
laryngophthisis
laryngoplasty
laryngoplegia
laryngoptosis
laryngoscope
commissure l.

laryngoscopic
laryngoscopist
laryngoscopy
direct l.
fiberoptic l.
indirect l.
suspension l.
transnasal fiberoptic l.

laryngospasm
laryngospastic reflex
laryngostenosis
laryngostomy
laryngostroboscope
laryngotomy
complete l.
inferior l.
median l.
superior l.

laryngotracheal
l. diphtheria
l. diverticulum
l. groove

laryngotracheitis
laryngotracheobronchitis
laryngotracheoesophageal cleft
laryngotracheoplasty
larynx, pl. **larynges**
artificial l.
Cooper-Rand artificial l.
fibroelastic membrane of l.

lase
Lasègue
L. sign
L. syndrome

laser
argon l.
continuous wave l.
l. corepraxy
excimer l.
l. iridectomy
l. iridotomy
krypton l.
KTP l.
l. microscope
Nd:YAG l.
l. photocoagulator
l. plume
pulsed l.
pumped l.
Q-switched l.

L

NOTES

529

laser *(continued)*
  quasi-continuous wave l.
  l. trabeculoplasty
laser-assisted in situ keratomileusis (LASIK)
lasering
Lash
  L. casein hydrolysate-serum medium
  L. operation
LASIK
  laser-assisted in situ keratomileusis
L-asparaginase
  Erwinia L-a.
Lassa
  L. hemorrhagic fever
  L. virus
lassitude
last menstrual period (LMP)
lata
  fascia l.
latah
Latarget
  L. nerve
  L. vein
late
  l. apical systolic murmur
  l. auditory-evoked response
  l. benign syphilis
  l. cyanosis
  l. deceleration
  l. diastole
  l. diastolic murmur
  l. dumping syndrome
  l. latent syphilis
  l. luteal phase dysphoria
  l. luteal phase dysphoric disorder
  l. reaction
  l. replicating chromosome
  l. rickets
  l. seizure
  l. systole
latebra
latency
  absolute l.
  l. period
  l. phase
  proximal l.
  sleep l.
  terminal l.
latent
  l. adrenocortical insufficiency
  l. allergy
  l. carcinoma
  l. carrier
  l. content
  l. diabetes
  l. empyema
  l. energy

  l. gout
  l. heat
  l. homosexuality
  l. hyperopia
  l. image
  l. infection
  l. learning
  l. membrane protein
  l. microbism
  l. neurosyphilis
  l. nystagmus
  l. period
  l. rat virus
  l. reflex
  l. scarlatina
  l. schizophrenia
  l. stage
  l. syphilis
  l. typhoid
  l. zone
late-phase response
laterad
lateral
  l. abdominal region
  l. aberrant thyroid carcinoma
  l. aberration
  l. alveolar abscess
  l. ampullar nerve
  l. amygdaloid nucleus
  l. aperture
  l. arcuate ligament
  l. aspect
  l. atlantoaxial joint
  l. atlantoepistrophic joint
  l. atrial branch
  l. atrial vein
  l. axillary lymph node
  l. basal branch
  l. basal bronchopulmonary segment
  l. basal segmental artery
  l. bicipital groove
  l. border
  l. bronchopulmonary segment
  l. calcaneal branch
  l. canthus
  l. cartilage
  l. cartilaginous plate
  l. central palmar space
  l. cerebellomedullary cistern
  l. cerebral fissure
  l. cerebral fossa
  l. cerebral sulcus
  l. cervical nucleus
  l. cervical region
  l. circumflex femoral artery
  l. circumflex femoral vein
  l. collateral ligament
  l. column
  l. compartment

l. condylar inclination
l. condyle
l. cord
l. corticospinal tract
l. costal branch
l. costotransverse ligament
l. cricoarytenoid muscle
l. crus
l. cuneate nucleus
l. cuneiform bone
l. curvature
l. cutaneous branch
l. decubitus radiograph
l. direct vein
l. division
l. dorsal cutaneous nerve
l. dorsal nucleus
l. epicondylar crest
l. epicondylar ridge
l. epicondyle
l. excursion
l. fasciculus proprius
l. femoral cutaneous nerve
l. femoral tuberosity
l. fillet
l. flank incision
l. frontobasal artery
l. funiculus
l. geniculate body
l. geniculate nucleus
l. ginglymus
l. glossoepiglottic fold
l. great muscle
l. ground bundle
l. habenular nucleus
l. head
l. hermaphroditism
l. horn
l. humeral epicondylitis
l. hypothalamic area
l. hypothalamic region
l. illumination
l. incisor
l. inferior genicular artery
l. inferior hepatic area
l. inguinal fossa
l. jugular lymph node
l. lacunar lymph node
l. lake
l. lemniscus
l. limb
l. lingual swelling

l. lip
l. lithotomy
l. longitudinal arch
l. longitudinal stria
l. malleolar artery
l. malleolar branch
l. malleolar facet
l. malleolar ligament
l. malleolar network
l. malleolar subcutaneous bursa
l. malleolar surface
l. malleolus
l. malleolus bursa
l. mammary branch
l. margin
l. medullary branch
l. medullary lamina
l. medullary syndrome
l. meniscus
l. mesoderm
l. midpalmar space
l. movement
l. myocardial infarction
l. nasal artery
l. nasal branch
l. nasal fold
l. nasal process
l. nasal prominence
l. nystagmus
l. oblique radiograph
l. occipital artery
l. occipital sulcus
l. occipitotemporal gyrus
l. occlusion
l. olfactory gyrus
l. orbitofrontal artery
l. palpebral commissure
l. palpebral ligament
l. palpebral raphe
l. parabrachial nucleus
l. patellar retinaculum
l. pectoral nerve
l. pelvic wall triangle
l. pericardial lymph node
l. pericuneate nucleus
l. periodontal abscess
l. periodontal cyst
l. pharyngeal space
l. pinch
l. plantar artery
l. plantar nerve
l. pole

NOTES

L

531

lateral *(continued)*
l. posterior nucleus
l. preoptic nucleus
l. projection
l. proprius bundle
l. pterygoid muscle
l. pterygoid plate
l. puboprostatic ligament
l. pyelography
l. pyramidal fasciculus
l. pyramidal tract
l. ramus radiograph
l. raphespinal tract
l. recess
l. rectus incision
l. rectus muscle
l. recumbent position
l. reticular nucleus
l. reticulospinal tract
l. root
l. rotation
l. sacral artery
l. sacral branch
l. sacral crest
l. sacral vein
l. sacrococcygeal ligament
l. segmental artery
l. semicircular canal
l. septal nucleus
l. sinus
l. skull radiograph
l. spinal sclerosis
l. spinothalamic tract
l. splanchnic artery
l. striate artery
l. superior genicular artery
l. superior hepatic area
l. superior olivary nucleus
l. supraclavicular nerve
l. supracondylar crest
l. supracondylar ridge
l. supraepicondylar ridge
l. sural cutaneous nerve
l. talocalcaneal ligament
l. tarsal artery
l. tarsal strip procedure
l. temporomandibular ligament
l. thalamic peduncle
l. thoracic artery
l. thoracic vein
l. thyrohyoid ligament
l. umbilical fold
l. umbilical ligament
l. vaginal wall smear
l. vastus muscle
l. ventral hernia
l. ventricle
l. vertigo
l. vestibular nucleus

l. vestibulospinal tract
l. wall
l. zone
laterales
lacunae l.
lateralis
funiculus l.
malleolus l.
meniscus l.
laterality
crossed l.
lateralization
lateriflection
lateriflexion
lateris
nevus unius l.
lateroabdominal
laterodeviation
lateroduction
lateroflexion, lateroflection
lateroposition
lateropulsion
laterotorsion
laterotrusion
lateroversion
latex
l. agglutination test
l. fixation test
lathe
lathyrism
lathyrogen
latina
Actinomadura l.
Latin square
latissimus dorsi muscle
latitude film
lato
sensu l.
lattice
l. corneal dystrophy
l. degeneration
latticed layer
latum
condyloma l.
Diphyllobothrium l.
latus
metatarsus l.
Latzko cesarean section
laudable pus
laudanine
laudanosine
laudanum
laughing gas
laughter reflex
Laugier hernia
Laumonier ganglion
Launois-Bensaude syndrome
Launois-Cléret syndrome
laurel fever

Laurence-Moon syndrome
Laurer canal
lauric acid
Lauth
    L. canal
    L. ligament
    L. violet
LAV
    lymphadenopathy-associated virus
lavage
    antral l.
    bronchoalveolar l. (BAL)
Lavdovsky nucleoid
law
    Alexander l.
    all or none l.
    Ångström l.
    Arndt l.
    Arrhenius l.
    l. of association
    Avogadro l.
    Baer l.
    Baruch l.
    Beer l.
    Beer-Lambert l.
    Behring l.
    Bell l.
    Bell-Magendie l.
    Bernoulli l.
    Berthollet l.
    biogenetic l.
    Blagden l.
    Bowditch l.
    Boyle l.
    Broadbent l.
    Bunsen-Roscoe l.
    Charles l.
    l. of contiguity
    Coppet l.
    Courvoisier l.
    Dale-Feldberg l.
    Dalton l.
    Dalton-Henry l.
    Descartes l.
    Donders l.
    Draper l.
    Dulong-Petit l.
    Einthoven l.
    Elliott l.
    Faraday l.
    Farr l.
    Fechner-Weber l.

Ferry-Porter l.
Flatau l.
Galton l.
Gay-Lussac l.
Godélier l.
Gompertz l.
Graham l.
Grasset l.
Guldberg-Waage l.
Haeckel l.
Halsted l.
Hamburger l.
Hardy-Weinberg l.
Heidenhain l.
Hellin l.
Henry l.
Herring l.
Hess l.
Hilton l.
Hooke l.
inverse square l.
isodynamic l.
Jackson l.
Koch l.
Lambert l.
Landouzy-Grasset l.
Lapicque l.
Laplace l.
Le Chatelier l.
Listing l.
Louis l.
Magendie l.
Marey l.
Marfan l.
Mariotte l.
mass l.
Meltzer l.
Mendeléeff l.
Mendel first l.
Mendel second l.
Müller l.
Nasse l.
Neumann l.
Newton l.
Ochoa l.
Pascal l.
Poiseuille l.
Profeta l.
Raoult l.
Ricco l.
Rosenbach l.
Sherrington l.

L

NOTES

law *(continued)*
 l. of similars
 Snell l.
 Spallanzani l.
 Stokes l.
 Thoma l.
 van't Hoff l.
 Vogel l.
 Weber l.
 Weber-Fechner l.
 Weigert l.
 Williston l.
 Wolff l.
Lawrence-Seip syndrome
lawrencium
Lawson operation
laxation
laxative
 l. abuse
 bulk-producing l.
 diphenylmethane l.
 emollient l.
 stimulant l.
 stool-softening l.
 surfactant l.
laxity
 valgus l.
 varus l.
layer
 ameloblastic l.
 anterior elastic l.
 anterior limiting l.
 bacillary l.
 basal l.
 basal cell l.
 l. of Bechterew
 blastodermic l.
 Bowman l.
 brown l.
 cambium l.
 Chievitz l.
 choriocapillary l.
 choroid capillary l.
 circular l.
 claustral l.
 clear l.
 conjunctival l.
 corneal l.
 deep l.
 elastic l.
 enamel l.
 ependymal l.
 episcleral l.
 epithelial choroid l.
 epitrichial l.
 external nuclear l.
 fatty l.
 fibromusculocartilagenous l.
 fibrous l.

 fillet l.
 fusiform l.
 ganglionic cell l.
 germ l.
 germinative l.
 glomerular l.
 granular l.
 half-value l. (HVL)
 Henle fiber l.
 Henle nervous l.
 horny l.
 Huxley l.
 infragranular l.
 inner limiting l.
 inner nuclear l.
 inner plexiform l.
 intermediate white l.
 investing l.
 Kölliker l.
 lacunar-molecular l.
 Langhans l.
 latticed l.
 longitudinal l.
 long pitch helicoidal l.
 malpighian l.
 mantle l.
 marginal l.
 medullary l.
 membranous l.
 meningeal l.
 Meynert l.
 middle gray l.
 molecular l.
 multiform l.
 Nitabuch l.
 odontoblastic l.
 osteogenetic l.
 pigmented l.
 piriform neuron l.
 posterior limiting l.
 prevertebral l.
 prickle cell l.
 Purkinje cell l.
 spinous l.
 still l.
 subendocardial l.
 subendothelial l.
 visceral l.
layered keratoplasty
lazaret
lazaretto
LBBB
 left bundle branch block
LCA
 left carotid artery
LCAT
 lecithin-cholesterol acyltransferase
 LCAT deficiency

L-chain
    L-c. disease
    L-c. myeloma
LCM
    left costal margin
L-D
    Leishman-Donovan
    L-D body
LDL
    low-density lipoprotein
    LDL receptor disorder
L-dopa
    levodopa
L+ dose
LE
    lupus erythematosus
    LE body
    LE cell
    LE cell test
    LE phenomenon
Le
    L. antigen
    L. Bel-van't Hoff rule
    L. blood group
    L. Chatelier law
    L. Chatelier principle
    L. Fort amputation
    L. Fort III craniofacial dysjunction
    L. Fort I, II, III fracture
    L. Fort osteotomy
    L. Fort sound
leaching
lead
    ABC l.'s
    l. acetate
    l. anemia
    augmented l.
    aVF l.
    aVL l.
    aVR l.
    bipolar l.
    black l.
    l. carbonate
    CB l.
    CF l.
    chest l.
    l. chromate
    CL l.
    l. colic
    CR l.
    direct l.
    l. encephalitis

    l. encephalopathy
    esophageal l.
    l. gout
    l. hydroxide stain
    indirect l.
    intracardiac l.
    limb l.
    l. line
    l. monoxide
    l. neuropathy
    l. oxide yellow
    pacemaker l.
    l. palsy
    l. paralysis
    l. poisoning
    precordial l.
    l. stomatitis
    l. sulfide
    l. tetraethyl
    l. tetroxide
    unipolar l.
leader sequence
leading
    l. ancestor
    l. edge
lead-pipe
    l.-p. colon
    l.-p. rigidity
leaflet
leak point pressure
lean body mass
leapfrog position
Lear complex
learned
    l. drive
    l. helplessness
learning
    l. disability
    incidental l.
    insight l.
    latent l.
    rote l.
    l. set
    state-dependent l.
    l. theory
least
    l. confusion circle
    l. splanchnic nerve
    l. squares
    l. squares estimator
leather-bottle stomach

L

NOTES

Leber
    L. hereditary optic atrophy
    L. idiopathic stellate neuroretinitis
    L. idiopathic stellate retinopathy
    L. plexus
lecithal
lecithin acyltransferase
lecithinase A, B, C, D
lecithin-cholesterol
    l.-c. acyltransferase (LCAT)
    l.-c. transferase
lecithin/sphingomyelin ratio
lecithoblast
lecithoprotein
LeCompte
    L. maneuver
    L. operation
lectin
    l. glycohistochemistry
    mitogenic l.
    l. pathway molecule
lectularia
    Acanthia l.
Ledermann formula
ledge
    dental l.
    enamel l.
leech
leeching
Leede-Rumpel phenomenon
Lee ganglion
LEEP
    loop electrocautery excision procedure
    loop electrosurgical excision procedure
Leeuwenhoek canal
leeway space
Lee-White method
left
    l. anterior descending (LAD)
    l. anterior descending artery
    l. anterior lateral hepatic segment
    l. anterior oblique (LAO)
    l. atrioventricular orifice
    l. atrioventricular valve
    l. atrium
    l. auricle
    l. auricular appendage
    l. axis deviation
    l. bundle branch
    l. bundle branch block (LBBB)
    l. carotid artery (LCA)
    l. circumflex coronary artery
    l. colic artery
    l. colic flexure
    l. colic lymph node
    l. colic vein
    l. coronary artery
    l. coronary vein
    l. costal margin (LCM)

    deviation to the l.
    l. fibrous ring
    l. fibrous trigone
    l. frontoanterior (LFA)
    l. frontoposterior (LFP)
    l. frontotransverse (LFT)
    l. gastric artery
    l. gastric lymph node
    l. gastric vein
    l. gastroepiploic artery
    l. gastroepiploic lymph node
    l. gastroepiploic vein
    l. gastroomental artery
    l. gastroomental lymph node
    l. gastroomental vein
    l. heart
    l. heart bypass
    l. hepatic artery
    l. hepatic duct
    l. hepatic vein
    l. inferior pulmonary vein
    l. lateral division
    l. liver
    l. lower lobe (LLL)
    l. lower quadrant (LLQ)
    l. lumbar lymph node
    l. main bronchus
    l. marginal artery
    l. medial division
    l. medial hepatic segment
    l. mentoanterior (LMA)
    l. mentoposterior (LMP)
    l. mentotransverse (LMT)
    l. occipitoanterior (LOA)
    l. occipitoposterior (LOP)
    l. occipitotransverse (LOT)
    l. outer quadrant (LOQ)
    l. ovarian vein
    l. posterior lateral hepatic segment III
    l. posterior oblique (LPO)
    l. pulmonary artery
    l. sacroanterior (LSA)
    l. sacroposterior (LSP)
    l. sacrotransverse (LST)
    l. sagittal fissure
    shift to the l.
    l. superior intercostal vein
    l. superior pulmonary vein
    l. suprarenal vein
    l. testicular vein
    l. triangular ligament
    l. umbilical vein
    l. upper extremity (LUE)
    l. upper lobe (LUL)
    l. upper quadrant (LUQ)
    l. ventricle
    l. ventricular assist device (LVAD)
    l. ventricular diastolic pressure

l. ventricular ejection fraction
l. ventricular ejection time (LVET)
l. ventricular end-diastolic pressure
l. ventricular enlargement
l. ventricular failure
l. ventricular myomectomy
l. ventricular systolic pressure
l. ventricular volume reduction
  surgery
left-footed
left-handed
left-sided
l.-s. appendicitis
l.-s. heart failure
left-sidedness
bilateral l.-s.
left-to-right shunt
left-ventricular assist device
leg
l. of antihelix
elephant l.
l. phenomenon
legal
l. blindness
l. dentistry
l. medicine
l. psychiatry
L. test
Legendre sign
Legg-Calvé-Perthes disease
Legg disease
Legg-Perthes disease
Legionella
L. bozemanii
L. dumoffii
L. feeleii
L. gormanii
L. longbeachae
L. micdadei
L. pneumophila
L. wadsworthii
legionellosis
Legionnaires disease
legumin
leguminivorous
Leigh disease
Leiner disease
leiodermia
leiomyofibroma
leiomyoma
l. cutis
vascular l.

leiomyomatosis peritonealis disseminata
leiomyomectomy
leiomyosarcoma
leiotrichous
Leipzig yellow
Leishman
L. chrome cell
L. stain
Leishman-Donovan (L-D)
L.-D. body
Leishmania
L. braziliensis braziliensis
L. braziliensis guyanensis
L. donovani
L. furunculosa
L. major
leishmaniasis
acute cutaneous l.
American l.
anergic l.
anthroponotic cutaneous l.
canine l.
chronic cutaneous l.
cutaneous l.
diffuse cutaneous l.
disseminated cutaneous l.
dry cutaneous l.
infantile l.
lupoid l.
mucocutaneous l.
nasopharyngeal l.
New World l.
visceral l.
zoonotic cutaneous l.
leishmanin test
leishmaniosis
leishmanoid
dermal l.
Lejeune syndrome
Lembert suture
lemic
Leminorella
lemmoblast
lemmocyte
lemniscal trigone
lemniscorum
decussatio l.
lemniscus
acoustic l.
auditory l.
gustatory l.

NOTES

537

lemniscus *(continued)*
  lateral l.
  medial l.
lemon
  l. sign
  l. yellow
Lendrum phloxine-tartrazine stain
Lenègre
  L. disease
  L. syndrome
length
  arch l.
  available arch l.
  crown-heel l. (CHL)
  crown-rump l. (CRL)
  greatest l.
length-breadth index
lengthening reaction
length-height index
Lenhossék process
lenitive
Lennert
  L. classification
  L. lymphoma
Lennox-Gastaut syndrome
Lennox syndrome
Lenoir facet
lens, pl. **lenses**
  achromatic l.
  acoustic l.
  aplanatic l.
  apochromatic l.
  aspheric l.
  astigmatic l.
  bandage contact l.
  biconcave l.
  biconvex l.
  bifocal l.
  capsule of l.
  l. capsule
  cataract l.
  l. clock
  compound l.
  concave l.
  concavoconcave l.
  concavoconvex l.
  contact l.
  convex l.
  convexoconcave l.
  convexoconvex l.
  corneal l.
  crystalline l.
  cylindrical l.
  decentered l.
  dislocation of l.
  double concave l.
  double convex l.
  eye l.
  field l.

foldable intraocular l.
Fresnel l.
Hruby l.
hydrophilic l.
immersion l.
lighthouse l.
meniscus l.
minus l.
multifocal l.
omnifocal l.
photochromic l.
l. pit
l. placode
planoconcave l.
planoconvex l.
safety l.
spherical l.
l. stars
l. suture
trial lenses
trifocal l.
l. vesicle
lensectomy
lens-induced uveitis
lensometer
lensopathy
lente insulin
lenticonus
lenticula
lenticular
  l. ansa
  l. apophysis
  l. astigmatism
  l. bone
  l. capsule
  l. colony
  l. fasciculus
  l. fossa
  l. ganglion
  l. knife
  l. loop
  l. nucleus
  l. papilla
  l. process
  l. progressive disease
  l. vesicle
lenticularis
  dystonia l.
lenticulo-optic
lenticulopapular
lenticulostriate artery
lenticulothalamic
lenticulus
lentiform bone
lentigines, electrocardiographic abnormalities, ocular hypertelorism, pulmonary stenosis, abnormalities of genitalia, retardation of growth, and deafness (LEOPARD)

lentiginosis
> centrofacial l.
> generalized l.

lentiglobus

lentigo
> l. maligna
> senile l.
> l. simplex

lentis
> chalcosis l.
> cortex l.
> ectopia l.
> equator l.
> radii l.
> vortex l.

lentivirus

lentogenic

lentula

lentulo

lentum
> *Eubacterium l.*

leonine facies

leontiasis

LEOPARD
> lentigines, electrocardiographic abnormalities, ocular hypertelorism, pulmonary stenosis, abnormalities of genitalia, retardation of growth, and deafness
> LEOPARD syndrome

leopard
> l. bane
> l. fundus
> l. retina

Leopold maneuver

Lepehne-Pickworth stain

leper

lepidic

Lepore
> hemoglobin L.
> L. thalassemia

lepothrix

lepra cell

leprae
> *Mycobacterium l.*

leprechaunism

leprid

leproma

lepromatous leprosy

lepromin
> l. reaction
> l. test

leprosarium

leprosery

leprostatic

leprosy
> anesthetic l.
> l. bacillus
> borderline l.
> cutaneous l.
> dimorphous l.
> dry l.
> histoid l.
> indeterminate l.
> intermediate l.
> lepromatous l.
> Lucio l.
> macular l.
> nodular l.
> spotted l.
> trophoneurotic l.
> tuberculoid l.

leprotic

leprotica
> alopecia l.

leprous neuropathy

leptandra

leptin

leptocephalous

leptocephaly

leptochromatic

leptocyte

leptocytosis

leptodactylous

leptomeningeal
> l. carcinoma
> l. carcinomatosis
> l. cyst
> l. fibrosis
> l. space

leptomeningitis
> basilar l.

leptomeninx, pl. **leptomeninges**

leptomere

leptomonad

leptonema

leptophonia

leptophonic

leptopodia

leptoprosopia

leptoprosopic

leptorrhine

leptoscope

leptosomatic

L

NOTES

leptosomic
Leptospira
leptospiral jaundice
leptospire
leptospirosis
    anicteric l.
leptospiruria
leptotene
leptothricosis
Leptotrichia buccalis
Leptotrombidium akamushi
lergotrile
Leri
    L. pleonosteosis
    L. sign
Leriche
    L. operation
    L. syndrome
Leri-Weill
    L.-W. disease
    L.-W. syndrome
Lermoyez syndrome
Lerner homeostasis
LES
    lower esophageal sphincter
lesbian
lesbianism
Lesch-Nyhan syndrome
Leser-Trélat sign
lesion
    anular l.
    Baehr-Lohlein l.
    Bankart l.
    benign lymphoepithelial l.
    Bracht-Wächter l.
    caviar l.
    coin l.
    Dieulafoy l.
    diffuse l.
    disseminated l.
    doughnut l.
    Duret l.
    focal l.
    Ghon primary l.
    gross l.
    high-grade squamous
      intraepithelial l. (HGSIL, HSIL)
    Hill-Sachs l.
    histologic l.
    indiscriminate l.
    Janeway l.
    Lohlein-Baehr l.
    lower motor neuron l.
    low-grade squamous
      intraepithelial l. (LGSIL, LSIL)
    Mallory-Weiss l.
    organic l.
    partial l.
    sessile l.

    SLAP l.
    systemic l.
    target l.
    total l.
    trophic l.
lesser
    l. alar cartilage
    l. arterial circle
    l. circulation
    l. cul-de-sac
    l. curvature
    l. horn of hyoid
    l. internal cutaneous nerve
    l. multangular bone
    l. occipital nerve
    l. omentum
    l. palatine artery
    l. palatine canal
    l. palatine foramen
    l. palatine nerve
    l. pancreas
    l. pelvis
    l. peritoneal cavity
    l. peritoneal sac
    l. rhomboid muscle
    l. sciatic notch
    l. splanchnic nerve
    l. superficial petrosal nerve
    l. supraclavicular fossa
    L. triangle
    l. trochanter
    l. tubercle
    l. tuberosity
    l. tympanic spine
    l. vestibular gland
    l. wing
    l. zygomatic muscle
Lesshaft triangle
let-down reflex
lethal
    clinical l.
    l. coefficient
    l. dose
    l. dwarfism
    l. equivalent
    l. factor
    l. gene
    genetic l.
    l. midline granuloma
    l. mutation
lethality rate
lethargic
    l. hypnosis
    l. stupor
lethargy
letter blindness
Letterer-Siwe disease
leucine
leucine-induced hypoglycemia

leucine-sensitive hypoglycemia
leucinosis
leucinuria
leucocelaenus
    Aedes l.
leucocidin
leucocyte
leucocytosis
leucoderma
leucoharmine
leucoline
leucoma
leucomethylene blue
leuconychia
leuco patent blue
leucopenia
leucoplakia
leucopoiesis
leucotomy
leucovorin
    calcium l.
    l. calcium
Leudet tinnitus
leuenkephalin
leukanemia
leukapheresis
leukemia
    acute lymphocytic l. (ALL)
    acute promyelocytic l.
    adult T-cell l.
    aleukemic l.
    basophilic l.
    basophilocytic l.
    chronic granulocytic l.
    chronic myelocytic l.
    chronic myelogenous l. (CML)
    chronic myeloid l.
    l. cutis
    embryonal l.
    eosinophilic l.
    eosinophilocytic l.
    granulocytic l.
    hairy cell l.
    l. inhibitory factor
    leukemic l.
    leukopenic l.
    lymphatic l.
    lymphoblastic l.
    lymphocytic l.
    lymphoid l.
    mast cell l.
    mature cell l.

    megakaryocytic l.
    meningeal l.
    micromyeloblastic l.
    mixed cell l.
    monocytic l.
    myeloblastic l.
    myelocytic l.
    myelogenic l.
    myelogenous l.
    myeloid l.
    natural killer cell l.
    plasma cell l.
    Rieder cell l.
    smoldering l.
    stem cell l.
    subleukemic l.
leukemic
    l. erythrocytosis
    l. hyperplastic gingivitis
    l. leukemia
    l. myelosis
    l. reticulosis
    l. retinitis
    l. retinopathy
leukemid
leukemogen
leukemogenesis
leukemogenic
leukemoid reaction
leukin
leukoagglutinin
leukobilin
leukoblast
leukoblastosis
leukochloroma
leukocidin
leukocoria
leukocytactic
leukocytal
leukocytaxia
leukocytaxis
leukocyte
    acidophilic l.
    l. adherence assay test
    l. adhesion deficiency
    agranular l.
    l. bactericidal assay test
    basophilic l.
    l. common antigen
    l. cream
    cystinotic l.
    endothelial l.

NOTES

leukocyte *(continued)*
    eosinophilic l.
    l. esterase test
    filament polymorphonuclear l.
    globular l.
    granular l.
    hyaline l.
    l. inclusion
    l. interferon
    mast l.
    neutrophilic l.
    oxyphilic l.
    polymorphonuclear l.
    polynuclear l.
leukocythemia
leukocytic
    l. pyrogen
    l. sarcoma
leukocytoblast
leukocytoclasis
leukocytoclastic vasculitis
leukocytogenesis
leukocytoid
leukocytolysin
leukocytolysis
leukocytolytic
leukocytoma
leukocytometer
leukocytopenia
leukocytoplania
leukocytopoiesis
leukocytosis
    absolute l.
    agonal l.
    basophilic l.
    digestive l.
    distribution l.
    emotional l.
    eosinophilic l.
    lymphocytic l.
    physiologic l.
    relative l.
leukocytosis-promoting factor
leukocytotactic
leukocytotaxia
leukocytotoxin
leukocyturia
leukoderma
    acquired l.
    syphilitic l.
leukodermatous
leukodontia
leukodystrophia
leukodystrophy
    adrenal l.
    cerebral l.
    globoid cell l.
    metachromatic l.
leukoedema

leukoencephalitis
    acute epidemic l.
    acute necrotizing hemorrhagic l.
leukoencephalopathy
    acute necrotizing hemorrhagic l.
    progressive multifocal l.
leukoerythroblastic anemia
leukoerythroblastosis
leukokinetic
leukokinetics
leukokoria
leukokraurosis
leukolysin
leukolysis
leukolytic
leukoma
    adherent l.
leukomatous
leukomyelitis
leukomyelopathy
leukon
leukonecrosis
leukonychia
leukopathia
    acquired l.
    congenital l.
leukopathy
leukopedesis
leukopenia
    basophilic l.
    eosinophilic l.
    histiocytic l.
    lymphocytic l.
    monocytic l.
    sclerosing l.
leukopenic
    l. factor
    l. index
    l. leukemia
    l. myelosis
leukoplakia
    hairy l.
    l. vulvae
leukopoiesis
leukopoietic
leukoprotease
leukoriboflavin
leukorrhagia
leukorrhea
    menstrual l.
leukorrheal
leukosis
leukotactic
leukotaxia
leukotaxine
leukotaxis
leukotic
leukotome
leukotomy

leukotoxin
leukotrichia
leukotriene receptor antagonist
leukotrienes
leupeptin
leuprolide acetate
leurocristine
Lev
    L. disease
    L. syndrome
Levaditi stain
levallorphan tartrate
levamisole
levansucrase
levarterenol bitartrate
levator
    l. anguli oris muscle
    l. ani muscle
    l. cushion
    l. hernia
    l. labii superioris muscle
    l. palati muscle
    l. palpebrae superioris muscle
    l. prostatae muscle
    l. scapulae muscle
    l. swelling
    l. veli palatini muscle
levatores
    l. costarum breves muscle
    l. costarum longi muscle
Levay antigen
LeVeen shunt
Level-7
    Health L.-7 (HL-7)
level
    acoustic reference l.
    l. of aspiration
    background l.
    Clark l.
    l. of consciousness
    hearing l.
    loudness discomfort l.
    saturation sound pressure l.
    sensation l.
    sensory acuity l.
    treble increase at low l.'s
    uncomfortable l.
level-dependent frequency response
lever
    dental l.
leverage

Levey-Jennings chart
Levin tube
levitation
levoatrio-cardinal vein
levocardia
levocardiogram
levocarnitine
levoclination
levocycleduction
levocycloduction
levodopa (L-dopa)
levoduction
levoform
levoglucose
levogram
levogyrate
levogyrous
levonordefrin
levophacetoperane
levophobia
levopropoxyphene napsylate
levorotation
levorotatory
levorphanol tartrate
levotorsion
levoversion
Levret forceps
levulan
levulic acid
levulin
levulinate
    calcium l.
levulinic acid
levulosan
levulose
levulosemia
levulosuria
Lewis
    L. acid
    L. base
    L. blood group
lewisite
Lewy
    L. body
    L. body dementia
lexical
Leyden
    L. ataxia
    L. crystal
    L. neuritis
Leyden-Möbius muscular dystrophy

L

NOTES

543

Leydig
    L. cell
    L. cell tumor
leydigarche
LFA
    left frontoanterior
Lf dose
LFP
    left frontoposterior
LFT
    left frontotransverse
LGSIL
    low-grade squamous intraepithelial lesion
LH
    luteinizing hormone
Lhermitte sign
LH/FSH-RF
    luteinizing hormone/follicle-stimulating
    hormone-releasing factor
LH-RF
    luteinizing hormone-releasing factor
LH-RH
    luteinizing hormone-releasing hormone
liberator
    histamine l.
liberomotor
libidinization
libidinous
libido
    bisexual l.
    ego l.
    object l.
    l. theory
Libman-Sacks
    L.-S. endocarditis
    L.-S. syndrome
Liborius method
library
    cDNA l.
    expression l.
    gene l.
    genomic l.
    l. screening
lice (*pl. of* louse)
licensed
    l. practical nurse
    l. vocational nurse
lichen
    l. amyloidosis
    l. myxedematosus
    l. nitidus
    l. nuchae
    l. obtusus
    l. planopilaris
    l. planus
    l. planus annularis
    l. planus follicularis
    l. planus hypertrophicus
    l. planus-like keratosis

    l. planus verrucosus
    l. ruber moniliformis
    l. ruber planus
    l. sclerosus et atrophicus
    l. scrofulosorum
    l. simplex chronicus
    l. spinulosus
    l. striatus
    tropical l.
    l. tropicus
    l. urticatus
lichenification
lichenin
lichenoid
    l. amyloidosis
    l. dermatosis
    l. eczema
    l. keratosis
lid
    l. crutch spectacles
    granular l.
    lower l.
    l. reflex
lid-closure reaction
Liddell-Sherrington reflex
lidoflazine
lie
    l. detector
    longitudinal l.
    oblique l.
    transverse l.
    unstable l.
Lieberkühn
    crypt of L.
    L. follicle
    L. gland
Liebermann-Burchard
    L.-B. reaction
    L.-B. test
Liebermeister rule
Liebig theory
lien
    l. accessorius
    l. mobilis
lienal artery
lienculus
lienectomy
lienomedullary
lienomyelogenous
lienopancreatic
lienophrenic ligament
lienorenal ligament
lienteric diarrhea
lientery
lienunculus
Liesegang ring
Lieutaud
    L. body
    L. triangle

L. trigone
L. uvula
life

change of l.
l. cycle
l. events
expectation of l.
l. instinct
quality of l.
l. stress
l. table
life-belt cataract
lifespan development
Li-Fraumeni cancer syndrome
ligament

accessory plantar l.
accessory volar l.
acromioclavicular l.
alar l.
alveolodental l.
anococcygeal l.
anterior costotransverse l.
anterior cruciate l.
anterior longitudinal l.
anterior meniscofemoral l.
anterior sacrococcygeal l.
anterior sacroiliac l.
anterior sacrosciatic l.
anterior sternoclavicular l.
anterior talofibular l.
anterior talotibial l.
anterior tibiofibular l.
anterior tibiotalar l.
anular l.
apical l.
Arantius l.
arcuate popliteal l.
arcuate pubic l.
arterial l.
auricular l.
Bardinet l.
Barkow l.
Bellini l.
Berry l.
Bertin l.
Bichat l.
bifurcate l.
bifurcated l.
Bigelow l.
Botallo l.
Bourgery l.
broad l.

Brodie l.
Burns l.
calcaneocuboid l.
calcaneofibular l.
calcaneonavicular l.
calcaneotibial l.
Caldani l.
Campbell l.
Camper l.
capsular l.
cardinal l.
caroticoclinoid l.
carpometacarpal l.
caudal l.
ceratocricoid l.
cervical l.
check l.
chondroxiphoid l.
ciliary l.
Civinini l.
Clado l.
coccygeal l.
collateral l.
Colles l.
conoid l.
Cooper l.
coracoacromial l.
coracoclavicular l.
coracohumeral l.
corniculopharyngeal l.
coronary l.
costoclavicular l.
costocolic l.
costotransverse l.
costoxiphoid l.
cotyloid l.
Cowper l.
cricoarytenoid l.
cricopharyngeal l.
cricosantorinian l.
cricotracheal l.
crucial l.
cruciate l.
cruciform l.
crural l.
Cruveilhier l.
cuboideonavicular l.
cuneocuboid interosseous l.
cuneometatarsal interosseous l.
cuneonavicular l.
cystoduodenal l.
deep dorsal sacrococcygeal l.

L

NOTES

ligament *(continued)*

deep posterior sacrococcygeal l.
deep transverse metacarpal l.
deep transverse metatarsal l.
deltoid l.
Denonvilliers l.
dentate l.
denticulate l.
Denucé l.
diaphragmatic l.
dorsal calcaneocuboid l.
dorsal carpal l.
dorsal carpometacarpal l.
dorsal cuboideonavicular l.
dorsal cuneocuboid l.
dorsal cuneonavicular l.
dorsal intercuneiform l.
dorsal metacarpal l.
dorsal metatarsal l.
dorsal radiocarpal l.
dorsal sacroiliac l.
dorsal tarsal l.
dorsal tarsometatarsal l.
duodenorenal l.
epihyal l.
external collateral l.
extracapsular l.
falciform l.
fallopian l.
Ferrein l.
fibular collateral l.
Flood l.
fundiform l.
gastrocolic l.
gastrodiaphragmatic l.
gastrolienal l.
gastrophrenic l.
gastrosplenic l.
genital l.
genitoinguinal l.
Gerdy l.
Gillette suspensory l.
Gimbernat l.
gingivodental l.
glenohumeral l.
glenoid l.
glossoepiglottic l.
Günz l.
hammock l.
Helmholtz axis l.
Hensing l.
hepatocolic l.
hepatoduodenal l.
hepatoesophageal l.
hepatogastric l.
hepatorenal l.
Hesselbach l.
Hey l.
Holl l.

Hueck l.
Humphry l.
Hunter l.
hyalocapsular l.
hyoepiglottic l.
hypsiloid l.
iliofemoral l.
iliolumbar l.
iliopectineal l.
iliotrochanteric l.
inferior calcaneonavicular l.
inferior pubic l.
inferior transverse scapular l.
infundibuloovarian l.
infundibulopelvic l.
inguinal l.
intercarpal l.
interclavicular l.
interclinoid l.
intercornual l.
intercostal l.
intercuneiform l.
interfoveolar l.
internal collateral l.
interosseous cuneocuboid l.
interosseous cuneometatarsal l.
interosseous metacarpal l.
interosseous metatarsal l.
interosseous sacroiliac l.
interosseous talocalcaneal l.
interosseous tibiofibular l.
interspinous l.
intertransverse l.
intraarticular sternocostal l.
intracapsular l.
ischiocapsular l.
ischiofemoral l.
jugal l.
Krause l.
laciniate l.
lacunar l.
Lannelongue l.
lateral arcuate l.
lateral collateral l.
lateral costotransverse l.
lateral malleolar l.
lateral palpebral l.
lateral puboprostatic l.
lateral sacrococcygeal l.
lateral talocalcaneal l.
lateral temporomandibular l.
lateral thyrohyoid l.
lateral umbilical l.
Lauth l.
left triangular l.
lienophrenic l.
lienorenal l.
Lisfranc l.
Lockwood l.

longitudinal l.
long plantar l.
lumbocostal l.
Luschka l.
Mackenrodt l.
Mauchart l.
Meckel l.
medial arcuate l.
medial canthal l.
medial collateral l.
medial palpebral l.
medial puboprostatic l.
medial talocalcaneal l.
medial umbilical l.
median arcuate l.
median cricothyroid l.
median thyrohyoid l.
median umbilical l.
meniscofemoral l.
metatarsal interosseous l.
middle costotransverse l.
middle umbilical l.
nuchal l.
palmar radiocarpal l.
palmar ulnocarpal l.
patellar l.
pectineal l.
periodontal l.
phrenicocolic l.
plantar calcaneonavicular l.
popliteal l.
posterior cruciate l.
pulmonary l.
radiate l.
radiocarpal l.
reflected inguinal l.
rhomboid l.
round l.
serous l.
Simonart l.
spiral l.
splenorenal l.
suspensory l.
sutural l.
synovial l.
talofibular l.
tarsometatarsal l.
tibial collateral l.
transverse carpal l.
transverse perineal l.
trapezoid l.
uterovesical l.

vocal l.
Y-shaped l.
ligamentopexis
ligamentopexy
ligamentous ankylosis
ligamentum deltoidcum
ligand
addressin l.
Fas l.
ligand-binding site
ligand-gated channel
ligandin
ligase
acetate-CoA l.
acetyl-CoA l.
aminoacid-tRNA l.
butyrate-CoA l.
l. chain reaction
DNA l.
ligate
ligation
blunt-end l.
enzyme-catalyzed l.
tubal l.
ligator
ligature
elastic l.
intravascular l.
l. sign
suture l.
l. wire
light
l. adaptation
l. bath
l. cell
l. chain
l. chain-related amyloidosis
cold l.
cone of l.
l. difference
l. differential threshold
glare of l.
l. green SF yellowish
infrared l.
invisible l.
l. liquid petrolatum
l. metal
l. micrograph
l. microscope
minimum l.
polarized l.
pupils equal, react to l. (PERL)

L

NOTES

light *(continued)*
 l. reflex
 l. sense
 l. sleep
 stray l.
 l. therapy
 l. treatment
 l. wire appliance
 Wood l.
light-activated resin
light-adapted eye
light-cured resin
lightening
lighthouse lens
light-meromyosin
light-near dissociation
lightning
 l. seizure
 l. strip
light-touch palpation
ligneous
 l. conjunctivitis
 l. struma
 l. thyroiditis
lignieresii
 Actinobacillus l.
lignin
lignoceric acid
Likert scale
Lillie
 L. allochrome connective tissue stain
 L. azure-eosin stain
 L. ferrous iron stain
 L. sulfuric acid Nile blue stain
limb
 ampullary membranous l.
 anacrotic l.
 l. bud
 inferior l.
 lateral l.
 l. lead
 long l.
 lower l.
 medial l.
 l. myokymia
 phantom l.
 upper l.
limbal incision
limb-girdle muscular dystrophy
limbi *(pl. of* limbus)
limbic
 l. lobe
 l. system
limb-kinetic apraxia
limbus, pl. **limbi**
 corneal l.
lime
 air-slaked l.

 chlorinated l.
 l. water
limen, pl. **limina**
 difference l.
limerence
liminal
 l. stimulus
 l. trait
liminometer
limit
 critical l.
 dextrin l.
 dose equivalent l.
 elastic l.
 Hayflick l.
 short-term exposure l.
 l. testing
 tolerance l.
 within normal l.'s (WNL)
limited neck dissection
limiting
 l. angle
 compression l.
 l. decision
 l. membrane
 l. sulcus
limnemia
limnemic
limnology
limophthisis
limosum
 Eubacterium l.
LINAC
 linear accelerator
lincomycin
lincosamide antibiotic
lincture
linctus
lindane
Lindau
 L. disease
 L. tumor
Lindner body
line
 absorption l.
 acanthomeatal l.
 accretion l.
 alveolonasal l.
 Amberg lateral sinus l.
 Amici l.
 l. angle
 anocutaneous l.
 anterior axillary l.
 anterior junction l.
 anterior median l.
 arcuate l.
 arterial l.
 axillary l.
 Baillarger l.

base l.
basinasal l.
Beau l.
l. of Bechterew
bismuth l.
black l.
l. of Blaschko
blue l.
Brödel bloodless l.
Burton l.
Camper l.
cell l.
cement l.
cervical l.
Chamberlain l.
Chaussier l.
choroid l.
Clapton l.
cleavage l.
Conradi l.
Correra l.
costal l.
costoclavicular l.
costophrenic septal l.
Crampton l.
Daubenton l.
demarcation l.
l. of demarcation
Dennie l.
dentate l.
developmental l.
Douglas l.
Eberth l.
Egger l.
Ehrlich-Türk l.
epiphysial l.
established cell l.
Farre l.
Feiss l.
Ferry l.
l. of fixation
Fleischner l.
Fraunhofer l.
fulcrum l.
Futcher l.
l. of Gennari
germ l.
gingival l.
glabellar frown l.
gluteal l.
Granger l.
growth arrest l.

Gubler l.
gum l.
Haller l.
Hampton l.
Harris l.
Head l.
Hensen l.
highest nuchal l.
high lip l.
Hilton white l.
His l.
Holden l.
Hudson-Stähli l.
Hunter l.
Hunter-Schreger l.
iliopectineal l.
incremental l.
inferior nuchal l.
inferior temporal l.
infracostal l.
intercondylar l.
intermediate l.
interspinal l.
intertrochanteric l.
intertubercular l.
iron l.
isoelectric l.
Kaes l.
l. of Kaes
Kerley A, B, C l.
Kilian l.
Langer l.
Lanz l.
lead l.
Looser l.
low lip l.
M l.
Mach l.
mammary l.
mammillary l.
McKee l.
median l.
Mees l.
mercurial l.
Meyer l.
midaxillary l.
midclavicular l. (MCL)
middle axillary l.
midsternal l.
milk l.
mucogingival l.
Muehrcke l.

L

NOTES

line *(continued)*
    Nélaton l.
    nipple l.
    Ogston l.
    Ohngren l.
    orbitomeatal l.
    Owen l.
    l. pairs
    pectinate l.
    pectineal l.
    Reid base l.
    Salter incremental l.
    semilunar l.
    Sergent white l.
    Shenton l.
    l. spectrum
    l. spread function
    sternal l.
    Stocker l.
    superior temporal l.
    terminal l.
    l. test
    trapezoid l.
    Ullmann l.
    vibrating l.
    white l.
    Z l.
    l. of Zahn
    Zöllner l.
linea, pl. **lineae**
    l. alba
    l. alba hernia
    lineae atrophicae
    l. nigra
linear
    l. absorption coefficient
    l. acceleration
    l. accelerator (LINAC)
    l. amplification
    l. amputation
    l. atrophy
    l. craniectomy
    l. energy transfer
    l. epidermal nevus
    l. IgA bullous disease in children
    l. incision
    l. phonocardiograph
    l. scleroderma
    l. skull fracture
linearity
linebreeding
lined flap
liner
    cavity l.
Lineweaver-Burk
    L.-B. equation
    L.-B. plot
Lingelsheimia
    L. anitrata

Ling method
lingua, pl. **linguae**
    l. cerebelli
    l. fissurata
    folia linguae
    l. frenata
    l. geographica
    l. nigra
    pityriasis linguae
    l. plicata
lingual
    l. aponeurosis
    l. arch
    l. artery
    l. bar
    l. bone
    l. branch
    l. crypt
    l. embrasure
    l. flange
    l. follicle
    l. frenulum
    l. gingiva
    l. gingival papilla
    l. gland
    l. goiter
    l. gyrus
    l. hemiatrophy
    l. hemorrhoid
    l. herpes
    l. interdental papilla
    l. lobe
    l. lymph node
    l. mucosa
    l. muscle
    l. nerve
    l. occlusion
    l. paralysis
    l. plate
    l. plexus
    l. quinsy
    l. rest
    l. salivary gland depression
    l. septum
    l. splint
    l. surface of tooth
    l. tonsil
    l. vein
lingual-facial-buccal dyskinesia
linguiform
lingula, pl. **lingulae**
lingular
    l. artery
    l. bronchus
    l. vein
lingulectomy
linguloides
    Diphyllobothrium l.
linguocervical ridge

linguoclination
linguoclusion
linguodistal
linguofacial arterial trunk
linguogingival
    l. fissure
    l. groove
    l. ridge
linguo-occlusal
linguopapillitis
linguoplate
linguoversion
liniment
    camphor l.
lining cell
linin network
linitis plastica
linkage
    l. analysis
    l. disequilibrium
    genetic l.
    l. group
    l. map
    l. marker
    medical record l.
    sex l.
linked
linker
    l. DNA
    l. scanning
linking number
linoleate
linoleic acid
linolenic acid
linolic acid
linseed oil
Linton operation
lion-jaw bone-holding forceps
LIP
    lymphocytic interstitial pneumonia
    lymphoid interstitial pneumonia
lip
    acetabular l.
    l. adhesion operation
    anterior l.
    articular l.
    cleft l.
    double l.
    external l.
    glenoidal l.
    Hapsburg l.

    inner l.
    internal l.
    junction of l.'s
    large pudendal l.
    lateral l.
    lower l.
    medial l.
    l. pit
    l. reading
    l. reflex
    l. sulcus
lipancreatin
liparocele
lipase
    diacylglycerol l.
    diglyceride l.
    lipoprotein l.
    l. test
    triacylglycerol l.
lipectomy
lipedema
lipedematous alopecia
lipemia
    alimentary l.
    diabetic l.
    l. retinalis
lipemic retinopathy
lipid
    l. A
    anisotropic l.
    anular l.
    brain l.
    compound l.'s
    l. granulomatosis
    l. histiocytosis
    isotropic l.
    l. keratopathy
    l. pneumonia
lipidemia
lipid-mobilizing hormone
lipidolytic
lipidosis
    cerebral l.
    ganglioside l.
    glycolipid l.
lipoamide
    l. dehydrogenase
    l. disulfide
    l. reductase NADH
lipoarthritis
lipoate acetyltransferase

L

NOTES

lipoatrophia
   l. annularis
   l. circumscripta
lipoatrophic diabetes
lipoatrophy
   insulin l.
lipoblast
lipoblastoma
lipoblastomatosis
lipocardiac
lipocatabolic
lipoceratous
lipocere
lipochondria
lipochondrodystrophy
lipochrome
lipoclasis
lipoclastic
lipocrit
lipocyte
lipodermoid
lipodieresis
lipodystrophy
   congenital total l.
   familial partial l.
   insulin l.
   membranous l.
lipoedema
lipofectin
lipofection
lipoferous
lipofibroma
lipofuscin
lipofuscinosis
   ceroid l.
lipogenesis
lipogenic
lipogenous diabetes
lipogranuloma
lipogranulomatosis
   disseminated l.
lipohemia
lipoic acid
lipoid
   l. dermatoarthritis
   l. granuloma
   l. granulomatosis
   l. nephrosis
   l. pneumonia
   l. proteinosis
   l. theory
lipoidemia
lipoidosis
   cerebroside l.
   galactosylceramide l.
lipoinjection
lipolipoidosis
lipolysis
lipolytic

lipoma
   atypical l.
   pleomorphic l.
   spindle cell l.
lipomatoid
lipomatosa
   macrodystrophia l.
lipomatosis
   encephalocraniocutaneous l.
   mediastinal l.
lipomatous
   l. hypertrophy
   l. infiltration
   l. polyp
lipomeningocele
lipomucopolysaccharidosis
liponucleoprotein
lipopenia
lipopenic
lipopeptid
lipopeptide
lipophage
lipophagic granuloma
lipophagy
lipophanerosis
lipophil
lipophilic
lipophosphodiesterase I, II
lipopolysaccharide
lipoprotein
   l. electrophoresis
   high-density l. (HDL)
   intermediate density l. (IDL)
   l. lipase
   low-density l. (LDL)
   malondialdehyde-modified low-
     density l.
   l. polymorphism
lipoprotein-associated coagulation
   inhibitor (LACI)
lipoprotein-X
liposarcoma
liposis
lipositol
liposoluble
liposome
liposuction
   tumescent l.
   wet-technique l.
liposuctioning
lipothiamide pyrophosphate
lipotrophic
lipotrophy
lipotropic
   l. factor
   l. pituitary hormone
lipotropin
lipotropy
lipovaccine

lipovitellin
lipoxenous
lipoxeny
lipoxidase
lipoxygenase
lipoyl dehydrogenase
lipping
lippitude
Lipschütz cell
lipuria
lipuric
liquefacient
liquefaction
    l. degeneration
    l. necrosis
liquefactive necrosis
liquefied phenol
liquescent
liquid
    l. air
    Cotunnius l.
    l. crystal thermography
    l. extract
    l. glucose
    l. human serum
    l. paraffin
    l. petroleum
    l. pitch
    l. scintillator
    l. ventilation
liquid-liquid chromatography
liquor
    l. amnii
    l. cerebrospinalis
    l. cotunnii
    l. entericus
    l. folliculi
    malt l.
liquoris
liquorrhea
Lisch nodule
Lisfranc
    L. amputation
    L. injury
    L. joint
    L. ligament
    L. operation
    L. tubercle
Lison-Dunn stain
lisping
lispro insulin
lissamine rhodamine B 200

Lissauer
    L. bundle
    L. column
    L. fasciculus
    L. marginal zone
    L. tract
lissencephalia
lissencephalic
lissencephaly
lissive
lissosphincter
lissotrichic
lissotrichous
Lister
    L. dressing
    L. method
    L. tubercle
Listeria
    L. denitrificans
    L. grayi
    L. monocytogene
listeria meningitis
listeriosis
listerism
listing
    l. gait
    L. law
    L. reduced eye
Liston
    L. knife
    L. shear
lisuride
litem
    guardian ad l.
liter
literal agraphia
literature
    gray l.
lithagogue
litharge
lithectomy
lithiasis conjunctivae
lithic acid
lithium
    l. bromide
    l. carbonate
    l. carmine
    l. citrate
    l. tungstate
lithocholic acid
lithoclast
lithogenesis

L

NOTES

lithogenic
lithogenous
lithogeny
lithokelyphos
litholabe
litholapaxy
litholysis
litholyte
litholytic
lithomyl
lithonephritis
lithopedion
lithopedium
lithotome
lithotomist
lithotomy
    high l.
    lateral l.
    marian l.
    median l.
    perineal l.
    l. position
lithotresis
lithotripsy, lithotrity
    electrohydraulic shock wave l.
    extracorporeal shock wave l.
      (ESWL)
    ultrasonic l.
lithotriptic
lithotriptor
lithotriptoscopy
lithotrite
lithotrity (var. of lithotripsy)
lithotroph
lithuresis
lithuria
litigious paranoia
litmus
little
    l. ACTH
    L. area
    L. disease
    L. League elbow
    L. Leaguer's elbow
    L. League shoulder
    l. toe
littoral cell
Littré
    L. gland
    L. hernia
Littré-Richard hernia
Litzmann obliquity
live
    l. birth
    l. oral poliovirus vaccine
livebirth
liveborn infant
livedo
    lupus l.

    postmortem l.
    l. reticularis
    l. telangiectatica
    l. vasculitis
livedoid dermatitis
liver
    l. acinus
    l. breath
    l. bud
    cardiac l.
    l. cell carcinoma
    desiccated l.
    duodenal impression on l.
    esophageal impression on l.
    fatty l.
    l. filtrate factor
    l. flap
    frosted l.
    l. function
    gastric impression on l.
    hobnail l.
    l. kidney syndrome
    lardaceous l.
    left l.
    l. palm
    polycystic l.
    right l.
    right lobe of l.
    l. spot
    l. starch
liver-shod clamp
livetin
livid
livida
    asphyxia l.
lividity
    postmortem l.
living
    activities of daily l. (ADL)
    l. anatomy
    l. related allograft
    l. unrelated allograft
    l. will
livor
lixivium
LLETZ
    large loop excision of transformation
    zone
L-L factor
LLL
    left lower lobe
Lloyd reagent
LLQ
    left lower quadrant
LMA
    left mentoanterior
LMP
    last menstrual period
    left mentoposterior

LMT
　left mentotransverse
LNPF
　lymph node permeability factor
LOA
　left occipitoanterior
loa
　　Loa l.
load
　　electronic pacemaker l.
　　genetic l.
　　viral l.
load-and-shift maneuver
loading
　　axial l.
　　carbohydrate l.
　　l. dose
　　glycogen l.
Loa loa
lobar
　　l. atelectasis
　　l. emphysema
　　l. pneumonia
　　l. sclerosis
lobate
lobatum
　　hepar l.
lobe
　　anterior l.
　　azygos l.
　　caudate l.
　　cerebral l.
　　cuneiform l.
　　ear l.
　　falciform l.
　　flocculonodular l.
　　frontal l.
　　glandular l.
　　Home l.
　　insular l.
　　kidney l.
　　left lower l. (LLL)
　　left upper l. (LUL)
　　limbic l.
　　lingual l.
　　middle l.
　　nervous l.
　　occipital l.
　　parietal l.
　　posterior l.
　　l. of prostate
　　pyramidal l.

　　quadrate l.
　　Spigelius l.
　　temporal l.
lobectomy
lobelia
lobeline sulfate
lobitis
Loboa loboi
Lobo disease
loboi
　　Loboa l.
lobomycosis
lobopodium
lobose
lobotomy
lobous
Lobry de Bruyn-van Ekenstein transformation
Lobstein ganglion
lobster-claw deformity
lobular
　　l. capillary hemangioma
　　l. carcinoma
　　l. carcinoma in situ
　　l. glomerulonephritis
　　l. neoplasia
lobulate
lobulated tongue
lobule
　　ansiform l.
　　anterior lunate l.
　　biventer l.
　　biventral l.
　　central l.
　　conical l.
　　cortical l.
　　crescentic l.
　　gracile l.
　　hepatic l.
　　inferior parietal l.
　　inferior semilunar l.
　　portal l.
　　primary pulmonary l.
　　quadrangular l.
lobulet, lobulette
lobus caudatus
LOCA
　low osmolar contrast agent
local
　　l. anaphylaxis
　　l. anemia
　　l. anesthesia

NOTES

L

local (*continued*)
l. anesthetic
l. anesthetic reaction
l. asphyxia
l. bloodletting
l. death
l. epilepsy
l. excitatory state
l. flap
l. glomerulonephritis
l. hormone
l. immunity
l. sign
l. stimulant
l. symptom
l. syncope
l. tetanus
l. tic
localization
l. agnosia
auditory l.
cerebral l.
germinal l.
localization-related epilepsy
localized
l. amnesia
l. mucinosis
l. nodular tenosynovitis
l. osteitis fibrosa
l. pemphigoid
l. peritonitis
l. scleroderma
localizing
l. electrode
l. symptom
locant
locator
lochia
l. alba
l. rubra
l. sanguinolenta
l. serosa
lochial
lochiometra
lochiorrhagia
lochiorrhea
loci (*pl. of* locus)
lock
English l.
l. finger
heparin l.
sliding l.
l. stitch
lock-and-key model
locked
l. bite
l. facets
l. knee
l. twins

locked-in syndrome
Locke-Ringer solution
Locke solution
locking suture
lockjaw, lock-jaw
lock-stitch suture
Lockwood ligament
LOCM
low osmolar contrast medium
locomotor ataxia
locomotorial
locomotorium
locomotory
locular
loculate
loculated
l. empyema
l. pleural effusion
loculation syndrome
loculus, pl. **loculi**
locum
l. tenant
l. tenens
locus, pl. **loci**
l. caeruleus
l. cinereus
complex l.
l. of control
l. ferrugineus
genetic l.
marker l.
l. niger
locust gum
Lo dose
Loeb deciduoma
Loeffler
L. bacillus
L. blood culture medium
L. caustic stain
L. methylene blue
L. syndrome I, II
Loevit cell
Loewenthal
L. bundle
L. reaction
L. tract
Löffler
L. disease
L. parietal fibroplastic endocarditis
L. syndrome
logagnosia
logagraphia
logamnesia
Logan bow
logaphasia
logarithm
logarithmic
l. phase
l. phonocardiograph

logasthenia
logetronography
logistic
    l. curve
    l. model
logit transformation
lognormal distribution
logopedia
logopedics
logoplegia
logorrhea
logospasm
logotherapy
Lohlein-Baehr lesion
Lohmann reaction
loiasis
loliism
Lombard voice-reflex test
lomustine
long
    l. adductor muscle
    l. association fiber
    l. axis
    l. axis view
    l. bone
    l. buccal nerve
    l. central artery
    l. chain
    l. ciliary nerve
    l. cone technique
    l. crus of incus
    l. extensor muscle
    l. fibular muscle
    l. flexor muscle
    L. formula
    l. gyrus
    l. head
    l. incubation hepatitis
    l. interspersed element
    l. leg brace
    l. levatores costarum muscle
    l. limb
    l. palmar muscle
    l. peroneal muscle
    l. pitch helicoidal layer
    l. plantar ligament
    l. posterior ciliary artery
    l. process of malleus
    l. pulse
    l. QT syndrome
    l. radial extensor muscle

    l. root of ciliary ganglion
    l. saphenous nerve
    l. saphenous vein
    l. sight
    l. slow distance training
    l. subscapular nerve
    l. terminal repeat sequences
    l. thoracic artery
    l. thoracic nerve
    l. thoracic vein
    l. vinculum
long-acting thyroid stimulator
longbeachae
    Legionella l.
longevity
longissimus
    l. capitis muscle
    l. cervicis muscle
    l. thoracis muscle
longitudinal
    l. aberration
    l. arc
    l. arch
    l. band
    l. canal
    l. cerebral fissure
    l. dissociation
    l. duct
    l. fold
    l. fracture
    l. incision
    l. layer
    l. lie
    l. ligament
    l. method
    l. oval pelvis
    l. pontine bundle
    l. pontine fasciculus
    l. pontine fiber
    l. pregnancy
    l. relaxation
    l. section
    l. study
    l. sulcus
    l. tear
    l. vertebral venous sinus
longitudinalis
    arcus pedis l.
longitype
long-leg arthropathy
Longmire operation

NOTES

long-term
l.-t. care facility
l.-t. memory
longus
l. capitis muscle
l. colli muscle
Lon protease
loop
afferent l.
Biebl l.
bulboventricular l.
capillary l.
cervical l.
cruciform l.'s
cutting l.
D l.
displacement l.
l. diuretic
efferent l.
l. electrocautery excision procedure (LEEP)
l. electrosurgical excision procedure (LEEP)
l. excision
gamma l.
Gerdy interatrial l.
Granit l.
hairpin l.
Henle l.
Hyrtl l.
lenticular l.
memory l.
Meyer-Archambault l.
nephronic l.
l. resection
l. stoma
loose
l. associations
l. body
l. cartilage
l. skin
loosening of associations
loose-packed position
Looser
L. line
L. zone
LOP
left occipitoposterior
lop-ear, lop ear
lophodont
lophotrichate
lophotrichous
lopremone
LOQ
left outer quadrant
Lorain disease
Lorain-Lévi
L.-L. dwarfism

L.-L. infantilism
L.-L. syndrome
lordoscoliosis
lordosis
cervical l.
l. cervicis
l. colli
l. lumbalis
lumbar l.
lordotic
l. albuminuria
l. pelvis
l. position
Lorenzo oil
Lorenz sign
Loschmidt number
loss
acoustic trauma hearing l.
boilermaker's hearing l.
conductive hearing l.
functional visual l.
hearing l.
industrial hearing l.
low-tone hearing l.
mixed hearing l.
neural hearing l.
noise-induced hearing l.
occupational hearing l.
retrocochlear hearing l.
sensorineural hearing l.
LOT
left occipitotransverse
Lotheissen operation
loudness discomfort level
Lou Gehrig disease
Louis
L. angle
L. law
Louis-Bar syndrome
loupe
binocular l.
louping-ill virus
louse, pl. **lice**
biting l.
chewing l.
feather l.
l. fly
sea l.
louse-borne typhus
lousy
lova
Dracunculus l.
Lovén reflex
Lovibond
L. angle
L. profile sign
low
l. convex
l. forceps delivery

l. grade astrocytoma
l. lip line
l. malignant potential tumor
l. molecular weight kininogen
l. molecular weight protein
l. osmolar contrast agent (LOCA)
l. osmolar contrast medium (LOCM)
l. output failure
l. salt syndrome
l. sodium syndrome
l. spinal anesthesia
l. wine
low-calorie diet
low-density
l.-d. lipoprotein (LDL)
l.-d. lipoprotein receptor
low-egg-passage vaccine
Löwenberg
L. canal
L. forceps
L. scala
Lowenstein-Jensen culture medium
lower
l. abdominal periosteal reflex
l. airway
l. alveolar point
l. dental arcade
l. esophageal sphincter (LES)
l. extremity
l. eyelid
l. jaw
l. lid
l. limb
l. lip
l. lobe bronchus
l. motor neuron
l. motor neuron dysarthria
l. motor neuron lesion
l. pole
l. respiratory tract smear
l. ridge slope
l. right quadrant (LRQ)
L. ring
l. sternal border (LSB)
L. tubercle
l. uterine segment
l. uterine segment cesarean section
lowest
l. lumbar artery
l. splanchnic nerve
l. thyroid artery

Lowe syndrome
Lowe-Terrey-MacLachlan syndrome
low-fat diet
low-frequency transduction
low-grade squamous intraepithelial lesion (LGSIL, LSIL)
Lown-Ganong-Levine syndrome
low-pass filter
low-pitched rhonchi
low-purine diet
low-residue diet
Lowry-Folin assay
Lowry protein assay
low-salt diet
Lowsley tractor
low-tension glaucoma
low-tone hearing loss
loxoscelism
lozenge
LP
lumbar puncture
L-phase variant
LPO
left posterior oblique
LR
lactated Ringer
L-radiation
Lr dose
LRF
luteinizing hormone-releasing factor
LRH
luteinizing hormone-releasing hormone
LRQ
lower right quadrant
LRS
lactated Ringer solution
LSA
left sacroanterior
LSB
lower sternal border
LSIL
low-grade squamous intraepithelial lesion
LSP
left sacroposterior
LST
left sacrotransverse
Lu
L. antigen
L. blood group
Lubarsch crystal
lubricating cream
Lucas groove

L

NOTES

lucidification
lucid interval
lucidity
lucidum
    stratum l.
luciferase
luciferins
lucifugal
lucimycin
Lucio
    L. leprosy
    L. leprosy phenomenon
lucipetal
lückenschädel
Lücke test
Lucké virus
Luc operation
Ludwig
    L. angina
    L. angle
    L. ganglion
    L. labyrinth
    L. nerve
    L. stromuhr
LUE
    left upper extremity
Luer-Lok syringe
Luer syringe
lues venerea
luetic mask
Luft
    L. disease
    L. potassium permanganate fixative
Lugol iodine solution
Lukes-Collins classification
LUL
    left upper lobe
luliberin
lumbago
    ischemic l.
lumbale
    trigonum l.
lumbales
    vertebra l.
lumbalis
    costa l.
    lordosis l.
lumbar
    l. appendicitis
    l. artery
    l. branch
    l. cistern
    l. fascia
    l. flexure
    l. ganglion
    l. hernia
    l. iliocostal muscle
    l. interspinal muscle
    l. lordosis

    l. lymphatic plexus
    l. lymphatic trunk
    l. lymph node
    l. myelogram
    l. nephrectomy
    l. nephrotomy
    l. nervous plexus
    l. puncture (LP)
    l. puncture needle
    l. quadrate muscle
    l. region
    l. rheumatism
    l. rib
    l. rotator muscle
    l. segment
    l. spine
    l. splanchnic nerve
    l. triangle
    l. vein
    l. vertebra
lumbarization
lumboabdominal
lumbocostal
    l. ligament
    l. triangle
lumbocostoabdominal triangle
lumbodorsal fascia
lumboiliac
lumboinguinal nerve
lumbosacral
    l. angle
    l. enlargement
    l. joint
    l. nerve trunk
    l. nervous plexus
lumbotomy incision
lumbrical muscle
lumbricidal
lumbricide
lumbricoid
lumbricoides
    Ascaris l.
lumbricosis
lumbricus
lumbus
lumen
    false l.
    true l.
lumichrome
lumiflavin
luminal
luminalis
luminance
luminescence
luminiferous
luminophore
luminous
    l. flux

l. intensity
l. retinoscope
lumirhodopsin
lumisterol
lumpectomy
lumpy jaw
lunacy
Luna-Ishak stain
lunar
    l. caustic
    l. periodicity
lunate
    l. bone
    l. fissure
    l. sulcus
    l. surface
lunatic
lunatomalacia
Lundh meal
lung
    air-conditioner l.
    bird-breeder's l.
    bird-fancier's l.
    black l.
    l. blast
    brown l.
    l. bud
    butterfly l.
    cardiac l.
    cheese worker's l.
    collier's l.
    l. compliance
    cystic l.
    end-stage l.
    farmer's l.
    fibroid l.
    l. fibroma
    l. fluke disease
    harvester l.
    honeycomb l.
    hyperlucent l.
    iron l.
    malt-worker's l.
    l. marking
    mason's l.
    miner's l.
    pump l.
    quiet l.
    shock l.
    silo-filler's l.
    trench l.
    unilateral hyperlucent l.

l. unit
l. volume reduction surgery
wet l.
white l.
l. window
lungworms
lunula, pl. **lunulae**
lunule
    azure l.
    l. of nail
Lunyo virus
lupiform
lupinidine
lupinosis
lupoid
    l. hepatitis
    l. leishmaniasis
    l. sycosis
lupous
lupulin
lupus
    l. anticoagulant
    l. band test
    chilblain l.
    discoid l.
    drug-induced l.
    l. erythematosus (LE)
    l. erythematosus cell
    l. erythematosus cell test
    l. erythematosus, neonatal
    l. erythematosus panniculitis
    l. erythematosus profundus
    l. livedo
    l. miliaris disseminatus faciei
    l. nephritis
    l. pernio
    l. serpiginosus
    l. vulgaris
lupus-like syndrome
LUQ
    left upper quadrant
Luschka
    L. bursa
    L. cartilage
    L. cystic gland
    L. duct
    foramen of L.
    L. joint
    L. ligament
    L. sinus
    L. tonsil
Luse body

NOTES

lusitropic
lusitropy
lusoria
    arteria l.
luteal
    l. cell
    l. phase
    l. phase defect
    l. phase deficiency
lutecium
lutein cell
luteinization
luteinized unruptured follicle
luteinizing
    l. hormone (LH)
    l. hormone/follicle-stimulating
    hormone-releasing factor (LH/FSH-RF)
    l. hormone-releasing factor (LH-RF, LRF)
    l. hormone-releasing hormone (LH-RH, LRH)
    l. principle
luteinoma
Lutembacher syndrome
luteogenic
luteohormone
luteol
luteolin
luteolysin
luteolysis
luteolytic
luteoma
luteoplacental shift
luteotropic, luteotrophic
    l. hormone
luteotropin
lutetium
luteum
    atretic corpus l.
luteus
    Micrococcus l.
luting agent
lutropin
lututrin
Lutz-Splendore-Almeida disease
luxatio
    l. erecta
    l. perinealis
luxation
    Malgaigne l.
Luxol fast blue
luxus
Luys body
LVAD
    left ventricular assist device
LVET
    left ventricular ejection time

LW
    lacerating wound
lyase
    cystine l.
    heparin l.
    hyaluronate l.
    hyaluronic l.
    isocitrate l.
    lactoylglutathione l.
lycanthropy
lycoctonine
lycopene
lycopenemia
lycoperdonosis
lycophora
lycopodium
Lyell
    L. disease
    L. syndrome
Lyme
    L. arthritis
    L. borreliosis
    L. disease
lymph
    aplastic l.
    blood l.
    l. capillary
    l. cell
    l. circulation
    l. cord
    l. corpuscle
    corpuscular l.
    croupous l.
    dental l.
    l. drainage
    l. embolism
    euplastic l.
    fibrinous l.
    l. follicle
    l. gland
    inflammatory l.
    intercellular l.
    intravascular l.
    l. node
    l. node permeability factor (LNPF)
    l. nodule
    l. sac
    l. scrotum
    l. sinus
    l. space
    tissue l.
    vaccine l.
    vaccinia l.
    l. varix
    l. vessel
lymphadenectomy
lymphadenitis
    dermatopathic l.

mesenteric l.
regional granulomatous l.
lymphadenocele
lymphadenography
lymphadenoid
lymphadenoma
lymphadenopathy
angioimmunoblastic l.
bulky l.
dermatopathic l.
immunoblastic l.
sinus histiocytosis with massive l.
lymphadenopathy-associated virus (LAV)
lymphadenosis
benign l.
lymphadenotomy
lymphadenovarix
lymphagogue
lymphangeitis
lymphangial
lymphangiectasia
lymphangiectasis
cavernous l.
cystic l.
intestinal l.
lymphangiectatic
lymphangiectomy
lymphangiitis
lymphangioendothelioma
lymphangiography
lymphangioleiomyomatosis
lymphangiology
lymphangioma
cavernous l.
lymphangiomatous
lymphangiomyomatosis
lymphangion
lymphangiophlebitis
lymphangioplasty
lymphangiosarcoma
lymphangiotomy
lymphangitic carcinomatosis
lymphangitis
indurated l.
lymphapheresis
lymphatic
afferent l.
l. angina
l. corpuscle
l. duct
l. edema
efferent l.

l. filariasis granuloma
l. fistula
l. follicle
l. leukemia
l. nevus
l. node
l. nodule
l. plexus
l. ring
l. sarcoma
l. sinus
l. stroma
l. system
l. tissue
l. valvule
l. vessel
lymphatica
vasa l.
lymphaticostomy
lymphatics
lymphaticus
folliculus l.
lymphatitis
lymphatology
lymphatolysis
lymphatolytic
lymphectasia
lymphedema
congenital l.
hereditary l.
l. praecox
lymphedematous keratoderma
lymphemia
lymphization
lymphoblast
lymphoblastic
l. leukemia
l. lymphoma
lymphoblastoma
giant follicular l.
lymphoblastosis
lymphocele
lymphocerastism
lymphocinesia
lymphocinesis
lymphocyst
lymphocytapheresis
lymphocyte
atypical l.
B l.
l. function associated antigen
Rieder l.

NOTES

lymphocyte *(continued)*
> T l.
> l. transformation

lymphocyte-mediated cytotoxicity
lymphocythemia
lymphocytic
> l. adenohypophysitis
> l. choriomeningitis
> l. choriomeningitis virus
> l. hypophysitis
> l. infiltration
> l. interstitial pneumonia (LIP)
> l. interstitial pneumonitis
> l. leukemia
> l. leukemoid reaction
> l. leukocytosis
> l. leukopenia
> l. series
> l. thyroiditis

lymphocytoblast
lymphocytoma
lymphocytopenia
lymphocytopoiesis
lymphocytosis
> neutrophilic l.

lymphocytotoxic antibody
lymphocytotoxicity
> cell-mediated l. (CML)

lymphoderma
lymphoduct
lymphoepithelial cyst
lymphoepithelioma
lymphogenesis
lymphogenic
lymphogenous
> l. embolism
> l. metastasis

lymphoglandula
lymphogranuloma
> l. benignum
> l. inguinale
> l. malignum
> venereal l.
> l. venereum
> l. venereum antigen
> l. venereum virus

lymphogranulomatosis
lymphography
lymphohistiocytosis
> familial erythrophagocytic l. (FEL)
> familial hemophagocytic l. (FHL)

lymphoid
> l. cell
> l. corpuscle
> l. hemoblast
> l. hypophysitis
> l. interstitial pneumonia (LIP)
> l. leukemia
> l. nodule

> l. polyp
> l. series
> l. system
> l. tissue

lymphoidectomy
lymphoidocyte
lymphokine
lymphokinesis
lympholeukocyte
lymphology
lymphoma
> adult T-cell l.
> anaplastic large cell l.
> benign l.
> Burkitt l.
> chronic lymphocytic l.
> diffuse small cleaved cell l.
> extranodal marginal zone l.
> follicular predominantly large
>   cell l.
> follicular predominantly small
>   cleaved cell l.
> histiocytic l.
> Hodgkin l.
> immunoblastic l.
> large cell l.
> Lennert l.
> lymphoblastic l.
> malignant l.
> mantle cell l.
> marginal zone l.
> Mediterranean l.
> nodular l.
> non-Hodgkin l.
> poorly differentiated lymphocytic l.
> T-cell–rich, B-cell l.
> well-differentiated lymphocytic l.

lymphomatoid
> l. granulomatosis
> l. papulosis
> l. polyposis
> l. vasculitis

lymphomatosa
> angina l.

lymphomatosis
lymphomatous
lymphomyxoma
lymphonodus
lymphopathia
lymphopathy
lymphopenia
lymphoplasmacellular disorder
lymphoplasmapheresis
lymphopoiesis
lymphopoietic
lymphoproliferative syndrome
lymphoreticulosis
> benign inoculation l.

lymphorrhagia

lymphorrhea
lymphorrhoid
lymphosarcoma
    fascicular l.
    sclerosing l.
lymphoscntlgraphy
lymphosis
lymphostasis
lymphostatic verrucosis
lymphotaxis
lymphotoxicity
lymphotoxin
lymphotrophy
lymphuria
Lynch syndrome
lynestrenol
lyoenzyme
lyolysis
Lyon hypothesis
lyonization
lyophil, lyophile
lyophilic colloid
lyophilization
lyophobe
lyophobic colloid
lyosorption
lyotropic series
lypressin
lyre of David
lysate
lyse
lysemia
lysergamide
lysergic acid
lysergide
lysergol
lysin
lysine decarboxylase
lysinemia
lysinium
lysinogen
lysinogenic
lysinuria

lysinuric protein intolerance
lysis
    bystander l.
lysocephalin
lysogen
lysogenesis
lysogenic
    l. bacterium
    l. induction
    l. strain
lysogenicity
lysogenization
lysogeny
lysokinase
lysolecithin
lysolecithinase
lysolecithin-lecithin acyltransferase
lysophosphatidic
    l. acid
    l. acid acyltransferase
lysophosphatidylcholine
lysophosphatidylserine
lysophospholipase
lysosomal disease
lysosome
    definitive l.
    primary l.
    secondary l.
lysostaphin
lysotype
lysozyme
lyssa
Lyssavirus
    Australian bat L.
lysyl
Lyt antigen
lytic
lyxitol
lyxoflavin
lyxose
lyxulose
lyze

NOTES

M
    M antigen
    M band
    M cell
    M concentration
    M line
    M phase
    M protein
    M shell
MAB
    monoclonal antibody
Macchiavello stain
MacConkey agar
macerate
macerated fetus
maceration
Macewen
    M. sign
    M. symptom
    M. triangle
Mach
    M. band
    M. effect
    M. line
    M. number
Machado-Guerreiro test
Machado-Joseph disease
machine
    anesthesia m.
    heart-lung m.
machinery murmur
Machupo virus
Mackay-Marg tonometer
Mackenrodt ligament
Mackenzie
    M. amputation
    M. polygraph
Maclagan thymol turbidity test
Macleod
    M. rheumatism
    M. syndrome
maclurin
MacNeal tetrachrome blood stain
macrencephalia
macrencephaly
macroadenoma
macroaggregated albumin
macroamylase
macroamylasemia
macrobacterium
macrobiosis
macrobiote
macrobiotic diet
macrobiotics
macroblast

macroblepharon
macrobrachia
macrocardia
macrocephalia (*var. of* macrocephaly)
macrocephalic
macrocephalous
macrocephaly, macrocephalia
macrocheilia
macrocheiria
macrochemistry
macrochilia
macrochiria
macrochylomicron
macrocnemia
macrococcus
macrocolon
macroconidium
macrocornea
macrocranium
macrocryoglobulin
macrocryoglobulinemia
macrocyst
macrocyte
macrocythemia
    hyperchromatic m.
macrocytic
    m. achylic anemia
    m. hyperchromia
macrocytosis
macrodactylia, macrodactylism,
    macrodactyly
macrodont
macrodontia
macrodontism
macrodystrophia lipomatosa
macroencephalon
macroerythroblast
macroerythrocyte
macroesthesia
macrofollicular adenoma
macrogamete
macrogametocyte
macrogamont
macrogamy
macrogastria
macrogenitosomia
    m. praecox
    m. praecox suprarenalis
macroglia cell
macroglobulin
macroglobulinemia
    Waldenström m.
macroglossia
macrognathia
macrography

M

macrogyria
macrolabia
macroleukoblast
macrolide antibiotic
macrolides
macromastia
macromazia
macromelanosome
macromelia
macromere
macromerozoite
macromineral
macromolecular chemistry
macromolecule
macromonocyte
macromyeloblast
macronormoblast
macronormochromoblast
macronucleus
macronutrient
macronychia
macroorchidism
macroparasite
macropathology
macropenis
macrophage
    activated m.
    alveolar m.
    armed m.
    m. colony-stimulating factor (M-CSF)
    fixed m.
    free m.
    Hansemann m.
    inflammatory m.
    m. inflammatory protein (MIP)
    m. migration inhibition test
    tangible body m.
macrophage-activating factor (MAF)
macrophagocyte
macrophallus
macrophthalmia
macropodia
macropolycyte
macropromyelocyte
macroprosopia
macroprosopous
macropsia
macrorhinia
macroscelia
macroscopic
    m. anatomy
    m. sphincter
macroscopy
macrosigmoid
macrosis
macrosmatic
macrosomia
macrosplanchnic

macrospore
macrostereognosis
macrostomia
macrotia
macrotome
macrotrauma
macula, pl. maculae
    m. adherens
    m. atrophica
    m. cerulea
    m. corneae
    m. densa
    false m.
    m. flava
    heterotopia maculae
    honeycomb m.
macular
    m. amyloidosis
    m. area
    m. artery
    m. atrophy
    m. coloboma
    m. corneal dystrophy
    m. degeneration
    m. drusen
    m. erythema
    m. evasion
    m. fasciculus
    m. leprosy
    m. pucker
    m. retinal dystrophy
    m. retinopathy
maculate
maculatum
    Amblyomma m.
macule
    ash-leaf m.
maculocerebral
maculoerythematous
maculopapule
maculopathy
    bull's-eye m.
    cystoid m.
    familial pseudoinflammatory m.
mad
    m. cow disease
    M. Hatter syndrome
madarosis
Maddox rod
Madelung
    M. deformity
    M. disease
    M. neck
Madlener operation
madre
    buba m.
Madura
    M. boil
    M. foot

madurae
    Actinomadura m.
maduromycosis
MAF
    macrophage-activating factor
Maffucci syndrome
Magendie
    foramen of M.
    M. law
    M. space
Magendie-Hertwig
    M.-H. sign
    M.-H. syndrome
magenstrasse
magenta tongue
maggot
    cheese m.
magical thinking
magic forceps
Magill forceps
magistral
magma
    magnesia m.
    m. reticulare
magna
    coxa m.
    lacuna m.
Magnan
    M. sign
    M. trombone movement
magnesia
    calcined m.
    m. magma
    milk of m.
magnesium
    m. benzoate
    m. carbonate
    m. chloride
    m. citrate
    m. hydroxide
    m. lactate
    m. oxide
    m. peroxide
magnet
    m. reaction
    m. reflex
    superconducting m.
magnetic
    m. attraction
    m. field
    m. field gradient
    m. implant
    m. inertia
    m. resonance angiography (MRA)
    m. resonance imaging
    m. resonance spectroscopy
magnetism
    animal m.
magnetocardiography
magnetoencephalogram
magnetoencephalography
magnetogyric ratio
magnetometer
magneton
    Bohr m.
    electron m.
magnetotherapy
magnification
    m. angiography
    m. radiography
magnitude
    average pulse m.
    m. image
magnocellular
magnum
magnus
Mahaim fiber
ma-huang
MAI
    Mycobacterium avium-intracellulare
maidenhair tree
maidenhead
maidism
Maier sinus
mainstream aerosol
mainstreaming
maintainer
maintenance
    m. dose
    m. drug therapy
    m. medication
maise oil
Maisonneuve fracture
Maissiat band
maize factor
Majocchi granuloma
major
    m. agglutinin
    m. alar cartilage
    m. amblyoscope
    m. amputation
    aphthae m.
    m. arterial circle
    m. calix

M

NOTES

major *(continued)*
- m. circulus arteriosus
- m. connector
- m. depression
- m. depressive disorder
- m. duodenal papilla
- m. epilepsy
- m. fissure
- m. forceps
- forceps m.
- globus m.
- m. groove
- m. hippocampus
- hippocampus m.
- m. histocompatibility complex
- m. hypnosis
- *Leishmania m.*
- m. mood disorder
- m. motor seizure
- m. operation
- pelvis justo m.
- m. salivary gland
- m. sublingual duct
- m. surgery
- thalassemia m.
- m. tranquilizer

majus
- labium m.
- os multangulum m.

Makeham hypothesis

mal
- m. de la rosa
- m. del pinto
- m. de Meleda
- m. de mer
- grand m.
- m. morado
- petit m.
- m. rosso

mala

malabsorption
- enterocyte cobalamin m.
- fructose m.
- hereditary folate m.
- m. syndrome

Malacarne
- M. pyramid
- M. space

malachite green

malacia

malacic

malacoplakia

malacosis

malacotic

malacotomy

malactic

maladie
- m. de Roger
- m. des jambes

maladjustment

malady

malagma

malaise

malakoplakia

malalignment

malar
- m. arch
- m. bone
- m. flush
- m. fold
- m. foramen
- m. fracture
- m. lymph node
- m. point
- m. process
- m. tuberosity

malaria
- acute m.
- airport m.
- algid m.
- autochthonous m.
- benign tertian m.
- bilious remittent m.
- cerebral m.
- chronic m.
- m. comatosa
- double tertian m.
- dysenteric algid m.
- falciparum m.
- gastric algid m.
- induced m.
- intermittent m.
- malariae m.
- malignant tertian m.
- quartan m.
- quotidian m.
- therapeutic m.
- vivax m.

malariae
- m. malaria
- *Plasmodium m.*

malarial
- m. cachexia
- m. crescent
- m. fever
- m. hemoglobinuria
- m. knob
- m. periodicity
- m. pigment
- m. pigment stain

malariology

malariotherapy

malarious

Malassez epithelial rests

Malassezia
- M. *furfur*
- M. *ovalis*
- M. *pachydermatis*

malassimilation
malate
    m. dehydrogenase
    m. synthase
malate-aspartate shuttle
malate-condensing enzyme
malathion
malaxation
malayanum
    Echinostoma m.
maldigestion
Maldonado-San Jose stain
male
    m. breast
    m. external genitalia
    genetic human m.
    m. gonad
    m. hermaphroditism
    m. homosexuality
    m. hypogonadism
    m. internal genitalia
    m. pattern alopecia
    m. pattern baldness
    m. pseudohermaphroditism
    m. sterility
    m. urethra
maleate
    dexbrompheniramine m.
    dexchlorpheniramine m.
    enalapril m.
    ergometrine m.
    ergonovine m.
    mepyramine m.
Malecot catheter
maleic acid
malemission
maleruption
maleylacetoacetate
malformation
    Arnold-Chiari m.
    cystic adenomatoid m.
    mermaid m.
    Michel m.
    vascular m.
    venous m.
malfunction
Malgaigne
    M. amputation
    M. fossa
    M. hernia
    M. luxation
    M. triangle

Malherbe calcifying epithelioma
malic
    m. acid
    m. acid dehydrogenase
    m. enzyme
maligna
    lentigo m.
malignancy
malignant
    m. anemia
    m. atrophic papulosis
    m. bubo
    m. carcinoid syndrome
    m. catarrhal fever virus
    m. ciliary epithelioma
    m. dysentery
    m. dyskeratosis
    m. endocarditis
    m. exophthalmos
    m. external otitis
    m. fibrous histiocytoma
    m. glaucoma
    m. granuloma
    m. hepatoma
    m. histiocytosis
    m. hyperphenylalaninemia
    m. hyperpyrexia
    m. hypertension
    m. hyperthermia
    m. jaundice
    m. lentigo melanoma
    m. lymphoma
    m. malnutrition
    m. melanoma in situ
    m. meningioma
    m. midline reticulosis
    m. mixed mesodermal tumor
    (MMMT)
    m. mixed müllerian tumor
    (MMMT)
    m. mole syndrome
    m. myopia
    m. neoplasm
    m. nephrosclerosis
    m. neutropenia
    m. pustule
    m. scleritis
    m. smallpox
    m. stupor
    m. teratoma
    m. tertian fever

M

NOTES

malignant (*continued*)
    m. tertian malaria
    m. tertian malarial parasite
malignum
    lymphogranuloma m.
malinger
malingerer
malingering
malinterdigitation
Mall
    M. formula
    M. ridge
malleable
mallear
    m. fold
    m. prominence
    m. stripe
mallebrin
mallei (*pl. of* malleus)
mallei
    Burkholderia m.
malleoincudal
malleolar
    m. articular surface
    m. groove
    m. stria
    m. sulcus
malleolus, pl. **malleoli**
    external m.
    inner m.
    internal m.
    lateral m.
    m. lateralis
    medial m.
    m. medialis
    outer m.
    tibial m.
    ulnar m.
malleotomy
mallet finger
malleus, pl. **mallei**
    hallux m.
    long process of m.
    m. shear
Mallory
    M. aniline blue stain
    M. body
    M. collagen stain
    M. iodine stain
    M. phloxine stain
    M. phosphotungstic acid
      hematoxylin stain
    M. trichrome stain
    M. triple stain
Mallory-Weiss
    M.-W. lesion
    M.-W. syndrome
    M.-W. tear

malnutrition
    malignant m.
malocclusion
    Angle classification of m.
malomaxillary suture
malonate semialdehyde
malondialdehyde-modified low-density
  lipoprotein
Maloney bougie
malonic acid
malonyl-CoA
malpighian
    m. body
    m. capsule
    m. cell
    m. corpuscle
    m. gland
    m. glomerulus
    m. layer
    m. nodule
    m. pyramid
    m. rete
    m. stigma
    m. stratum
    m. tubule
    m. tuft
    m. vesicle
malposition
malpractice
malpresentation
malrotation
MALT
    mucosa-associated lymphoid tissue
malt
    m. liquor
    m. sugar
Malta fever
maltase
    acid m.
maltese cross
maltobiose
MALToma
maltose
maltotetrose
malt-worker's lung
malum
    m. articulorum senilis
    m. perforans pedis
    m. venereum
malunion
mamanpian
mamelon
mamelonated
mamelonation
mamelonné
    état m.
mamillation
mamillothalamic tract
mamma, pl. **mammae**

m. accessoria
m. erratica
m. masculina
m. virilis
mammal
mammalgia
Mammalia
mammaplasty
augmentation m.
reconstructive m.
reduction m.
mammary
m. adenocarcinoma
m. branch
m. calculus
m. duct
m. duct ectasia
m. fistula
m. fold
m. gland
m. line
m. neuralgia
m. plexus
m. region
m. ridge
m. souffle
mammectomy
mammiform
mammilla
mammillaplasty
mammillare
mammillaria
mammillary
m. artery
m. body
m. duct
m. line
m. process
m. suture
m. tubercle
mammillate
mammillated
mammillation
mammilliform
mammillitis
mammillotegmental fasciculus
mammillothalamic fasciculus
mammogram
mammography
mammoplasty
mammosomatotroph cell adenoma
mammotomy

mammotroph
mammotrophic
mammotrophin
mammotropic
m. factor
m. hormone
mammotropin
managed care
management
airway m.
case m.
component m.
critical incident stress m.
Manchester
M. operation
M. ovoid
manchette
Manchurian
M. hemorrhagic fever
M. typhus
mandatory
m. breath
m. minute ventilation
mandelate
calcium m.
methenamine m.
mandelic acid
Mandelin reagent
mandelytropine
mandible
mandibula, pl. mandibulae
biventer mandibulae
mandibular
m. arch
m. axis
m. canal
m. cartilage
m. condyle
m. dental arcade
m. dentition
m. disc
m. foramen
m. fossa
m. glide
m. guide prosthesis
m. hinge position
m. joint
m. lymph node
m. movement
m. nerve
m. notch
m. process

NOTES

mandibular *(continued)*
    m. protraction
    m. reflex
    m. retraction
    m. symphysis
    m. tongue
    m. torus
mandibularis
    arcus dentalis m.
    torus m.
mandibulectomy
mandibuloacral
    m. dysostosis
    m. dysplasia
mandibulofacial
    m. dysostosis
    m. dysotosis syndrome
    m. dysplasia
mandibulomaxillary fixation
mandibulo-oculofacialis
    dyscephalia m.-o.
mandibulo-oculofacial syndrome
mandibulopharyngeal
mandibulum
mandragora
mandrake
mandrel, mandril
mandrill
mandrin
maneuver
    Adson m.
    Barlow m.
    Bill m.
    Bracht m.
    Brandt-Andrews m.
    Buzzard m.
    Credé m.
    Dix-Hallpike m.
    doll's head m.
    Ejrup m.
    Hampton m.
    Heimlich m.
    Hillis-Müller m.
    Hueter m.
    Jendrassik m.
    key-in-lock m.
    LeCompte m.
    Leopold m.
    load-and-shift m.
    Mauriceau m.
    Mauriceau-Levret m.
    McDonald m.
    McRoberts m.
    Mendelsohn m.
    Müller m.
    Ortolani m.
    Phalen m.
    Pinard m.
    Prague m.

    Ritgen m.
    Scanzoni m.
    Sellick m.
    Toynbee m.
    Valsalva m.
    Zavanelli m.
manganese
manganic
manganous
manganum
mange
    demodectic m.
mango dermatitis
mangrove fly
mania
    acute m.
    periodical m.
maniacal
manic
    m. episode
    m. excitement
    m. psychosis
manic-depressive
    m.-d. disorder
    m.-d. illness
    m.-d. psychosis
manicky
manifest
    m. content
    m. hyperopia
    m. strabismus
    m. tetany
    m. vector
manifestation
    behavioral m.
manifesting
    m. carrier
    m. heterozygote
manikin
maniphalanx
mannan
manna sugar
Mann-Bollman fistula
manner
    aggressive m.
mannerism
mannite
mannitol
Mannkopf sign
Mann methyl blue-eosin stain
mannoheptulose
mannomustine
mannosamine
mannosan
mannose
mannose-binding protein
mannosidase
mannoside
mannosidosis

mannuronic acid
Mann-Williamson
    M.-W. operation
    M.-W. ulcer
man-of-war
    Portuguese m.-o.-w.
manometer
    aneroid m.
    dial m.
    differential m.
    mercurial m.
manometric
manometry
    esophageal m.
manoptoscope
manoscopy
Manson
    M. disease
    M. eye worm
    M. schistosomiasis
mansonelliasis
mansonellosis
mansoni
    Diphyllobothrium m.
    Schistosoma m.
    schistosomiasis m.
mansonoides
    Diphyllobothrium m.
Mantel-Haenszel test
mantle
    brain m.
    m. cell lymphoma
    m. layer
    m. radiotherapy
    m. sclerosis
    m. zone
Mantoux
    M. pit
    M. test
manual
    m. English
    m. lymph drainage
    m. pelvimetry
    m. ventilation
    m. visual method
manubriosternal
    m. joint
    m. junction
    m. symphysis
manubrium, pl. **manubria**
manudynamometer
manus

many-tailed dressing
MAP
    microtubule-associated protein
map
    choroplethic m.
    chromosomal m.
    chromosome m.
    conformational m.
    contig m.
    cytogenetic m.
    m. distance
    fate m.
    genetic m.
    isodemographic m.
    linkage m.
    physical m.
    spot m.
map-dot-fingerprint dystrophy
maple
    m. bark disease
    m. sugar
    m. syrup urine
    m. syrup urine disease
maplike skull
mapping
    cardiac m.
    chromosome m.
    m. function
    gene m.
maprotiline
Marañón sign
marantic
    m. atrophy
    m. edema
    m. endocarditis
    m. thrombosis
    m. thrombus
marasmic
    m. kwashiorkor
    m. thrombosis
    m. thrombus
marasmoid
marasmus
marathon group psychotherapy
marble
    m. bone
    m. bone disease
    m. skin
Marburg
    M. virus
    M. virus disease
Marcacci muscle

M

NOTES

marcescens
    endonuclease *Serratia m.*
march
    m. fracture
    m. hemoglobinuria
Marchand
    M. adrenal
    M. rest
    M. wandering cell
Marchant zone
Marchi
    M. fixative
    M. reaction
    M. stain
    M. tract
Marchiafava-Bignami disease
Marchiafava-Micheli
    M.-M. anemia
    M.-M. syndrome
marcid
Marcille triangle
Marcus
    M. Gunn phenomenon
    M. Gunn pupil
    M. Gunn sign
    M. Gunn syndrome
Marcy operation
Marek disease virus
marenostrin
Marey law
Marfan
    M. disease
    M. law
    M. syndrome
marfanoid
margarine disease
Margaropus winthemi
margin
    acetabular m.
    anterior palpebral m.
    articular m.
    cavity m.
    cervical m.
    ciliary m.
    corneal m.
    costal m.
    falciform m.
    fibular m.
    free m.
    frontal m.
    gingival m.
    incisal m.
    inferior m.
    inferolateral m.
    inferomedial m.
    infraorbital m.
    intercostal m. (ICM)
    interosseous m.
    lacrimal m.
    lambdoid m.
    lateral m.
    left costal m. (LCM)
    mastoid m.
    medial m.
    orbital m.
    right costal m. (RCM)
    m. of safety
    supraorbital m.
marginal
    m. abscess
    m. arcade
    m. artery
    m. atrial branch
    m. blepharitis
    m. crest
    m. fasciculus
    m. gingivitis
    m. gyrus
    m. integrity of amalgam
    m. keratitis
    m. layer
    m. mandibular branch
    m. ray
    m. ridge
    m. ring ulcer
    m. sinus
    m. sphincter
    m. sulcus
    m. tentorial branch
    m. tubercle
    m. zone
    m. zone lymphoma
marginalis
    alopecia m.
    keratoelastoidosis m.
marginata
    placenta m.
margination
marginatum
    eczema m.
    erythema m.
marginatus
    Dermacentor m.
marginoplasty
marian lithotomy
Marie ataxia
Marie-Robinson syndrome
Marie-Strümpell disease
marijuana
marine
    m. pharmacology
    m. soap
Marine-Lenhart syndrome
Marinesco-Garland syndrome
Marinesco-Sjögren syndrome
Marinesco succulent hand
marinobufotoxin

marinum
  Mycobacterium m.
Marion disease
Mariotte
  M. blind spot
  M. bottle
  M. experiment
  M. law
mariposia
marital
  m. counseling
  m. therapy
Marjolin ulcer
mark
  alignment m.
  port-wine m.
  strawberry m.
marked
  m. fetal bradycardia
  m. rhonchi
marker
  allotypic m.
  cell surface m.
  m. chromosome
  DNA m.
  m. enzyme
  genetic m.
  linkage m.
  m. locus
  oncofetal m.
  polymorphic genetic m.
  m. trait
  tumor m.
  m. X syndrome
marking
  lung m.
Markov process
Marme reagent
marmorata
  cutis m.
marmorated
marmoset virus
marmot
Maroteaux-Lamy syndrome
Marquis reagent
marriage therapy
marrow
  bone m.
  m. canal
  m. cell
  gelatinous bone m.
marrow-lymph gland

marrow-mesenchyme connection
Marseilles fever
marsh
  m. fever
  m. gas
Marshall
  M. method
  M. oblique vein
  M. syndrome
  M. test
  M. vestigial fold
Marshallagia marshalli
marshalli
  Marshallagia m.
Marshall-Marchetti-Krantz operation
Marshall-Marchetti test
marshmallow root
marsupialization
marsupial notch
marsupium
Martegiani
  M. area
  M. funnel
Martin
  M. bandage
  M. disease
  M. tube
Martin-Bell syndrome
Martin-Gruber anastomosis
Martinotti cell
martius yellow
Martorell syndrome
Maryland coma scale
masculina
  mamma m.
masculine
  m. pelvis
  m. protest
  m. uterus
masculinity
masculinity-femininity scale
masculinization
masculinize
masculinus
mask
  BLB m.
  ecchymotic m.
  entrainment m.
  Hutchinson m.
  laryngeal m.
  luetic m.
  partial rebreathing m.

M

NOTES

mask *(continued)*
    m. of pregnancy
    tracheostomy m.
masked
    m. epilepsy
    m. gout
    m. hyperthyroidism
    m. hysteria
    m. virus
masking
    m. dilemma
    m. level difference
masklike face
Maslow hierarchy
masochism
masochist
masochistic personality
Mason-Pfizer virus
mason's lung
MASS
    mitral valve prolapse, aortic anomalies, skeletal and skin changes
    MASS syndrome
mass
    m. action principle
    m. action theory
    apperceptive m.
    discrete m.
    fat-free body m.
    filar m.
    m. hysteria
    m. infection
    injection m.
    inner cell m.
    intermediate m.
    m. law
    lean body m.
    molar m.
    molecular m.
    m. movement
    m. number
    m. peristalsis
    m. radiography
    m. reflex
    relative molecular m.
    sclerotic cemental m.
    m. screening
    m. sociogenic illness
    m. spectrograph
mass-action ratio
massage
    cardiac m.
    carotid sinus m.
    closed chest m.
    deep tissue m.
    external cardiac m.
    gingival m.
    heart m.
    on-site m.
    open chest m.
    prostatic m.
    seated m.
    sports m.
    Swedish m.
    m. therapy
Masselon spectacles
masseter
    m. muscle
    m. reflex
masseteric
    m. artery
    m. fascia
    m. nerve
    m. tuberosity
    m. vein
masseur
masseuse
massicot
massive
    m. bowel resection syndrome
    m. collapse
Masson
    M. argentaffin stain
    M. trichrome stain
Masson-Fontana ammoniac silver stain
massotherapy
MAST
    military antishock trousers
mast
    m. cell
    m. cell leukemia
    m. leukocyte
mastadenitis
mastadenoma
Mastadenovirus
mastalgia
mastatrophia
mastatrophy
mastauxe
mastectomy
    extended radical m.
    modified radical m.
    radical m.
    simple m.
    subcutaneous m.
master
    m. cast
    m. eye
    m. gland
    m. patient index
    M. 2-step exercise test
mastery motive
masticate
masticating
    m. cycle
    m. surface
mastication
    force of m.

masticator
>m. nerve
>m. space

masticatory
>m. apparatus
>m. diplegia
>m. force
>m. muscle
>m. nucleus
>m. silent period
>m. spasm
>m. surface
>m. system

mastigote

mastitis
>chronic cystic m.
>cystic m.
>gargantuan m.
>glandular m.
>granulomatous m.
>interstitial m.
>lactational m.
>m. neonatorum
>plasma cell m.
>stagnation m.
>submammary m.
>suppurative m.

mastoccipital

mastocyte

mastocytogenesis

mastocytoma

mastocytosis
>diffuse cutaneous m.

mastodynia

mastoid
>m. abscess
>m. air cell
>m. angle
>m. antrum
>m. artery
>m. bone
>m. border
>m. branch
>m. canaliculus
>m. cortex
>m. emissary vein
>m. empyema
>m. fontanelle
>m. foramen
>m. fossa
>m. groove
>m. incision

>m. lymph node
>m. margin
>m. notch
>m. process
>m. sinus
>m. wall

mastoidal

mastoidectomy
>combined approach m.
>complete m.
>conservative m.
>cortical m.
>modified radical m.
>radical m.
>simple m.

mastoideum
>tegmen m.

mastoiditis

mastoncus

mastooccipital

mastoparietal

mastopathy

mastopexy

mastoplasia

mastoplasty

mastoptosis

mastorrhagia

mastosquamous

mastosyrinx

mastotomy

masturbate

masturbation

MAT
>multifocal atrial tachycardia

mat
>m. burn
>m. gold

match
>color m.

matched groups

matching
>afterload m.
>impedance m.

mater
>arachnoid m.
>arachnoidea m.
>cranial arachnoid m.
>cranial dura m.
>cranial pia m.
>dura m.
>spinal arachnoid m.
>spinal pia m.

M

NOTES

materia
    m. alba
    m. medica
material
    base m.
    by-product m.
    certified reference m.
    coarse m.
    contrast m.
    cross-reacting m. (CRM)
    dental m.
    genetic m.
    impression m.
maternal
    m. cotyledon
    m. death
    m. death rate
    m. deprivation syndrome
    m. dystocia
    m. immunity
    m. inheritance
    m. morbidity
    m. mortality ratio
    m. placenta
maternal-fetal medicine
maternity hospital
mathematical
    m. chaos
    m. determinant
    m. genetics
    m. model
mating
    assortative m.
    cross m.
    m. isolate
    random m.
matrass
matrical
matricaria
matricial
matricide
matrilineal
matrix
    amalgam m.
    m. band
    bone m.
    m. calculus
    cartilage m.
    cell m.
    cytoplasmic m.
    external m.
    m. Gla protein
    identity m.
    m. metalloproteinase
    mitochondrial m.
    m. mitochondrialis
    m. retainer
    territorial m.

    m. unguis
    m. vesicle
matruchotii
    Corynebacterium m.
matter
    gray m.
    white m.
mattress suture
maturate
maturation
    m. arrest
    m. factor
    m. index
    m. value
mature
    m. bacteriophage
    m. cataract
    m. cell leukemia
    m. neutrophil
    m. ovarian follicle
    m. teratoma
maturity-onset diabetes
matutinal epilepsy
Mauchart ligament
Maurer
    M. cleft
    M. dot
Mauriac syndrome
Mauriceau-Levret maneuver
Mauriceau maneuver
Mauthner sheath
maxilla
maxillaris
    arcus dentalis m.
    hiatus m.
maxillary
    m. advancement
    m. angle
    m. antrum
    m. artery
    m. dental arcade
    m. dentition
    m. eminence
    m. gland
    m. hiatus
    m. nerve
    m. plexus
    m. process
    m. protraction
    m. sinus
    m. sinus mucocele
    m. sinus radiograph
    m. surface
    m. tuberosity
    m. vein
maxillectomy
maxillitis
maxillodental

maxillofacial
    m. prosthesis
    m. prosthetic
maxillojugal
maxillomandibular
    m. disharmony
    m. fixation
    m. record
    m. registration
    m. relation
    m. traction
maxillopalatine
maxillotomy
maxilloturbinal
maximal
    m. Histalog test
    m. oxygen consumption
    m. oxygen uptake
    m. permissible dose
    m. stimulus
    m. thymectomy
Maxim-Gilbert sequencing
Maximow stain
maximum
    m. breathing capacity (MBC)
    m. expiratory flow rate (MEFR)
    m. expiratory flow volume (MEFV)
    m. expiratory pressure
    glucose transport m.
    m. hospital benefit
    m. inspiratory pressure
    m. intensity projection (MIP)
    m. likelihood estimator
    m. medical benefit
    m. occipital point
    m. permissible dose
    m. power output
    repetition m.
    m. temperature
    m. tolerated dose
    transport m.
    m. urea clearance
    m. velocity
    m. voluntary ventilation
May
    M. apple
    M. apple root
Mayaro virus
Maydl hernia
Mayer
    M. hemalum stain
    M. mucicarmine stain
    M. mucihematein stain
    M. pessary
    M. reflex
Mayer-Rokitansky-Küster-Hauser syndrome
May-Grünwald stain
May-Hegglin anomaly
mayidism
Mayo
    M. bunionectomy
    M. operation
    M. stand
    M. vein
Mayo-Robson
    M.-R. point
    M.-R. position
May-White syndrome
mazamorra
Mazzoni corpuscle
Mazzotti
    M. reaction
    M. test
MBC
    maximum breathing capacity
Mc antigen
McArdle
    M. disease
    M. syndrome
McArdle-Schmid-Pearson disease
McArthur operation
McBurney
    M. incision
    M. operation
    M. point
    M. sign
McCall culdoplasty procedure
McCarey-Kaufmann media
McCarthy reflex
McCrea sound
McCune-Albright syndrome
McDonald maneuver
McGoon technique
MCH
    mean corpuscular hemoglobin
MCHC
    mean corpuscular hemoglobin concentration
mCi
    millicurie
McIndoe operation
McKee line

M

NOTES

McKusick metaphysial dysplasia
MCL
    midclavicular line
McMurray test
McNemar test
McPhail test
MCR
    metabolic clearance rate
McRoberts maneuver
M-CSF
    macrophage colony-stimulating factor
MCV
    mean corpuscular volume
McVay operation
MDF
    myocardial depressant factor
MDNCF
    monocyte-derived neutrophil chemotactic factor
M:E
    myeloid-erythrocyte
    M:E ratio
meadow grass dermatitis
Meadows syndrome
meal
    barium m.
    Boyden m.
    Lundh m.
    test m.
    m. worm
mean
    arithmetic m.
    m. calorie
    m. corpuscular hemoglobin (MCH)
    m. corpuscular hemoglobin concentration (MCHC)
    m. corpuscular volume (MCV)
    m. electrical axis
    m. foundation plane
    geometric m.
    harmonic m.
    m. manifest vector
    m. pulmonary arterial pressure
    m. temperature
measles
    atypical m.
    black m.
    m. convalescent serum
    3-day m.
    German m.
    hemorrhagic m.
    m. immune globulin human
    m. immunoglobulin
    m., mumps, and rubella (MMR)
    m., mumps, and rubella vaccine
    m. virus
    m. virus vaccine
measly

measure
    Geneva lens m.
measured intelligence
measurement
    end-point m.
    kinetic m.
    skinfold m.
meatal
    m. cartilage
    m. incision
    m. spine
meatometer
meatoplasty
meatorrhaphy
meatoscope
meatoscopy
meatotome
meatotomy
meatus
    acoustic m.
    m. acusticus externus
    auditory m.
    external acoustic m.
    external auditory m.
    external urinary m.
    fishmouth m.
    internal acoustic m.
    internal auditory m.
    nasal m.
    m. nasi
    m. nasopharyngeus
    m. urinarius
    urinary m.
mebanazine
mebendazole
Mecca balsam
mechanical
    m. antidote
    m. corepraxy
    m. dysmenorrhea
    m. efficiency
    m. heart
    m. ileus
    m. intelligence
    m. jaundice
    m. strabismus
    m. vector
    m. ventilation
    m. vertigo
mechanically balanced occlusion
mechanicoreceptor
mechanics
    body m.
mechanism
    association m.
    countercurrent m.
    defense m.
    double displacement m.
    Douglas m.

Duncan m.
feedback m.
gating m.
immunologic m.
immunological m.
pinchcock m.
proprioceptive m.
reentrant m.
Schultze m.
speech m.
mechanism-based inhibitor
mechanistic school
mechanobullous disease
mechanocardiography
mechanocyte
mechanoelectric transduction
mechanophobia
mechanoreceptor
mechanoreflex
mechanotherapy
mèche
mecism
Meckel
    M. band
    M. cartilage
    M. cavity
    M. diverticulum
    M. ganglion
    M. ligament
    M. plane
    M. scan
    M. space
    M. syndrome
Meckel-Gruber syndrome
Mecke reagent
meclastine
meclofenoxate
mecometer
meconate
meconial colic
meconic acid
meconin
meconiorrhea
meconium
    m. aspiration
    m. aspiration syndrome
    m. blockage syndrome
    m. ileus
    m. peritonitis
    m. plug
media (*pl. of* medium)
mediad

medial
    m. accessory olivary nucleus
    m. amygdaloid nucleus
    m. angle
    m. antebrachial cutaneous nerve
    m. anterior thoracic nerve
    m. arcuate ligament
    m. arteriole
    m. arteriosclerosis
    m. atrial vein
    m. basal branch
    m. basal bronchopulmonary segment
    m. basal segmental artery
    m. bicipital groove
    m. border
    m. brachial cutaneous nerve
    m. bronchopulmonary segment
    m. calcaneal branch
    m. canthal ligament
    m. canthic fold
    m. canthus
    m. cartilaginous plate
    m. central nucleus
    m. cerebral surface
    m. circumflex femoral artery
    m. circumflex femoral vein
    m. clunial nerve
    m. collateral artery
    m. collateral ligament
    m. commisural artery
    m. compartment
    m. condyle
    m. cord
    m. crural cutaneous branch
    m. crural cutaneous nerve
    m. crus
    m. cuneiform bone
    m. dorsal cutaneous nerve
    m. dorsal nucleus
    m. eminence
    m. epicondylar crest
    m. epicondylar ridge
    m. epicondyle
    m. epicondylitis
    m. femoral circumflex artery
    m. femoral tuberosity
    m. fillet
    m. forebrain bundle
    m. frontal gyrus
    m. frontobasal artery
    m. geniculate body
    m. geniculate nucleus

NOTES

M

medial (*continued*)

m. great muscle
m. habenular nucleus
m. head
m. inferior genicular artery
m. inguinal fossa
m. lacunar lymph node
m. lemniscus
m. limb
m. lip
m. longitudinal arch
m. longitudinal bundle
m. longitudinal fasciculus
m. longitudinal stria
m. lumbar intertransversarii muscle
m. lumbar intertransverse muscle
m. lumbocostal arch
m. magnocellular nucleus
m. malleolar artery
m. malleolar branch
m. malleolar facet
m. malleolar network
m. malleolar subcutaneous bursa
m. malleolus
m. mammary branch
m. margin
m. medullary branch
m. medullary lamina
m. meniscectomy
m. meniscus
m. midpalmar space
m. nasal branch
m. nasal fold
m. nasal process
m. nasal prominence
m. occipital artery
m. occipitotemporal gyrus
m. olfactory gyrus
m. orbitofrontal artery
m. palpebral commissure
m. palpebral ligament
m. parabrachial nucleus
m. patellar retinaculum
m. pectoral nerve
m. pericuneate nucleus
m. plantar artery
m. plantar nerve
m. pole
m. popliteal nerve
m. posterior cervical
  intertransversarii muscle
m. preoptic nucleus
m. pterygoid muscle
m. pterygoid plate
m. puboprostatic ligament
m. rectus muscle
m. reticulospinal tract
m. root
m. rotator

m. segmental artery
m. septal nucleus
m. striate artery
m. sulcus
m. superior genicular artery
m. superior olivary nucleus
m. supraclavicular nerve
m. supracondylar crest
m. supracondylar ridge
m. supraepicondylar ridge
m. sural cutaneous nerve
m. talocalcaneal ligament
m. tarsal artery
m. tubercle
m. umbilical fold
m. umbilical ligament
m. vastus muscle
m. ventral nucleus
m. venule
m. vestibular nucleus
m. vestibulospinal tract
m. wall
m. zone

medialis

malleolus m.
meniscus m.

medialization

median

m. antebrachial vein
m. anterior maxillary cyst
m. aperture
m. arcuate ligament
m. artery
m. atlantoaxial joint
m. bar
m. basilic vein
m. callosal artery
m. cephalic vein
m. commissural artery
m. conjugate
m. cricothyroid ligament
m. cubital vein
m. effective dose
m. eminence
m. glossoepiglottic fold
m. groove
m. incision
m. laryngotomy
m. line
m. lithotomy
m. longitudinal raphe
m. mandibular point
m. maxillary anterior alveolar cleft
m. nerve
m. palatal cyst
m. palatine suture
m. plane
m. preoptic nucleus
m. raphe cyst

m. retruded relation
m. rhinoscopy
m. rhomboid glossitis
m. sacral artery
m. sacral crest
m. sacral vein
m. section
m. sternotomy
m. sulcus
m. thyrohyoid ligament
m. tongue bud
m. umbilical fold
m. umbilical ligament

mediana
arteria m.

mediastinal
m. abscess
m. artery
m. branch
m. crunch
m. emphysema
m. fibrosis
m. lipomatosis
m. pleura
m. pleurisy
m. space
m. surface
m. vein
m. window

mediastinitis
fibrosing m.
fibrous m.
idiopathic fibrous m.

mediastinography
gaseous m.

mediastinopericarditis
mediastinoscope
mediastinoscopy
anterior m.
extended m.

mediastinotomy
anterior m.

mediastinum
anterior m.
m. anterius
inferior m.
m. inferius
m. medium
middle m.
posterior m.
superior m.

m. superius
m. testis

mediate
m. auscultation
m. percussion
m. transfusion

mediation
mediator complex
medica
materia m.

medicable
medical
m. anatomy
m. assistant
m. biophysics
m. care
m. corps
m. diathermy
m. director
m. ethics
m. examiner
m. genetics
m. jurisprudence
m. model
m. mycology
m. pathology
m. psychology
m. record
m. record linkage
m. selection
m. transcriptionist
m. treatment

medicament
medicamentosa
acne m.
alopecia m.
dermatitis m.
dermatosis m.
stomatitis m.
urticaria m.

medicamentosus
Cushing syndrome m.

medicate
medication
ionic m.
maintenance m.

medicator
medicephalic
medicinal
m. charcoal
m. chemistry
m. eruption

M

NOTES

medicinal *(continued)*
    m. scarlet red
    m. soft soap
    m. zinc peroxide
medicine
    adolescent m.
    aerospace m.
    alternative m.
    aviation m.
    behavioral m.
    clinical m.
    complementary m.
    defensive m.
    desmoteric m.
    electrodiagnostic m.
    evidence-based m.
    experimental m.
    family m.
    fetal m.
    folk m.
    forensic m.
    geriatric m.
    holistic m.
    hyperbaric m.
    internal m.
    legal m.
    maternal-fetal m.
    military m.
    neonatal m.
    nuclear m.
    occupational m.
    osteopathic m.
    patent m.
    perinatal m.
    physical m.
    podiatric m.
    preventive m.
    proprietary m.
    psychosomatic m.
    rehabilitation m.
    socialized m.
    sports m.
    tropical m.
medicobiologic
medicobiological
medicochirurgical
medicolegal
medicomechanical
medicophysical
medicopsychology
Medicus
    Cumulative Index M.
medinensis
    Dracunculus m.
mediocarpal
medioccipital
mediocolic sphincter
mediodens
mediodorsal nucleus

mediolateral
medionecrosis
mediopubic reflex
mediotarsal amputation
mediotrusion
mediotype
medisect
Mediterranean
    M. erythematous fever
    M. exanthematous fever
    M. lymphoma
    M. spotted fever
mediterranei
    Nocardia m.
medium, pl. **media**
    Acanthamoeba m.
    active m.
    aerotitis media
    m. artery
    auris media
    Balamuth aqueous egg yolk
      infusion m.
    barotitis media
    bilateral otitis media (BOM)
    Boeck and Drbohlav Locke-egg-
      serum m.
    clearing m.
    complete m.
    contrast m.
    culture m.
    Czapek-Dox m.
    dispersion m.
    Dorset culture egg m.
    Eagle basal m.
    Eagle minimum essential m.
    Endo m.
    external m.
    growth m.
    high osmolar contrast m. (HOCM)
    Lash casein hydrolysate-serum m.
    Loeffler blood culture m.
    Lowenstein-Jensen culture m.
    low osmolar contrast m. (LOCM)
    McCarey-Kaufmann media
    mediastinum m.
    mounting m.
    Mueller-Hinton m.
    nutrient m.
    otitis media
    reflux otitis media
    secretory otitis media
    serous otitis media
    Simmons citrate m.
    transport m.
    tunica media
    m. vein
medium-chain
    m.-c. acyl-CoA dehydrogenase

m.-c. acyl-CoA dehydrogenase
deficiency
medius
medphalan
medrogestone
medroxyprogesterone acetate
medrylamine
medrysone
medulla, pl. **medullae**
m. oblongata
renal m.
m. renalis
m. spinalis
suprarenal m.
medullar
medullare
osteoma m.
medullaris
conus m.
substantia m.
medullary
m. callus
m. carcinoma
m. cavity
m. center
m. chemoreceptor
m. cone
m. cord
m. fold
m. groove
m. lamina
m. layer
m. membrane
m. plate
m. pyramid
m. pyramidotomy
m. ray
m. reticulospinal tract
m. sarcoma
m. sheath
m. space
m. spinal artery
m. sponge kidney
m. stria
m. substance
m. teniae
m. tube
medullated nerve fiber
medullation
medullectomy
medullization
medulloarthritis

medulloblastoma
desmoplastic m.
melanotic m.
medullocell
medulloepithelioma
adult m.
embryonal m.
medullomyoblastoma
medullopontine sulcus
medusae
caput m.
Medusa head
Meeh-Dubois formula
Meeh formula
Mees
M. line
M. stripe
Meesman dystrophy
mefenamic acid
mefexamide
mefloquine
MEFR
maximum expiratory flow rate
MEFV
maximum expiratory flow volume
megabacterium
megabladder
megacalycosis
megacardia
megacaryoblast
megacaryocyte
megacephalia
megacephalic
megacephalous
megacephaly
megacin
megacoccus
megacolon
acquired m.
congenital m.
m. congenitum
idiopathic m.
toxic m.
megacycle
megacystic syndrome
megacystis
megacystitis-megaureter syndrome
megacystitis-microcolon-intestinal
hypoperistalsis syndrome
megadactylia
megadactylism
megadactyly

M

NOTES

587

megadolichocolon
megadont
megadontism
megadyne
megaesophagus
megagamete
megagnathia
megahertz (MHz)
megakaryoblast
megakaryocyte
megakaryocytic leukemia
megalecithal
megalgia
megaloblast
megaloblastic anemia
megalocardia
megalocephaly, megalocephalia
megalocheiria, megalochiria
megalocornea
megalocystis
megalocyte
megalocythemia
megalocytic anemia
megalocytosis
megalodactylia, megalodactylism,
    megalodactyly
megalodont
megalodontia
megaloencephalic
megaloencephalon
megaloencephaly
megaloenteron
megalogastria
megaloglossia
megalographia
megalohepatia
megalokaryocyte
megalomania
megalomaniac
megalomelia
megalophthalmos
    anterior m.
megalopodia
megalosplanchnic
megalosplenia
megalospore
megalosyndactyly, megalosyndactylia
megaloureter
megalourethra
megamerozoite
meganucleus
megapoietin
megaprosopia
megaprosopous
megarectum
megaseme
megasigmoid
megasomia
megaspore

megathrombocyte
megaureter
megavolt
megavoltage
megestrol acetate
meglitinide
meglumine
    iodoxamate m.
megohm
megophthalmus
megoxycyte
megoxyphil
megoxyphile
meibomian
    m. blepharitis
    m. cyst
    m. gland
    m. sty
meibomianitis
meibomianum
    hordeolum m.
meibomitis
Meige disease
Meigs syndrome
Meinicke test
meiosis
meiotic
    m. division
    m. drive
    m. phase
Meischer syndrome
Meissner
    M. corpuscle
    M. plexus
melagra
melalgia
melamine
    m. formaldehyde
    m. resin
melancholia
    agitated m.
    hypochondriacal m.
    involutional m.
    stuporous m.
melancholic
melancholy
melanedema
melanemia
melaniferous
melanimon
    Aedes m.
melanin
    artificial m.
    factitious m.
melaninogenica
    Prevotella m.
melaninogenicus
    Bacteroides m.
melanism

melanoacanthoma
melanoameloblastoma
melanoblast
melanocyte
melanocyte-stimulating hormone
melanocytoma
melanodendrocyte
melanoderma
 parasitic m.
 senile m.
melanodermatitis
melanodermic
melanogen
melanogenemia
melanogenesis
melanoglossia
melanoid
melanokeratosis
melanoleukoderma colli
melanoliberin
melanoma
 acral lentiginous m.
 amelanotic m.
 benign juvenile m.
 Cloudman m.
 desmoplastic malignant m.
 Harding-Passey m.
 malignant lentigo m.
 minimal deviation m.
 subungual m.
melanomatosis
melanonychia
melanopathy
melanophage
melanophore
melanophore-expanding principle
melanoplakia
melanoprotein
melanorrhagia
melanorrhea
melanosis
 m. coli
 Riehl m.
melanosome
 giant m.
melanostatin
melanotic
 m. carcinoma
 m. freckle
 m. medulloblastoma
 m. neuroectodermal tumor

 m. pigment
 m. progonoma
melanotonin
melanotrichous
melanotroph
melanotropin, melanotrophin
 m. release-inhibiting hormone
 (MIH)
melanotropin-releasing
 m.-r. factor
 m.-r. hormone
melanuria
melanuric
melarsoprol
melas
 icterus m.
melasma
 m. gravidarum
 m. universale
melatonin
Meleda
 mal de M.
melena
 m. neonatorum
 m. spuria
 m. vera
melenemesis
Meleney
 M. gangrene
 M. ulcer
melengestrol acetate
meletin
melibiase
melibiose
melicera
meliceris
melioidosis
melissic acid
melissophobia
melitensis
 Brucella m.
melitis
melitose
melitriose
melittin
Melkersson-Rosenthal syndrome
mellitum, pl. **melliti**
mellitus
 diabetes m. (DM)
 insulin-dependent diabetes m.
 (IDDM)

M

NOTES

mellitus *(continued)*
    non-insulin-dependent diabetes m.
      (NIDDM)
Melnick-Needles
    M.-N. osteodysplasty
    M.-N. syndrome
melodidymus
melomania
melomelia
melon-seed body
meloplasty
melorheostosis
meloschisis
melotia
melphalan
melting
    m. point
    m. temperature
Meltzer law
Meltzer-Lyon test
member
    inferior m.
membra (*pl. of* membrum)
membrana, pl. **membranae**
    m. adventitia
    m. decidua
    m. serosa
    m. vitellina
membranacea
    placenta m.
membrane
    adamantine m.
    allantoid m.
    alveolar-capillary m.
    alveolocapillary m.
    alveolodental m.
    anal m.
    anterior atlantooccipital m.
    arachnoid m.
    atlantooccipital m.
    m. attack complex
    Barkan m.
    basement m.
    basilar m.
    Bichat m.
    Bogros serous m.
    m. bone
    Bowman m.
    Bruch m.
    Brunn m.
    bucconasal m.
    buccopharyngeal m.
    cell m.
    chorioallantoic m.
    choroid m.
    cloacal m.
    closing m.
    Corti m.
    cricothyroid m.

cricotracheal m.
cricovocal m.
croupous m.
deciduous m.
Descemet m.
diphtheritic m.
double m.
drum m.
Duddell m.
dysmenorrheal m.
egg m.
elastic m.
embryonic m.
enamel m.
m. enzyme
epipapillary m.
epiretinal m.
exocelomic m.
m. expansion theory
external intercostal m.
extraembryonic m.
false m.
fenestrated m.
fertilization m.
fetal m.
fibrous m.
Fielding m.
flaccid m.
germ m.
germinal m.
glassy m.
glial limiting m.
Henle fenestrated elastic m.
Heuser m.
Hunter m.
Huxley m.
hyaline m.
hyaloid m.
hymenal m.
hyoglossal m.
inner m.
intercostal m.
internal intercostal m.
interosseous m.
ivory m.
Jackson m.
keratogenous m.
limiting m.
medullary m.
mitochondrial m.
mucous m.
Nitabuch m.
nuclear m.
olfactory m.
ovular m.
peridental m.
periodontal m.
placental m.
plasma m.

postsynaptic m.
m. potential
presynaptic m.
pupillary m.
Reissner m.
reticular m.
round window m.
m. rupture
Ruysch m.
secondary tympanic m.
serous m.
m. stripping
synovial m.
tectorial m.
Toldt m.
tympanic m.
undulating m.
undulatory m.
unit m.
vestibular m.
vitreous m.
Wachendorf m.
yolk m.
membrane-coating granule
membranectomy
membranelle
membraniform
membranocartilaginous
membranoid
membranoproliferative glomerulonephritis
membranous
m. adhesion
m. ampulla
m. cataract
m. cochlea
m. conjunctivitis
m. dysmenorrhea
m. glomerulonephritis
m. labyrinth
m. labyrinthectomy
m. lamina
m. laryngitis
m. layer
m. lipodystrophy
m. neurocranium
m. ossification
m. pharyngitis
m. rhinitis
m. septum
m. urethra

m. viscerocranium
m. wall
membrum, pl. **membra**
memory
affect m.
anterograde m.
m. B, T cell
long-term m.
m. loop
Ribot law of m.
screen m.
short-term m.
m. span
visual m.
MEN
multiple endocrine neoplasia
MEN1
multiple endocrine neoplasia, type 1
MEN2A
multiple endocrine neoplasia, type 2A
menacme
Menangle virus
menaphthone
menaquinone
menarche
menarcheal
menarchial
Mendel
M. first law
M. instep reflex
M. second law
Mendel-Bechterew reflex
Mendeléeff law
mendelevium
mendelian
m. character
m. genetics
m. inheritance
m. ratio
m. trait
mendelism
mendelizing
Mendelsohn maneuver
Ménétrier
M. disease
M. syndrome
Menge pessary
Mengo
M. encephalitis
M. virus

M

NOTES

Ménière
    M. disease
    M. syndrome
meningeal
    m. branch
    m. carcinoma
    m. carcinomatosis
    m. headache
    m. hernia
    m. layer
    m. leukemia
    m. neurosyphilis
    m. plexus
    m. vein
meningeocortical
meningeorrhaphy
meninges (*pl. of* meninx)
meningioangiomatosis
meningioma
    cutaneous m.
    fibrous m.
    malignant m.
    mesodermal m.
    psammomatous m.
meningiomatosis
meningis
meningisepticum
    Flavobacterium m.
meningism
meningitic streak
meningitidis
    Neisseria m.
meningitis
    basilar m.
    cerebrospinal m.
    eosinophilic m.
    epidemic cerebrospinal m.
    epidural m.
    external m.
    internal m.
    listeria m.
    meningococcal m.
    Mollaret m.
    occlusive m.
    otitic m.
    serous m.
    suppurative m.
    tuberculous m.
    typhoid m.
meningocele
meningococcal meningitis
meningococcemia
    acute fulminating m.
meningococcus
meningocortical
meningocyte
meningoencephalitis
    acute primary hemorrhagic m.
    biundulant m.

    eosinophilic m.
    herpetic m.
meningoencephalocele
meningoencephalomyelitis
meningoencephalopathy
meningomyelitis
meningomyelocele
meningo-osteophlebitis
meningoradicular
meningoradiculitis
meningorrhachidian
meningorrhagia
meningosis
meningotyphoid fever
meningovascular
    m. neurosyphilis
    m. syphilis
meninguria
meninx, pl. **meninges**
    m. fibrosa
    m. primitiva
    m. tenuis
    m. vasculosa
meniscectomy
    medial m.
menisci (*pl. of* meniscus)
meniscitis
meniscocyte
meniscofemoral ligament
meniscopexy
meniscorrhaphy
meniscotome
meniscus, pl. **menisci**
    articular m.
    m. articularis
    converging m.
    diverging m.
    lateral m.
    m. lateralis
    m. lens
    medial m.
    m. medialis
    m. sign
    tactile m.
    m. tactus
Menkes syndrome
menocelis
menometrorrhagia
menopausal syndrome
menopause
    premature m.
menophania
menorrhagia
menorrhalgia
menoschesis
menostaxis
menotropins
menouria
menoxenia

menses
menstrual
    m. age
    m. colic
    m. cycle
    m. dermatosis
    m. edema
    m. extraction abortion
    m. leukorrhea
    m. migraine
    m. molimina
    m. period
    m. sclerosis
menstrualis
    decidua m.
menstruant
menstruate
menstruation
    anovular m.
    anovulational m.
    retained m.
    retrograde m.
    vicarious m.
menstruum
mensual
mensuration
mental
    m. aberration
    m. age
    m. apparatus
    m. artery
    m. blind spot
    m. branch
    m. canal
    m. chronometry
    m. deficiency
    m. disease
    m. disorder
    m. disturbance
    m. foramen
    m. health
    m. hospital
    m. hygiene
    m. illness
    m. image
    m. impairment
    m. impression
    m. nerve
    m. point
    m. process
    m. protuberance
    m. region

    m. retardation
    m. scotoma
    m. spine
    m. status
    m. symphysis
    m. tubercle
mentalis muscle
mentality
mentation
menthane
menthol
    camphorated m.
menthyl salicylate
menti (*pl. of* mentum)
mentis
    compos m.
mentoanterior
    m. fetal position
    left m. (LMA)
mentolabial
    m. furrow
    m. sulcus
mentolabialis
menton
mentoplasty
mentoposterior
    left m. (LMP)
    m. position
mentotransverse
    m. fetal position
    left m. (LMT)
mentum, pl. **menti**
menyanthes
mephenesin
mephenytoin
mephitic
mephobarbital
meprobamate
meptazinol
mepyramine maleate
mepyrapone
mEq, meq
    milliequivalent
mer
    mal de m.
meralgia paresthetica
meralluride
merbromin
mercaptal
mercaptan
    methyl m.
mercaptoacetic acid

NOTES

M

mercaptoethanol
mercaptol
mercaptolactate-cysteine disulfiduria
mercaptomerin sodium
mercapturic
   m. acid
   m. acid pathway
Mercier
   M. bar
   M. sound
   M. valve
mercocresol
mercumatilin
mercuramide
mercurial
   m. diuretic
   m. line
   m. manometer
   m. necrosis
   m. stomatitis
mercurialentis
mercurialism
mercuric salicylate
mercurochrome
mercurophen
mercurophylline sodium
mercurous
   m. chloride
   m. iodide
mercury
   ammoniated m.
   m. arc
   m. bichloride
   m. biniodide
   m. deutoiodide
   m. perchloride
   m. poisoning
   m. protoiodide
   m. subsalicylate
   m. vapor lamp
Merendino technique
Meretoja syndrome
meridian
meridional
   m. aberration
   m. amblyopia
   m. cleavage
   m. fiber
merispore
meristematic
meristic
Merkel
   M. cell tumor
   M. corpuscle
   M. filtrum ventriculi
   M. fossa
   M. muscle
   M. tactile cell
   M. tactile disc

mermaid malformation
meroacrania
meroanencephaly
meroblastic cleavage
merocrine gland
merodiastolic
merogastrula
merogenesis
merogenetic
merogenic
merogony
meromelia
meromicrosomia
meromyosin
meront
merorachischisis
merorrhachischisis
merosmia
merosporangium
merosystolic
merotomy
merozoite
merozygote
merphalan
Merrifield
   M. knife
   M. synthesis
mersalyl theophylline
Méry gland
Merzbacher-Pelizaeus disease
mesad
mesal
mesameboid
mesangial
   m. cell
   m. nephritis
   m. proliferative glomerulonephritis
mesangiocapillary glomerulonephritis
mesangium
   extraglomerular m.
mesaortitis
mesareic, mesaraic
mesarteritis
mesaticephalic
mesatipellic pelvis
mesatipelvic
mesaxon
mescal button
mescaline
mesectoderm
mesencephalic
   m. corticonuclear fiber
   m. flexure
   m. nucleus
   m. tegmentum
   m. tract
   m. vein
mesencephalitis
mesencephalon

mesencephalotomy
mesenchyma
mesenchymal
    m. cell
    m. epithelium
    m. tissue
mesenchyme
    interzonal m.
mesenchymoma
mesenteric
    m. adenitis
    m. artery occlusion
    m. gland
    m. hernia
    m. lymphadenitis
    m. lymph node
    m. portion
    m. thrombosis
    m. vein
mesenterica
    tabes m.
mesentericoparietal
    m. fossa
    m. recess
mesenteriopexy
mesenteriorrhaphy
mesenteriplication
mesenteritis
mesenterium
mesenteroaxial volvulus
mesenteron
mesentery
mesethmoid bone
mesh graft
meshwork
    trabecular m.
mesiad
mesial
    m. angle
    m. caries
    m. displacement
    m. occlusion
    m. surface
mesiobuccal
mesiobucco-occlusal
mesiobuccopulpal
mesiocervical
mesioclusion
mesiodens
mesiodistal
mesiodistocclusal (MOD)
mesiogingival

mesiognathic
mesioincisal
mesiolabial
    mesiolingual m.
mesiolingual mesiolabial
mesiolinguo-occlusal
mesiolinguopulpal
mesio-occlusal
mesio-occlusion
mesioplacement
mesiopulpal
mesioversion
mesmerism
mesmerize
mesoappendix
mesoarium
mesobilane
mesobilene
mesobilirubin
mesobilirubinogen
mesobiliviolin
mesoblast
mesoblastema
mesoblastemic
mesoblastic
    m. nephroma
    m. segment
mesocardium
    dorsal m.
mesocarpal
mesocaval shunt
mesocecal
mesocecum
mesocephalic
mesocephalous
Mesocestoides
mesocolic
    m. hernia
    m. lymph node
    m. tenia
mesocolon
    ascending m.
    descending m.
    sigmoid m.
    transverse m.
mesocolopexy
mesocoloplication
meso compound
mesocord
mesocuneiform
meso-cystine

M

NOTES

mesoderm
    branchial m.
    extraembryonic m.
    gastral m.
    intermediate m.
    intraembryonic m.
    lateral m.
mesodermal
    m. factor
    m. meningioma
mesodermic
mesodiastolic
mesodont
mesoduodenal
mesoduodenum
mesoenteriolum
mesoepididymis
mesogaster
mesogastric zone
mesogastrium
    dorsal m.
mesogenic
mesoglia
mesoglial cell
mesogluteal
mesogluteus
mesognathic
mesognathion
mesognathous
mesoileum
meso-inositol
mesojejunum
mesolobus
mesolymphocyte
mesomelia
mesomelic dwarfism
mesomere
mesomeric
mesomerism
mesometanephric carcinoma
mesometrium
mesomorph
mesomorphic
meson
mesonephric
    m. adenocarcinoma
    m. duct
    m. fold
    m. rest
    m. ridge
    m. tissue
    m. tubule
mesonephroid tumor
mesonephroma
mesonephros
mesoneuritis
meso-ontomorph
mesopexy
mesophil

mesophile
mesophilic
mesophlebitis
mesophragma
mesophryon
mesopic perimetry
mesopneumonium
mesoporphyrins
mesoprocton
mesoprosopic
mesopulmonum
mesorchial
mesorchium
mesorectum
mesorrhaphy
mesorrhine
mesosalpinx
mesoscapulae
    delta m.
mesoscope
mesoseme
mesosigmoid
mesosigmoiditis
mesosigmoidopexy
mesosomatous
mesosome
mesosomia
mesostenium
mesosternum
mesosystolic
mesotarsal
mesotendineum
mesotendon
mesothelial cell
mesothelioma
    benign m.
mesothelium
mesothorium
mesotropic
mesotympanum
mesouranic
mesovarian border
mesovarium
messenger
    first m.
    m. RNA
messengerlike RNA
mestanolone
mestenediol
mestranol
mesulphen
mesuranic
mesylate
    deferoxamine m.
    desferrioxamine m.
    dihydroergotoxine m.
    fonazine m.
MET
    metabolic equivalent

metaanalysis
metabasis
metabiosis
metabisulfite test
metabolic
    m. acidosis
    m. alkalosis
    m. calculus
    m. clearance rate (MCR)
    m. coma
    m. craniopathy
    m. disease
    m. encephalopathy
    m. equivalent (MET)
    m. indican
    m. mucinosis
    m. pool
metabolimeter
metabolin
metabolism
    basal m.
    carbohydrate m.
    electrolyte m.
    energy m.
    fat m.
    first-pass m.
    inborn error of m.
    intermediary m.
    protein m.
metabolite
metabolize
metabolized vitamin D milk
metabotropic receptor
metacarpal
    m. bone
    m. index
    m. vein
metacarpectomy
metacarpi (*pl. of* metacarpus)
metacarpohypothenar reflex
metacarpophalangeal
    m. articulation
    m. joint
metacarpothenar reflex
metacarpus, pl. **metacarpi**
    ossa metacarpi
metacentric chromosome
metacercaria
metacestode
metachloral
metachromasia

metachromatic
    m. body
    m. granule
    m. leukodystrophy
    m. stain
metachromatism
metachroming
metachromophil, metachromophile
metachronous
metachrosis
metacone
metaconid
metacontrast
metaconule
metacresol
metacryptozoite
metadysentery
metafacial angle
metaherpetic keratitis
metahypophysial diabetes
metaicteric
metainfective
metakinesia
metakinesis
metal
    alkali earth m.
    Babbitt m.
    base m.
    m. base
    basic m.
    colloidal m.
    d'Arcet m.
    m. fume fever
    fusible m.
    heavy m.
    m. insert teeth
    m. interface
    light m.
    m. object
metaldehyde
metallic
    m. foreign body
    m. rale
metallocyanide
metalloenzyme
metalloflavodehydrogenase
metalloflavoenzyme
metalloflavoprotein
metalloid
metallophilia
metallophobia
metalloporphyrin

M

NOTES

metalloprotein
metalloproteinase
   matrix m.
metallothionein
metaluetic
metamer
metamere
metameric nervous system
metamerism
metamorphopsia
metamorphosis
   complete m.
   fatty m.
   heterometabolous m.
   holometabolous m.
   incomplete m.
metamorphotic
metamyelocyte
metanephric
   m. blastema
   m. bud
   m. cap
   m. diverticulum
   m. duct
   m. tubule
metanephrine
metanephrogenic tissue
metanephrogenous
metanephros
metaneutrophil, metaneutrophile
metanil yellow
metaperiodic acid
metaphase
metaphosphoric acid
metaphysial, metaphyseal
   m. dysostosis
   m. dysplasia
   m. fibrous cortical defect
metaphysis
metaphysitis
metaplasia
   agnogenic myeloid m.
   apocrine m.
   autoparenchymatous m.
   Barrett m.
   intestinal m.
   myeloid m.
   squamous m.
metaplasis
metaplasm
metaplastic
   m. anemia
   m. carcinoma
   m. ossification
   m. polyp
metaplexus
metapophysis
metapore
metaprotein

metaproterenol sulfate
metapsychology
metapyretic
metapyrocatechase
metarhodopsin
metarteriole
metarubricyte
metastable
metastasis, pl. metastases
   biochemical m.
   calcareous m.
   contact m.
   hematogenous m.
   in-transit m.
   lymphogenous m.
   nodular m.
   pleural m.
   retrograde m.
   tumor node m. (TNM)
metastasize
metastasizing septicemia
metastatic
   m. abscess
   m. calcification
   m. carcinoid syndrome
   m. carcinoma
   m. choroiditis
   m. mumps
   m. myelitis
   m. neoplasm
   m. ophthalmia
   m. pneumonia
   m. retinitis
metasternum
metastrongyle
metasyphilis
metasyphilitic
metatarsal
   m. artery
   m. bone
   m. interosseous ligament
   m. reflex
metatarsalgia
metatarsectomy
metatarsophalangeal
   m. articulation
   m. joint
metatarsus, pl. metatarsi
   m. adductovarus
   m. adductus
   m. atavicus
   m. latus
   ossa metatarsi
   m. varus
metathalamus
metathesis
metatroph
metatrophic
metatropic dwarfism

metatypical
metaxalone
metazoonosis
Metchnikoff theory
metel
    Datura m.
metencephalic
metencephalon
Metenier sign
metenkephalin
meteorism
meteoropathy
meteorotropic
meter
    m. angle
    potential acuity m.
meter-candle
metered-dose inhaler
metergasia
metergoline
meter-kilogram-second (MKS, mks)
    m.-k.-s. system
    m.-k.-s. unit
metestrum
metestrus
methacholine
    m. challenge test
    m. chloride
methacrylate
    methyl m.
    m. resin
methacrylic acid
methallenestril
methamphetamine base
methampyrone
methandienone
methandriol
methandrostenolone
methane
methanogen
methanol fixative
methantheline bromide
methapyrilene
methaqualone
metharbital
methargen
methazolamide
methemalbumin
methemalbuminemia
methemoglobin
    cyanide m.

methemoglobinemia
    acquired m.
    congenital m.
    enterogenous m.
    hereditary m.
methemoglobinuria
methenamine
    m. hippurate
    m. mandelate
    m. salicylate
    m. silver stain
methenamine-silver
methene
methergoline
methicillin sodium
methimazole
methiodal sodium
methionine
    active m.
methionine-activating enzyme
methionyl dipeptidase
methisazone
methitural
methocarbamol
method
    Abbott m.
    Abell-Kendall m.
    activated sludge m.
    Altmann-Gersh m.
    Anel m.
    Antyllus m.
    aristotelian m.
    Ashby m.
    auxanographic m.
    Barraquer m.
    Beck m.
    Bier m.
    Billings m.
    Born m.
    Brasdor m.
    Callahan m.
    capture-recapture m.
    Charters m.
    Chayes m.
    chloropercha m.
    closed-circuit m.
    Cobb m.
    combined m.'s
    confrontation m.
    cooled-knife m.
    copper sulfate m.
    correlational m.

M

NOTES

method *(continued)*
    Credé m.
    cross-sectional m.
    Deaver m.
    definitive m.
    Dick m.
    diffusion m.
    disc sensitivity m.
    double antibody m.
    Edman m.
    Eggleston m.
    Eicken m.
    encu m.
    ensu m.
    experimental m.
    Fick m.
    flash m.
    flotation m.
    fusion temperature wire m.
    Gärtner m.
    Gerota m.
    glucose oxidase m.
    Gruber m.
    Hamilton-Stewart m.
    Hammerschlag m.
    hexokinase m.
    Hilton m.
    Hirschberg m.
    Hung m.
    immunofluorescence m.
    impedance m.
    indicator dilution m.
    indophenol m.
    introspective m.
    ITO m.
    Johnson m.
    Keating-Hart m.
    Kety-Schmidt m.
    Kjeldahl m.
    Lamaze m.
    Langendorff m.
    Lee-White m.
    Liborius m.
    Ling m.
    Lister m.
    longitudinal m.
    manual visual m.
    Marshall m.
    micro-Astrup m.
    micro-Kjeldahl m.
    microsphere m.
    Moore m.
    Nikiforoff m.
    open circuit m.
    oral auditory m.
    Pachon m.
    Purmann m.
    rhythm m.

    Roux m.
    Scarpa m.
    Schede m.
    Theden m.
    Wardrop m.
    Westergren m.
    Wilson m.
methodism
methodology
methohexital sodium
methonium compound
methophenazine
methopholine
methopterin
methorphinan
methoserpidine
methotrexate
methotrimeprazine
methoxsalen
methoxychlor
methoxyflurane
methoxyl
methsuximide
methyclothiazide
methyl
    active m.
    m. alcohol
    m. aldehyde
    angular m.
    m. blue
    m. bromide
    m. chloride
    m. green
    m. green-pyronin stain
    m. hydroxybenzoate
    m. isobutyl ketone
    m. mercaptan
    m. methacrylate
    m. nicotinate
    m. orange
    m. red
    m. salicylate
    m. violet
    m. yellow
methylase
    dam m.
    deoxyadenosine m.
methylate
methylated spirit
methylation
methylbenzene
methyl-CCNU
methylcellulose
methylchloroform
methylcitrate
methylcobalamin
methyldichloroarsine
methyldopa

methylene
    m. blue
    m. blue test
methylenophil, methylenophile
methylenophilic
methylenophilous
methylglucamine
methylglyoxalase
methylhexaneamine
methylkinase
methylmalonate semialdehyde
methylmalonic acid
methylmercury
methylmorphine
methylol riboflavin
methylose
methylparaben
methylpentose
methylsulfate
    diphemanil m.
methyl-tert-butyl ether
methyltransferase
metmyoglobin
metocurine iodide
metolazone
metonymy
metopagus
metopic
    m. point
    m. suture
metopion
metopism
metopoplasty
metoposcopy
metoprolol tartrate
metoxenous
metoxeny
metratonia
metratrophia
metratrophy
metria
metric system
metrifonate
metriocephalic
metritis
metrizamide
metrizoate sodium
metrocyte
metrodynamometer
metrodynia
metrofibroma

metrolymphangitis
metronidazole
metronoscope
metroparalysis
metropathia hemorrhagica
metropathic
metropathy
metroperitoneal fistula
metroperitonitis
metrophlebitis
metroplasty
metrorrhagia
metrorrhea
metrosalpingitis
metrosalpingography
metroscope
metrostaxis
metrostenosis
metrotomy
metrotrophic test
metyrapone
metyrosine
Meulengracht diet
Mev
    1 million electron-volts
mevalonate kinase
mevalonic
    m. acid
    m. aciduria
mevinolin
Mexican
    M. hat cell
    M. hat corpuscle
    M. spotted fever
    M. tea
    M. typhus
mexiletine
Meyenburg
    M. complex
    M. disease
Meyenburg-Altherr-Uehlinger syndrome
Meyer
    M. cartilage
    M. line
    M. reagent
    M. sinus
Meyer-Archambault loop
Meyer-Betz
    M.-B. disease
    M.-B. syndrome
Meyerhof oxidation quotient

M

NOTES

Meyer-Overton
  M.-O. rule
  M.-O. theory
Meyer-Schwickerath
Meynert
  M. cell
  M. commissure
  M. decussation
  M. layer
mezlocillin sodium
mg
  milligram
Mg antigen
MGUS
  monoclonal gammopathy of unknown
  significance
MHA-TP test
MHz
  megahertz
MI
  myocardial infarction
miasma theory
Mibelli
  M. angiokeratoma
  M. disease
MIC
  minimal inhibitory concentration
micatosis
micdadei
  Legionella m.
micellar
micelle
Michaelis
  M. complex
  M. constant
Michaelis-Gutmann body
Michaelis-Menten
  M.-M. constant
  M.-M. equation
  M.-M. hypothesis
Michel
  M. malformation
  M. spur
miconazole nitrate
micracoustic
micrencephalia
micrencephalous
micrencephaly
microabscess
  Munro m.
  Pautrier m.
microabsorption spectroscopy
microadenoma
microaerobion
microaerophil, microaerophile
microaerophilic
microaerophilous
microaerosol
microaggregate

microalbuminuria
microanalysis
microanastomosis
microanatomist
microanatomy
microaneurysm
microangiography
microangiopathic hemolytic anemia
microangiopathy
microangioscopy
microarteriography
micro-Astrup method
microatelectasis
microbalance
microbe
microbial
  m. associate
  m. collagenase
  m. genetics
  m. persistence
  m. RNase II
  m. vitamin
microbic
microbicidal
microbicide
microbiologic
microbiologist
microbiology
microbiotic
microbism
  latent m.
microblast
microblepharia
microblepharism
microblepharon
microbody
microbrachia
microbrenner
microcalcifications
microcardia
microcentrum
microcephalia
microcephalic
microcephalism
microcephalous
microcephaly
  encephaloclastic m.
microcheilia, microchilia
microcheiria, microchiria
microchemistry
microchilia (*var. of* microcheilia)
microchimerism
microchiria (*var. of* microcheiria)
microcide
microcinematography
microcirculation
micrococcal
  m. endonuclease
  m. nuclease

Micrococcus
    M. conglomeratus
    M. luteus
    M. varians
microcolitis
microcolon
microcolony
microconidium
microcoria
microcornea
microcoulomb
microcoustic
microcrystalline cellulose
microcurie
microcyst
microcystic
    m. disease
    m. epithelial dystrophy
microcyte
microcythemia
microcytic anemia
microcytosis
microdactylous
microdactyly, microdactylia
microdermatome
microdialysis
microdissection
microdont
microdontia
microdontism
microdose
microdrepanocytic anemia
microdrepanocytosis
microdysgenesia
microelectric wave
microelectrode
microelement
microencephaly
microerythrocyte
microetching technique
microevolution
microfibril
microfilament
microfilaremia
microfilaria
microfilarial sheath
microfilm
microflora
microfold cell
microfollicular
    m. adenoma
    m. goiter

microgamete
microgametocyte
microgamont
microgamy
microgastria
microgcnia
microgenitalism
microglandular adenosis
microglia cell, microglial cell
microgliacyte
microglioma
microgliomatosis
microgliosis
microglobulin
microglossia
micrognathia with peromelia
microgonioscope
microgram
micrograph
    electron m.
    light m.
micrography
microgyria
microhemagglutination-*Treponema*
    pallidum test
microhematocrit concentration
microhepatia
microheterogeneity
microhistology
microhm
microincineration
microincision
microinjector
microinvasion
microinvasive carcinoma
microkatal
micro-Kjeldahl method
microkymatotherapy
microlecithal egg
microlesion
microleukoblast
microliter
microlith
microlithiasis
    pulmonary alveolar m.
micrology
micromanipulation
micromanipulator
micromazia
micromelia
micromelic dwarfism
micromere

M

NOTES

micromerozoite
micrometastasis
micrometastatic disease
micrometer
    caliper m.
    filar m.
micrometry
micromicrogram
micromicron
microminerals
micromolar
micromole
micromotoscope
micromyelia
micromyeloblast
micromyeloblastic leukemia
micron
microneedle
microneme
micronic
micronodular
micronucleus
micronutrients
micronychia
micronystagmus
micro-ohm
microorganism
microparasite
micropathology
micropenis
microphage
microphagocyte
microphallus
microphobia
microphone
microphonia
microphonic
    cochlear m.
microphonoscope
microphony
microphotograph
microphthalmia
    colobomatous m.
microphthalmos
microphthalmoscope
micropipette, micropipet
microplania
microplasia
microplethysmography
micropodia
micropolariscope
micropore
microprecipitation test
microprobe
micropromyelocyte
microprosopia
micropsia
micropuncture
micropyle

microradiography
microrefractometer
microrespirometer
microsaccades
microscintigraphy
microscope
    binocular m.
    color-contrast m.
    comparator m.
    compound m.
    confocal m.
    dark-field m.
    dissecting m.
    electron m.
    fluorescence m.
    flying spot m.
    infrared m.
    interference m.
    laser m.
    light m.
    operating m.
    optical m.
    phase m.
    phase-contrast m.
    scanning electron m.
    simple m.
    single m.
    stereoscopic m.
    stroboscopic m.
    surgical m.
    ultraviolet m.
    x-ray m.
microscopic
    m. anatomy
    m. field
    m. hematuria
    m. polyangiitis
    m. section
    m. sphincter
microscopical
microscopically controlled surgery
microscopy
    electron m.
    epiluminescence m.
    fluorescence m.
    immersion m.
    immune electron m.
    immunofluorescence m.
    phase-contrast m.
    scanning electron m.
    surface m.
    television m.
microseme
microside
microsmatic
microsome
microsomia
microspectrophotometry
microspectroscope

microsphere method
microspherocytosis
microsphygmy
microsphyxia
microsplanchnic
microsplenia
microsporidian keratoconjunctivitis
microsporidiasis
microsporidiosis
Microsporum
    M. audouinii
    M. canis
    M. ferrugineum
    M. fulvum
    M. gallinae
    M. gypseum
    M. nanum
    M. persicolor
    M. vanbreuseghemi
microstethophone
microstethoscope
microstomia
microsurgery
microsuture
microsyringe
microthelia
microti
    Babesia m.
microtia
microtine
microtome
    freezing m.
    rocking m.
    rotary m.
    sliding m.
microtomy
microtonometer
microtrauma
microtropia
microtubule
microtubule-associated protein (MAP)
microtubule-organizing center
microvascular anastomosis
microvesicle
microvillus inclusion disease
microvivisection
microvolt
microwave therapy
microwelding
microxyphil
microzoon
micrurgical

miction
micturate
micturating cystourethrogram
micturition
    m. reflex
    m. syncope
MID
    minimal infecting dose
midaxillary line
midbody
midbrain
    tectum of m.
    m. tegmentum
    m. vesicle
midcarpal joint
midclavicular line (MCL)
middiastolic murmur
middle
    m. atlantoepistrophic joint
    m. axillary line
    m. cardiac vein
    m. carpal joint
    m. cerebellar peduncle
    m. cerebral artery
    m. cervical cardiac nerve
    m. cervical fascia
    m. cervical ganglion
    m. clinoid process
    m. cluneal nerve
    m. colic artery
    m. colic lymph node
    m. colic vein
    m. collateral artery
    m. constrictor muscle
    m. costotransverse ligament
    m. cranial fossa
    m. cuneiform bone
    m. ear
    m. esophageal constriction
    m. ethmoidal air cell
    m. ethmoidal sinus
    m. finger
    m. fossa approach
    m. frontal convolution
    m. frontal gyrus
    m. frontal sulcus
    m. genicular artery
    m. glossoepiglottic fold
    m. gray layer
    m. hemorrhoidal artery
    m. hemorrhoidal plexus
    m. hemorrhoidal vein

NOTES

M

middle *(continued)*
    m. hepatic vein
    m. kidney
    m. latency response
    m. lobar artery
    m. lobe
    m. lobe branch
    m. lobe bronchus
    m. lobe syndrome
    m. lobe vein
    m. macular arteriole
    m. mediastinum
    m. meningeal artery
    m. meningeal artery groove
    m. meningeal branch
    m. meningeal nerve
    m. meningeal vein
    m. nasal concha
    m. pain
    m. palatine suture
    m. palmar space
    m. phalanx
    m. piece
    m. radioulnar joint
    m. rectal artery
    m. rectal lymph node
    m. rectal nervous plexus
    m. rectal vein
    m. sacral artery
    m. sacral lymphatic plexus
    m. scalene muscle
    m. superior alveolar branch
    m. supraclavicular nerve
    m. suprarenal artery
    m. talar articular surface
    m. temporal artery
    m. temporal branch
    m. temporal convolution
    m. temporal gyrus
    m. temporal sulcus
    m. temporal vein
    m. thyroid vein
    m. transverse rectal fold
    m. trunk
    m. turbinated bone
    m. umbilical fold
    m. umbilical ligament
middle-ear effusion
midforceps delivery
midgastric transverse sphincter
midge
midget bipolar cell
midgracile
midgut
midlife crisis
midline
    m. incision
    m. lethal granuloma

    m. malignant reticulosis granuloma
    m. myelotomy
midmenstrual
midoccipital
midpain
midpalmar space
midplane
midpoint
    temperature m.
midriff
midsagittal
    m. plane
    m. section
midsection
midsigmoid sphincter
midsternal line
midsternum
midtarsal joint
midwife
midwifery
Miescher
    M. elastoma
    M. granuloma
    M. tube
MIF
    migration-inhibitory factor
mifepristone
mignon lamp
migraine
    abdominal m.
    acephalgic m.
    basilar m.
    classic m.
    common m.
    complicated m.
    fulgurating m.
    Harris m.
    hat band m.
    hemiplegic m.
    menstrual m.
    ocular m.
    retinal m.
    m. without headache
migraine-related vestibulopathy
migrans
    cutaneous larva m.
    erythema chronicum m.
    keratitis linearis m.
    larva m.
migrating
    m. abscess
    m. teeth
migration
    branch m.
    epithelial m.
    m. inhibition test
    m. inhibitory factor test
migration-inhibitory factor (MIF)

migratory
 m. cell
 m. pneumonia
MIH
 melanotropin release-inhibiting hormone
mika operation
Mikulicz
 M. aphthae
 M. cell
 M. clamp
 M. disease
 M. drain
 M. operation
 M. procedure
 M. syndrome
Mikulicz-Vladimiroff amputation
mild
 m. fetal bradycardia
 m. mercurial ointment
 m. silver protein
Miles operation
milestone
 developmental m.
miliaria
 m. alba
 apocrine m.
 m. crystallina
 m. profunda
 m. rubra
miliaris
 acne necrotica m.
miliary
 m. abscess
 m. aneurysm
 m. embolism
 m. fever
 m. pattern
 m. tuberculosis
milieu
 m. intérieur
 m. interne
 m. therapy
military
 m. antishock trousers (MAST)
 m. medicine
milium
 colloid m.
milk
 acidophilus m.
 m. anemia
 m. of bismuth
 buddeized m.

m. of calcium
certified pasteurized m.
condensed m.
m. corpuscle
m. crust
m. cyst
m. dentition
m. duct
m. factor
m. fever
fortified vitamin D m.
m. gland
irradiated vitamin D m.
lactobacillary m.
m. let-down reflex
m. line
m. of magnesia
metabolized vitamin D m.
modified m.
m. ridge
m. sickness
skim m.
skimmed m.
m. spot
m. sugar
m. of sulfur
m. tooth
vitamin D m.
witch's m.
milk-alkali syndrome
milk-ejection reflex
milkers'
 m. node
 m. nodule
 m. nodule virus
Milkman syndrome
milkpox
milk-ring test
milky
 m. ascites
 m. urine
mill
 m. fever
 m. wheel murmur
Millard-Gubler syndrome
milled-in
 m.-i. curve
 m.-i. path
miller
 m. asthma
 M. chemoparasitic theory
Miller-Abbott tube

NOTES

607

millet seed
milliampere
milliampere-impulse
milliampere-second
millibar
millicurie (mCi)
milliequivalent (mEq, meq)
milligram (mg)
millilambert
milliliter
millimeter (mm)
millimicron
millimole (mmol)
milling-in
1 million electron-volts (Mev)
milliosmole
millipede
millisecond (ms, msec)
millivolt (mV)
Millner needle
Millon
    M. reaction
    M. reagent
Millon-Nasse test
milphosis
milrinone
Milroy disease
mimesis
mimetic
    m. convulsion
    m. muscle
    m. paralysis
mimic gene
mimicus
    Vibrio m.
mimmation
Minamata disease
mind blindness
mind-reading
mineral
    m. oil
    m. water
    m. wax
mineralization
mineralocoid
mineralocorticoid
mineralotropic
miner's
    m. asthma
    m. cramps
    m. disease
    m. elbow
    m. lung
    m. nystagmus
    m. phthisis
Minerva jacket
miniature
    m. scarlet fever
    m. stomach

minicore-multicore myopathy
minilaparotomy
minimal
    m. air
    m. alveolar concentration
    m. amplitude nystagmus
    m. anesthetic concentration
    m. brain dysfunction
    m. deviation melanoma
    m. infecting dose (MID)
    m. inhibitory concentration (MIC)
    m. lethal dose (MLD, mld)
    m. reacting dose
minimal-change
    m.-c. disease
    m.-c. nephrotic syndrome
minimally invasive surgery
minimi
    abductor digiti m.
minimum
    m. data set
    m. light
    m. light threshold
    m. protein requirement
    m. temperature
minimyosin
minithoracotomy
mink enteritis virus
Minnesota
    M. Multiphasic Personality
    Inventory (MMPI)
    M. Multiphasic Personality
    Inventory test
minocycline
minor
    m. agglutinin
    m. alar cartilage
    m. amputation
    aphthae m.
    m. arterial circle
    m. calix
    chorea m.
    m. connector
    m. duodenal papilla
    m. fissure
    forceps m.
    m. forceps
    globus m.
    m. groove
    hippocampus m.
    m. hippocampus
    m. histocompatibility complex
    m. hypnosis
    m. hysteria
    m. motor seizure
    m. operation
    pelvis justo m.
    m. salivary gland
    m. sublingual duct

m. surgery
thalassemia m.
m. tranquilizer
Minot-Murphy diet
minus
labium m.
m. lens
m. strand
minute
counts per m. (cpm)
m. output
m. ventilation
m. volume
minutissimum
Corynebacterium m.
minutum
Eubacterium m.
miodidymus
miodymus
miolecithal
miopragia
miopus
miosis
irritative m.
paralytic m.
miosphygmia
miostagmin reaction
miotic
MIP
macrophage inflammatory protein
maximum intensity projection
miracidium
Mirchamp sign
mire
mirex
Mirizzi syndrome
mirror
concave m.
convex m.
m. drill
m. haploscope
head m.
m. image
m. image dextrocardia
m. speech
mirror-image cell
mirror-writing
miryachit
MIS
müllerian inhibiting substance
misandry
misanthropy

miscarriage
miscegenation
miscible
misdiagnosis
misdirection phenomenon
mismatch repair
misogamy
misogyny
misopedia
misopedy
misoprostol
missed
m. abortion
m. labor
m. period
missense
m. mutation
m. suppression
missiles
mistletoe
Mitchell
M. disease
M. procedure
M. treatment
mitchellae
Aedes m.
mite-born typhus
mite typhus
mithramycin
mithridatism
miticidal
miticide
mitigate
mitis
prurigo m.
mitochondrial
m. biogenesis
m. chromosome
m. disorder
m. gene
m. matrix
m. membrane
m. myopathy
m. sheath
mitochondrialis
matrix m.
mitochondrion
mitogen
mitogenesis
mitogenetic
mitogenic lectin
mitomycin

NOTES

mitoplast
mitosis
    heterotype m.
mitotane
mitotic
    m. cycle
    m. division
    m. figure
    m. index
    m. period
    m. rate
    m. spindle
mitral
    m. anulus
    m. area
    m. cell
    m. click
    m. commissurotomy
    m. facies
    m. gradient
    m. incompetence
    m. insufficiency
    m. murmur
    m. opening snap
    m. orifice
    m. prosthesis
    m. regurgitation
    m. stenosis
    m. tap
    m. valve
    m. valve prolapse
    m. valve prolapse, aortic anomalies, skeletal and skin changes (MASS)
    m. valve prolapse syndrome
    m. valvotomy
    m. valvulitis
    m. valvuloplasty
mitrale
    P m.
mitralization
Mitrofanoff principle
Mitsuda
    M. antigen
    M. reaction
Mitsuo phenomenon
mittelschmerz
Mittendorf dot
mix
    case m.
mixed
    m. agglutination reaction
    m. agglutination test
    m. aphasia
    m. astigmatism
    m. beat
    m. cell leukemia
    m. chancre
    m. connective-tissue disease

    m. discrete-continuous random variable
    m. drug abuse
    m. esotropia
    m. expired gas
    m. function oxygenase
    m. gland
    m. glioma
    m. glycerides
    m. hearing loss
    m. hemorrhoid
    m. hyperlipemia
    m. hyperlipidemia
    m. hypoglycemia
    m. infection
    m. lymphocyte culture
    m. lymphocyte culture reaction
    m. lymphocyte culture test
    m. mesodermal tumor
    m. nerve
    m. nevus
    m. paralysis
    m. thrombus
    m. tocopherols concentrate
mixotrophy
Mixter clamp
mixture
    Basham m.
    Bordeaux m.
    extemporaneous m.
Miyagawa body
MKS, mks
    meter-kilogram-second
    MKS unit
MLD, mld
    minimal lethal dose
mm
    millimeter
M1, M2 antigen
MMMT
    malignant mixed mesodermal tumor
    malignant mixed müllerian tumor
M-mode echocardiography
mmol
    millimole
MMPI
    Minnesota Multiphasic Personality Inventory
MMR
    measles, mumps, and rubella
MM virus
M'Naghten rule
MND
    motor neuron disease
mneme
mnemenic
mnemic
    m. hypothesis
    m. theory

mnemism
mnemonic
mnemonics
MNSs
    MNSs antigen
    MNSs blood group
MoAb
    monoclonal antibody
mobile
    cor m.
    m. end
    m. part
    punctum m.
    m. spasm
mobilis
    Klebsiella m.
    lien m.
mobilization
    stapes m.
mobilize
Mobitz block
Möbius
    M. sign
    M. syndrome
MOD
    mesiodistocclusal
modal
    m. alteration
    m. frequency
    m. pitch
modality
model
    additive m.
    animal m.
    Armitage-Doll m.
    Bingham m.
    biomedical m.
    biopsychosocial m.
    cloverleaf m.
    computer m.
    concerted m.
    cooperativity m.
    fluid mosaic m.
    m. game
    genetic m.
    independent living m.
    induced fit m.
    KNF m.
    Koshland-Némethy-Filmer m.
    lock-and-key m.
    logistic m.
    mathematical m.

    medical m.
    pathologic m.
    Reed-Frost m.
    Sartwell incubation m.
modeling
    m. composition
    m. compound
    m. plastic
moderate hypothermia
moderator
    m. band
    m. variable
modern genetics
modification
    behavior m.
    chemical m.
    covalent m.
modified
    m. acid-fast stain
    m. milk
    m. radical hysterectomy
    m. radical mastectomy
    m. radical mastoidectomy
    m. smallpox
    m. trichrome stain
    m. zinc oxide-eugenol cement
modifier
    biologic response m.
    effect m.
    m. gene
modiolus labii
modular prosthesis
modulation
    biochemical m.
    m. transfer function
modulator
    selective estrogen receptor m.
modulus
    bulk m.
    Young m.
Moeller
    M. glossitis
    M. grass bacillus
mofebutazone
Mogen clamp
mogiarthria
mogilalia
mogiphonia
Mohr
    M. pipette
    M. syndrome

NOTES

M

Mohrenheim
>   M. fossa
>   M. space

Mohs
>   M. chemosurgery
>   M. fresh tissue chemosurgery technique
>   M. micrographic surgery
>   M. procedure
>   M. scale

moiety
moist
>   m. gangrene
>   m. necrosis
>   m. papule
>   m. rale

moisture
Mokola virus
molal
molality
molar
>   m. absorbancy index
>   m. absorption coefficient
>   m. absorptivity
>   m. behavior
>   m. concentration
>   m. extinction coefficient
>   first m.
>   first permanent m.
>   m. gland
>   m. mass
>   Moon m.
>   mulberry m.
>   m. pregnancy
>   second m.
>   sixth-year m.
>   third m.
>   m. tooth
>   m. tubercle
>   twelfth-year m.

molariform
molaris
>   dens m.

molarity
mold guide
molding
>   border m.
>   compression m.
>   injection m.

mole
>   Breus m.
>   carneous m.
>   cystic m.
>   fleshy m.
>   m. fraction
>   hairy m.
>   hydatid m.
>   hydatidiform m.
>   invasive m.

molecular
>   m. behavior
>   m. biology
>   m. biophysics
>   m. disease
>   m. dispersed solution
>   m. dispersion
>   m. dissociation theory
>   m. distillation
>   m. epidemiology
>   m. formula
>   m. genetics
>   m. heat
>   m. layer
>   m. mass
>   m. movement
>   m. pathology
>   m. rotation
>   m. sieve
>   m. weight
>   m. weight ratio

molecularity
molecule
>   accessory m.
>   adhesion m.
>   cell adhesion m.
>   chimeric m.
>   class I, II m.
>   costimulatory m.
>   endothelial-leukocyte adhesion m.
>   lectin pathway m.

molilalia
molimen
molimina
>   menstrual m.

Molisch test
Mollaret meningitis
molle
>   fibroma m.
>   heloma m.

Moll gland
mollities
Molluscipoxvirus
molluscous
molluscum
>   m. body
>   m. conjunctivitis
>   m. contagiosum
>   m. contagiosum virus
>   m. corpuscle

mollusk
Moloney
>   M. test
>   M. virus

molt
molybdate
molybdenic
molybdenous

molybdenum
    m. cofactor
    m. target tube
molybdenum-99
molybdic acid
molybdous
molysmophobia
moment
    dipole m.
momism
monad
Monakow
    M. bundle
    M. fascia
    M. nucleus
    M. stria
    M. syndrome
    M. tract
monamide
monamine
monaminuria
monangle
monarda
monarthric
monarthritis
monarticular
monaster
monathetosis
monatomic
monaural
Mönckeberg
    M. arteriosclerosis
    M. calcification
    M. degeneration
    M. sclerosis
Mondini
    M. dysplasia
    M. hearing impairment
Mondor disease
monesthetic
Monge disease
mongolian spot
mongolism
    translocation m.
monilethrix
monilial
moniliasis
moniliforme
    Eubacterium m.
moniliform hair
moniliformis
    lichen ruber m.

moniliid
monitor
    cardiac m.
    electronic fetal m.
    Holter m.
    home m.
    transcutaneous blood gas m.
monoamelia
monoamide
monoamine
    m. hypothesis
    m. oxidase inhibitor
monoaminergic
monoamniotic twin
monobasic
monoblast
monobrachius
    acephalus m.
monochorea
monochorionic diamnionic placenta
monochromatic
    m. aberration
    m. radiation
monochromatism
    blue cone m.
monochromatophil
monochromatophile
monoclonal
    m. antibody (MAB, MoAb)
    m. gammopathy
    m. gammopathy of unknown
      significance (MGUS)
    m. immunoglobulin
monocrotic
monocrotism
monocular diplopia
monocyte
    m. chemoattractant protein
    m. function test
monocyte-derived neutrophil chemotactic factor (MDNCF)
monocytic
    m. leukemia
    m. leukopenia
monocytogene
    Listeria m.
monocytoid cell
monocytopenia
monocytosis
monodactylism
monodactyly
monofixation syndrome

M

NOTES

monogametic
monogamy
monogenesis
monogenetic
monogenic
monogenous
monohydric alcohol
monolayers
monolocular
monomania
monomelic
monomer
monomeric
monomorphic
monomyoplegia
monomyositis
mononeural
mononeuralgia
mononeuric
mononeuritis
mononeuropathy
mononuclear phagocyte system
mononucleosis
    infectious m.
mononucleotide
    flavin m.
    nicotinamide m.
monooxygenase
monoparesis
monoparesthesia
monopathic
monopathy
monophasia
monophasic
monophosphate
    adenosine m. (AMP)
monophthalmos
monophyletic
monoplegia
monopodia
monopolar cautery
monopus
    acephalus m.
monorchid
monorchidic
monorchism
monosaccharide
monosodium glutamate
monosomia
monosomic
monosomy
monospasm
monostotic
monostratal
monosymptomatic
monosynaptic
monothermia
monotrichous
monovalence

monovalency
monovalent
monoxenic culture
monoxenous
monoxide
    barium m.
    carbon m. (CO)
    dinitrogen m.
    lead m.
monozygotic twins
monozygous
Monro doctrine
mons pubis
monster
    Gila m.
Monteggia fracture
Montevideo unit
Montgomery
    M. follicle
    M. tubercle
monticulus
montis
mood
    m. stabilizing agent
    m. swing
mood-congruent hallucination
mood-incongruent hallucination
moon
    m. face
    M. molar
Moore
    M. lightning streak
    M. method
Mooren ulcer
morado
    mal m.
Moraxella
morbidity
    maternal m.
    m. rate
morbid obesity
morbific
morbilli
morbilliform
Morbillivirus
    equine *M.*
morbillorum
    Gemella m.
morbus
morcellated nephrectomy
morcellation operation
mordant
Morel ear
Morgagni
    M. cataract
    M. column
    M. disease
    M. foramen hernia
    M. globule

M. prolapse
M. retinaculum
M. sinus
M. syndrome
morgagnian cyst
morgan
Morganella morganii
morganii
    Morganella m.
    Proteus m.
morgue
moria
moribund
Mörner test
morning
    m. after pill
    m. sickness
Moro reflex
morphea
morphine sulfate
morphogenesis
morphogenetic movement
morphologic
morphology
morphometric
morphometry
morphosis
mortality rate
mortar
mortification
mortified
mortis
    rigor m.
mortise joint
Morton
    M. neuralgia
    M. syndrome
    M. toe
mortuary
morula
morulation
Morvan
    M. chorea
    M. disease
mosaic
    m. inheritance
    m. pattern
    m. wart
mosaicism
    cellular m.
    chromosome m.
    gene m.

germinal m.
gonadal m.
moshkovskii
    Entamoeba m.
Mosler sign
mosquito
    m. clamp
    m. forceps
moss
    club m.
    Iceland m.
    Irish m.
    M. tube
Mosso
    M. ergograph
    M. sphygmomanometer
Motais operation
mote
    blood m.
mother
    m. cell
    m. cyst
    surrogate m.
    m. yaw
motile scotoma
motility
    ocular m.
motion
    brownian m.
    continuous passive m. (CPM)
    equation of m.
    range of m.
    m. sickness
motivation
    extrinsic m.
    intrinsic m.
motive
    achievement m.
    mastery m.
motofacient
motoneuron
motor
    m. aphasia
    m. area
    m. ataxia
    m. cortex
    m. decussation
    m. endplate
    m. fiber
    m. image
    m. nerve
    m. neuron

M

NOTES

motor *(continued)*
    m. neuron disease (MND)
    m. paralysis
    m. plate
    m. point
    m. speech center
    m. unit
    m. urgency
    m. vehicle accident (MVA)
mottled enamel
mottling
mounding
mount
    wet m.
mountain sickness
mounting medium
mouse
    joint m.
mouse-tooth forceps
mouth
    carp m.
    denture sore m.
    m. prop
    tapir m.
    trench m.
mouth-to-mouth
    m.-t.-m. breathing
    m.-t.-m. respiration
    m.-t.-m. resuscitation
movable
    m. joint
    m. spleen
movement
    active m.
    adversive m.
    ameboid m.
    assistive m.
    associated m.
    Bennett m.
    border tissue m.
    bowel m.
    brownian m.
    brownian-Zsigmondy m.
    cardinal ocular m.
    choreic m.
    ciliary m.
    circus m.
    cogwheel ocular m.
    compensatory m.
    conjugate m.
    decomposition of m.
    disconjugate m.
    dissociation m.
    drift m.
    dynamic m.
    m. economy
    fetal m.
    fixational ocular m.
    flick m.

    free mandibular m.
    functional mandibular m.
    fusional m.
    hinge m.
    illusion of m.
    intermediary m.'s
    lateral m.
    Magnan trombone m.
    mandibular m.
    mass m.
    molecular m.
    morphogenetic m.
    nonrapid eye m.
    paradoxical vocal cord m.
    passive m.
    rapid eye m.'s
    streaming m.
    m. system
    vermicular m.
Mowry colloidal iron stain
Moynihan operation
MRA
    magnetic resonance angiography
ms, msec
    millisecond
M2 segment
mucicarmine
muciform
mucihematein
mucilage
mucilaginous
mucin
    gastric m.
mucinase
mucinogen
mucinoid
mucinosa
    alopecia m.
mucinosis
    cutaneous focal m.
    follicular m.
    localized m.
    metabolic m.
    papular m.
    secondary m.
mucinous carcinoma
mucocele
    ethmoid sinus m.
    frontal sinus m.
    lacrimal m.
    maxillary sinus m.
    suppurating m.
mucociliary
    m. clearance
    m. clearance rate
    m. transport
mucocutaneous
    m. hemorrhoid
    m. junction

m. leishmaniasis
m. lymph node syndrome
mucoenteritis
mucoepidermoid
mucogingival line
mucoid degeneration
mucolytic
mucomembranous enteritis
mucoperiosteal
mucoperiosteum
mucopolysaccharidase
mucopolysaccharide
mucopolysaccharidosis
mucopolysacchariduria
mucoprotein
Tamm-Horsfall m.
mucopurulent
mucormycosis
mucosa
alveolar m.
bronchial m.
buccal m.
esophageal m.
gastric m.
gingival m.
laryngeal m.
lingual m.
mucosa-associated lymphoid tissue (MALT)
mucosae
muscularis m.
mucosal
m. hernia
m. wave
mucosanguineous
mucosanguinolent
mucosectomy
mucoserous cell
mucotome
mucous
m. cell
m. colitis
m. connective tissue
m. cyst
m. gland
m. hypersecretion
m. membrane
m. plug
m. plugging
m. stool
m. tunic

mucus
m. blanket
glairy m.
mud fever
Muehrcke line
Mueller electronic tonometer
Mueller-Hinton medium
mulberry molar
Mules operation
mule-spinner's cancer
muliebris
corpus spongiosum urethrae m.
dartos m.
Müller
M. duct
M. fixative
M. law
M. maneuver
M. sign
M. tubercle
müllerian
m. duct
m. inhibiting substance (MIS)
multangular bone
multiarticular
multiaxial joint
multicolony-stimulating factor
multicuspidate
multicystic ameloblastoma
multidrug resistance
multifactorial inheritance
multifid
multifidus muscle
multifilament suture
multifocal
m. atrial tachycardia (MAT)
m. lens
multiformat camera
multiforme
erythema m.
giant cell glioblastoma m.
glioblastoma m.
granuloma m.
multiformis
Haverhillia m.
multiform layer
multigravida
multi-infection
multilamellar body
multilobar
multilobate placenta
multilobed

M

NOTES

multilobular
multilocal
multilocular cyst
multilocularis
    Echinococcus m.
multinodular goiter
multinodulate
multinuclear
multinucleate
multipara
    grand m.
multiparity
multiparous
multiple
    m. ego states
    m. endocrine deficiency syndrome
    m. endocrine neoplasia (MEN)
    m. endocrine neoplasia 1, 2, 3
    m. endocrine neoplasia, type 1
      (MEN1)
    m. endocrine neoplasia, type 2A
      (MEN2A)
    m. epiphysial dysplasia
    m. fission
    m. fracture
    m. intestinal polyposis
    m. marker screen
    m. mucosal neuroma syndrome
    m. myeloma
    m. myositis
    m. neuritis
    m. neuromas
    m. personality
    m. pregnancy
    m. puncture tuberculin test
    m. sclerosis
    m. stain
    m. system atrophy
    m. vision
multiple-gated acquisition scan
multiplex
    dysostosis m.
    dysplasia epiphysialis m.
    myeloma m.
    myoclonus m.
    xanthoma m.
multiplicative division
multiplier
    countercurrent m.
multipolar
    m. cell
    m. neuron
multistrand suture
multisynaptic
multisystem disease
multivalence
multivalency
multivalent vaccine

multocida
    Pasteurella m.
mummification
mummified
    m. fetus
    m. pulp
mumps
    metastatic m.
    m. pancreatitis
    m. skin test antigen
    m. virus
mundi
    anima m.
Munro
    M. microabscess
    M. point
Munson sign
mural
    m. abscess
    m. endocarditis
    m. thrombosis
    m. thrombus
muramidase
murine typhus
murmur
    accidental m.
    anemic m.
    aneurysmal m.
    aortic m.
    arterial m.
    atriosystolic m.
    Austin Flint m.
    bellows m.
    bicuspid m.
    blowing m.
    brain m.
    Cabot-Locke m.
    cardiac m.
    cardiopulmonary m.
    cardiorespiratory m.
    Carey Coombs m.
    Cole-Cecil m.
    continuous m.
    cooing m.
    Coombs m.
    crescendo m.
    Cruveilhier-Baumgarten m.
    diamond-shaped m.
    diastolic m. (DM)
    Duroziez m.
    dynamic m.
    early diastolic m.
    ejection m.
    endocardial m.
    extracardiac m.
    Flint m.
    Fräntzel m.
    friction m.
    functional m.

Gibson m.
Graham Steell m.
Hamman m.
hemic m.
Hodgkin-Key m.
holosystolic m.
hourglass m.
innocent m.
inorganic m.
late apical systolic m.
late diastolic m.
machinery m.
middiastolic m.
mill wheel m.
mitral m.
obstructive m.
organic m.
pansystolic m.
pericardial m.
presystolic m.
pulmonary m.
pulmonic m.
regurgitant m.
Roger m.
sea gull m.
Steell m.
stenosal m.
Still m.
systolic m.
tricuspid m.
venous m.
vesicular m.

Murphy
    M. button
    M. drip
    M. percussion
    M. sign
Murray Valley encephalitis
Musca
muscae volitantes
muscaria
    Amanita m.
muscarine
muscarinic agonist
muscle
    abdominal external oblique m.
    abdominal internal oblique m.
    abductor digiti minimi m.
    abductor hallucis m.
    abductor pollicis brevis m.
    abductor pollicis longus m.
    accessory flexor m.

adductor brevis m.
adductor hallucis m.
adductor longus m.
adductor magnus m.
adductor minimus m.
adductor pollicis m.
Albinus m.
anconeus m.
anorectoperineal m.
antagonistic m.
anterior auricular m.
anterior cervical
  intertransversarii m.
anterior cervical intertransverse m.
anterior rectus m.
anterior scalene m.
anterior serratus m.
anterior tibial m.
anterior tibiofascial m.
antigravity m.
antitragicus m.
appendicular m.
arrector pili m.
articular m.
articularis cubiti m.
articularis genus m.
aryepiglottic m.
auricular m.
auricularis anterior m.
auricularis posterior m.
auricularis superior m.
axial m.
axillary arch m.
Bell m.
biceps brachii m.
biceps femoris m.
bipennate m.
Bochdalek m.
Bowman m.
brachial m.
brachialis m.
brachioradial m.
brachioradialis m.
branchiomeric m.
Braune m.
bronchoesophageal m.
bronchoesophageus m.
Brücke m.
buccinator m.
bulbocavernosus m.
bulbospongiosus m.
cardiac m.

M

NOTES

muscle *(continued)*

Casser perforated m.
ceratocricoid m.
ceratoglossus m.
cervical iliocostal m.
cervical interspinal m.
cervical longissimus m.
cervical rotator m.
cheek m.
chin m.
chondroglossus m.
ciliary m.
coccygeal m.
coccygeus m.
Coiter m.
compressor urethra m.
m. contraction headache
coracobrachial m.
coracobrachialis m.
corrugator cutis m.
corrugator supercilii m.
cowl m.
Crampton m.
cremaster m.
cricopharyngeus m.
cricothyroid m.
cruciate m.
cutaneous m.
dartos m.
deep flexor m.
deep transverse perineal m.
deltoid m.
depressor anguli oris m.
depressor labii inferioris m.
depressor septi m.
depressor supercilii m.
detrusor m.
digastric m.
dilator pupillae m.
dorsal interossei interosseous m.
dorsal sacrococcygeal m.
Dupré m.
Duverney m.
elevator m.
m. energy technique
epicranial m.
epicranius m.
erector spinae m.
extensor carpi radialis brevis m.
extensor carpi radialis longus m.
extensor carpi ulnaris m.
extensor digiti minimi m.
extensor digitorum m.
extensor digitorum brevis m.
extensor digitorum longus m.
extensor hallucis brevis m.
extensor hallucis longus m.
extensor indicis m.
extensor pollicis brevis m.

extensor pollicis longus m.
external intercostal m.
external oblique m.
external obturator m.
external pterygoid m.
external sphincter m.
extraocular m.
extrinsic m.
facial m.
femoral m.
m. fiber
fibularis brevis m.
fibularis longus m.
fibularis tertius m.
fixator m.
flat m.
flexor accessorius m.
flexor carpi radialis m.
flexor carpi ulnaris m.
flexor digiti minimi brevis m.
flexor digitorum brevis m.
flexor digitorum longus m.
flexor digitorum profundus m.
flexor digitorum superficialis m.
flexor hallucis brevis m.
flexor hallucis longus m.
flexor pollicis brevis m.
flexor pollicis longus m.
frontalis m.
fusiform m.
Gantzer m.
gastrocnemius m.
gastrointestinal smooth m.
Gavard m.
genioglossal m.
genioglossus m.
geniohyoid m.
gluteus maximus m.
gluteus medius m.
gluteus minimus m.
gracilis m.
great adductor m.
greater pectoral m.
greater posterior rectus m.
greater psoas m.
greater rhomboid m.
greater zygomatic m.
Guthrie m.
hamstring m.
4-headed m.
helicis major m.
helicis minor m.
m. hemoglobin
Horner m.
Houston m.
hyoglossal m.
hyoglossus m.
iliac m.
iliacus minor m.

iliococcygeal m.
iliococcygeus m.
iliocostal m.
iliocostalis cervicis m.
iliocostalis lumborum m.
iliocostalis thoracis m.
iliopsoas m.
index extensor m.
inferior constrictor m.
inferior gemellus m.
inferior lingual m.
inferior longitudinal m.
inferior oblique m.
inferior posterior serratus m.
inferior rectus m.
inferior tarsal m.
infrahyoid m.
infraspinatus m.
innermost intercostal m.
intermediate great m.
intermediate vastus m.
internal intercostal m.
internal oblique m.
internal obturator m.
internal pterygoid m.
internal sphincter m.
interosseous m.
interspinal m.
interspinales cervicis m.
interspinales lumborum m.
interspinales thoracis m.
intertransversarii m.
intertransverse m.
intrinsic m.
involuntary m.
ischiocavernous m.
Jung m.
Kohlrausch m.
Landström m.
Langer m.
lateral cricoarytenoid m.
lateral great m.
lateral pterygoid m.
lateral rectus m.
lateral vastus m.
latissimus dorsi m.
lesser rhomboid m.
lesser zygomatic m.
levator anguli oris m.
levator ani m.
levatores costarum breves m.
levatores costarum longi m.

levator labii superioris m.
levator palati m.
levator palpebrae superioris m.
levator prostatae m.
levator scapulae m.
lcvator vcli palatini m.
lingual m.
long adductor m.
long extensor m.
long fibular m.
long flexor m.
longissimus capitis m.
longissimus cervicis m.
longissimus thoracis m.
long levatores costarum m.
long palmar m.
long peroneal m.
long radial extensor m.
longus capitis m.
longus colli m.
lumbar iliocostal m.
lumbar interspinal m.
lumbar quadrate m.
lumbar rotator m.
lumbrical m.
Marcacci m.
masseter m.
masticatory m.
medial great m.
medial lumbar intertransversarii m.
medial lumbar intertransverse m.
medial posterior cervical
  intertransversarii m.
medial pterygoid m.
medial rectus m.
medial vastus m.
mentalis m.
Merkel m.
middle constrictor m.
middle scalene m.
mimetic m.
multifidus m.
mylohyoid m.
nasal m.
nasalis m.
obturator externus m.
obturator internus m.
occipitofrontal m.
occipitofrontalis m.
omohyoid m.
opponens digiti minimi m.
opponens pollicis m.

M

NOTES

muscle *(continued)*

orbicularis oculi m.
orbicularis oris m.
orbital m.
orbitalis m.
palatoglossus m.
palatopharyngeal m.
palatopharyngeus m.
palmar interosseous m.
papillary m.
pectinate m.
pectineal m.
pectineus m.
peroneus tertius m.
piriform m.
piriformis m.
plantar interosseous m.
plantaris m.
m. plate
platysma m.
pleuroesophageal m.
popliteal m.
popliteus m.
procerus m.
pronator quadratus m.
pronator teres m.
pubococcygeal m.
pubococcygeus m.
puboprostatic m.
puborectal m.
puborectalis m.
pubovaginal m.
pubovaginalis m.
pubovesical m.
pubovesicalis m.
pyramidal auricular m.
pyramidalis m.
quadratus femoris m.
quadratus labii superioris m.
quadratus lumborum m.
quadratus plantae m.
quadriceps femoris m.
radial flexor m.
rectococcygeal m.
rectococcygeus m.
rectourethralis m.
rectouterine m.
rectovesical m.
rectovesicalis m.
rectus abdominis m.
rectus capitis anterior m.
rectus capitis lateralis m.
rectus capitis posterior major m.
rectus capitis posterior minor m.
rectus femoris m.
red m.
Reisseisen m.
risorius m.
rotatores m.

salpingopharyngeus m.
sartorius m.
scalenus medius m.
scalenus minimus m.
semimembranosus m.
semispinalis capitis m.
semispinalis cervicis m.
semispinalis thoracis m.
semitendinosus m.
serratus anterior m.
m. serum
short adductor m.
short extensor m.
short flexor m.
short radial extensor m.
skeletal m.
smaller posterior rectus m.
smooth m.
soleus m.
m. spasm
sphincter m.
spinal m.
spinalis capitis m.
spinalis cervicis m.
spinalis thoracis m.
splenius capitis m.
splenius cervicis m.
stapedius m.
sternal m.
sternalis m.
sternocleidomastoid m.
sternohyoid m.
sternomastoid m.
sternothyroid m.
striated m.
styloglossus m.
stylohyoid m.
stylopharyngeal m.
stylopharyngeus m.
subclavian m.
subclavius m.
subcostal m.
subscapular m.
subscapularis m.
superficial flexor m.
superficial transverse perineal m.
superior auricular m.
superior constrictor m.
superior gemellus m.
superior oblique m.
superior rectus m.
supinator m.
supraspinatus m.
supraspinous m.
suspensory m.
synergistic m.
temporal m.
temporalis m.
temporoparietal m.

temporoparietalis m.
tensor fasciae latae m.
tensor tympani m.
tensor veli palati m.
teres major m.
teres minor m.
third peroneal m.
thoracic longissimus m.
thyroarytenoid m.
thyroepiglottic m.
thyroepiglottidean m.
thyrohyoid m.
tibialis anterior m.
tibialis posterior m.
m. tone
trachealis m.
tragicus m.
transverse m.
transversospinal m.
transversospinalis m.
transversus abdominis m.
transversus menti m.
transversus nuchae m.
transversus thoracis m.
trapezius m.
triangular m.
triceps brachii m.
triceps surae m.
ulnar extensor m.
ulnar flexor m.
uvular m.
vastus intermedius m.
vastus lateralis m.
vastus medialis m.
vertical m.
vocal m.
vocalis m.
voluntary m.
white m.
zygomaticus major m.
muscle-bound
muscle-sparing thoracotomy
muscle-splitting incision
muscular
m. asthenopia
m. atrophy
m. coat
m. dystrophy
m. endurance
m. power
m. relaxant
m. rigidity

m. sense
m. tissue
m. triangle
m. tunic
muscularis mucosae
muscularity
musculature
musculi (*pl. of* musculus)
musculoaponeurotic
musculocutaneous nerve
musculomembranous
musculophrenic
m. artery
m. vein
musculorum
lacuna m.
musculoskeletal
musculospiral paralysis
musculotendinous
musculotropic
musculotubal canal
musculus, pl. **musculi**
m. attollens aurem
m. attollens auriculam
m. attrahens aurem
m. attrahens auriculam
m. quadratus labii superioris
m. thyrohyoideus
m. tibiofascialis anterior
m. tibiofascialis anticus
mushroom poisoning
musical rhonchi
musicotherapy
Musset sign
mussitation
Mussy
Guéneau de M.
mustache dressing
mustard
black m.
hemisulfur m.
Mustard operation
mutagen
frameshift m.
mutagenesis
cassette m.
insertional m.
mutagenic
mutant
active m.
amber m.
auxotrophic m.

M

NOTES

mutant *(continued)*
    cold-sensitive m.
    conditional-lethal m.
    conditionally lethal m.
    deficiency m.
    m. gene
    inactive m.
mutase
    ketone-aldehyde m.
mutation
    addition m.
    addition-deletion m.
    amber m.
    back m.
    deletion m.
    frameshift m.
    induced m.
    lethal m.
    missense m.
    neutral m.
    point m.
    m. rate
    somatic m.
    spontaneous m.
    suppressor m.
    transition m.
    transversion m.
mute
mutilans
    arthritis m.
    keratoma hereditarium m.
mutilating keratoderma
mutilation
mutism
    akinetic m.
    elective m.
mutualism
mutualist
mutual resistance
mV
    millivolt
MVA
    motor vehicle accident
myalgia
    epidemic m.
myalgic encephalomyelitis
myasthenia
    m. angiosclerotica
    m. gravis
myasthenic
    m. facies
    m. syndrome
myatonia congenita
myatony
mycelian
mycelium
    aerial m.
mycete
mycetism

mycetismus
mycetogenetic
mycetogenic
mycetoma
mycid
mycobacteria
    atypical m.
    Runyon group I–IV m.
mycobacteriosis
Mycobacterium
    M. avium
    M. avium-intracellulare (MAI)
    M. avium-intracellulare complex
    M. bovis
    M. chelonae
    M. kansasii
    M. leprae
    M. marinum
    M. scrofulaceum
    M. tuberculosis
    M. vaccae
mycodermatitis
mycoides
    Mycoplasma m.
mycologist
mycology
    medical m.
mycophage
Mycoplasma
    M. hominis
    M. mycoides
    M. pharyngis
    M. pneumoniae
mycoplasmal pneumonia
mycosis fungoides
mycotic
    m. aneurysm
    m. keratitis
    m. stomatitis
mycotoxicosis
mycotoxin
mycovirus
mydriasis
    alternating m.
    amaurotic m.
    bounding m.
    paralytic m.
    spinal m.
mydriatic
myectomy
myectopia
myectopy
myelapoplexy
myelatelia
myelencephalon
myelin
    m. sheath
    Weigert stain for m.
myelinated

myelination
myelinolysis
    central pontine m.
myelitic
myelitis
    acute necrotizing m.
    acute transverse m.
    ascending m.
    bulbar m.
    concussion m.
    demyelinated m.
    Foix-Alajouanine m.
    funicular m.
    metastatic m.
    subacute necrotizing m.
myeloblast
myeloblastemia
myeloblastic leukemia
myeloblastoma
myeloblastosis
myelocele
myelocyst
myelocystic
myelocystocele
myelocystomeningocele
myelocyte
myelocythemia
myelocytic leukemia
myelocytoma
myelocytomatosis
myelocytosis
myelodysplasia
myelodysplastic syndrome
myelofibrosis
myelogenesis
myelogenetic
myelogenic leukemia
myelogenous leukemia
myelogone
myelogonium
myelogram
    cervical m.
    lumbar m.
myelography
    computer-assisted m. (CAM)
myeloid
    m. leukemia
    m. metaplasia
    m. sarcoma
    m. series
    m. tissue
myeloid-erythrocyte (M:E)

myeloidosis
myelokathexis
myelolipoma
myeloma
    amyloidosis of multiple m.
    Bence Jones m.
    endothelial m.
    giant cell m.
    L-chain m.
    multiple m.
    m. multiplex
    plasma cell m.
myelomalacia
    angiodysgenetic m.
myelomatosis
myelomeningocele
myelomere
myeloneuritis
myelonic
myelopathic anemia
myelopathy
    carcinomatous m.
    compressive m.
    diabetic m.
    radiation m.
myelopetal
myelophthisic anemia
myelophthisis
myeloplast
myelopoiesis
myelopoietic
myeloproliferative syndrome
myeloradiculitis
myeloradiculodysplasia
myeloradiculopathy
myelorrhagia
myelorrhaphy
myelosclerosis
myelosis
    aleukemic m.
    chronic erythremic m.
    chronic nonleukemic m.
    erythremic m.
    funicular m.
    leukemic m.
    leukopenic m.
myelotomy
    Bischof m.
    commissural m.
    midline m.
myelotoxic
myenteric plexus

M

NOTES

myenteron
myesthesia
myiasis
    accidental m.
    African furuncular m.
    aural m.
    human botfly m.
    intestinal m.
mylohyoid
    m. muscle
    m. nerve
myoarchitectonic
myoblast
myoblastic
myoblastoma
    granular cell m.
myobradia
myocardia (*pl. of* myocardium)
myocardial
    m. abscess
    m. bridging
    m. depressant factor (MDF)
    m. disease
    m. dysfunction
    m. hibernation
    m. hypertrophy
    m. infarction (MI)
    m. insufficiency
    m. oxygen consumption
    m. stiffness
    m. tension
myocardiograph
myocardiopathy
    alcoholic m.
    chagasic m.
myocarditis
    acute isolated m.
    chronic m.
    Fiedler m.
    giant cell m.
    idiopathic m.
    indurative m.
    rheumatic m.
    tuberculoid m.
    tuberculous m.
myocardium, pl. **myocardia**
    hibernating m.
myocele
myocellulitis
myocerosis
myoclonia
    fibrillary m.
myoclonic
    m. absence
    m. astatic epilepsy
    m. attack
    m. seizure
myoclonica
    dyssynergia cerebellaris m.

myoclonus
    benign infantile m.
    m. epilepsy
    epileptic m.
    intention m.
    m. multiplex
    nocturnal m.
    postural m.
    spinal m.
    stimulus sensitive m.
myocutaneous
myocyte
    Anitschkow m.
myocytolysis
myocytoma
myodemia
myodynia
myodystony
myodystrophia
myodystrophy
myoedema
myoelastic
myoendocarditis
myoepithelial
myoepithelioma
myoepithelium
myofascial
myofascitis
myofibril
myofibroblast
myofibroma
myofibromatosis
    infantile m.
myofibrosis
myofibrositis
myofilament
myofunctional therapy
myogenesis
myogenetic
myogenic
    m. paralysis
    m. torticollis
myogenous
myoglobin
    carbonmonoxy m.
myoglobinuria
    familial m.
    idiopathic m.
    paroxysmal m.
    traumatic m.
myoglobulin
myoglobulinuria
myogram
myograph
myographic
myography
myoid cell
myokinesimeter

myokymia
    facial m.
    generalized m.
    hereditary m.
    limb m.
myolipoma
myology
    descriptive m.
myolysis
    cardiotoxic m.
myoma
myomalacia
myomatous
myomectomy
    abdominal m.
    left ventricular m.
myomelanosis
myomere
myometer
myometrial
myometritis
myometrium
myonecrosis
myoneme
myoneural
    m. blockade
    m. blocking agent
    m. junction
myopalmus
myoparalysis
myoparesis
myopathic scoliosis
myopathy
    carcinomatous m.
    centronuclear m.
    distal m.
    dysthyroid m.
    endocrine m.
    minicore-multicore m.
    mitochondrial m.
    ocular m.
    proximal myotonic m.
    steroid m.
myopericarditis
myopia
    axial m.
    curvature m.
    degenerative m.
    index m.
    malignant m.
    pathologic m.

    primary m.
    prodromal m.
myopic
    m. astigmatism
    m. crescent
    m. reflex
myoplasm
myoplastic
myoplasty
myorrhaphy
myorrhexis
myosalpinx
myosarcoma
myosclerosis
myosin filament
myositic
myositis
    cervical m.
    epidemic m.
    m. epidemica acuta
    m. fibrosa
    infectious m.
    interstitial m.
    multiple m.
    m. ossificans
myospasm
    cervical m.
myospasmus
myotactic
myotasis
myotatic
    m. contraction
    m. irritability
    m. reflex
myotenositis
myotenotomy
myotherapy
myotome
myotomy
    cricopharyngeal m.
    Heller m.
myotonia congenita
myotonic
    m. chondrodystrophy
    m. dystrophy
    m. response
myotonoid
myotonus
myotony
myotrophy
myotube
myringa

M

NOTES

myringectomy
myringitis
    bullous m.
myringoplasty
myringosclerosis
myringostapediopexy
myringotomy
myrinx
myrmecia
mysophilia
mysophobia
myxadenoma
myxasthenia
myxedema
    circumscribed m.
    congenital m.
    infantile m.
    pituitary m.
    pretibial m.
myxedematoid
myxedematosus
    lichen m.

myxedematous
myxochondrofibrosarcoma
myxochondroma
myxocyte
myxoedema
myxofibroma
myxofibrosarcoma
myxoid cyst
myxolipoma
myxoma
    atrial m.
myxomatodes
    fibroma m.
myxomatosis
myxomatous
myxomembranous colitis
myxopapillary ependymoma
myxopapilloma
myxopoiesis
myxosarcoma

N
    newton
        N terminus
nabothian
        n. cyst
        n. follicle
nacreous
NADH
        fumarate reductase NADH
        lipoamide reductase NADH
NADP+
        alcohol dehydrogenase NADP+
NADPH
        enoyl-ACP reductase NADPH
Naegeli syndrome
naeslundii
        Actinomyces n.
Naffziger operation
Nägele
        N. obliquity
        N. pelvis
        N. rule
Nagel test
nail
        n. bed
        egg shell n.
        n. fold
        half and half n.
        hippocratic n.
        ingrown n.
        Küntscher n.
        lunule of n.
        n. nipper
        pincer n.
        n. pit
        n. plate
        shell n.
        n. skin
        spoon n.
Nair buffered methylene blue stain
Nakagawa
        angioblastoma of N.
Nakanishi stain
naked virus
nalidixic acid
name
        generic n.
        nonproprietary n.
        proprietary n.
        trivial n.
Nance-Insley syndrome
Nance-Sweeney chondrodysplasia
nanism
nanocephalic
nanocephalous

nanocephaly
nanocormia
nanogram
nanomelia
nanometer
nanometre
nanum
        Microsporum n.
naphtha
        coal tar n.
naphthol yellow S
napsylate
        levopropoxyphene n.
narcissism
narcoanalysis
narcohypnia
narcohypnosis
narcolepsy
narcosis
        adsorption theory of n.
        CO_2 n.
        intravenous n.
        nitrogen n.
        n. paralysis
narcosynthesis
narcotherapy
narcotic
        n. agonist
        n. agonist-antagonist
        n. blockade
        n. poison
        n. reversal
naris, pl. **nares**
        anterior n.
        external n.
        internal n.
narrow-angle glaucoma
narrowband
narrowing
        discrete n.
nasal
        n. bone
        n. capsule
        n. cavity
        n. congestion
        n. crest
        n. deformity
        n. emission
        n. escape
        n. flaring
        n. fracture
        n. herpes
        n. meatus
        n. muscle
        n. pit

N

nasal *(continued)*
    n. point
    n. reflex
    n. septal cartilage
    n. septum
    n. speculum
    n. spine
    n. tampon
    n. turbinate
    n. vestibule
nasalis muscle
nascent
nasi
    agger n.
    ala n.
    cavum n.
    columella n.
    dorsum n.
    granulosis rubra n.
    meatus n.
nasoalveolar cyst
nasoantral
nasociliary nerve
nasoendoscope
nasoendoscopy
nasofrontal vein
nasogastric tube
nasolabial lymph node
nasolacrimal
    n. canal
    n. duct
nasomaxillary fracture
nasooral
nasopalatine
    n. cyst
    n. nerve
nasopharyngeal
    n. airway
    n. carcinoma
    n. leishmaniasis
nasopharyngeus
    meatus n.
nasopharyngolaryngoscope
nasopharyngoscopy
nasopharynx
nasosinusitis
nasotracheal tube
Nasse law
nata
    pro re n.
natality
natimortality
natremia
natriferic
natrium
natriuresis
natriuretic
natural
    n. abortion

    n. antibody
    n. dye
    n. immunity
    n. killer (NK)
    n. killer cell
    n. killer cell leukemia
    n. pitch
    n. resistance
    n. selection
naturales
    per vias n.
naturopathic
naturopathy
nausea
    epidemic n.
    n. gravidarum
    n. and vomiting (N&V)
    n., vomiting, and diarrhea (NVD)
nauseant
nauseate
nauseated
nauseous
Nauta stain
navel
navicular
    n. abdomen
    n. arthritis
    n. bone
    n. cell
    n. fossa
navigator echo
n-capric acid
n-caproic acid
N-carbamoylaspartic acid
Nd:YAG
    neodymium-yttrium-aluminum-garnet
    Nd:YAG laser
near-and-far suture
near point
near-point reaction
nearsightedness
nearthrosis
nebula
nebulizer
    jet n.
    ultrasonic n.
necatoriasis
neck
    buffalo n.
    bull n.
    dental n.
    Madelung n.
    stiff n.
    webbed n.
necklace
    Casal n.
neck-righting reflex
necrobiotic
necrocytosis

necrogenica
    verruca n.
necrogenic wart
necrology
necrolysis
    toxic epidermal n.
necromania
necrophagous
necrophilia
necrophilism
necrophilous
necrophobia
necropsy
necrose
necrosis
    acute massive liver n.
    acute retinal n. (ARN)
    aseptic n.
    avascular n.
    bridging hepatic n.
    caseation n.
    caseous n.
    central n.
    cheesy n.
    coagulation n.
    colliquative n.
    contraction band n.
    cystic medial n.
    embolic n.
    epiphysial aseptic n.
    fat n.
    fibrinoid n.
    focal n.
    gangrenous n.
    glomerular n.
    hyaline n.
    ischemic n.
    laminar cortical n.
    liquefaction n.
    liquefactive n.
    mercurial n.
    moist n.
    pressure n.
    progressive emphysematous n.
    progressive outer retinal n.
    radiation n.
    scrotal fat n.
    septic n.
    simple n.
    superficial n.
    total n.
    transmural n.

    tubular n.
    zonal n.
necrospermia
necrotic
    n. arachnidism
    n. cirrhosis
    n. inflammation
    n. pulp
necroticans
    enteritis n.
necrotizing
    n. arteriolitis
    n. enterocolitis
    n. inflammation
    n. keratitis
    n. ulcerative gingivitis
    n. vasculitis
necrotomy
needle
    aneurysm n.
    artery n.
    aspirating n.
    atraumatic n.
    n. bath
    n. biopsy
    biopsy n.
    butterfly n.
    cataract n.
    cutting n.
    Deschamps n.
    discission n.
    electrosurgical n.
    Emmet n.
    exploring n.
    n. forceps
    Francke n.
    Frazier n.
    Gillmore n.
    Hagedorn n.
    hypodermic n.
    knife n.
    lumbar puncture n.
    Millner n.
    popoff n.
    Salah sternal puncture n.
needle-carrier
needle-driver
needle-holder
needling
Neer impingement sign
negation
    delusion of n.

NOTES

N

negative
    n. accommodation
    n. anergy
    n. base excess
    n. convergence
    n. electrode
    n. end-expiratory pressure
    false n.
    n. myoclonic seizure
    n. pressure ventilation
    n. scotoma
    n. stain
    n. symptom
negativism
negatron
neglect
    visual n.
Negri body
Neisseria
    N. gonorrhoeae
    N. meningitidis
neisseria
Neisser-Wechsberg phenomenon
Nélaton
    N. catheter
    N. line
Nelson syndrome
nematocyst
nematodiasis
    cerebrospinal n.
nematoid
neoadjuvant therapy
neoantigen
neoarthrosis
neobladder
neoblastic
neocystostomy
neocyte
neodymium
neodymium-yttrium-aluminum-garnet
    (Nd:YAG)
neogenesis
neogenetic
neokinetic
neologism
neomembrane
neon
neonatal
    n. anemia
    n. diagnosis
    n. hepatitis
    n. herpes
    n. hyperbilirubinemia
    n. hypocalcemia (NHC)
    n. intensive care unit (NICU)
    lupus erythematosus, n.
    n. medicine
    n. mortality rate
    n. neutropenia

    n. pneumonia
    n. seizure
    n. tetany
neonate
neonatologist
neonatology
neonatorum
    acne n.
    anemia n.
    anoxia n.
    asphyxia n.
    blennorrhea n.
    dermatitis exfoliativa n.
    edema n.
    erythema toxicum n.
    icterus n.
    impetigo n.
    mastitis n.
    melena n.
    ophthalmia n.
    sclerema n.
    tetanus n.
neoneurotization
neoplasia
    cervical intraepithelial n.
    lobular n.
    multiple endocrine n. (MEN)
    prostatic intraepithelial n.
    vaginal intraepithelial n.
    vulvar intraepithelial n.
neoplasm
    adrenal n.
    benign n.
    histoid n.
    malignant n.
    metastatic n.
    Revised European-American
        Classification of Lymphoid N.'s
        (REAL)
    stromal cell n.
    trophoblastic n.
    vascular n.
neoplastic
neopterin
neostriatum
neothalamus
neovascularization
    choroidal n.
    classic choroidal n.
    occult choroidal n.
neper
nephelometry
nephralgia
nephrectomy
    abdominal n.
    laparoscopic n.
    lumbar n.
    morcellated n.
    posterior n.

radical n.
simple n.
nephrelcosis
nephric
nephritic syndrome
nephritis
acute interstitial n.
analgesic n.
antibasement membrane n.
antikidney serum n.
chronic n.
focal n.
glomerular n.
hemorrhagic n.
hereditary n.
immune complex n.
interstitial n.
lupus n.
mesangial n.
salt-losing n.
serum n.
suppurative n.
transfusion n.
tubulointerstitial n.
nephritogenic
nephrocalcinosis
nephrocardiac
nephrocele
nephrocystosis
nephrogenetic
nephrogenic
n. ascites
n. cord
n. diabetes insipidus
nephrogenous albuminuria
nephrogram
nephrography
nephroid
nephrolithiasis
nephrolithotomy
nephrology
nephrolysis
nephrolytic
nephroma
mesoblastic n.
nephromegaly
nephron
nephronic loop
nephropathia
nephropathy
acute hypokalemic n.
analgesic n.

Balkan n.
Danubian endemic familial n.
diabetic n.
hypokalemic n.
IgA n.
IgM n.
nephropexy
nephrophthisis
familial juvenile n.
nephroptosis, nephroptosia
nephropyosis
nephrorrhaphy
nephrosclerosis
arterial n.
arteriolar n.
benign n.
malignant n.
nephrosclerotic
nephroscope
nephrosis
acute lobar n.
amyloid n.
chronic n.
congenital n.
familial n.
hemoglobinuric n.
hypoxic n.
lipoid n.
toxic n.
nephrostogram
nephrostomy tube
nephrotic syndrome
nephrotomogram
nephrotomography
nephrotomy
abdominal n.
anatrophic n.
lumbar n.
nephrotoxic
nephrotoxicity
nephrotoxin
nephrotrophic, nephrotropic
nephrotuberculosis
nephroureterectomy
nephroureterocystectomy
Neptune girdle
neptunium
Néri sign
Nernst equation
nerve
abdominopelvic splanchnic n.
abducens n.

N

NOTES

nerve *(continued)*
abducent n.
accelerator n.
accessory phrenic n.
acoustic n.
afferent n.
Andersch n.
anococcygeal n.
anterior ampullary n.
anterior antebrachial n.
anterior auricular n.
anterior crural n.
anterior ethmoidal n.
anterior femoral cutaneous n.
anterior interosseous n.
anterior labial n.
anterior scrotal n.
anterior superior alveolar n.
anterior supraclavicular n.
anterior tibial n.
aortic n.
Arnold n.
articular n.
auditory n.
augmentor n.
auriculotemporal n.
autonomic n.
n. avulsion
axillary n.
baroreceptor n.
Bell respiratory n.
n. block
n. block anesthesia
Bock n.
buccal n.
buccinator n.
cardiopulmonary splanchnic n.
caroticotympanic n.
carotid sinus n.
cavernous n.
centrifugal n.
centripetal n.
cervical splanchnic n.
circumflex n.
coccygeal n.
cochlear n.
common fibular n.
common palmar digital n.
common peroneal n.
common plantar digital n.
n. conduction
cranial n.
crural interosseous n.
cubital n.
cutaneous cervical n.
Cyon n.
dead n.
n. decompression
deep fibular n.

deep peroneal n.
deep petrosal n.
deep temporal n.
dental n.
depressor n.
dorsal digital n.
dorsal interosseous n.
dorsal lateral cutaneous n.
dorsal medial cutaneous n.
dorsal scapular n.
efferent n.
eighth cranial n.
eleventh cranial n.
esodic n.
excitor n.
excitoreflex n.
exodic n.
external carotid n.
external respiratory n.
external saphenous n.
external sheath of optic n.
external spermatic n.
facial n.
femoral n.
fifth cranial n.
first cranial n.
fourth cranial n.
fourth lumbar n.
frontal n.
furcal n.
Galen n.
gangliated n.
ganglionated n.
genitocrural n.
genitofemoral n.
glossopharyngeal n.
great auricular n.
greater occipital n.
greater palatine n.
greater splanchnic n.
greater superficial petrosal n.
great sciatic n.
hemorrhoidal n.
Hering sinus n.
hypogastric n.
hypoglossal n.
iliohypogastric n.
ilioinguinal n.
inferior alveolar n.
inferior anal n.
inferior cervical cardiac n.
inferior clunial n.
inferior dental n.
inferior gluteal n.
inferior hemorrhoidal n.
inferior laryngeal n.
inferior lateral brachial
   cutaneous n.
inferior maxillary n.

inferior rectal n.
infraorbital n.
infratrochlear n.
inhibitory n.
inner sheath of optic n.
intercarotid n.
intercostal n.
intercostobrachial n.
intercostohumeral n.
intermediary n.
intermediate dorsal cutaneous n.
intermediate supraclavicular n.
internal carotid n.
internal saphenous n.
internal sheath of optic n.
interosseous n.
Jacobson n.
jugular n.
lacrimal n.
Latarget n.
lateral ampullar n.
lateral dorsal cutaneous n.
lateral femoral cutaneous n.
lateral pectoral n.
lateral plantar n.
lateral supraclavicular n.
lateral sural cutaneous n.
least splanchnic n.
lesser internal cutaneous n.
lesser occipital n.
lesser palatine n.
lesser splanchnic n.
lesser superficial petrosal n.
lingual n.
long buccal n.
long ciliary n.
long saphenous n.
long subscapular n.
long thoracic n.
lowest splanchnic n.
Ludwig n.
lumbar splanchnic n.
lumboinguinal n.
mandibular n.
masseteric n.
masticator n.
maxillary n.
medial antebrachial cutaneous n.
medial anterior thoracic n.
medial brachial cutaneous n.
medial clunial n.
medial crural cutaneous n.

medial dorsal cutaneous n.
medial pectoral n.
medial plantar n.
medial popliteal n.
medial supraclavicular n.
medial sural cutaneous n.
median n.
mental n.
middle cervical cardiac n.
middle cluneal n.
middle meningeal n.
middle supraclavicular n.
mixed n.
motor n.
musculocutaneous n.
mylohyoid n.
nasociliary n.
nasopalatine n.
ninth cranial n.
obturator n.
oculomotor n.
olfactory n.
ophthalmic n.
optic n.
parasympathetic n.
perineal n.
phrenic n.
n. plexus
pneumogastric n.
posterior auricular n.
posterior interosseous n.
pressor n.
pterygoid n.
pudendal n.
radial n.
saccular n.
sacral splanchnic n.
saphenous n.
sciatic n.
second cranial n.
secretory n.
sensory n.
seventh cranial n.
sixth cranial n.
somatic n.
spinal n.
subclavian n.
subcostal n.
sublingual n.
suboccipital n.
superior alveolar n.
supraorbital n.

N

NOTES

nerve *(continued)*
    suprascapular n.
    supratrochlear n.
    sural n.
    sympathetic n.
    temporomandibular n.
    tenth cranial n.
    terminal n.
    third cranial n.
    thoracic cardiac n.
    thoracic spinal n.
    thoracodorsal n.
    tibial n.
    transverse cervical n.
    trigeminal n.
    trochlear n.
    twelfth cranial n.
    tympanic n.
    ulnar n.
    utricular n.
    utriculoampullar n.
    vaginal n.
    vagus n.
    vascular n.
    vasomotor n.
    vertebral n.
    vestibular n.
    vestibulocochlear n.
    zygomatic n.
nervimotor
nervonic acid
nervosa
    anorexia n.
    bulimia n.
nervous
    n. bladder
    n. breakdown
    n. indigestion
    n. lobe
    n. system
    n. tinnitus
nervousness
nest
    Brunn n.
    cell n.
    epithelial n.
    isogenous n.
nested polymerase chain reaction
net
    Chiari n.
    chromidial n.
Netherton syndrome
nettle
    sea n.
Nettleshop-Falls albinism
network
    acromial arterial n.
    arteriolar n.
    articular vascular n.

    calcaneal arterial n.
    chromatin n.
    cytokine n.
    dorsal carpal n.
    dorsal venous n.
    lateral malleolar n.
    linin n.
    medial malleolar n.
    Purkinje n.
Neufeld
    N. capsular swelling
    N. reaction
Neumann law
neural
    n. arch
    n. crest
    n. crest syndrome
    n. fold
    n. foramen
    n. groove
    n. hearing loss
    n. plate
    n. spine
neuralgia
    atypical facial n.
    atypical trigeminal n.
    cranial n.
    epileptiform n.
    facial n.
    Fothergill n.
    geniculate n.
    glossopharyngeal n.
    hallucinatory n.
    Hunt n.
    idiopathic n.
    intercostal n.
    mammary n.
    Morton n.
    red n.
    Sluder n.
    sphenopalatine n.
    trifacial n.
    trigeminal n.
neuralgic
    n. amyotrophy
    n. headache
neuraminic acid
neuranagenesis
neurapophysis
neurapraxia
neurasthenia
    angioparalytic n.
    angiopathic n.
    gastric n.
neurasthenic
neuraxis
neurectasis, neurectasia
neurectomy
    gastric n.

presacral n.
vestibular n.
neurectopia, neurectopy
neurenteric cyst
neurergic
neurexeresis
neurilemma cell
neurilemoma
acoustic n.
Antoni type A, B n.
neurimotor
neurinoma
acoustic n.
neuritic
n. atrophoderma
n. plaque
neuritis
adventitial n.
ascending n.
axial n.
brachial n.
central n.
descending n.
Eichhorst n.
endemic n.
fallopian n.
interstitial n.
intraocular n.
Leyden n.
multiple n.
optic n.
parenchymatous n.
retrobulbar n.
segmental n.
senile n.
syphilitic n.
toxic n.
traumatic n.
neuroanastomosis
neuroanatomy
neuroarthropathy
neuroblast
neuroblastoma
neurocardiac
neurochemistry
neurochorioretinitis
neurochoroiditis
neurocladism
neurocranium
cartilaginous n.
membranous n.
neurocristopathy

neurocyte
neurocytolysis
neurocytoma
neurodendrite
neurodermatitis
neurodermatosis
neurodevelopmental treatment
neurodynamic
neurodynia
neuroectoderm
neuroectodermal
neuroencephalomyelopathy
neuroendocrine
neuroendocrinology
neuroepithelial
neuroepithelium
neurofibril
neurofibrillar
neurofibroma
plexiform n.
neurofibromatosis
abortive n.
central type n.
incomplete n.
neurofilament
neuroganglion
neurogenesis
neurogenetic
neurogenic
n. arthritis
n. bladder
n. claudication
n. torticollis
n. tumor
neurogenous
neuroglia
peripheral n.
protoplasmic n.
Weigert stain for n.
neurogliacyte
neuroglial
neurogliar
neurogliomatosis
neurogram
neurohistology
neurohormone
neurohypophysial
neuroid
neurolemma cell
neuroleptanalgesia
neuroleptanesthesia

N

NOTES

neuroleptic
> n. agent
> n. malignant syndrome

neurolinguistic programming
neurological intensive care unit (NICU)
neurologist
neurology
neurolysin
neurolysis
> trigeminal n.

neurolytic
neuroma
> acoustic n.
> amputation n.
> n. cutis
> false n.
> fibrillary n.
> multiple n.'s
> plexiform n.
> n. telangiectodes
> traumatic n.

neuromalacia
neuromatosa
> elephantiasis n.

neuromatosis
neuromere
neuromuscular spindle
neuromyasthenia
> epidemic n.

neuromyelitis optica
neuromyopathy
> carcinomatous n.

neuron
> autonomic motor n.
> bipolar n.
> gamma motor n.
> ganglionic motor n.
> Golgi type I, II n.
> intercalary n.
> internuncial n.
> lower motor n.
> motor n.
> multipolar n.
> unipolar n.

neuronal
neurone
neuronevus
neuronitis
> vestibular n.

neuronopathy
> sensory n.
> X-linked recessive bulbospinal n.

neuronophage
neuronophagia
neuronophagy
neuron-specific enolase
neurooncology
neuroophthalmology
neurootology

neuropacemaker
neuroparalysis
neuroparalytic
> n. keratitis
> n. keratopathy

neuropathia epidemica
neuropathic
> n. arthropathy
> n. bladder
> n. joint

neuropathogenesis
neuropathology
neuropathy
> acute sensory motor axonal n.
> acute sensory-motor axonal n.
> asymmetric motor n.
> auditory n.
> brachial plexus n.
> compression n.
> dapsone n.
> diabetic n.
> diphtheritic n.
> entrapment n.
> familial amyloid n.
> giant axonal n.
> Graves optic n.
> heavy metal n.
> hereditary hypertrophic n.
> hereditary sensory radicular n.
> hypertrophic interstitial n.
> ischemic optic n.
> isoniazid n.
> lead n.
> leprous n.
> vitamin B12 n.

neuropeptide
neuropharmacology
neurophysin
neurophysiology
neuropil, neuropile
neuroplasm
neuroplasty
neuroplegic
neuropodia
neuropore
> anterior n.
> caudal n.
> cranial n.

neuropsychiatry
neuropsychologic disorder
neuropsychopathy
neuroradiology
neuroregulator
neuroretinitis
> diffuse unilateral subacute n. (DUSN)
> Leber idiopathic stellate n.

neurorrhaphy
neurosarcocleisis

neurosarcoidosis
neuroscience
neurosecretion
neurosecretory
neurosis, pl. **neuroses**
    accident n.
    anxiety n.
    battle n.
    cardiac n.
    character n.
    combat n.
    compensation n.
    compulsion n.
    compulsive n.
    conversion hysteria n.
    depressive n.
    experimental n.
    fright n.
    gastric n.
    hypochondriacal n.
    hysterical n.
    transference n.
    traumatic n.
    war n.
neurosplanchnic
neurosurgeon
neurosurgery
    functional n.
neurosuture
neurosyphilis
    asymptomatic n.
    latent n.
    meningeal n.
    meningovascular n.
    paretic n.
    tabetic n.
neurotendinous spindle
neurotensin
neurothekeoma
neurotic
    n. anxiety
    n. atrophy
    n. disorder
neurotization
neurotmesis
neurotomy
neurotonic
neurotoxic
neurotoxin
neurotransmitter
    adrenergic n.
    cholinergic n.

neurotripsy
neurotrophic keratitis
neurotrophy
neurotropic
neurotropy, **neurotropism**
neurotubule
neurovaccine
neurovascular bundle
neurovirus
neurovisceral
neuroviscerolipidosis
    familial n.
neurula, pl. **neurulae**
Neusser granule
neuter
neutral
    n. mutation
    n. occlusion
    n. stain
neutralization
    n. plate
    n. test
neutralizing antibody
neutroclusion
neutron
    epithermal n.
neutropenia
    congenital n.
    idiopathic n.
    malignant n.
    neonatal n.
    periodic n.
    primary splenic n.
neutrophil, **neutrophile**
    band n.
    hypersegmented n.
    immature n.
    juvenile n.
    mature n.
neutrophil-activating
    n.-a. factor
    n.-a. protein
neutrophilia
neutrophilic
    n. dermatosis
    n. leukocyte
    n. lymphocytosis
neutrotaxis
nevoid
nevus, pl. **nevi**
    acquired n.
    balloon cell n.

NOTES

N

nevus *(continued)*
 basal cell n.
 bathing trunk n.
 Becker n.
 blue n.
 blue rubber-bleb n.
 capillary n.
 n. cell
 cellular blue n.
 comedo n.
 n. comedonicus
 compound n.
 congenital n.
 dysplastic n.
 epithelioid cell n.
 erectile n.
 fatty n.
 faun tail n.
 flame n.
 n. flammeus
 giant n.
 giant pigmented n.
 hairy n.
 halo n.
 hard n.
 inflammatory linear verrucous epidermal n.
 intradermal n.
 Ito n.
 Jadassohn n.
 junction n.
 linear epidermal n.
 lymphatic n.
 mixed n.
 n. pigmentosus
 n. pilosus
 soft n.
 spider n.
 n. spilus
 Spitz n.
 strawberry n.
 Sutton n.
 n. unius lateris
 Unna n.
 n. vascularis
 n. vasculosus
 verrucous n.
 vulvar n.
new
 N. Hampshire rule
 N. World leishmaniasis
 N. York Heart Association classification
 N. York virus
newborn
 congenital epulis of n.
Newcastle-Manchester bacillus
Newcomer fixative

Newton
 N. disc
 N. law
newton (N)
newtonian constant of gravitation
newton-meter
nexin
nexus
NHC
 neonatal hypocalcemia
niacin
niacinamide
niche
 enamel n.
 Haudek n.
nicking
 arteriovenous n.
Nick procedure
Nicolle stain
nicotinamide
 n. adenine dinucleotide
 n. adenine dinucleotide phosphate
 n. mononucleotide
nicotinate
 methyl n.
nicotine
nicotinic acid
nictitation
NICU
 neonatal intensive care unit
 neurological intensive care unit
nidal
nidation
NIDDM
 non-insulin-dependent diabetes mellitus
nidulans
 Aspergillus n.
nidus avis
Niemann-Pick
 N.-P. C1 disease
 N.-P. cell
Niemann splenomegaly
niger
 Aspergillus n.
 locus n.
night
 n. blindness
 n. soil
 n. terrors
 n. vision
nightmare
nightshade
 deadly n.
nightstick fracture
nigra
 linea n.
 lingua n.
 substantia n.

nigricans
    acanthosis n.
nigrificans
    Clostridium n.
    Desulfotomaculum n.
nigripalpus
    Culex n.
nigrities
nigromaculis
    Aedes n.
nigrosin
nigrosine
nigrostriatal
nigrum
    catechu n.
    pigmentum n.
nihilism
nihonkaiense
    Diphyllobothrium n.
Nikiforoff method
Nikolsky sign
nil per os
nine
    rule of n.'s
ninhydrin reaction
ninth cranial nerve
niobium
Nipah virus
nipper
    nail n.
nipple
    accessory n.
    aortic n.
    cyclist's n.'s
    invaginated n.
    n. line
    n. shield
Nissen fundoplication
Nissl
    N. body
    N. granule
    N. stain
    N. substance
nit
Nitabuch
    N. layer
    N. membrane
    N. stria
niter
    cubic n.
nitidus
    lichen n.

nitrate
    fused silver n.
    miconazole n.
nitric
    n. acid
    n. oxide
nitridation
nitride
nitrification
nitrile
nitrite
    amyl n.
    isobutyl n.
nitrituria
nitrofurantoin
nitrogen
    n. balance
    blood urea n. (BUN)
    n. cycle
    n. distribution
    n. equivalent
    filtrate n.
    n. group
    heavy n.
    n. lag
    n. narcosis
    nonprotein n.
    n. partition
    undetermined n.
    urea n.
    urinary n.
nitrogenase
nitrogenous
nitroprusside test
nitrosyl
nitrous
    n. acid
    n. oxide
nitryl
NK
    natural killer
    NK cell
NKA
    no known allergies
NKDA
    no known drug allergies
N-methyltransferase
    guanidinoacetate N.-m.
NNRTI
    nonnucleoside reverse transcriptase
    inhibitor

NOTES

N

no

n. evidence of recurrence
n. evidence of recurrent disease
n. known allergies (NKA)
n. known drug allergies (NKDA)
n. significant abnormality

Noack syndrome
nobelium
noble

n. gas
N. position
N. stain

Nocardia

N. *asteroides*
N. *caviae*
N. *farcinica*
N. *mediterranei*
N. *nova*
N. *orientalis*
N. *otitidiscaviarum*
N. *transvalensis*

nocardiosis

granulomatous n.

nocebo
nociceptive
nociceptor
nocifensor
nociperception
nocturia
nocturnal

n. amblyopia
n. dyspnea
n. enuresis
n. myoclonus

nocturnus

angor n.
pavor n.

nodal

n. point
n. tachycardia

nodding spasm
node

abdominal lymph n.
accessory nerve lymph n.
anorectal lymph n.
anterior axillary lymph n.
anterior deep cervical lymph n.
anterior jugular lymph n.
anterior mediastinal lymph n.
anterior superficial cervical
  lymph n.
anterior tibial lymph n.
apical axillary lymph n.
appendicular lymph n.
atrioventricular n.
AV n.
axillary lymph n.
Babès n.
brachial lymph n.

brachiocephalic lymph n.
bronchopulmonary lymph n.
buccal lymph n.
buccinator n.
carinal lymph n.
celiac lymph n.
central axillary lymph n.
central superior mesenteric
  lymph n.
n. of Cloquet
colic lymph n.
common iliac lymph n.
coronary n.
cubital lymph n.
cystic n.
cystic lymph n.
deep anterior cervical lymph n.
deep inguinal lymph n.
deep lateral cervical lymph n.
deep parotid lymph n.
delphian n.
Dürck n.
external iliac lymph n.
facial lymph n.
fibular lymph n.
Flack n.
foraminal lymph n.
gastroduodenal lymph n.
gluteal lymph n.
Haygarth n.
Heberden n.
hemal n.
hemolymph n.
Hensen n.
hepatic lymph n.
hilar lymph n.
humeral axillary lymph n.
ileocolic lymph n.
inferior epigastric lymph n.
inferior mesenteric lymph n.
inferior phrenic lymph n.
inferior tracheobronchial lymph n.
infraauricular deep parotid
  lymph n.
infraauricular subfascial parotid
  lymph n.
intercostal lymph n.
interiliac lymph n.
intermediate lacunar lymph n.
intermediate lumbar lymph n.
internal iliac lymph n.
interpectoral lymph n.
intraglandular deep parotid
  lymph n.
intrapulmonary lymph n.
jugulodigastric lymph n.
juguloomohyoid lymph n.
juxtaesophageal pulmonary
  lymph n.

juxtaintestinal mesenteric lymph n.
Keith and Flack n.
Koch n.
lateral axillary lymph n.
lateral jugular lymph n.
lateral lacunar lymph n.
lateral pericardial lymph n.
left colic lymph n.
left gastric lymph n.
left gastroepiploic lymph n.
left gastroomental lymph n.
left lumbar lymph n.
lingual lymph n.
lumbar lymph n.
lymph n.
lymphatic n.
malar lymph n.
mandibular lymph n.
mastoid lymph n.
medial lacunar lymph n.
mesenteric lymph n.
mesocolic lymph n.
middle colic lymph n.
middle rectal lymph n.
milkers' n.
nasolabial lymph n.
Osler n.
parietal lymph n.
primitive n.
proximal deep inguinal lymph n.
Ranvier n.
n. of Ranvier
retroauricular lymph n.
Rosenmüller n.
sentinel lymph n.
shotty n.
signal lymph n.
sinoatrial n.
sinuatrial n.
Virchow n.
visceral lymph n.

nodi (*pl. of* nodus)

nodosa
arteritis n.
arthritis n.
endophthalmitis ophthalmia n.
periarteritis n.
polyarteritis n.
trichorrhexis n.

nodose rheumatism

nodosity

nodosum
amnion n.
erythema n.

nodosus
Bacteroides n.
Dichelobacter n.

nodous

nodular
n. amyloidosis
n. arteriosclerosis
n. fasciitis
n. leprosy
n. lymphoma
n. metastasis
n. vasculitis

nodularis
prurigo n.

nodulate

nodulated

nodulation

nodule
aggregated lymphatic n.
aggregated lymphoid n.
Albini n.
apple jelly n.
Arantius n.
Aschoff n.
Babès n.
benign rheumatoid n.
Bianchi n.
Bohn n.
Busacca n.
Caplan n.
cold n.
Dalen-Fuchs n.
discrete n.
enamel n.
Gamna-Gandy n.
Gandy-Gamna n.
gastric lymphoid n.
Hoboken n.
hot n.
Jeanselme n.
juxtaarticular n.
laryngeal lymphoid n.
Lisch n.
lymph n.
lymphatic n.
lymphoid n.
malpighian n.
milkers' n.
rheumatoid n.

NOTES

N

nodule *(continued)*
    Schmorl n.
    singer's n.
    Sister Joseph n.
    speaker's n.
    vocal n.
nodulous
nodus, pl. **nodi**
noise
    n. pollution
    white n.
noise-induced hearing loss
nomenclature
    binary n.
    binomial n.
    Cleland n.
    Palmer dental n.
    universal dental n.
    Zsigmondy dental n.
nominal aphasia
nomogram
    blood volume n.
    cartesian n.
    d'Ocagne n.
nomotopic
non–A-E hepatitis
nonbacterial verrucous endocarditis
noncommunicating
    n. hydrocele
    n. hydrocephalus
noncompetitive inhibition
nonconjugative plasmid
noncontained disc herniation
noncovalent bond
nondepolarizing block
nondisjunction
    primary n.
    secondary n.
nonelectrolyte
nonessential amino acid
nonfenestrated forceps
nonfluency
nonfluent aphasia
non-Hodgkin lymphoma
nonimmune serum
non-insulin-dependent diabetes mellitus (NIDDM)
noninvasive
nonionic contrast agent
nonisolated proteinuria
nonlamellar bone
nonmedullated fiber
nonnucleoside reverse transcriptase inhibitor (NNRTI)
nonnutrient
    bioactive n.
nonobstructive
    n. appendicitis
    n. jaundice

nonoral communication
nonossifying fibroma
nonosteogenic fibroma
nonparametric
nonpenetrance
nonpenetrant trait
nonpenetrating wound
nonpitting edema
nonpropositional speech
nonproprietary name
nonprotein nitrogen
nonrapid eye movement
nonreassuring fetal status
nonrebreathing anesthesia
nonresponsive tumor
nonrigid connector
nonsecretor
nonsense triplet
nonsexual generation
nonshivering thermogenesis
nonspecific
    n. building-related illnesses
    n. immunity
    n. protein
nonsteroidal antiinflammatory drug (NSAID)
nonstress test
nonsuppressible insulinlike activity
nonthrombocytopenic purpura
nontoxic goiter
nontropical sprue
nonunion
nonvalent
nonverbal communication
nonviable
nonvital pulp
nonweightbearing exercise
Noonan syndrome
noose suture
noradrenaline
no-reflow phenomenon
norepinephrine
norleucine
norma, pl. **normae**
normal
    n. antibody
    n. antitoxin
    n. concentration
    cupric acetate n.
    n. distribution
    n. human plasma
    n. human serum albumin
    n. occlusion
    n. opsonin
    n. pressure hydrocephalus
    n. range
    n. saline
    n. serum
    n. solution

n. temperature
upper limit of n. (ULN)
n. value
normalization
normal-tension glaucoma
normoblast
normocapnia
normochromia
normochromic anemia
normocytic anemia
normocytosis
normoglycemia
normoglycemic
normokalemia
normokalemic periodic paralysis
normokaliemia
normotensive
normothermia
normotonic
normovolemia
Norrie disease
Norris corpuscle
North American blastomycosis
Northern blot analysis
Norton operation
Norwalk virus
Norwood operation
NOS
not otherwise specified
nose
artificial n.
brandy n.
cleft n.
copper n.
dog n.
external n.
hammer n.
saddle n.
nosebleed
nosepiece
nosoacusis
nosocomial disease
nosogenic
nosologic
nosology
nosomania
nosonomy
nosophilia
nosophobia
nosopoietic
nosotaxy
nostalgia

nostras
influenza n.
nostril
internal n.
nostrum
notal
notancephalia
notanencephalia
notch
acetabular n.
anacrotic n.
angular n.
antegonial n.
anterior cerebellar n.
aortic n.
auricular n.
cardiac n.
cardial n.
Carhart n.
clavicular n.
coracoid n.
costal n.
cotyloid n.
dicrotic n.
digastric n.
ethmoidal n.
fibular n.
frontal n.
greater sciatic n.
hamular n.
Hutchinson crescentic n.
iliosciatic n.
inferior thyroid n.
interarytenoid n.
interclavicular n.
intercondylar n.
intercondyloid n.
intertragic n.
intervertebral n.
ischiatic n.
jugular n.
Kernohan n.
lacrimal n.
lesser sciatic n.
mandibular n.
marsupial n.
mastoid n.
parotid n.
semilunar n.
trochlear n.
vertebral n.
notencephalocele

N

NOTES

Nothnagel syndrome
notice
　advance beneficiary n.
notifiable disease
notochord
notochordal
not otherwise specified (NOS)
nourishment
nova
　Nocardia n.
novo
　de n.
novyi
　Clostridium n.
Novy and MacNeal blood agar
noxious
NPH insulin
NSAID
　nonsteroidal antiinflammatory drug
N-sulfatase
　heparan N-s.
nuchae
　cutis rhomboidalis n.
　erythema n.
　fascia n.
　lichen n.
nuchal
　n. arm
　n. cord
　n. ligament
　n. plane
　n. rigidity
Nuck
　canal of N.
nuclear
　n. aplasia
　n. cataract
　n. envelope
　n. family
　n. inclusion body
　n. jaundice
　n. magnetic resonance
　n. medicine
　n. medicine technologist
　n. membrane
　n. ophthalmoplegia
　n. RNA
　n. spindle
　n. stain
nuclear:cytoplasmic ratio
nuclease
　azotobacter n.
　micrococcal n.
nucleate
nucleated
nucleation
　heterogeneous n.
　homogeneous n.
nuclei (*pl. of* nucleus)

nucleic acid
nucleiform
nucleocapsid
nucleofugal
nucleohistone
nucleoid
　Lavdovsky n.
nucleolar
nucleoliform
nucleoloid
nucleolonema
nucleolus
　chromatin n.
　false n.
nucleon
nucleopetal
nucleophil, nucleophile
nucleophilic
nucleoplasm
nucleoprotein
nucleorrhexis
nucleosidase
　adenosine n.
nucleoside
nucleosome
nucleotidase
nucleotide
　adenine n.
　diphosphopyridine n.
　flavin n.
　triphosphopyridine n.
nucleotidylexotransferase
　DNA n.
nucleotidyltransferase
nucleotoxin
nucleus, pl. nuclei
　abducens n.
　accessory cuneate n.
　accessory olivary n.
　amygdaloid n.
　anterior hypothalamic n.
　anterior interpositus n.
　anterior olfactory n.
　anterior periventricular n.
　anteromedial n.
　anteroventral n.
　arcuate n.
　auditory n.
　autonomic visceral motor nuclei
　basal n.
　basket n.
　Bechterew n.
　benzene n.
　Blumenau n.
　branchiomotor n.
　Burdach n.
　caudal pontine reticular n.
　caudate n.
　central amygdaloid n.

centromedian n.
cerebellar n.
Clarke n.
cortical amygdaloid n.
cuneate n.
cunciform n.
Deiters n.
dentate n.
descending n.
diploid n.
dorsal accessory olivary n.
dorsal lateral geniculate n.
dorsal premammillary n.
dorsal septal n.
dorsal thoracic n.
dorsal vagal n.
dorsolateral n.
dorsomedial hypothalamic n.
droplet n.
Edinger-Westphal n.
emboliform n.
endolemniscal n.
endopeduncular n.
external cuneate n.
facial motor n.
fastigial n.
filiform n.
gametic n.
gelatinous n.
germ n.
gigantocellular n.
globosus n.
gonad n.
gracile n.
Gudden tegmental n.
gustatory n.
habenular n.
hypoglossal n.
inferior olivary n.
inferior salivary n.
inferior salivatory n.
inferior vestibular n.
intercalated n.
intermediolateral n.
intermediomedial n.
interpeduncular n.
interpositus n.
interstitial amygdaloid n.
intralaminar n.
Klein-Gumprecht shadow n.
lateral amygdaloid n.
lateral cervical n.

lateral cuneate n.
lateral dorsal n.
lateral geniculate n.
lateral habenular n.
lateral parabrachial n.
lateral pericuneate n.
lateral posterior n.
lateral preoptic n.
lateral reticular n.
lateral septal n.
lateral superior olivary n.
lateral vestibular n.
lenticular n.
masticatory n.
medial accessory olivary n.
medial amygdaloid n.
medial central n.
medial dorsal n.
medial geniculate n.
medial habenular n.
medial magnocellular n.
medial parabrachial n.
medial pericuneate n.
medial preoptic n.
medial septal n.
medial superior olivary n.
medial ventral n.
medial vestibular n.
median preoptic n.
mediodorsal n.
mesencephalic n.
Monakow n.
oculomotor n.
n. of origin
pontine n.
raphe n.
red n.
n. of solitary tract
somatic motor n.
tegmental n.
terminal n.
vestibular n.
vestibulocochlear n.
nuclide
null
    n. cell
    n. hypothesis
nulligravida
nullipara
nulliparity
nulliparous
numb chin syndrome

NOTES

number
atomic mass n.
Avogadro n.
Brinell hardness n.
CT n.
dibucaine n.
electronic n.
fluoride n.
gold n.
Hehner n.
Hogben n.
Hounsfield n.
hydrogen n.
iodine n.
Kestenbaum n.
Knoop hardness n.
Koettstorfer n.
linking n.
Loschmidt n.
Mach n.
mass n.
stoichiometric n.
turnover n.
nummular
n. eczema
n. psoriasis
n. sputum
nummularis
keratitis n.
nurse
dry n.
flight n.
general duty n.
graduate n.
head n.
home health n.
hospital n.
infection control n.
licensed practical n.
licensed vocational n.
scrub n.
nursemaid's elbow
nurse-midwife
certified n.-m.
nursing
n. audit
n. diagnosis
n. facility
n. history
n. home
primary n.
nut
betel n.
nutans
spasmus n.
nutation
nutraceutical
nutrient
n. artery

n. canal
essential n.
n. foramen
n. medium
n. vessel
nutrition
total parenteral n. (TPN)
nutritive equilibrium
nutriture
Nuttall operation
N&V
nausea and vomiting
NVD
nausea, vomiting, and diarrhea
nyctalgia
nyctalopia
nycterine
nyctohemeral
nyctophilia
nyctophobia
nympha
nymphectomy
nymphitis
nymphomania
nymphomaniacal
nymphoncus
nymphotomy
nystagmic
nystagmiform
nystagmograph
nystagmography
nystagmoid
nystagmus
amaurotic n.
benign positional n.
Bruns n.
caloric n.
cervical n.
compressive n.
congenital n.
conjugate n.
convergence-retraction n.
deviational n.
dissociated n.
downbeat n.
dysjunctive n.
end-point n.
fast component of n.
fixation n.
galvanic n.
gaze paretic n.
incongruent n.
irregular n.
jerky n.
labyrinthine n.
latent n.
lateral n.
miner's n.
minimal amplitude n.

optokinetic n.
oscillating n.
pendular n.
periodic alternating n.
positional n.
rebound n.
rotational n.
rotatory n.

seesaw n.
spontaneous n.
unilateral n.
upbeat n.
vertical n.
vestibular n.
voluntary n.

nyxis

NOTES

N

ω (*var. of* omega)

O

    O agglutinin
    O antigen
    O shell

oat

    o. cell
    o. cell carcinoma

oath

    Hippocratic O.

obdormition

obeliac

obelion

Ober test

obese

obesity

    android o.
    gynecoid o.
    hypothalamic o.
    hypothyroid o.
    morbid o.
    simple o.

object

    o. choice
    good o.
    o. libido
    metal o.
    o. relationship
    transitional o.

objective

    achromatic o.
    apochromatic o.
    o. assessment data
    immersion o.
    o. sensation
    o. sign
    o. symptom
    o. tinnitus

obligate

    o. aerobe
    o. anaerobe
    o. parasite

oblique

    o. amputation
    o. diameter
    o. fiber
    o. fracture
    o. hernia
    left anterior o. (LAO)
    left posterior o. (LPO)
    o. lie
    o. pelvis
    o. ridge
    o. section
    o. vein

obliquity

    Litzmann o.
    Nägele o.

obliterans

    arteriosclerosis o.
    arteritis o.
    balanitis xerotica o.
    bronchiolitis fibrosa o.
    bronchitis o.
    endarteritis o.
    pericarditis o.
    thromboangiitis o.

obliterating

    o. arteritis
    o. endarteritis

obliteration

    osteoplastic o.

obliterative

    o. bronchitis
    o. pericarditis

oblongata

    medulla o.

obsession

    impulsive o.
    inhibitory o.

obsessive-compulsive disorder

obstetric

    o. conjugate
    o. hand
    o. palsy
    o. paralysis

obstetrical

    o. binder
    o. forceps
    o. hand

obstetrician

obstetrics

obstinate

obstipation

obstipum

    abdomen o.

obstructed

    o. labor
    o. testis

obstruction

    airway o.
    bronchial o.
    closed loop o.
    duodenal o.
    extrathoracic airway o.
    intrathoracic airway o.
    ureteropelvic junction o.

obstructive

    o. anuria
    o. dysmenorrhea

O

obstructive *(continued)*
   o. hydrocephalus
   o. jaundice
   o. murmur
   o. sleep apnea
   o. thrombus
   o. uropathy
   o. ventilatory defect
obtund
obtundation
obturans
   keratosis o.
obturating embolism
obturation
obturator
   o. artery
   o. branch
   o. canal
   o. crest
   o. externus muscle
   o. foramen
   o. hernia
   o. internus muscle
   o. nerve
   o. sign
   o. vein
obtuse
obtusion
obtusus
   lichen o.
Occam razor
occasional rhonchi
occidentalis
   Dermacentor o.
occipital
   o. artery
   o. bone
   o. cerebral vein
   o. lobe
   o. lobe epilepsy
   o. pole
   o. sinus
   o. spur
occipitalis
   forceps o.
occipitalization
occipitis
occipitoanterior
   o. fetal position
   left o. (LOA)
occipitofacial
occipitofrontal
   o. diameter
   o. muscle
occipitofrontalis muscle
occipitomental diameter
occipitoposterior
   left o. (LOP)
   o. position

occipitotransverse
   left o. (LOT)
   o. position
occiput
occlude
occlusal
   o. analysis
   o. equilibration
   o. film
   o. force
   o. imbalance
   o. plane
   o. position
occlusion
   abnormal o.
   acentric o.
   afunctional o.
   anterior o.
   balanced o.
   bimaxillary protrusive o.
   buccal o.
   centric o.
   coronary o.
   curve of o.
   distal o.
   eccentric o.
   edge-to-edge o.
   end-to-end o.
   functional o.
   gliding o.
   hyperfunctional o.
   labial o.
   lateral o.
   lingual o.
   mechanically balanced o.
   mesenteric artery o.
   mesial o.
   neutral o.
   normal o.
   pathogenic o.
   physiologic o.
   protrusive o.
   retrusive o.
   skeletal o.
   o. trauma
   traumatic o.
   traumatogenic o.
   working o.
occlusive
   o. dressing
   o. ileus
   o. meningitis
occult
   o. blood
   o. carcinoid
   o. choroidal neovascularization
   o. cleft palate
   o. fracture

o. PEEP
o. posterior laryngeal cleft
occulta
spina bifida o.
occupational
o. acne
o. behavior
o. disease
o. hearing loss
o. medicine
o. role
o. science
o. therapy (OT)
Ochoa law
ochratoxin A
ochre codon
Ochrobactrum
ochrometer
ochronosis
exogenous o.
ochronotic
octafluoropropane
ocular
o. albinism
o. albinism 1, 2, 3
o. cicatricial pemphigoid
compensating o.
o. flutter
o. humor
Huygens o.
o. hypertelorism
o. hypotony
o. larva migrans granuloma
o. migraine
o. motility
o. myopathy
o. prosthesis
o. tension
o. vertigo
ocularis
angor o.
ocularist
oculi (*pl. of* oculus)
oculist
oculocutaneous
oculodynia
oculofacial
oculography
oculogyria
oculogyric

oculomotor
o. nerve
o. nucleus
oculonasal
oculopharyngeal dystrophy
oculoplethysmography
oculopneumoplethysmography
oculopupillary
oculosympathetic
oculozygomatic
oculus, pl. **oculi**
abducens oculi
adnexa oculi
camera oculi
Dracunculus oculi
equator bulbi oculi
fundus oculi
Oddi
sphincter of O.
odontalgia
odontalgic
odontectomy
odontoblast
odontoblastic layer
odontoblastoma
odontoclast
odontodysplasia
odontogenesis
odontogenic
o. cyst
o. keratocyst
odontogeny
odontoid process
odontology
forensic o.
odontolysis
odontolyticus
Actinomyces o.
odontoma
ameloblastic o.
complex o.
compound o.
odontoneuralgia
odontonomy
odontopathy
odontoplasty
odontosis
odontotomy
odynacusis
odynometer
odynophagia
oedipal phase

O

NOTES

oedipism
Oedipus complex
oenology
oersted
oesophagostomiasis
oestradiol
oestriol
oestrogen
oestrone
oestrus
officer
> house o.

official formula
off label indication
off-vertical rotation
Ofuji disease
Ogilvie
> O. operation
> O. syndrome

Ogino-Knaus rule
Ogston line
Oguchi disease
Ogura operation
OHI-S
> Simplified Oral Hygiene Index

ohm
ohne Hauch
Ohngren line
oidiomycin
oil
> allspice o.
> almond o.
> apple o.
> arachis o.
> aromatic castor o.
> beech o.
> benne o.
> betula o.
> birch tar o.
> bitter almond o.
> bitter orange peel o.
> cacao o.
> cade o.
> cajeput o., cajuput oil
> camphorated o.
> cassia o.
> castor o.
> chaulmoogra o.
> checkerberry o.
> chloriodized o.
> cinnamon o.
> clove o.
> coal o.
> cod liver o.
> corn o.
> cottonseed o.
> croton o.
> dill o.
> o. emulsion adjuvant

essential o.
estragon o.
ethereal o.
ethiodized o.
eucalyptus o.
expressed mustard o.
fatty o.
fixed o.
flaxseed o.
fusel o.
garlic o.
gaultheria o.
gingili o.
gynocardia o.
halibut liver o.
hydnocarpus o.
iodized o.
joint o.
jojoba o.
juniper berry o.
linseed o.
Lorenzo o.
maise o.
mineral o.
red o.
volatile o.

ointment
> blue o.
> eye o.
> hydrophilic o.
> mild mercurial o.

OKT
> Ortho-Kung T
> OKT cell

Oldfield syndrome
oleaginous
oleate
olecrani
> fossa o.

olecranon spur
olefin
oleoresin
> ginger o.

olfaction
olfactoria
> fila o.
> hyperesthesia o.

olfactory
> o. agnosia
> o. amnesia
> o. aura
> o. bulb
> o. epithelium
> o. foramen
> o. gland
> o. hallucination
> o. hypoesthesia
> o. membrane
> o. nerve

o. peduncle
o. receptor
o. receptor cell
o. sulcus
oligemia
oligemic
oligoamnios
oligoclonal band
oligocystic
oligodactyly, oligodactylia
oligodendria
oligodendrocyte
oligodendroglia
oligodendroglioma
anaplastic o.
oligodipsia
oligodontia
oligodynamic
oligogalactia
oligohydramnios
oligomenorrhea
oligomerization
oligomorphic
oligonucleotide
oligopnea
oligoptyalism
oligoria
oligosaccharide
oligospermatism
oligospermia
oligosynaptic
oligotrophia, oligotrophy
oligozoospermia
oliguria
olivary
olive
inferior o.
o. ring
o. wire
olivifugal
olivipetal
olivopontocerebellar
Ollier
O. graft
O. incision
O. theory
Ollier-Thiersch graft
Olmsted syndrome
omega, ω
interferon o.
omega-oxidation theory
Omenn syndrome

omental
o. appendix
o. bursa
o. flap
o. foramen
o. graft
o. hernia
omentectomy
omentitis
omentofixation
omentopexy
omentoplasty
omentorrhaphy
omentosplenopexy
omentum
gastrocolic o.
gastrohepatic o.
gastrosplenic o.
greater o.
lesser o.
omnifocal lens
omnivorous
omohyoid muscle
omphalectomy
omphalelcosis
omphalic
omphalitis
omphalocele
omphaloenteric
omphalomesenteric duct
omphalophlebitis
omphalorrhagia
omphalorrhea
omphalorrhexis
omphalosite
omphalospinous
omphalotomy
onanism
onchocercoma
oncocytic
o. adenoma
o. carcinoma
o. hepatocellular tumor
oncofetal
o. antigen
o. marker
oncogene
ras o.
oncogenesis
oncogenic virus
oncogenous
oncologist

O

NOTES

oncology
    radiation o.
oncolysis
oncolytic
oncornavirus
oncosis
oncostatin M
oncotic pressure
oncotomy
oncotropic
oncovirus
Ondine curse
oneiric
oneirism
oneirodynia
oneirophrenia
oneiroscopy
ongoing assessment
on-off phenomenon
onomatomania
onomatophobia
on-site massage
ontogenesis
ontogenetic
ontogenic
ontogeny
onychalgia
onychatrophia
onychatrophy
onychauxis
onychectomy
onychia
onychitis
onychoclasis
onychodystrophy
onychograph
onychogryposis
onychoheterotopia
onychoid
onycholysis
onychoma
onychomadesis
onychomalacia
onychomycosis
onychopathic
onychopathy
onychophagy, onychophagia
onychoplasty
onychorrhexis
onychoschizia
onychosis
onychotillomania
onychotomy
onyx
oocyst
oocyte
    primary o.
    secondary o.
oogenesis

oogenetic
oogonium
ookinesis, ookinesia
ookinete
oolemma
oophorectomy
oophoritis
oophorocystectomy
oophorocystosis
oophorohysterectomy
oophoron
oophoropexy
oophoroplasty
oophorostomy
oophorotomy
ooplasm
ootid
O&P
    ova and parasites
opacification
opacity
    vitreous o.
opal codon
opalescent dentin
opaque
open
    o. biopsy
    o. bite
    o. chain compound
    o. chest massage
    o. circuit method
    o. circuit spirometry
    o. comedo
    o. dislocation
    o. drainage
    o. drop anesthesia
    o. flap
    o. fracture
    o. head injury
    o. heart surgery
    o. hospital
    keep vein o. (KVO)
    o. operation
    o. pneumothorax
    o. reduction
    o. tenotomy
    o. tuberculosis
    o. wound
open-angle glaucoma
open-circuit nitrogen wash-out
opening
    access o.
    aortic o.
    cardiac o.
    caval o.
    esophageal o.
    external o.
    femoral o.
    ileocecal o.

internal acoustic o.
internal urethral o.
lacrimal o.
pharyngeal o.
saphenous o.
o. snap
tympanic o.
open-packed position
operable
operant
operate
operating microscope
operation
Abernethy o.
Allarton o.
Altemeier o.
Anson-McVay o.
Appolito o.
Arlt o.
arterial switch o.
Auchincloss o.
Ball o.
Barkan o.
Bassini o.
Battista o.
Baudelocque o.
Baynton o.
Belsey Mark o.
Bernard o.
Billroth o. I, II
Bircher o.
Blalock-Hanlon o.
Blalock-Taussig o.
bloodless o.
Bose o.
Bozeman o.
Brenner o.
Bricker o.
Brock o.
Brunschwig o.
buttonhole o.
Caldwell-Luc o.
Carmody-Batson o.
cesarean o.
Chaput o.
Cheyne o.
commando o.
concrete o.
Cotte o.
Cotting o.
cricoid split o.
Crile-Matas o.

Czerny o.
Dana o.
Dandy o.
Daviel o.
debulking o.
decompression o.
Dohlman o.
Doyle o.
Drummond-Morison o.
Dupuy-Dutemps o.
Eagleton o.
Ekehorn o.
Elliot o.
Emmet o.
endolymphatic shunt o.
Estes o.
Estlander o.
exploratory o.
fenestration o.
filtering o.
Finney o.
flap o.
Fontan o.
formal o.
Fothergill o.
Frazier-Spiller o.
Fredet-Ramstedt o.
Freund o.
Gilliam o.
Gillies o.
Gil-Vernet o.
Glenn o.
Graefe o.
Gritti o.
Grondahl-Finney o.
Gussenbauer o.
Hahn o.
Halsted o.
Handley o.
Hartmann o.
Heaney o.
Heaton o.
Heller o.
Hey Groves o.
Hill o.
Hochenegg o.
Hoffa o.
Hofmeister o.
Hummelsheim o.
Hunter o.
interval o.
Jaboulay o.

O

NOTES

operation *(continued)*
    Jackson-Babcock o.
    Jacobaeus o.
    Jansen o.
    Kader-Senn o.
    Kasai o.
    Kazanjian o.
    Keen o.
    Keller-Madlener o.
    Kelly o.
    Killian o.
    Koerte-Ballance o.
    Kondoleon o.
    Kraske o.
    Krönlein o.
    Ladd o.
    Lahey o.
    Lambrinudi o.
    Lane o.
    Laroyenne o.
    Lash o.
    Lawson o.
    LeCompte o.
    Leriche o.
    Linton o.
    lip adhesion o.
    Lisfranc o.
    Longmire o.
    Lotheissen o.
    Luc o.
    Madlener o.
    major o.
    Manchester o.
    Mann-Williamson o.
    Marcy o.
    Marshall-Marchetti-Krantz o.
    Mayo o.
    McArthur o.
    McBurney o.
    McIndoe o.
    McVay o.
    mika o.
    Mikulicz o.
    Miles o.
    minor o.
    morcellation o.
    Motais o.
    Moynihan o.
    Mules o.
    Mustard o.
    Naffziger o.
    Norton o.
    Norwood o.
    Nuttall o.
    Ogilvie o.
    Ogura o.
    open o.
    Owen o.
    Patey o.
    Payne o.
    Peet o.
    Physick o.
    Pirogoff o.
    Pollock o.
    Pólya o.
    Pomeroy o.
    Portmann interposition o.
    Potts o.
    Putti-Platt o.
    Ramstedt o.
    Rashkind o.
    Rastelli o.
    Récamier o.
    Ridell o.
    Ripstein o.
    Roux-en-Y o.
    Saenger o.
    Scarpa o.
    Schlatter o.
    Schroeder o.
    Schuchardt o.
    Scott o.
    second-look o.
    seton o.
    Smith o.
    Smith-Gibson o.
    Smith-Indian o.
    Soave o.
    State o.
    Stoffel o.
    Stookey-Scarff o.
    string o.
    Sturmdorf o.
    subcutaneous o.
    Syme o.
    talc o.
    Tanner o.
    Tansini o.
    Taussig o.
    Taussig-Morton o.
    Thomas o.
    Travel o.
    Trendelenburg o.
    Treves o.
    Urban o.
    van Buren o.
    Vermale o.
    Verneuil o.
    Waters o.
    Watson o.
    Wertheim o.
    Whipple o.
    Whitehead o.
    Wise o.
    Witzel o.
    Zimmerman o.

operative
operator **gene**

opercular
operculitis
operculum
operon
> Lac o.

ophiasis
ophritis
ophryon
ophryosis
ophthalmia
> catarrhal o.
> caterpillar-hair o.
> Egyptian o.
> gonorrheal o.
> granular o.
> metastatic o.
> o. neonatorum
> purulent o.
> sympathetic o.

ophthalmic
> o. artery
> o. nerve
> o. solution
> o. vesicle

ophthalmica
> zona o.

ophthalmicus
> herpes zoster o.

ophthalmodynamometer
> Bailliart o.

ophthalmodynamometry
ophthalmofunduscope
ophthalmolith
ophthalmologist
ophthalmology
ophthalmomalacia
ophthalmometer
ophthalmomycosis
ophthalmopathy
> endocrine o.
> external o.
> Graves o.
> internal o.

ophthalmoplegia
> basal o.
> chronic progressive external o. (CPEO)
> congenital o.
> diabetic o.
> exophthalmic o.
> o. externa
> external o.

fascicular o.
fibrotic o.
o. interna
internal o.
internuclear o. (INO)
nuclear o.
orbital o.
Parinaud o.
total o.
wall-eyed bilateral internuclear o.

ophthalmoplegic
ophthalmoscope
> binocular o.
> demonstration o.
> direct o.
> indirect o.

ophthalmoscopic
ophthalmoscopy
> direct o.
> indirect o.

ophthalmovascular
opiate receptor
opiocortin
opioid antagonist
opiomelanocortin
opisthenar
opisthotonic
opisthotonos
opisthotonus
Opitz
> O. BBB syndrome
> O. G syndrome

opium
> Boston o.
> denarcotized o.
> deodorized o.
> granulated o.
> gum o.

Oppenheim
> O. disease
> O. reflex

opponens
> o. digiti minimi muscle
> o. pollicis muscle

opportunistic
oppositional defiant disorder
opsin
opsinogen
opsiuria
opsoclonus
opsogen
opsomania

NOTES

O

opsonic index
opsonin
 immune o.
 normal o.
 specific o.
opsonization
opsonocytophagic
opsonometry
optic
 o. activity
 o. ataxia
 o. axis
 o. canal
 o. capsule
 o. chiasm
 o. cup
 o. decussation
 o. density
 o. disc
 o. foramen
 o. isomerism
 o. nerve
 o. neuritis
 o. papilla
 o. radiation
 o. rotation
 o. rotatory dispersion
 o. tract
optica
 hyperesthesia o.
 neuromyelitis o.
 radiatio o.
optical
 o. aberration
 o. activity
 o. density
 o. esophagoscope
 o. image
 o. isomerism
 o. keratoplasty
 o. microscope
 o. rotation
optician
opticianry
opticociliary
opticopupillary
optimal pitch
optimum dose
optokinetic nystagmus
optometer
optometrist
optometry
optomyometer
orad
oral
 o. antibiotic
 o. auditory method
 o. biology
 o. cavity

 o. contraceptive
 o. defensiveness
 o. hygiene
 o. motor apraxia
 o. pathology
 o. phase
 o. poliovirus vaccine
 o. surgeon
 o. surgery
 o. vestibule
oralis
 Bacteroides o.
orality
orange
 acridine o.
 Agent O.
 methyl o.
 o. wood
ora serrata retinae
orbicular
orbiculare
orbicularis
 o. oculi muscle
 o. oris muscle
 zona o.
orbiculus ciliaris
orbit
 floor of o.
orbital
 o. cavity
 o. cellulitis
 o. gyrus
 o. margin
 o. muscle
 o. ophthalmoplegia
 o. plane
 o. process
orbitalis muscle
orbitography
orbitomeatal
 o. line
 o. plane
orbitonasal cleft
orbitonometer
orbitonometry
orbitopathy
 dysthyroid o.
 Graves o.
orbitostat
orbitotomy
Orbivirus
orcein
orchalgia
orchialgia
orchica
 adiposis o.
orchidectomy
orchidic
orchidometer

orchidopexy
orchiectomy
orchiepididymitis
orchiocele
orchiopathy
orchiopexy
orchioplasty
orchiotomy
orchitic
orchitis
orcini
　　Diphyllobothrium o.
ordinate
orexigenic
organ
　　accessory o.
　　annulospiral o.
　　auditory o.
　　Chievitz o.
　　circumventricular o.
　　Corti o.
　　critical o.
　　o. culture
　　dental o.
　　enamel o.
　　end o.
　　external female genital o.
　　external male genital o.
　　floating o.
　　genital o.
　　Golgi tendon o.
　　gustatory o.
　　internal female genital o.
　　internal male genital o.
　　intromittent o.
　　Jacobson o.
　　otolithic o.
　　sense o.
　　spiral o.
　　supernumerary o.
　　target o.
　　vestibular o.
　　vestigial o.
organelle
　　cell o.
organic
　　o. acid
　　o. brain syndrome
　　o. chemistry
　　o. compound
　　o. contracture
　　o. delusion

o. disease
o. evolution
o. hearing impairment
o. lesion
o. mental disorder
o. murmur
o. paralysis
o. vertigo
organism
　　calculated mean o.
　　defective o.
　　fastidious o.
　　hypothetical mean o.
　　pleuropneumonia-like o.
organization
　　exclusive provider o.
　　health maintenance o. (HMO)
　　peer-review o.
　　preferred provider o. (PPO)
organize
organized thrombus
organizer
organogel
organogenesis
organogenetic
organogenic
organogeny
organoid tumor
organomegaly
organomercurial
organometallic
organon
organophosphate
organotrophic
organotropic
organotropism
organ-specific antigen
orgasm
orgasmic
orgastic
orientalis
　　Nocardia o.
oriental sore
orientation
　　sexual o.
　　topographical o.
　　visual o.
orienting
　　o. reflex
　　o. response
orifice
　　anal o.

NOTES

O

orifice *(continued)*
    aortic o.
    cardiac o.
    cardial o.
    esophagogastric o.
    external urethral o.
    filling internal urethral o.
    gastroduodenal o.
    golf-hole ureteral o.
    hymenal o.
    ileal o.
    ileocecal o.
    internal urethral o.
    left atrioventricular o.
    mitral o.
    pyloric o.
    tricuspid o.
    ureteric o.
    vaginal o.
orificial
orificium
origin
    bleeding of undetermined o. (BUO)
    fever of unknown o. (FUO)
    nucleus of o.
oris
    Bacteroides o.
    cavum o.
    fetor o.
    labia o.
Ormond disease
ornithine
ornithinuria
Ornithodoros
ornithosis
orodigitofacial dysostosis
orofacial
orolingual
oronasal fistula
oropharyngeal
    o. airway
    o. gonorrhea
oropharynx
Oropouche fever
orosomucoid
orotate
orotic acid
orotidine
orotracheal tube
Oroya fever
orphan
    chicken embryo lethal o. (CELO)
    o. disease
    o. drug
    o. product
    o. receptor
    o. virus
Orr incision

Orth
    O. fixative
    O. stain
orthesis
orthetics
orthochorea
orthochromatic
orthocytosis
orthodeoxia
orthodontics
orthodontist
orthodromic
orthognathia
orthognathic
orthognathous
orthograde degeneration
orthokeratology
orthokeratosis
Ortho-Kung T (OKT)
orthomechanical
orthomolecular
Orthomyxoviridae
orthopedics
    dental o.
    functional jaw o.
orthopedic surgery
orthopercussion
orthophoria
orthophoric
orthophosphate
    inorganic o.
orthophosphoric acid
orthopnea
    2-pillow o.
    3-pillow o.
orthopneic
orthopsychiatry
orthoptic
orthoptics
Orthoreovirus
orthoscope
orthosis
    ankle-foot o.
    cervical o.
    cervicothoracic o.
    knee-ankle-foot o.
    pneumatic o.
    resting o.
    spinal o.
    static o.
    therapeutic o.
    thoracolumbosacral o.
    wrist-hand o.
orthostatic
    o. congestion
    o. dyspnea
    o. hypotension
    o. purpura
    o. tachycardia

orthotics
orthotist
orthotonos
orthotonus
orthotopic ureterocele
orthotropic
Ortolani maneuver
os, pl. ossa
    external o.
    histological internal o.
    o. incisivum
    incompetent cervical o.
    o. intermetatarseum
    ossa metacarpi
    ossa metatarsi
    o. multangulum majus
    nil per o.
    per o.
    o. scaphoideum
    o. trigonum
oscheal
oscheitis
oscheohydrocele
oscheoplasty
oscillating
    o. nystagmus
    o. vision
oscillation wave
oscillatory potential
oscillometer
oscillometric
oscillometry
oscillopsia
oscilloscope
    cathode ray o.
osculum
Osgood-Schlatter disease
Osler
    O. disease
    O. node
Osler-Vaquez disease
osmic acid
osmics
osmidrosis
osmium
osmolality
    calculated serum o.
osmolar
osmolarity
osmole
osmometry
osmoreceptor

osmoregulatory
osmoscope
osmose
osmosis
    reverse o.
osmotic
    o. diuresis
    o. diuretic
    o. fragility
    o. pressure
osphresis
osphretic
ossa (*pl. of* os)
ossein, osseine
osseocartilaginous
osseointegration
osseomucin
osseous
    o. hydatid cyst
    o. lacuna
    o. spiral lamina
    o. tissue
ossicle
    Andernach o.
    auditory o.
    Bertin o.
    epactal o.
    Kerckring o.
ossicular
    o. chain
    o. reconstruction
    o. system
ossiculectomy
ossiculotomy
ossiculum
ossiferous
ossificans
    myositis o.
ossification
    cartilaginous o.
    center of o.
    ectopic o.
    endochondral o.
    intramembranous o.
    membranous o.
    metaplastic o.
    periosteal o.
ossific center
ossify
osteal
ostealgia
ostealgic

NOTES

O

ostearthritis
    interphalangeal o.
ostectomy
ostein, osteine
osteitic
osteitis
    alveolar o.
    caseous o.
    central o.
    condensing o.
    cortical o.
    o. deformans
    o. fibrosa cystica
    focal condensing o.
    hematogenous o.
    o. pubis
    sclerosing o.
ostempyesis
osteoanagenesis
osteoarthritis
    endemic o.
    erosive o.
    hyperplastic o.
osteoarthropathy
    hypertrophic pulmonary o.
    idiopathic hypertrophic o.
osteoarthrosis
osteoblast
osteoblastic
osteoblastoma
osteocartilaginous
osteochondral fracture
osteochondritis dissecans
osteochondrodystrophy
osteochondroma
osteochondrosarcoma
osteochondrosis
osteoclasis, osteoclasia
osteoclast activating factor
osteoclastic
osteoclastoma
osteocranium
osteocystoma
osteocyte
osteodentin
osteodermia
osteodiastasis
osteodynia
osteodysplasty
    Melnick-Needles o.
osteodystrophia
osteodystrophy
    Albright hereditary o.
    renal o.
osteoectasia
osteofibroma
osteofibrosis
osteogen

osteogenesis
    distraction o.
    endochondral o.
    o. imperfecta
    o. imperfecta congenita
    o. imperfecta tarda
    periosteal o.
osteogenetic
    o. fiber
    o. layer
osteogenic
    o. osteomalacia
    o. sarcoma
osteogenous
osteogeny
osteoid osteoma
osteokinematics
osteology
osteolysis
osteolytic
osteoma
    compact o.
    o. cutis
    dental o.
    giant osteoid o.
    ivory o.
    o. medullare
    osteoid o.
    o. spongiosum
osteomalacia
    infantile o.
    juvenile o.
    osteogenic o.
    renal tubular o.
    senile o.
osteomalacic pelvis
osteomatoid
osteomere
osteomyelitis
    chronic diffuse sclerosing o.
    chronic focal sclerosing o.
    Garré o.
osteomyelodysplasia
osteon, osteone
osteonecrosis
osteopath
osteopathia hemorrhagica infantum
osteopathic
    o. manipulative therapy
    o. medicine
    o. physician
osteopathy
    alimentary o.
osteopenia
osteoperiostitis
osteopetrosis
osteophage
osteophlebitis
osteophyma

osteophyte
osteoplastic
    o. bone flap
    o. obliteration
osteoplasty
osteopoikilosis
osteoporosis
    juvenile o.
osteoporotic
osteoprogenitor cell
osteoprotegerin
osteoradiology
osteoradionecrosis
osteorrhaphy
osteosarcoma
osteosclerosis
osteosclerotic
osteosis cutis
osteosuture
osteosynthesis
osteothrombosis
osteotome
osteotomy
    block o.
    chevron o.
    C sliding o.
    displacement o.
    Dwyer o.
    horizontal o.
    Le Fort o.
    pelvic o.
    subtrochanteric o.
osteotribe
osteotrite
ostia (*pl. of* ostium)
ostial
ostitic
ostitis
ostium, pl. ostia
    abdominal o.
    aortic o.
    o. ileale
    uterine o.
ostomate
ostomy
Ostwald solubility coefficient
OT
    occupational therapy
otalgia
    geniculate o.
otalgic

otic
    o. capsule
    o. ganglion
    o. vesicle
oticus
    herpes zoster o.
otitic
    o. abscess
    o. meningitis
otitidiscaviarum
    Nocardia o.
otitis
    adhesive o.
    o. externa
    o. interna
    malignant external o.
    o. media
    serous o.
otoacoustic emission
otocephaly
otoconia
otoconium
otocranial
otocranium
otocyst
otodynia
otoencephalitis
otogenic
otogenous
otolaryngologist
otolaryngology
otolithic
    o. crisis
    o. organ
otologic
otologist
otology
otomucormycosis
otomycosis
otopathy
otopharyngeal
otoplasty
otorhinolaryngology
otorrhea
    cerebrospinal fluid o.
otosclerosis
otoscope
    Siegle o.
otoscopy
    pneumatic o.
otospondylomegaepiphyseal dysplasia
otospongiosis

NOTES

O

665

otosteal
ototoxic
ototoxicity
    familial aminoglycoside o.
Otto disease
Ouchterlony technique
OURQ
    outer upper right quadrant
out
    acting o.
    salting o.
    working o.
outcome score
outer
    o. hair cell
    o. malleolus
    o. upper right quadrant (OURQ)
outflow
    aqueous o.
outlet
    o. forceps
    o. forceps delivery
    pelvic o.
    rule of o.
outpatient surgery
output
    cardiac o.
    intake and o. (I&O)
    maximum power o.
    minute o.
outstanding ear
ova (*pl. of* ovum)
oval
    o. amputation
    o. esophagoscope
    o. foramen
    o. window
ovalbumin
ovale
    centrum o.
    foramen o.
    patent foramen o.
    Plasmodium o.
ovalis
    anulus o.
    fossa o.
    Malassezia o.
ovalocyte
ovalocytosis
ovarialgia
ovarian
    o. agenesis
    o. artery
    o. cycle
    o. cyst
    o. follicle
    o. fossa
    o. hernia
    o. pregnancy

ovariectomy
ovarii
    rete o.
    struma o.
ovariocele
ovariocentesis
ovariocyesis
ovariohysterectomy
ovariorrhexis
ovariosalpingectomy
ovariosalpingitis
ovariostomy
ovariotomy
    abdominal o.
ovaritis
ovary
    polycystic o.
over-and-over suture
overanxious disorder
overbite
overcompensation
overcorrection
overdenture
overdetermination
overdominance
overdominant
overdrive
overflow
    o. incontinence
    o. wave
overjet
overjut
overlap
    horizontal o.
    vertical o.
overlapping sutures
overlay
    o. denture
    emotional o.
overload
    circulatory o.
    o. principle
overriding aorta
overshoot
overt homosexuality
overtraining syndrome
overtube
overuse syndrome
overwintering
ovicidal
oviducal
oviduct
oviductal
oviferous
oviform
ovigenesis
ovigenetic
ovigenic

ovoid
    fetal o.
    Manchester o.
ovoplasm
ovosiston
ovotestis
ovular membrane
ovulation
    anestrous o.
ovulational age
ovulatory
ovule
ovulocyclic
ovulum
ovum, pl. **ova**
    alecithal o.
    blighted o.
    centrolecithal o.
    fertilized o.
    isolecithal o.
    ova and parasite examination
    ova and parasites (O&P)
    Peters o.
Owen
    contour line of O.
    O. line
    O. operation
Owren disease
oxalate
    calcium o.
    o. calculus
    cerium o.
oxalemia
oxalic acid
oxaloacetic acid
oxalosuccinic acid
oxaluria
oxalylurea
oxazin dye
oxazolidinones
ox heart
oxidant
oxidase
    adrenaline o.
    amine o.
    amino acid o.
    ascorbate o.
    catechol o.
    coproporphyrinogen o.
    cytochrome c o.
    diamine o.
    direct o.

    dopa o.
    glucose o.
    homogentisic acid o.
    indirect o.
    indophenol o.
    sulfite o.
    urate o.
oxidation
    end o.
oxidation-reduction
oxidative phosphorylation
oxide
    acid o.
    antimonous o.
    antimony o.
    barium o.
    basic o.
    bismuth chloride o.
    calcium o.
    deuterium o.
    eserine o.
    ferric o.
    indifferent o.
    magnesium o.
    nitric o.
    nitrous o.
oxidize
oxidoreductase
oxime
    hexamethylpropyleneamine o.
oximeter
    cuvet o.
    pulse o.
oximetry
    finger o.
    pulse o.
oxycarbonate
    bismuth o.
oxycephalic
oxycephalous
oxycephaly
oxychloride
    bismuth o.
oxychromatic
oxyesthesia
oxygen
    o. affinity hypoxia
    o. capacity
    o. concentrator
    o. consumption
    o. content
    o. debt

NOTES

O

oxygen *(continued)*
    o. deficit
    heavy o.
    high pressure o.
    hyperbaric o.
    o. pulse
    o. toxicity
oxygenase
    mixed function o.
oxygenate
oxygenation
    apneic o.
    extracorporeal-membrane o.
    hyperbaric o.
oxygen-derived free radical
oxygeusia
oxyheme
oxyhemochromogen
oxyhemoglobin dissociation curve
oxyhydrase
    glucose o.

oxymyoglobin
oxyntic cell
oxyphil, oxyphile
    o. cell
oxyphilic
    o. carcinoma
    o. leukocyte
oxyphonia
oxytalan
oxytoca
    Klebsiella o.
oxytocia
oxytocic
oxytocin challenge test
oxyuriasis
oxyuricide
oxyurid
ozaenae
    Klebsiella pneumoniae o.
ozena
ozone

Ψ (*var. of* upsilon)

P
- P congenitale
- P mitrale
- P pulmonale
- P selectin
- P sinistrocardiale
- P wave

PA
- posteroanterior
- PA conduction time
- PA interval
- PA projection

P&A
- percussion and auscultation

Paas disease
pacchionian body
pacefollower
pacemaker
- artificial p.
- demand p.
- diaphragmatic p.
- ectopic p.
- electric cardiac p.
- electronic p.
- external p.
- fixed-rate p.
- p. lead
- runaway p.
- subsidiary atrial p.
- wandering p.

Pacheco parrot disease virus
Pachon
- P. method
- P. test

pachyblepharon
pachycephalic
pachycephalous
pachycephaly
pachycheilia, pachychilia
pachychromatic
pachydactyly
pachyderma laryngis
pachydermatis
- *Malassezia p.*

pachydermatocele
pachydermodactyly
pachyglossia
pachygyria
pachyleptomeningitis
pachymeningitis
- cerebral p.
- external p.
- hemorrhagic p.

- hypertrophic cervical p.
- purulent p.

pachymeningopathy
pachynsis
pachyntic
pachyonychia
pachyperiostitis
pachyperitonitis
pachypleuritis
pachysalpingitis
pachysalpingoovaritis
pachysomia
pachytene
pachyvaginalitis
pachyvaginitis
pacificum
- *Diphyllobothrium p.*

pacing
- p. catheter
- underdrive p.
- ventricular p.

pacinian corpuscle
pack
- cold p.
- dry p.
- hot p.
- ice p.

packed red cells (PRCs)
packing
- denture p.

pad
- abdominal p.
- dinner p.
- fat p.
- heel p.
- knuckle p.
- laparotomy p.
- retromolar p.

Pagenstecher circle
Paget
- P. cell
- P. disease

pagetoid cell
pain
- bearing-down p.
- expulsive p.
- false p.
- girdle p.
- growing p.
- hunger p.
- intermenstrual p.
- intractable p.
- labor p.
- lancinating p.
- middle p.

P

pain (*continued*)
   phantom limb p.
   psychogenic p.
   recrudescent p.
   referred p.
   somatic p.
   p. spot
   visceral p.
   writhing in p.
painful
   p. arc sign
   p. heel
pain-pleasure principle
pain-spasm-ischemia cycle
pain-spasm-pain cycle
paint
   carbol-fuchsin p.
   Castellani p.
pair
   base p.
   buffer p.
   chromosome p.
   conjugate acid-base p.
   line p.'s
pairing
   chromosome p.
palatal
   p. elevator
   p. index
   p. reflex
   p. shelf
palate
   bony p.
   Byzantine arch p.
   cleft p.
   falling p.
   Gothic p.
   hard p.
   occult cleft p.
   p. retractor
   soft p.
   submucous cleft p.
palatine
   p. bone
   p. crest
   p. gland
   p. process
   p. raphe
   p. reflex
   p. shelf
   p. spine
   p. tonsil
   p. uvula
   p. vein
palatinum
   velum p.
palatinus
   torus p.
palatitis

palatoethmoidal suture
palatoglossal arch
palatoglossus
   arcus p.
   p. muscle
palatognathous
palatomaxillary suture
palatonasal
palatopharyngeal
   p. arch
   p. muscle
palatopharyngeus
   arcus p.
   p. muscle
palatopharyngorrhaphy
palatoplasty
palatoplegia
palatorrhaphy
palatoschisis
paleokinetic
paleopathology
paleostriatal
paleostriatum
paleothalamus
palikinesia, palicinesia
palilalia
palindrome
palindromia
palindromic
palinopsia
paliphrasia
palladium
pallaesthesia
pallanesthesia
pallesthesia
pallesthetic
pallial
palliate
palliative
   p. surgery
   p. treatment
pallidal
pallidectomy
pallidoansotomy
pallidotomy
pallidum
   dorsal p.
   Treponema p.
pallidus
   globus p.
pallor
   cachectic p.
palm
   liver p.
palmar
   p. arch
   p. interosseous muscle
   p. pinch
   p. psoriasis

p. radiocarpal ligament
p. space
p. ulnocarpal ligament
palmaris
arcus p.
palmate fold
Palmer dental nomenclature
palmic
palmitate
ascorbyl p.
palmitoleic acid
palmitoyltransferase
carnitine p.
palmus
palpable
palpate
palpation
bimanual p.
light-touch p.
palpatory percussion
palpebral
p. artery
p. fissure
p. vein
palpebralis
epicanthus p.
palpebrarum
xanthelasma p.
palpitation
palsy
accommodative p.
Bell p.
birth p.
brachial birth p.
bulbar p.
cerebral p.
crutch p.
cyclist's p.
Dejerine-Klumpke p.
diver's p.
double elevator p.
Erb p.
extrapyramidal cerebral p.
facial p.
gaze p.
hammer p.
ischemic p.
Klumpke p.
lead p.
obstetric p.
pseudobulbar p.

ulnar p.
wasting p.
pamoate
cycloguanil p.
pampiniform plexus
panacea
panagglutinins
panangiitis
panarthritis
panatrophy
panbronchiolitis
diffuse p.
pancake kidney
pancarditis
Pancoast syndrome
pancolectomy
pancreas
accessory p.
anular p.
Aselli p.
dorsal p.
lesser p.
tail of p.
pancreatalgia
pancreatectomy
pancreatic
p. calculus
p. cystoduodenostomy
p. digestion
p. duct
p. pseudocyst
p. vein
pancreatica
achylia p.
diarrhea p.
pancreaticoduodenal vein
pancreaticoduodenectomy
pylorus-preserving p.
pancreaticus
hemosuccus p.
pancreatitis
acute hemorrhagic p.
calcareous p.
calcific p.
chronic fibrosing p.
chronic relapsing p.
mumps p.
purulent p.
pancreatoduodenectomy
pancreatoduodenostomy
pancreatogastrostomy
pancreatogenic

NOTES

P

671

pancreatogenous
pancreatography
pancreatolithectomy
pancreatolithiasis
pancreatolithotomy
pancreatolysis
pancreatolytic
pancreatopathy
pancreatorenal syndrome
pancreatotomy
pancreatropic
pancrelipase
pancytopenia
 congenital p.
 Fanconi p.
pandemic
panel
 urine drug p.
panencephalitis
 subacute sclerosing p.
panendoscope
panesthesia
pang
 breast p.
panhypopituitarism
panic
 p. attack
 p. disorder
 homosexual p.
panimmunity
panlobular emphysema
panmyelophthisis
panmyelosis
Panner disease
pannicular hernia
panniculectomy
panniculitis
 cytophagic histiocytic p.
 lupus erythematosus p.
 relapsing febrile nodular
  nonsuppurative p.
 scrotal p.
 subacute migratory p.
pannus
 corneal p.
 p. crassus
 p. siccus
 p. tenuis
panoramic
 p. radiograph
 p. tomography
 p. x-ray film
panotitis
pansinusitis
pansystolic murmur
pantalgia
pantaloon hernia
pantomogram
pantomograph

pantomography
pantoscopic tilt
pantothenate
 calcium p.
pantothenic acid
Panum area
PAP
 3'-phosphoadenosine 5'-phosphate
 PAP technique
Pap
 P. smear
 P. test
Papanicolaou stain
paper
 articulating p.
 chromatography p.
 p. chromatography
 filter p.
 high-quality filter p.
 p. mill worker's disease
papilla, pl. papillae
 acoustic p.
 basilar p.
 Bergmeister p.
 bile p.
 circumvallate papillae
 conical p.
 dental p.
 dentinal p.
 dermal p.
 excavatio p.
 filiform p.
 foliate p.
 fungiform p.
 gingival p.
 hair p.
 ileal p.
 incisive p.
 interdental p.
 interproximal p.
 lacrimal p.
 lenticular p.
 lingual gingival p.
 lingual interdental p.
 major duodenal p.
 minor duodenal p.
 optic p.
 parotid p.
 renal p.
 retrocuspid p.
 tactile p.
 urethral p.
 p. urethralis
 vallate p.
papillaris
 areola p.
papillary
 p. adenocarcinoma
 p. carcinoid

p. carcinoma
p. cystic adenoma
p. cystitis
p. hidradenoma
p. muscle
p. stasis
p. tumor
papillate
papillectomy
papilledema
papilliferum
hidradenoma p.
papilliform
papillitis
foliate p.
papilloadenocystoma
papillocarcinoma
papilloma
basal cell p.
duct p.
hard p.
Hopmann p.
intracystic p.
intraductal p.
inverted p.
squamous p.
urothelial p.
papillomatosis
florid oral p.
juvenile p.
laryngeal p.
recurrent respiratory p.
papillomatous
papillomavirus
human p. (HPV)
papilloretinitis
papillotomy
Pappenheimer body
papular
p. mucinosis
p. tuberculid
p. urticaria
papule
follicular p.
moist p.
piezogenic pedal p.
prurigo p.
pruritic urticarial p.
papuloerythematous
papulonecrotic tuberculid
papulopustular

papulosa
acne p.
papulosis
bowenoid p.
lymphomatoid p.
malignant atrophic p.
papulosquamous
papulosum
eczema p.
papulous vaginitis
papulovesicular
papyraceous
papyraceus
fetus p.
paraaortic body
paraballism
parabasal body
parabiosis
parabiotic
parabotulinum
Clostridium p.
parabulia
paracasein
paracenesthesia
paracentesis
paracentetic
paracentral fissure
paracervical
paracervix
paracholera
parachordal
parachroma
parachromatosis
parachute
p. mitral valve
p. reflex
paracicatricial emphysema
paracoccidioidal granuloma
Paracoccidioides brasiliensis
paracoccidioidin
paracoccidioidomycosis
paracolitis
paracone
paraconid
paracrine
paracusis, paracusia
false p.
paracystic
paracystitis
paracytic hemoptysis
paradidymis
paradipsia

NOTES

P

paradox
    lactate p.
    Weber p.
paradoxic
    p. pulse
    p. pupillary reflex
paradoxical
    p. contraction
    p. diaphragm phenomenon
    p. diplopia
    p. embolism
    p. extensor reflex
    p. pulse
    p. respiration
    p. sleep
    p. vocal cord movement
paradoxus
    pulsus p.
paraesophageal hernia
parafascicular thalamotomy
paraffin
    chlorinated p.
    hard p.
    liquid p.
paraffinoma
parafollicular cell
parafunction
paraganglioma
paraganglion
parageusia
parageusic
paraglottic space
Paragonimus **granuloma**
paragrammatism
paragraphia
parahaemolyticus
    Haemophilus p.
    Vibrio p.
parahippocampal gyrus
parahormone
parainfluenzae
    Haemophilus p.
parainfluenza virus
parakeratosis
parakinesia
parakinesis
paralalia
paralexia
paralgesia
parallactic
parallax
    binocular p.
    heteronymous p.
    homonymous p.
    p. test
parallergic
paralogia
paralogism

paralogy
paralysis, pl. **paralyses**
    acute ascending p.
    arsenical p.
    ascending p.
    brachial p.
    Brown-Séquard p.
    bulbar p.
    central p.
    compression p.
    crossed p.
    crutch p.
    diphtheritic p.
    diver's p.
    Duchenne-Erb p.
    Erb p.
    facial p.
    familial periodic p.
    faucial p.
    flaccid p.
    functional p.
    generalized p.
    ginger p.
    global p.
    glossolabiolaryngeal p.
    glossolabiopharyngeal p.
    glossopalatolabial p.
    glossopharyngeolabial p.
    Gubler p.
    hyperkalemic periodic p.
    hypokalemic periodic p.
    hysterical p.
    immune p.
    immunologic p.
    immunological p.
    jake p.
    Klumpke p.
    Landry p.
    lead p.
    lingual p.
    mimetic p.
    mixed p.
    motor p.
    musculospiral p.
    myogenic p.
    narcosis p.
    normokalemic periodic p.
    obstetric p.
    organic p.
    periodic p.
    peripheral facial p.
    phrenic p.
    pressure p.
    progressive bulbar p.
    pseudobulbar p.
    sensory p.
    sleep p.
    spinal p.
    supranuclear p.

tick p.
Todd postepileptic p.
tourniquet p.
vasomotor p.
wasting p.
Zenker p.
paralytic
p. abasia
p. dementia
p. facies
p. ileus
p. incontinence
p. miosis
p. mydriasis
paralytica
aphonia p.
dementia p.
paralyticus
ictus p.
paralyzant
paralyze
Paramecium
paramedic
paramedical
paramenia
paramesonephric duct
parameter
enzyme p.
infection transmission p.
parametrial
parametric
parametritic
parametritis
paramimia
paramnesia
paramyloidosis
paramyotonia
ataxic p.
p. congenita
congenital p.
paranasal
p. cartilage
p. sinus
p. sinus cholesteatoma
paraneoplasia
paraneoplastic
p. encephalomyelopathy
p. pemphigus
p. syndrome
paranephric
paranephros

paranoia
acute hallucinatory p.
alcoholic p.
litigious p.
paranoid
p. personality
p. schizophrenia
paranomia
paranuclear
paranucleate
paranucleus
paraoperative
paraparesis
paraparetic
paraperitoneal hernia
parapharyngeal abscess
paraphasia
central p.
paraphasic
paraphia
paraphilia
paraphimosis
paraplectic
paraplegia
ataxic p.
congenital spastic p.
flaccid p.
infantile spastic p.
Pott p.
toxic p.
paraplegic headache
parapraxia
paraprotein
paraproteinaemia
paraproteinemia
parapsia
parapsilosis
Candida p.
parapsoriasis
parapsychology
pararectal pouch
parareflexia
pararenal
pararosanilin
pararrhythmia
parasaccular hernia
parasinoidal
parasite
accidental p.
autistic p.
autochthonous p.
commensal p.

NOTES

P

parasite *(continued)*
    euroxenous p.
    facultative p.
    heterogenetic p.
    heteroxenous p.
    incidental p.
    inquiline p.
    malignant tertian malarial p.
    obligate p.
    ova and p.'s (O&P)
    specific p.
    spurious p.
    temporary p.
parasitemia
parasitic
    p. cyst
    p. fetus
    p. melanoderma
parasitica
    achromia p.
parasiticidal
parasiticide
parasiticum
    eczema p.
parasiticus
    janiceps p.
parasitism
parasitize
parasitogenic
parasitologist
parasitology
parasitosis
parasitotropic
parasitotropism
parasomnia
parastasis
parasternal hernia
parasympathetic
    p. ganglion
    p. nerve
parasympatholytic
parasympathomimetic
parasynapsis
parasynovitis
parasystole
parataxic distortion
paratenon
parathyroid
    p. gland
    p. hormone
    p. hormone-related peptide
    p. tetany
parathyroidectomy
parathyrotrophic
parathyrotropic
paratope
paratropicalis
    Haemophilus p.
paratyphoid fever

paraumbilical
    p. hernia
    p. vein
paraurethral duct
paravaginal hysterectomy
paravaginitis
paravertebral
    p. block
    p. ganglion
paravesical fossa
paraxial
paraxon
parenchyma
parenchymatitis
parenchymatous
    p. degeneration
    p. glossitis
    p. goiter
    p. hemorrhage
    p. neuritis
    p. salpingitis
parental generation
parent cyst
parenteral
parenteric fever
Parenti-Fraccaro syndrome
parepididymis
paresis
    divergence p.
    general p.
paresthesia
paresthetic
paresthetica
    cheiralgia p.
    meralgia p.
Paré suture
paretic
    p. dementia
    p. neurosyphilis
pareunia
paries
parietal
    p. bone
    p. cell
    p. fistula
    p. foramen
    p. hernia
    p. lobe
    p. lymph node
    p. pericardium
    p. thrombus
    p. wall
parietalis
    decidua p.
parietis
parietography
parietooccipital sulcus
Parinaud
    P. conjunctivitis

P. oculoglandular syndrome
P. ophthalmoplegia
parity
Park aneurysm
Parkes Weber syndrome
Parkinson
P. disease
P. facies
parkinsonian dysarthria
parkinsonism
postencephalitis p.
secondary p.
vascular p.
parolfactory sulci
paromphalocele
paronychia
paronychial
paroöphoron
parorchidium
parorexia
parosmia
parosteosis
parostosis
parotic
parotid
p. duct
p. gland
p. notch
p. papilla
p. vein
parotidectomy
parotiditis
epidemic p.
parotitis
parous
parovarian
paroxysm
paroxysmal
p. cold hemoglobinuria
p. hypersomnia
p. hypertension
p. myoglobinuria
p. nocturnal dyspnea (PND)
p. nocturnal hemoglobinemia
p. nocturnal hemoglobinuria
p. tachycardia
parrot
p. beak tear
P. disease
p. fever
Parry disease
pars, pl. **partes**

p. amorpha
p. granulosa
p. interarticularis
p. plana
p. tympanica
part
acromial p.
basal p.
basilar p.
cortical p.
cuneiform p.
distal p.
dorsal p.
flaccid p.
hidden p.
infraclavicular p.
infrasegmental p.
infundibular p.
inguinal p.
insular p.
intercartilaginous p.
intermediate p.
intersegmental p.
intralobar p.
intramural p.
intraocular p.
intrasegmental p.
iridial p.
laryngeal p.
mobile p.
parthenogenesis
partial
p. agglutinin
p. ankylosis
p. anomalous pulmonary venous
connection
p. antigen
p. birth
p. cricoid cleft
p. denture
p. hysterectomy
p. laryngectomy
p. left ventriculectomy
p. lesion
p. posterior laryngeal cleft
p. pressure
p. rebreathing mask
p. seizure
p. thromboplastin time (PTT)
p. volume
partial-thickness
p.-t. burn

NOTES

P

partial-thickness *(continued)*
    p.-t. flap
    p.-t. graft
particle
    alpha p.
    beta p.
    chromatin p.
    core p.
    Dane p.
    defective interfering p.
    electron transport p. (ETP)
    elementary p.
    kappa p.
particulate wear debris
partition
    p. chromatography
    nitrogen p.
partner
    contralateral p.
partogram
parturient canal
parturiometer
parturition
parvocellular
parvum
    Corynebacterium p.
    Cryptosporidium p.
    Eubacterium p.
Pascal law
passage
    blind p.
    bouton en p.
Passavant ridge
Passavoy factor
passive
    p. anaphylaxis
    p. atelectasis
    p. clot
    p. congestion
    p. hemagglutination
    p. hyperemia
    p. immunity
    p. movement
passive-aggressive personality
passivism
passivity
    delusion of p.
past
    p. medical history (PMH)
    p. surgical history (PSH)
paste
    dermatologic p.
    desensitizing p.
Pasteur effect
Pasteurella
    P. aerogenes
    P. multocida
    P. pseudotuberculosis
pasteurellosis

pasteurization
Pastia sign
pastil, pastille
patch
    butterfly p.
    cotton-wool p.
    p. dressing
    herald p.
    Hutchinson p.
    Peyer p.
    p. test
patella, pl. **patellae**
    p. alta
    p. baja
    ballotable p.
    chondromalacia patellae
    floating p.
    squinting p.
patellar
    p. apprehension sign
    p. ligament
    p. reflex
patellectomy
patelliform
patelloadductor reflex
patellofemoral
    p. joint
    p. stress syndrome
patency
patent
    p. foramen ovale
    p. medicine
Patey operation
path
    clinical p.
    condyle p.
    generated occlusal p.
    incisal p.
    milled-in p.
pathergy
pathfinder
pathic
pathobiology
pathoclisis
pathogen
    behavioral p.
pathogenesis
    drug p.
pathogenetic
pathogenicity
pathogenic occlusion
pathognomonic symptom
pathognomy
pathologic
    p. calcification
    p. diagnosis
    p. fracture
    p. model
    p. myopia

p. protein
p. retraction ring
pathological anatomy
pathologist
speech-language p.
pathology
anatomic p.
cellular p.
clinical p.
comparative p.
dental p.
functional p.
humoral p.
medical p.
molecular p.
oral p.
speech p.
speech-language p.
surgical p.
pathomimesis
pathophysiology
pathosis
pathway
auditory p.
complement p.
critical p.
Embden-Meyerhof p.
Embden-Meyerhof-Parnas p.
Entner-Douderoff p.
extrinsic coagulation p.
hexose monophosphate p.
intrinsic coagulation p.
lacrimal p.
mercapturic acid p.
pentose phosphate p.
reentrant p.
ubiquitin-protease p.
patient
p. advocate
recalcitrant p.
patient-controlled
p.-c. analgesia (PCA)
p.-c. anesthesia (PCA)
Patrick test
patrilineal
pattern
airspace-filling p.
airway p.
alveolar p.
ballerina-foot p.
butterfly p.
capsular p.

cusp and groove p.
p. distortion amblyopia
ground-glass p.
honeycomb p.
hourglass p.
interstitial p.
juvenile p.
miliary p.
mosaic p.
p. retinal dystrophy
rugal p.
patterned alopecia
pattern-sensitive epilepsy
patulous
pauciarticular
paucibacillary
paucisynaptic
Pauli exclusion principle
pause
apneic p.
compensatory p.
postextrasystolic p.
preautomatic p.
respiratory p.
p. signal
sinus p.
Pautrier microabscess
Pavlov reflex
pavor nocturnus
payer
third-party p.
Payne operation
Payr
P. clamp
P. sign
PCA
patient-controlled analgesia
patient-controlled anesthesia
PE
physical evaluation
physical examination
peak
biclonal p.
p. expiratory flow
p. flowmeter
p. flow rate (PFR)
juxtaphrenic p.
kilovolts p. (kVp)
pearl
Elschnig p.
enamel p.
epithelial p.

NOTES

P

pearl (*continued*)
    Epstein p.
    gouty p.
    P. index
    keratin p.
    Laënnec p.
peau d'orange
peccant
pecten
    anal p.
    p. analis
    p. pubis
pectenitis
pectenosis
pectinata
    zona p.
pectinate
    p. line
    p. muscle
    p. zone
pectineal
    p. hernia
    p. ligament
    p. line
    p. muscle
pectineus muscle
pectiniform
pectora (*pl. of* pectus)
pectoral
    p. girdle
    p. region
    p. vein
pectoralis
    fascia p.
    fremitus p.
pectoriloquy
    aphonic p.
pectoris
    angina p.
    angor p.
    variant angina p.
pectus, pl. **pectora**
    p. carinatum
    p. excavatum
pederasty
Pederson speculum
pedesis
pediatric
    p. dentist
    p. dentistry
    p. intensive care unit (PICU)
pediatrician
pediatrics
pedicel
pedicellate
pedicellation
pedicle
    p. clamp
    p. flap

pedicular
pediculate
pediculation
pediculicide
pediculosis pubis
pediculous
pediculus
pedigree analysis
pedis
    arcus p.
    dermatomycosis p.
    dorsum p.
    malum perforans p.
    tinea p.
pedodontics
pedodontist
pedodynamometer
pedomorphism
pedophilia
pedophilic
peduncle
    cerebellar p.
    cerebral p.
    inferior cerebellar p.
    inferior thalamic p.
    lateral thalamic p.
    middle cerebellar p.
    olfactory p.
    superior cerebellar p.
    thalamic p.
    ventral thalamic p.
peduncular
pedunculate
pedunculotomy
pedunculus
peel
    bitter orange p.
    face p.
peeling
    chemical p.
PEEP
    positive end-expiratory pressure
    intrinsic P.
    occult P.
peeping testis
peer review
peer-review organization
Peet operation
peg-and-socket suture
pegged tooth
Pel-Ebstein
    P.-E. disease
    P.-E. fever
peliosis
    bacterial p.
    p. hepatis

pellagra
    infantile p.
pellagrous
Pellegrini disease
pellet
pellicle
    acquired p.
    brown p.
    dental acquired p.
pelliertieri
    Actinomadura p.
pellucid
    p. marginal corneal degeneration
    p. zone
pellucida
    zona p.
peltation
pelves (*pl. of* pelvis)
pelvic
    p. axis
    p. cavity
    p. cellulitis
    p. diaphragm
    p. direction
    p. exenteration
    p. fascia
    p. ganglion
    p. girdle
    p. inflammatory disease (PID)
    p. inlet
    p. osteotomy
    p. outlet
    p. peritonitis
    p. plane
    p. pole
    p. region
    p. version
pelvicephalometry
pelvifixation
pelvilithotomy
pelvimeter
pelvimetry
    CT p.
    manual p.
pelvioplasty
pelviotomy
pelviperitonitis
pelvis, pl. **pelves**
    android p.
    anthropoid p.
    assimilation p.
    beaked p.

brachypellic p.
contracted p.
cordate p.
cordiform p.
Deventer p.
dolichopellic p.
dwarf p.
extrarenal p.
false p.
flat p.
frozen p.
funnel-shaped p.
greater p.
gynecoid p.
hardened p.
heart-shaped p.
inclination of p.
inverted p.
p. justo major
p. justo minor
juvenile p.
kyphoscoliotic p.
kyphotic p.
large p.
lesser p.
longitudinal oval p.
lordotic p.
masculine p.
mesatipellic p.
Nägele p.
oblique p.
osteomalacic p.
platypellic p.
platypelloid p.
Prague p.
pseudoosteomalacic p.
rachitic p.
renal p.
Rokitansky p.
rostrate p.
scoliotic p.
small p.
split p.
spondylolisthetic p.
true p.
pelvitomy
pelvivertebral angle
pelvocaliectasis
pemphigoid
    benign mucosal p.
    bullous p.
    cicatricial p.

NOTES

P

pemphigoid *(continued)*
> localized p.
> ocular cicatricial p.

pemphigus
> benign familial chronic p.
> Brazilian p.
> p. erythematosus
> p. foliaceus
> p. gangrenosus
> paraneoplastic p.
> p. vulgaris

Pendred syndrome
pendular nystagmus
pendulum
> cor p.

penes (*pl. of* penis)
penetrance
> genetic p.

penetrating
> p. corneal graft
> p. wound

penicillin
> aluminum p.

penicilliosis
penicillus
penile
> p. clamp
> p. hypospadias
> p. prosthesis
> p. raphe

penis, pl. **penes**
> bifid p.
> buried p.
> clubbed p.
> concealed p.
> crus p.
> dorsum p.
> foreskin of p.
> glans p.
> gryposis p.
> septum p.

penischisis
pennate
penniform
Penrose drain
pentose phosphate pathway
pentosuria
> alimentary p.
> essential p.

pentyl
penumbra
peplomer
peplos
pep pill
pepsinogen
peptic
> p. cell
> p. digestion

> p. esophagitis
> p. ulcer

peptidase
> dipeptidyl p.

peptide
> adrenocorticotropic p.
> anionic neutrophil-activating p.
>   (ANAP)
> p. antibiotic
> antigen p.
> atrial natriuretic p. (ANP)
> bitter p.
> p. bond
> bradykinin-potentiating p.
> calcitonin gene-related p.
> corticotropin-like intermediate-
>   lobe p.
> gastric inhibitory p.
> glucagonlike p.
> glucagonlike insulinotropic p.
> heterodetic p.
> heteromeric p.
> homodetic p.
> homomeric p.
> parathyroid hormone-related p.

peptidergic
peptidoglycan
peptidoid
peptidolytic
peptidyl dipeptidase A
peptogenic
peptogenous
peptolysis
peptolytic
peptone
peptonic
peptonization
per
> p. anum
> p. contiguum
> p. continuum
> p. os
> p. primam intentionem
> p. rectum
> p. tubam
> p. vias naturales

peracid
peracute
percept
perception
> depth p.
> extrasensory p. (ESP)
> figure-ground p.
> speech p.

perceptive
> p. deafness
> p. hearing impairment

perceptivity
perceptual processing

perchloride
    mercury p.
percolation
percuss
percussion
    p. and auscultation (P&A)
    auscultation and p. (A&P)
    auscultatory p.
    bimanual p.
    clavicular p.
    clear to auscultation and p.
      (CTAP)
    deep p.
    direct p.
    distal tingling on p.
    finger p.
    immediate p.
    mediate p.
    Murphy p.
    palpatory p.
    p. sound
    p. wave
percussor
percutaneous
    p. transhepatic cholangiography
    p. transluminal angioplasty (PTA)
    p. transluminal coronary angioplasty
      (PTCA)
perencephaly
perfect
    p. fungus
    p. stage
perfectionism
perfectionistic personality
perforated ulcer
perforating
    p. abscess
    p. appendicitis
    p. artery
    p. fiber
    p. ulcer
    p. vein
    p. wound
perforation
perforin
performance
    p. area
    p. component
    p. context
    p. intensity
perfringens
    Clostridium p.

perfuse
perfusion
    pulmonary p.
periadenitis mucosa necrotica recurrens
perianal incision
periangitis
periaortitis
periapical
    p. cemental dysplasia
    p. curettage
    p. film
    p. granuloma
    p. radiograph
periappendiceal abscess
periappendicitis
periareolar incision
periarterial
    p. plexus
    p. sympathectomy
periarteritis nodosa
periarthritis
periarticular abscess
peribronchiolitis
peribronchitis
pericardiac
pericardiacophrenic
    p. artery
    p. vein
pericardial
    p. cavity
    p. cyst
    p. decompression
    p. effusion
    p. fremitus
    p. friction
    p. murmur
    p. rub
    p. sinus
    p. symphysis
    p. vein
pericardicentesis
pericardiectomy
pericardiology
pericardioperitoneal
pericardiophrenic
pericardiopleural
pericardiorrhaphy
pericardiostomy
pericardiotomy
pericarditic
pericarditis
    acute fibrinous p.

NOTES

P

pericarditis *(continued)*
  adhesive p.
  bacterial p.
  carcinomatous p.
  chronic constrictive p.
  constrictive p.
  dry p.
  epistenocardiac p.
  fibrinous p.
  fibrous p.
  hemorrhagic p.
  internal adhesive p.
  p. obliterans
  obliterative p.
  postpericardiotomy p.
  p. with effusion
pericardium
  adherent p.
  bread-and-butter p.
  calcified p.
  dropsy of p.
  fibrous p.
  parietal p.
pericholangitis
perichondral bone
perichondrial
perichondritis
perichrome
pericolitis
pericolpitis
pericoronitis
pericostal suture
pericranitis
pericranium
pericystic
pericystitis
pericyte
pericytic venule
peridental membrane
periderm, periderma
peridesmitis
peridesmium
perididymitis
peridiverticulitis
periduodenitis
peridural anesthesia
periencephalitis
perienteritis
periesophagitis
perifolliculitis
perigastritis
periglottis
perihepatitis
periinfarction block
perijejunitis
perikaryon
perikymata
perilabyrinthitis

perilimbal incision
perilymph, perilympha
perilymphangitis
perilymphatic
  p. duct
  p. fistula
  p. gusher
  p. space
perimeningitis
perimeter
  arc p.
  Goldmann p.
perimetric
perimetritic
perimetritis
perimetry
  computed p.
  flicker p.
  kinetic p.
  mesopic p.
perimolysis
perimyelitis
perimyositis
perimysial
perimysiitis, perimysitis
perimysium
perinatal
  p. medicine
  p. septicemia
perinatologist
perinatology
perineal
  p. artery
  p. fascia
  p. hernia
  p. hypospadias
  p. lithotomy
  p. nerve
  p. prostatectomy
  p. raphe
  p. section
  p. sensation
  p. testis
perinealis
  luxatio p.
perineocele
perineoplasty
perineorrhaphy
perineoscrotal
perineostomy
perineotomy
perineovaginal
perinephrial
perinephritis
perinephrium
perineum
  anterior p.
  posterior p.

perineural
  p. anesthesia
  p. block
perineurial
perineuritis
period
  absolute refractory p.
  amblyogenic p.
  critical p.
  eclipse p.
  effective refractory p.
  ejection p.
  extrinsic incubation p.
  fertile p.
  functional refractory p.
  gap0 p.
  gap1 p.
  gap2 p.
  incubation p.
  induction p.
  intrapartum p.
  isoelectric p.
  isometric contraction p.
  isometric relaxation p.
  isovolumic p.
  last menstrual p. (LMP)
  latency p.
  latent p.
  masticatory silent p.
  menstrual p.
  missed p.
  mitotic p.
  p. polyserositis
  prepatent p.
  refractory p.
  synthesis p.
  Wenckebach p.
periodic
  p. alternating nystagmus
  p. disease
  p. hypersomnia
  p. neutropenia
  p. paralysis
periodical mania
periodicity
  diurnal p.
  filarial p.
  lunar p.
  malarial p.
periodization
periodontal
  p. disease

  p. ligament
  p. membrane
  p. probe
  p. trauma
periodontics
periodontist
periodontitis
  apical p.
  juvenile p.
periodontium
periodontoclasia
periodontosis
perionychium
perioophoritis
perioophorosalpingitis
perioperative
periorbit
periorbital cellulitis
periorchitis
periosteal
  p. band
  p. bud
  p. elevator
  p. graft
  p. ossification
  p. osteogenesis
periosteitis
periosteoma
periosteomyelitis
periosteophyte
periosteoplastic amputation
periosteosis
periosteotomy
periosteum
  alveolar p.
periostitis
periostosis
periovaritis
peripachymeningitis
peripancreatitis
peripherad
peripheral
  p. ageusia
  p. angiography
  p. apnea
  p. arteriosclerosis
  p. facial paralysis
  p. fusion
  p. nervous system
  p. neuroglia
  p. ossifying fibroma
  p. resistance

NOTES

P

peripheral (*continued*)
    p. scotoma
    p. T-cell lymphoma, unspecified
    p. uveitis
    p. venography
    p. vision
periphery
periphlebitis
periporitis
periproctitis
periprostatitis
peripylephlebitis
perirectal fistula
perirectitis
perirhizoclasia
perisalpingitis
perisalpingoovaritis
perisalpinx
periscapular incision
periscopic
perisigmoiditis
perispermatitis
perisplanchnitis
perisplenitis
perispondylitis
peristalsis
    mass p.
    reversed p.
peristaltic anastomosis
peristole
peristolic
peritectomy
peritendineum
peritendinitis, peritenontitis
perithelium
    Eberth p.
perithyroiditis
peritomy
peritoneal
    p. abscess
    p. button
    p. carcinoma
    p. cavity
    p. dialysis
    p. incision
    p. insufflation
peritonei
    pseudomyxoma p.
peritoneocentesis
peritoneoclysis
peritoneopericardial
peritoneopexy
peritoneoplasty
peritoneoscope
peritoneoscopy
peritoneotomy
peritoneovenous shunt

peritoneum
    urogenital p.
    p. urogenitale
peritonitis
    adhesive p.
    bacterial p.
    benign paroxysmal p.
    bile p.
    chemical p.
    chyle p.
    chylous p.
    circumscribed p.
    diaphragmatic p.
    diffuse p.
    fibrocaseous p.
    gas p.
    general p.
    localized p.
    meconium p.
    pelvic p.
    tuberculous p.
peritonization
peritonize
peritonsillar abscess
peritonsillitis
peritrichal
peritrichate
peritrichic
peritrichous
peritubular contractile cell
periureteritis
periurethritis
periuterine
perivaginitis
perivasculitis
perivesical
perivisceritis
PERL
    pupils equal, react to light
PERLA
    pupils equal, react to light and
    accommodation
permanent
    p. callus
    p. cartilage
    p. dentition
    p. stained smear examination
    p. threshold shift
    p. tooth
permeability
    p. coefficient
    p. constant
permeable
permease
permeate
permeation
pernicious
    p. anemia
    p. vomiting

pernio
> erythema p.
> lupus p.

perodactyly, perodactylia

peromelia, peromely
> micrognathia with p.

peroneal
> p. artery
> p. muscular atrophy
> p. retinaculum
> p. sign
> p. vein

peroneus tertius muscle

peroral endoscopy

peroxidase
> horseradish p.
> iodide p.

peroxide
> benzoyl p.
> hydrogen p.
> magnesium p.
> medicinal zinc p.

peroxisome

peroxyl

perpendicularis
> agger p.

PERRLA
> pupils equal, round, react to light and accommodation

persalt

persarum
> *Dracunculus p.*

persecution
> delusion of p.

persecutory delusion

perseveration

persicolor
> *Microsporum p.*

persistence
> lactase p.
> microbial p.

persistent
> p. anterior hyperplastic primary vitreous
> p. chronic hepatitis
> p. cloaca
> p. posterior hyperplastic primary vitreous
> p. truncus arteriosus
> p. vegetative state

persona

personal
> p. equation
> p. space

personality
> affective p.
> antisocial p.
> asthenic p.
> authoritarian p.
> avoidant p.
> basic p.
> borderline p.
> compulsive p.
> cyclothymic p.
> dependent p.
> p. disorder
> dual p.
> p. formation
> hysterical p.
> inadequate p.
> masochistic p.
> multiple p.
> paranoid p.
> passive-aggressive p.
> perfectionistic p.
> p. profile
> schizoid p.
> schizotypal p.
> schizotypical p.
> type A, B p.

perspiration
> insensible p.
> sensible p.

perstans
> acrodermatitis p.

pertactin

pertechnetate

pertenue
> *Treponema p.*

Perthes test

Pertik diverticulum

pertussis
> *Bordetella p.*
> diphtheria, tetanus, and acellular p. (DTaP)

peruana
> verruca p.
> verruga p.

peruviana
> verruca p.

Peruvian wart

pervasive developmental disorder

pervious

NOTES

pes
  p. anserinus
  p. cavus
  p. planus
pessary
  cube p.
  diaphragm p.
  doughnut p.
  Dumontpallier p.
  Gariel p.
  Hodge p.
  Mayer p.
  Menge p.
pesticide
pestilence
pestilential
pestle
petechia, pl. **petechiae**
  calcaneal p.
  Tardieu p.
petechial hemorrhage
Peters ovum
petiolate
petiolated
petiolus
petit
  P. hernia
  P. herniotomy
  P. lumbar triangle
  p. mal
Petri dish culture
petrifaction
petrificans
  urethritis p.
pétrissage
petrolatum
  p. gauze dressing
  heavy liquid p.
  hydrophilic p.
  light liquid p.
petroleum
  liquid p.
petromastoid
petrooccipital fissure
petrosa
petrosal
petrositis
petrosphenoid
petrosquamosal
petrosquamous
petrotympanic fissure
petrous
Petzval surface
Peyer patch
Peyronie disease
Peyrot thorax
Pfannenstiel incision
Pfeiffer
  P. bacillus

  P. phenomenon
  P. syndrome
PFR
  peak flow rate
PFT
  pulmonary function test
P-glycoprotein
pH
  blood pH
  critical pH
phacoanaphylactica
  endophthalmitis p.
phacoanaphylaxis
phacocele
phacoemulsification
phacoerysis
phacogenic glaucoma
phacoid
phacolysis
phacolytic
phacoma, phakoma
phacomalacia
phacomatosis
phacomorphic glaucoma
phacoscope
phage
  defective p.
  Lambda p.
phagedena
phagedenic ulcer
phagocyte
phagocytic
  p. index
  p. pneumonocyte
phagocytin
phagocytize
phagocytolysis
phagocytolytic
phagocytophilia
  Ehrlichia p.
phagocytose
phagocytosis
  induced p.
phagolysosome
phagosome
phagotype
phakic eye
phakoma (*var. of* phacoma)
phakomatosis
phalangeal
phalangectomy
phalanx, pl. **phalanges**
  distal p.
  middle p.
Phalen maneuver
phallectomy
phallic phase
phallocampsis
phallodynia

phalloides
    Amanita p.
phalloidin
phalloplasty
phallotomy
phallus
phanerosis
    fatty p.
phantasia
phantasm
phantasmagoria
phantastica
    pseudologia p.
phantom
    p. aneurysm
    p. corpuscle
    p. limb
    p. limb pain
    Schultze p.
    sensory p.
    p. tumor
pharmaceutic
pharmaceutical care
pharmaceutics
pharmacodiagnosis
pharmacodynamic
pharmacodynamics
pharmacoeconomics
pharmacoepidemiology
pharmacogenetics
pharmacogenomics
pharmacognosy
pharmacokinetic
pharmacokinetics
pharmacologic
pharmacological
pharmacologist
pharmacology
    biochemical p.
    marine p.
Pharmacopoeia
    British P.
pharmacotherapy
pharmakinetics
pharyngeal
    p. arch
    p. bursa
    p. cleft
    p. flap
    p. gonorrhea
    p. groove
    p. herpes

    p. opening
    p. reflex
    p. tonsil
    p. vein
pharyngectomy
pharynges (*pl. of* pharynx)
pharyngis
    lacuna p.
    Mycoplasma p.
pharyngismus
pharyngitic
pharyngitis
    atrophic p.
    gangrenous p.
    granular p.
    membranous p.
    viral p.
pharyngocele
pharyngoconjunctival fever
pharyngoepiglottic
pharyngoepiglottidean
pharyngoesophageal diverticulum
pharyngoglossal
pharyngolaryngeal
pharyngolaryngitis
pharyngolith
pharyngomycosis
pharyngonasal
pharyngoplasty
pharyngoplegia
pharyngoscope
pharyngoscopy
pharyngospasm
pharyngostenosis
pharyngotomy
    anterior p.
    external p.
    subhyoid p.
pharyngotympanic auditory tube
pharynx, pl. **pharynges**
    isthmus of p.
    laryngeal p.
phase
    anal p.
    aqueous p.
    arrest of active p.
    continuous p.
    coupling p.
    discontinuous p.
    dispersed p.
    dispersion p.
    eclipse p.

NOTES

P

phase *(continued)*
    eruptive p.
    external p.
    gap0 p.
    gap1 p.
    gap2 p.
    genital p.
    horizontal growth p.
    p. I, II block
    p. image
    in p.
    internal p.
    lag p.
    latency p.
    logarithmic p.
    luteal p.
    M p.
    meiotic p.
    p. microscope
    oedipal p.
    oral p.
    phallic p.
    radial growth p.
    vertical growth p.
    vulnerable p.
phase-contrast
    p.-c. microscope
    p.-c. microscopy
PH conduction time
Phemister graft
phenaceturic acid
phenocopy
phenol
    camphorated p.
    p. coefficient
    liquefied p.
phenoluria
phenomenon, pl. **phenomena**
    adhesion p.
    AFORMED p.
    Anrep p.
    aqueous influx p.
    Arias-Stella p.
    arm p.
    Arthus p.
    Ascher aqueous influx p.
    Aschner p.
    Ashman p.
    Aubert p.
    Austin Flint p.
    autoscopic p.
    Babinski p.
    Bell p.
    Bombay p.
    Bordet-Gengou p.
    brake p.
    breakaway p.
    breakoff p.
    Brücke-Bartley p.

Capgras p.
centralization p.
cervicolumbar p.
cogwheel p.
constancy p.
crowding p.
Cushing p.
Danysz p.
dawn p.
Debré p.
declamping p.
déjà vu p.
Dejerine hand p.
Denys-Leclef p.
d'Herelle p.
2-dimension–3-dimension p.
dip p.
Donath-Landsteiner p.
Doppler p.
Duckworth p.
Ehret p.
Ehrlich p.
erythrocyte adherence p.
escape p.
facialis p.
finger p.
flat-and-rise p.
Flynn p.
Friedreich p.
Galassi pupillary p.
Gallavardin p.
gap p.
Gärtner vein p.
generalized Shwartzman p.
Gengou p.
gestalt p.
Glover p.
Grasset p.
Grasset-Gaussel p.
Gunn p.
Hamburger p.
Hill p.
hip p.
hip-flexion p.
Hoffmann p.
Houssay p.
Hunt paradoxic p.
immune adherence p.
jaw-winking p.
Jod-Basedow p.
Köbner p.
Koch p.
Kohnstamm p.
Kühne p.
LE p.
Leede-Rumpel p.
leg p.
Lucio leprosy p.
Marcus Gunn p.

misdirection p.
Mitsuo p.
Neisser-Wechsberg p.
no-reflow p.
on-off p.
paradoxical diaphragm p.
Pfeiffer p.
pivot-shift p.
Pool p.
pseudo-Graefe p.
psi p.
Pulfrich p.
Purkinje p.
quellung p.
Raynaud p.
rebound p.
reclotting p.
Riddoch p.
Rust p.
satellite p.
Schüller p.
second-set p.
Shwartzman p.
Somogyi p.
Soret p.
springlike p.
staircase p.
Strümpell p.
Tullio p.
Tyndall p.
warm-up p.
phenotype
phenotypic value
phenozygous
phenyl
phenylacetic acid
phenylaceturic acid
phenylalaninase
phenylalanine
phenyldichloroarsine
phenylhydrazine hemolysis
phenylketonuria
phenyllactic acid
phenylpyruvic acid
phenylthiohydantoin
pheochrome
pheochromocyte
pheochromocytoma
pheresis
pheromone
Phialophora
Philadelphia chromosome

Phillips catheter
Phillipson reflex
philtrum
phimosis
phimotic
phlebectasia
phlebectomy
phlebitic
phlebitis
adhesive p.
septic p.
phleboclysis
drip p.
phlebogram
phlebograph
phlebography
phlebolith
phlebolithiasis
phlebomanometer
phlebophlebostomy
phleboplasty
phleborrhaphy
phlebosclerosis
phlebostasis
phlebostenosis
phlebothrombosis
phlebotomist
phlebotomize
Phlebotomus
phlebotomy
bloodless p.
phlegm
phlegmasia
phlegmatic
phlegmon
phlegmonous
p. abscess
p. adenitis
phloridzin glycosuria
phlorizin glycosuria
phlyctena
phlyctenar
phlyctenoid
phlyctenula
phlyctenular keratitis
phlyctenule
phlyctenulosis
phobia
school p.
simple p.
social p.

NOTES

P

691

phobia *(continued)*
    specific p.
    street p.
phobic
phobophobia
phocomelia
phocomely
phon
phonacoscope
phonacoscopy
phonal
phonasthenia
phonation
phonatory
phoneme
phonendoscope
phonendoskiascope
phonetic balance
phoniatrics
phonic
phonoangiography
phonocardiogram
phonocardiograph
    linear p.
    logarithmic p.
phonocardiography
phonocatheter
phonogram
phonometer
phonomyoclonus
phonopathy
phonophoresis
phonophotography
phonopsia
phonoreceptor
phonoscopy
phoresis
phoria
phoriascope
phoroscope
phosgene
phosphatase
    acid p.
    alkaline p.
    choline p.
    hexose p.
    phosphorylase p.
phosphate
    acetyl p.
    adenosine cyclic p.
    aluminum p.
    amphetamine p.
    amprotropine p.
    bone p.
    calcium monohydrogen p.
    codeine p.
    creatine p.
    d-amphetamine p.
    deoxyribose p.

    dexamphetamine sodium p.
    dextroamphetamine p.
    p. diabetes
    dihydrogen p.
    dipotassium p.
    disodium p.
    dolichol p.
    effervescent sodium p.
    energy-rich p.
    ferric p.
    glycerol p.
    guaiacol p.
    high-energy p.
    histamine p.
    inorganic p.
    nicotinamide adenine dinucleotide p.
    sodium p. 32P
5′-phosphate
    3′-phosphoadenosine 5′-p. (PAP)
6-phosphate
    glucose 6-p.
phosphatemia
phosphatic
phosphatide
    acetal p.
phosphatidylglycerol
phosphaturia
phosphene
phosphide
    hydrogen p.
3′-phosphoadenosine 5′-phosphate (PAP)
phosphoamidase
phosphoamide
phosphocreatine
phosphodiesterase
    sphingomyelin p.
phosphoenolpyruvic acid
phosphoglyceride
phosphokinase
    choline p.
    creatine p. (CPK)
phospholipase
phospholipid
phosphomutase
phosphonecrosis
phosphoprotein
phosphor
phosphorescence
phosphorescent
phosphoribosyltransferase
    adenine p.
phosphoric acid
phosphorism
phosphorolysis
phosphoroscope
phosphorous
phosphorus
    amorphous p.
phosphorus-32

phosphorylase
    glycogen p.
    p. phosphatase
phosphorylation
    oxidative p.
phosphosugar
phosphotungstic acid
photalgia
photic driving
photic-sneeze reflex
photism
photoablation
photoaging
photobiotic
photocatalyst
photochemical
photochemotherapy
photochromic lens
photocoagulation
photocoagulator
    laser p.
photodermatitis
photodetector
photodistribution
photodynamic
    p. sensitization
    p. therapy
photodynia
photoelectric
photofluorography
photofluoroscope
photofluoroscopy
photogastroscope
photogenic epilepsy
photogenous
photoinactivation
photoluminescent
photolyase
    deoxyribodipyrimidine p.
    dipyrimidine p.
photolysis
photolytic
photometer
    flame p.
    flicker p.
photomicrograph
photomicrography
photomicroscope
photomicroscopy
photomyoclonus
    hereditary p.
photon

photo-patch test
photoperceptive
photophobia
photophobic
photophoresis
    extracorporeal p.
photophthalmia
photopia
photopic
    p. adaptation
    p. eye
    p. vision
photopsia
photopsin
photopsy
photoptarmosis
photoradiation therapy
photoreaction
photoreactivation
photoreceptive
photoreceptor cell
photoretinitis
photoretinopathy
photoscan
photoscopy
photosensitisation
photosensitization
photostable
photostethoscope
photosynthesis
    bacterial p.
phototaxis
phototherapeutic keratectomy
phototherapy
phototimer
phototoxicity
phototropism
photuria
phrenalgia
phrenetic
phrenic
    p. ganglion
    p. nerve
    p. paralysis
phrenicectomy
phreniclasia
phrenicoabdominal branch
phrenicocolic ligament
phrenicoexeresis
phrenicogastric
phrenicohepatic
phrenicopleural fascia

NOTES

P

693

phrenicotomy
phrenicotripsy
phrenocardia
phrenoplegia
phrenoptosia
phrynoderma
phthisis
    aneurysmal p.
    bacillary p.
    grinder's p.
    miner's p.
    potter's p.
    pulmonary p.
phycomycosis
phylaxis
phyllodes
    cystosarcoma p.
phylloquinone
phylogenesis
phylogenetic
phylogenic
phylogeny
phylum
phyma
phymatosis
physaliform
physaliphora
    ecchordosis p.
physalis
physeal
physiatrics
physiatrist
physiatry
physical
    p. activity
    p. agent
    p. allergy
    p. conditioning
    p. diagnosis
    p. evaluation (PE)
    p. examination (PE)
    p. fitness
    history and p. (H&P)
    p. map
    p. medicine
    p. medicine and rehabilitation
    (PMR)
    p. sign
    p. therapist
    p. therapy
physic epilepsy
physician
    admitting p.
    attending p.
    family p.
    hospital-based p.
    p. office laboratory
    osteopathic p.
    primary care p.

physician-assisted suicide
Physick
    P. operation
    P. pouch
physicochemical
physics
physiogenic
physiognomy
physiologic
    p. amenorrhea
    p. antidote
    p. bradycardia
    p. chemistry
    p. congestion
    p. dead space
    p. gastrectomy
    p. homeostasis
    p. hypertrophy
    p. icterus
    p. jaundice
    p. leukocytosis
    p. occlusion
    p. rest position
    p. retina
    p. retraction ring
    p. saline
    p. scotoma
    p. sphincter
    p. unit
physiological drive
physiologist
physiology
    exercise p.
    general p.
    hominal p.
physiotherapeutic
physiotherapist
physiotherapy
physique
physocele
physometra
physopyosalpinx
phytoagglutinin
phytobezoar
phytochemical
phytodermatitis
phytohemagglutinin
phytoid
phytol
phytolectin
phytomitogen
phytophlyctodermatitis
phytophotodermatitis
phytotoxic
phytotoxin
pia
pia-arachnitis
pia-arachnoid
pial

piarachnoid
pica
Picchini syndrome
Pick
    P. atrophy
    P. body
    P. cell
    P. disease
Pickles chart
pickwickian syndrome
picogram
picokatal
picolinate
    chromium p.
picometer
picomole
picornavirus
picrocarmine stain
PICU
    pediatric intensive care unit
PID
    pelvic inflammatory disease
piebald
    p. eyelash
    p. skin
piebaldism
piebaldness
piece
    end p.
    Fab p.
    Fc p.
    middle p.
piecemeal
piedra
    black p.
    white p.
Pierre Robin syndrome
piesesthesia
piesimeter
    Hales p.
piesometer
piezogenic pedal papule
pig
    guinea p.
pigeon breast
piggyback
pigment
    bile p.
    chymotropic p.
    p. dispersion syndrome
    formalin p.
    hematogenous p.

    hepatogenous p.
    malarial p.
    melanotic p.
    respiratory p.
    visual p.
    wear-and-tear p.
pigmentary retinopathy
pigmentation
    arsenic p.
    exogenous p.
pigmented
    p. layer
    p. villonodular synovitis
    p. villonodular tenosynovitis
pigmentolysin
pigmentosa
    retinitis p.
    urticaria p.
pigmentosum
    xeroderma p.
pigmentosus
    nevus p.
pigmentum nigrum
pigtail
    p. appearance
    p. catheter
pilar
    p. cyst
    p. tumor
pilaris
    keratosis p.
    pityriasis rubra p.
pilary
pile
    sentinel p.
pileous gland
pili (*pl. of* pilus)
piliform
pill
    bread p.
    morning after p.
    pep p.
pillar
    anterior p.
    Corti p.
pillow splint
2-pillow orthopnea
3-pillow orthopnea
pill-rolling tremor
pilobezoar
pilocystic

NOTES

P

pilocytic astrocytoma
piloerection
piloid
pilojection
pilomatrixoma
pilomotor reflex
pilon fracture
pilonidal
    p. cyst
    p. sinus
pilorum
    cruces p.
    flumina p.
pilose
pilosebaceous
pilosus
    nevus p.
pilus, pl. pili
    F p.
    folliculus pili
    pili torti
pimelic acid
Pinard maneuver
pincement
pincer nail
pinch
    p. graft
    lateral p.
    palmar p.
    tip p.
pinchcock mechanism
pincushion distortion
pineal
    p. body
    p. gland
    p. stalk
pinealectomy
pinealocyte
pinealoma
    ectopic p.
    extrapineal p.
Pinel system
pineoblastoma
pinguecula, pinguicula
pinhole pupil
piniform
pink disease
pinkeye
pinna, pl. pinnae
pinnal
pinocyte
pinocytosis
pinosome
Pins
    P. sign
    P. syndrome
pinto
    mal del p.
pinworm

piperazine
    acefylline p.
Piper forceps
piperidine
pipette
    blowout p.
    graduated p.
    Mohr p.
piriform
    p. muscle
    p. neuron layer
piriformis muscle
Pirogoff
    P. amputation
    P. operation
Pirquet test
piscicida
    Flavobacterium p.
pisiform bone
pit
    anal p.
    auditory p.
    buccal p.
    central p.
    coated p.
    commissural p.
    gastric p.
    granular p.
    inferior costal p.
    iris p.
    lens p.
    lip p.
    Mantoux p.
    nail p.
    nasal p.
    preauricular p.
pitch
    Burgundy p.
    habitual p.
    liquid p.
    modal p.
    natural p.
    optimal p.
    p. wart
pithecoid
Pitres sign
pitted keratolysis
pitting edema
Pittsburgh
    P. pneumonia
    P. pneumonia agent
pituicyte
pituicytoma
pituitarism
pituitary
    p. adamantinoma
    p. amenorrhea
    p. cachexia
    desiccated p.

p. diverticulum
p. dwarfism
p. dystopia
p. gigantism
p. gland
p. gonadotropic hormone
p. growth hormone
p. myxedema
p. stalk
pityriasic
pityriasis
    p. alba
    p. linguae
    p. rosea
    p. rubra
    p. rubra pilaris
    p. versicolor
pityrodes
    alopecia p.
pityroid
pivot
    adjustable occlusal p.
    p. joint
pivot-shift
    p.-s. phenomenon
    p.-s. sign
PIVU
    pulmonary intensive care unit
pixel
PJ interval
place
    p. coding
    deep p.
    deserted p.
placebo
    active p.
placenta
    accessory p.
    p. accreta
    adherent p.
    anular p.
    battledore p.
    bidiscoidal p.
    chorioallantoic p.
    chorioamnionic p.
    p. circumvallata
    cotyledonary p.
    deciduate p.
    dichorionic diamnionic p.
    disperse p.
    Duncan p.
    endotheliochorial p.

endothelio-endothelial p.
epitheliochorial p.
p. fenestrata
fetal p.
p. fetalis
hemochorial p.
hemoendothelial p.
horseshoe p.
incarcerated p.
p. increta
labyrinthine p.
p. marginata
maternal p.
p. membranacea
monochorionic diamnionic p.
multilobate p.
p. previa
p. reflexa
Schultze p.
p. spuria
succenturiate p.
twin p.
varicose p.
placentae
    abruptio p.
placental
    p. barrier
    p. circulation
    p. dystocia
    p. growth hormone
    p. membrane
    p. pregnancy
    p. presentation
    p. transfusion syndrome
placentation
placentitis
placentoma
Placido da Costa disc
placode
    auditory p.
    epibranchial p.
    lens p.
plafond
plagiocephalic
plagiocephaly
plague
    ambulant p.
    ambulatory p.
    black p.
    bubonic p.
    glandular p.
    hemorrhagic p.

NOTES

P

plague *(continued)*
    larval p.
    pneumonic p.
plain film
plana
    cornea p.
    coxa p.
    pars p.
    verruca p.
    vertebra p.
plana *(pl. of* planum)
planar
    echo p.
Planck
    P. constant
    P. theory
plane
    Addison clinical p.
    Aeby p.
    auriculoinfraorbital p.
    axial p.
    axiolabiolingual p.
    axiomesiodistal p.
    bite p.
    Broca visual p.
    Camper p.
    canthomeatal p.
    coronal p.
    cove p.
    datum p.
    Daubenton p.
    equatorial p.
    eye-ear p.
    facial p.
    first parallel pelvic p.
    fourth parallel pelvic p.
    Frankfort horizontal p.
    frontal p.
    guide p.
    horizontal p.
    infraorbitomeatal p.
    interspinal p.
    interspinous p.
    intertubercular p.
    p. joint
    labiolingual p.
    mean foundation p.
    Meckel p.
    median p.
    midsagittal p.
    nuchal p.
    occlusal p.
    orbital p.
    orbitomeatal p.
    pelvic p.
    sagittal p.
    sternal p.
    subcostal p.
    supraorbitomeatal p.

    p. suture
    temporal p.
    transverse p.
planigraphy
planing
planning
    comprehensive discharge p.
planocellular
planoconcave lens
planoconvex lens
planography
planopilaris
    lichen p.
planovalgus
plantalgia
plantar
    p. arch
    p. calcaneonavicular ligament
    p. fasciitis
    p. fibromatosis
    p. interosseous muscle
    p. metatarsal artery
    p. reflex
    p. space
    p. wart
plantarflexion
plantaris
    keratosis palmaris et p.
    p. muscle
    pustulosis palmaris et p.
    verruca p.
plantarum
    Lactobacillus p.
plantigrade
planula, pl. **planulae**
    invaginate p.
planum, pl. **plana**
    xanthoma p.
planus
    lichen p.
    lichen ruber p.
    pes p.
    talipes p.
plaque
    atheromatous p.
    bacterial p.
    bacteriophage p.
    collagenous p.
    dental p.
    herald p.
    Hollenhorst p.
    neuritic p.
    Randall p.
    senile p.
    shagreen p.
plasma, plasm
    p. accelerator globulin
    antihemophilic p.
    blood p.

p. cell
p. cell leukemia
p. cell mastitis
p. cell myeloma
p. expander
p. fibronectin
fresh frozen p. (FFP)
p. membrane
normal human p.
p. protein
p. renin activity
p. scalpel
p. thromboplastin antecedent

plasmablast
plasmacellularis
balanitis circumscripta p.
plasmacrit test
plasmacyte
plasmacytoma
plasmacytosis
plasmakinin
plasmalemma
plasmalogen
plasmapheresis
plasmapheretic
plasmatic
plasmic
plasmid
bacteriocinogenic p.
conjugative p.
F p.
infectious p.
nonconjugative p.
resistance p.
plasmin
plasminogen activator
plasmodial
Plasmodium
P. falciparum
P. malariae
P. ovale
P. vivax
plasmogamy
plasmolysis
plasmolytic
plasmon
plasmorrhexis
plasmoschisis
plasmotropic
plasmotropism
plaster bandage

plastic
Bingham p.
p. envelope culture
modeling p.
p. pleurisy
p. surgery
plastica
linitis p.
plasticity
plastid
blood p.
plate
alar p.
amorphous selenium p.
anal p.
axial p.
basal p.
base p.
blood p.
bone p.
buttress p.
cardiogenic p.
cell p.
chorionic p.
cloacal p.
compression p.
cribriform p.
cutis p.
dorsal p.
dorsolateral p.
end p.
epiphysial p.
equatorial p.
ethmovomerine p.
flat p.
floor p.
foot p.
frontal p.
growth p.
horizontal p.
Kühne p.
lateral cartilaginous p.
lateral pterygoid p.
lingual p.
medial cartilaginous p.
medial pterygoid p.
medullary p.
motor p.
muscle p.
nail p.
neural p.
neutralization p.

NOTES

P

plate (*continued*)
    roof p., roofplate
    selenium p.
    stigmal p.
    ventral p.
plateau
    p. pressure
    p. pulse
platelet
    p. factor 3, 4
    hemolysis, elevated liver function, and low p.'s (HELLP)
    p. neutralization procedure
    p. tissue factor
platelet-activating factor
platelet-aggregating factor
plateletpheresis
platelike atelectasis
platform
    force p.
plating
    compression p.
platinum
platybasia
platycephaly
platyhelminth
Platyhelminthes
platypellic pelvis
platypelloid pelvis
platypnea
platysma muscle
platyspondylia
platyspondylisis
play
    speed p.
    p. therapy
pleasure principle
pledget
pleiotropia
pleiotropic gene
pleiotropy
    functional p.
pleocytosis
pleomastia
pleomazia
pleomorphic lipoma
pleomorphism
pleomorphous
pleonasm
pleonosteosis
    Leri p.
plessimeter
plessor
plethora
plethoric
plethysmograph
    body p.
    digital p.

plethysmography
    impedance p.
plethysmometry
pleura, pl. **pleurae**
    cervical p.
    costal p.
    diaphragmatic p.
    dome of p.
    mediastinal p.
pleural
    p. cavity
    p. effusion
    p. fluid
    p. fremitus
    p. metastasis
    p. pressure
    p. rub
    p. space
    p. tap
pleurapophysis
pleurectomy
pleurisy
    adhesive p.
    basal p.
    benign dry p.
    bilateral p.
    blocked p.
    chronic p.
    costal p.
    diaphragmatic p.
    diffuse p.
    double p.
    dry p.
    encysted p.
    epidemic benign dry p.
    epidemic diaphragmatic p.
    fibrinous p.
    hemorrhagic p.
    interlobular p.
    mediastinal p.
    plastic p.
    primary p.
    purulent p.
    serofibrinous p.
    serous p.
    visceral p.
    wet p.
pleuritic rub
pleuritis
pleurocele
pleurocentesis
pleurocentrum
pleuroclysis
pleurodesis
pleurodynia
    epidemic p.
pleuroesophageal muscle
pleurogenic
pleurogenous

pleurography
pleurohepatitis
pleurolith
pleurolysis
pleuropericardial rub
pleuropericarditis
pleuroperitoneal shunt
pleuropneumonectomy
pleuropneumonia-like organism
pleuropulmonary
pleurotomy
pleurovenous shunt
pleurovisceral
plexal
plexectomy
plexiform
    p. ameloblastoma
    p. neurofibroma
    p. neuroma
pleximeter
plexitis
    brachial p.
plexogenic
plexometer
plexopathy
plexor
plexus, pl. **plexus, plexuses**
    abdominal aortic p.
    acromial p.
    anterior coronary periarterial p.
    anular p.
    aortic lymphatic p.
    areolar venous p.
    arterial p.
    articular vascular p.
    ascending pharyngeal p.
    Auerbach p.
    autonomic p.
    axillary lymphatic p.
    basilar venous p.
    Batson p.
    brachial autonomic p.
    cardiac p.
    cardiac nervous p.
    cavernous nervous p.
    cavernous vascular p.
    celiac p.
    celiac lymphatic p.
    celiac nervous p.
    cervical p.
    choroid p.
    ciliary ganglionic p.

coccygeal p.
common carotid nervous p.
coronary p.
Cruveilhier p.
deep cardiac p.
deferential nervous p.
enteric nervous p.
esophageal nervous p.
Exner p.
external carotid nervous p.
external iliac lymphatic p.
external maxillary p.
facial p.
femoral nervous p.
gastric nervous p.
Haller p.
Heller p.
hemorrhoidal p.
hepatic nervous p.
iliac nervous p.
inferior dental nervous p.
inferior hemorrhoidal p.
inferior hypogastric nervous p.
inferior mesenteric nervous p.
inferior rectal nervous p.
inferior thyroid p.
inferior vesical venous p.
inguinal lymphatic p.
intermesenteric nervous p.
internal carotid nervous p.
internal carotid venous p.
internal mammary p.
internal maxillary p.
internal thoracic lymphatic p.
intracavernous p.
intraepithelial p.
intraparotid p.
ischiadic p.
Jacobson p.
Jacques p.
jugular lymphatic p.
Leber p.
lingual p.
lumbar lymphatic p.
lumbar nervous p.
lumbosacral nervous p.
lymphatic p.
mammary p.
maxillary p.
Meissner p.
meningeal p.
middle hemorrhoidal p.

NOTES

P

plexus *(continued)*
   middle rectal nervous p.
   middle sacral lymphatic p.
   myenteric p.
   nerve p.
   pampiniform p.
   periarterial p.
   pulmonary p.
   sacral p.
   Santorini p.
   scleral p.
   submucosal p.
   tympanic p.
plica, pl. **plicae**
plicata
   lingua p.
plicate
plicating suture
plication
plicotomy
ploidy
plot
   double-reciprocal p.
   Eadie-Hofstee p.
   funnel p.
   Hanes p.
   Hill p.
   Lineweaver-Burk p.
plug
   Dittrich p.
   epithelial p.
   laminated epithelial p.
   meconium p.
   mucous p.
plugger
   automatic p.
   back-action p.
   foot p.
plugging
   mucous p.
plumbism
plumbum
plume
   laser p.
Plummer-Vinson syndrome
pluriglandular
pluripotent
pluripotential
plutonium
plyometric training
PMH
   past medical history
PMI
   point of maximal impulse
   point of maximal intensity
PMR
   physical medicine and rehabilitation
PND
   paroxysmal nocturnal dyspnea

pneumarthrogram
pneumarthrography
pneumarthrosis
pneumatic
   p. antishock garment
   p. bone
   p. boot
   p. dilator
   p. orthosis
   p. otoscopy
   p. tonometer
pneumatization
pneumatocardia
pneumatocele
   extracranial p.
   intracranial p.
pneumatorrhachis
pneumatosis
pneumaturia
pneumoarthrography
pneumocardial
pneumocele
   extracranial p.
   intracranial p.
pneumocentesis
pneumocephalus
pneumococcal
pneumococcemia
pneumococcidal
pneumococcosis
pneumococcosuria
pneumococcus
   Fraenkel p.
pneumoconiosis
   asbestos p.
   bauxite p.
   coal worker's p.
   collagenous p.
   complicated p.
pneumocranium
Pneumocystis carinii
pneumocystography
pneumocystosis
pneumoderma
pneumodynamics
pneumogastric nerve
pneumogram
pneumograph
pneumography
pneumohemopericardium
pneumohemothorax
pneumohydrometra
pneumohydropericardium
pneumohydroperitoneum
pneumohydrothorax
pneumolith
pneumolithiasis
pneumomediastinum
pneumomyelography

pneumonectomy
pneumonia
    acute interstitial p.
    alcoholic p.
    anaerobic p.
    apex p.
    apical p.
    aspiration p.
    atypical p.
    bacterial p.
    bilious p.
    bronchial p.
    bronchiolitis obliterans with
      organizing p. (BOOP)
    caseous p.
    central p.
    chemical p.
    chronic eosinophilic p.
    community-acquired p.
    congenital p.
    core p.
    deglutition p.
    desquamative p.
    desquamative interstitial p.
    double p.
    embolic p.
    eosinophilic p.
    fibrous p.
    Friedländer bacillus p.
    gangrenous p.
    giant cell p.
    Hecht p.
    hospital-acquired p.
    hypostatic p.
    influenza p.
    influenzal virus p.
    interstitial plasma cell p.
    intrauterine p.
    lipid p.
    lipoid p.
    lobar p.
    lymphocytic interstitial p. (LIP)
    lymphoid interstitial p. (LIP)
    metastatic p.
    migratory p.
    mycoplasmal p.
    neonatal p.
    Pittsburgh p.
    primary atypical p.
    rheumatic p.
    septic p.
    usual interstitial p.

pneumoniae
    Chlamydia p.
    Klebsiella p.
    Mycoplasma p.
pneumonic plague
pneumonitis
    acute interstitial p.
    hypersensitivity p.
    lymphocytic interstitial p.
pneumonocele
pneumonocentesis
pneumonococcal
pneumonocyte
    granular p.
    phagocytic p.
pneumonopathy
    eosinophilic p.
pneumonopexy
pneumonorrhaphy
pneumonotomy
pneumoorbitography
pneumopericardium
    tension p.
pneumoperitoneum
pneumoperitonitis
pneumophila
    Legionella p.
pneumopleuritis
pneumopyelography
pneumopyothorax
pneumoradiography
pneumoretroperitoneum
pneumorrhachis
pneumotachogram
pneumotachograph
    Fleisch p.
pneumotachometer
pneumothorax
    artificial p.
    catamenial p.
    clicking p.
    extrapleural p.
    iatrogenic p.
    open p.
    spontaneous p.
    tension p.
    traumatic p.
    valvular p.
pneumotomy
pocket
    p. dosimeter
    gingival p.

NOTES

P

pocket *(continued)*
    infrabony p.
    intrabony p.
    Rathke p.
    retraction p.
    rheumatoid p.
    Seessel p.
pocketed calculus
pockmark
podagra
podalgia
podalic version
podarthritis
podedema
podiatric medicine
podiatrist
podiatry
podocyte
pododynamometer
pododynia
podogram
podomechanotherapy
podophyllum
    Indian p.
poeciloides
    Eubacterium p.
pogonion
poikiloblast
poikilocyte
poikilocythemia
poikilocytosis
poikiloderma
poikilothermal
poikilothermic
poikilothermous
point
    p. A, B
    absorbent p.
    alveolar p.
    p. angle
    anterior focal p.
    apophysary p.
    apophysial p.
    auricular p.
    axial p.
    boiling p.
    break-even p.
    Cannon p.
    Capuron p.
    cardinal p.
    p. of care
    central-bearing p.
    Clado p.
    clinical end p.
    cold-rigor p.
    congruent p.
    conjugate p.
    contact p.

    craniometric p.
    critical p.
    dew p.
    end p.
    p. epidemic
    equivalence p.
    far p.
    flash p.
    focal p.
    freezing p.
    fusing p.
    Guéneau de Mussy p.
    gutta-percha p.
    Hallé p.
    heat-rigor p.
    image p.
    incident p.
    incisal p.
    isoelectric p. (IEP)
    isoionic p.
    isosbestic p.
    J p.
    jugal p.
    lower alveolar p.
    malar p.
    p. of maximal impulse (PMI)
    p. of maximal intensity (PMI)
    maximum occipital p.
    Mayo-Robson p.
    McBurney p.
    median mandibular p.
    melting p.
    mental p.
    metopic p.
    motor p.
    Munro p.
    p. mutation
    nasal p.
    near p.
    nodal p.
    posterior focal p.
    pressure p.
    principal p.
    tender p.
    trigger p.
    Trousseau p.
    Valleix p.
    zygomaxillary p.
pointed condyloma
pointer
    hip p.
pointes
    torsade de p.
2-point gait
3-point gait
pointillage
Poiseuille
    P. law

P. space
P. viscosity coefficient
poison
    acrid p.
    arrow p.
    corrosive p.
    fish p.
    fugu p.
    narcotic p.
    puffer p.
poisoning
    acetaminophen p.
    acetanilid p.
    ackee p.
    bacterial food p.
    blood p.
    carbon disulfide p.
    carbon monoxide p.
    crotalaria p.
    cyanide p.
    Datura p.
    djenkol p.
    ergot p.
    food p.
    lead p.
    mercury p.
    mushroom p.
    scombroid p.
poisonous
poker spine
Poland syndrome
polar
    p. body
    p. cataract
    p. star
    p. temporal artery
polarity therapy
polarization
polarized light
pole
    abapical p.
    animal p.
    anterior p.
    apical p.
    cephalic p.
    frontal p.
    germinal p.
    inferior p.
    lateral p.
    lower p.
    medial p.
    occipital p.

    pelvic p.
    temporal p.
    twin p.'s
    vegetal p.
    vegetative p.
    vitelline p.
polecki
    Entamoeba p.
polioclastic
poliodystrophy
polioencephalitis
    inferior p.
polioencephalomeningomyelitis
polioencephalomyelitis
polioencephalopathy
poliomyelitis
    acute anterior p.
    acute bulbar p.
    chronic anterior p.
    p. virus
poliomyeloencephalitis
poliomyelopathy
poliosis
    ciliary p.
poliovirus
    p. hominis
    p. vaccine
Politzer
    P. bag
    P. luminous cone
politzerization
pollenosis
pollicization
pollinosis
Pollock operation
pollutant
pollution
    air p.
    noise p.
polonium
Pólya
    P. gastrectomy
    P. operation
polyacrylamide gel electrophoresis
polyadenitis
polyadenopathy
polyamine
polyangiitis
    microscopic p.
polyanion
polyarteritis nodosa
polyarthric

NOTES

P

705

polyarthritis
    epidemic p.
polyarticular
polyaxial joint
polybasic
polyblast
polychondritis
    chronic atrophic p.
    relapsing p.
polychromasia
polychromatic
    p. cell
    p. radiation
polychromatocyte
polychromatophil, polychromatophile
    p. cell
polychromatophilia
polychromatophilic
polychromemia
polyclinic
polyclonal gammopathy
polyclonia
polycoria
polycrotic
polycrotism
polycyesis
polycystic
    p. disease
    p. kidney
    p. liver
    p. ovary
    p. ovary syndrome
polycythemia
    benign p.
    compensatory p.
    p. hypertonica
    inappropriate p.
    primary p.
    relative p.
    p. rubra
    secondary p.
    p. vera
polycythemica
    hypertonia p.
polydactyly
polydipsia
    hysterical p.
polydrug abuse
polydysplasia
polyendocrinopathy
polyene antibiotic
polyenoic acid
polyergic
polyesthesia
polyethylene collar button
polygalactia
polygalacturonase
polygene
polygenic

polyglandular
polygraph
    Mackenzie p.
polygyria
polyhidrosis
polyhydramnios
polyhydric
polyleptic
polymastia
polymelia
polymenorrhea
polymenorrhoea
polymer
    cross-linked p.
polymerase
    p. chain reaction
    DNA p.
polymeria
polymeric
polymerization
polymerize
polymorphic genetic marker
polymorphism
    balanced p.
    corneal endothelial p.
    DNA p.
    fragment length p.
    genetic p.
    lipoprotein p.
    restriction fragment length p.
    restriction-site p.
polymorphocellular
polymorphonuclear leukocyte
polymorphous
    p. light eruption
    p. low-grade carcinoma
polymyalgia
polymyoclonus
polymyositis
polynesic
polynesiensis
    Aedes p.
polyneural
polyneuralgia
polyneuritic psychosis
polyneuritiformis
    heredopathia atactica p.
polyneuritis
    acute febrile p.
    acute idiopathic p.
    anemic p.
    chronic familial p.
    cranial p.
    infectious p.
    postinfectious p.
polyneuropathy
    acute inflammatory p.
    alcoholic p.
    arsenical p.

axonal p.
axon loss p.
buckthorn p.
chronic inflammatory
  demyelinating p. (CIDP)
critical illness p.
demyelinating p.
diabetic p.
isoniazid p.
progressive hypertrophic p.
polynuclear leukocyte
polynucleate
polynucleotidase
polynucleotide
polyodontia
polyoncosis, polyonchosis
polyonychia
polyopia, polyopsia
polyorchidism
polyorchism
polyostotic
polyotia
polyovular
polyovulatory
polyp
adenomatous p.
bleeding p.
bronchial p.
cardiac p.
cellular p.
cervical p.
choanal p.
cystic p.
dental p.
endocervical p.
endometrial p.
fibrinous p.
fibroepithelial p.
fibrous p.
fleshy p.
gelatinous p.
Hopmann p.
hydatid p.
hyperplastic p.
inflammatory p.
juvenile p.
laryngeal p.
lipomatous p.
lymphoid p.
metaplastic p.
regenerative p.

sessile p.
vascular p.
polypectomy
polypeptide
gastric inhibitory p. (GIP)
glucose-dependent insulinotropic p.
vasoactive intestinal p.
polyphagia
polypharmacy abuse
polyphenic gene
polyphobia
polyphrasia
polyphyletic
polyplastic
polyploid
polyploidy
polypnea
polypoid
p. adenocarcinoma
p. hyperplasia
polyporous
polyposa
decidua p.
enteritis p.
polyposis
familial adenomatous p. (FAP)
lymphomatoid p.
multiple intestinal p.
polypous
polyptychial
polypus
polyradiculitis
polyradiculomyopathy
polyradiculoneuropathy
acute inflammatory demyelinating p.
polyradiculopathy
diabetic p.
polyribosome
polysaccharide conjugated vaccine
polyserositis
familial paroxysmal p.
familial recurrent p.
period p.
recurrent p.
polysinusitis
polysome
polysomia
polysomic
polysomnogram
polysomnography
polysomy
polyspermia, polyspermism, polyspermy

NOTES

P

polysplenia
polystichia
polysubstance abuse
polysymbrachydactyly
polysynaptic
polysyndactyly
polytendinitis
polythelia
polytomography
polytrichia
polyuria
polyvalent
  p. allergy
  p. serum
  p. vaccine
pomade acne
Pomeroy operation
Pompe disease
ponceau de xylidine
Ponfick shadow
pons, pl. pontes
pontic
pontile apoplexy
pontine
  p. flexure
  p. nucleus
pontocerebellar fiber
pontomedullary groove
pool
  abdominal p.
  gene p.
  metabolic p.
  P. phenomenon
poorly differentiated lymphocytic
  lymphoma
popliteal
  p. artery
  p. fascia
  p. fossa
  p. groove
  p. ligament
  p. muscle
  p. space
  p. vein
popliteus muscle
popoff needle
population
  p. genetics
  growth rate of p.
pore
  alveolar p.
  auditory p.
  dilated p.
  external acoustic p.
  external auditory p.
  gustatory p.
  interalveolar p.
  internal acoustic p.

Kohn p.
sweat p.
porencephalia
porencephalic
porencephalitis
porencephalous
porencephaly
porokeratosis
  actinic p.
poroma
  eccrine p.
porosis
  cerebral p.
porosity
porous
porphobilin
porphobilinogen
porphyria
  acute intermittent p.
  congenital erythropoietic p.
  p. cutanea tarda
  erythropoietic p.
  hepatic p.
  hepatoerythropoietic p.
  intermittent acute p. (IAP)
  symptomatic p.
  variegate p.
porphyrin
porphyrinogens
porphyrinuria
port
  ancillary p.
portacaval shunt
portal
  anterior intestinal p.
  p. canal
  p. fissure
  p. hypertension
  p. hypophysial circulation
  p. lobule
  p. system
  p. triad
  p. vein
portal-systemic encephalopathy
portion
  mesenteric p.
  supravaginal p.
  vaginal p.
Portland
  hemoglobin P.
Portmann interposition operation
portobilioarterial
portoenterostomy
portogram
portography
portosystemic
Portuguese man-of-war

port-wine
    p.-w. mark
    p.-w. stain
position
    Adams p.
    Albert p.
    anatomic p.
    anatomical p.
    arm-extension p.
    Bonner p.
    Boyce p.
    Bozeman p.
    Casselberry p.
    centric p.
    close-packed p.
    coiled p.
    condylar hinge p.
    Depage p.
    dorsal decubitus p.
    dorsal elevated p.
    dorsal lithotomy p.
    dorsal recumbent p.
    dorsal rigid p.
    dorsosacral p.
    Duncan p.
    eccentric p.
    p. effect
    electrical heart p.
    Elliot p.
    emprosthotonos p.
    energy of p.
    English p.
    fetal p.
    flank p.
    Fowler p.
    frog-leg p.
    frontoanterior fetal p.
    frontoposterior fetal p.
    frontotransverse fetal p.
    Fuchs p.
    genucubital p.
    genufacial p.
    genupectoral p.
    head dependent p.
    heart p.
    hinge p.
    intercuspal p.
    knee-chest p.
    knee-elbow p.
    lateral recumbent p.
    leapfrog p.
    lithotomy p.
    loose-packed p.
    lordotic p.
    mandibular hinge p.
    Mayo-Robson p.
    mentoanterior fetal p.
    mentoposterior p.
    mentotransverse fetal p.
    Noble p.
    occipitoanterior fetal p.
    occipitoposterior p.
    occipitotransverse p.
    occlusal p.
    open-packed p.
    physiologic rest p.
    postural resting p.
    rest p.
    Rose p.
    sacroanterior p.
    sacroposterior fetal p.
    sacrotransverse fetal p.
    Scultetus p.
    semi-Fowler p.
    p. sense
    Simon p.
    Sims p.
    Stern p.
    terminal hinge p.
    Trendelenburg p.
    Valentine p.
positional
    p. nystagmus
    p. vertigo
positive
    p. accommodation
    p. anergy
    p. convergence
    p. end-expiratory pressure (PEEP)
    false p.
    p. pressure ventilation
    p. scotoma
    p. stain
    p. symptom
positive-negative pressure breathing
positron emission tomography
posologic
posology
postadrenalectomy syndrome
postauricular incision
postaxial
postbrachial
postcapillary venule
postcava

NOTES

postcaval
postcentral
  p. area
  p. gyrus
  p. sulcus
postcibal
postcoital
  p. contraception
  p. test
postcoitus
postcommissurotomy syndrome
postconcussional headache
postconcussion syndrome
postcordial
postcostal anastomosis
postcubital
postdate pregnancy
postductal
postencephalitis parkinsonism
posterior
  p. aphasia
  p. arch
  p. asynclitism
  p. auricular nerve
  p. blepharitis
  p. cerebral commissure
  p. chamber
  p. column
  p. compartment
  p. cord
  p. cruciate ligament
  p. elastic lamina
  p. embryotoxon
  p. focal point
  forceps p.
  p. fossa approach
  p. funiculus
  funiculus p.
  p. glandular branch
  p. hepatic segment I
  p. horn
  p. intercostal vein
  p. interosseous nerve
  p. labial branch
  p. labial commissure
  p. labial vein
  p. lacrimal crest
  p. laryngeal cleft
  p. leukoencephalopathy syndrome
  p. limiting layer
  p. lobe
  p. mediastinum
  p. nasal spine
  p. nephrectomy
  p. palatine suture
  p. perineum
  p. polymorphous corneal dystrophy
  p. ramus
  p. rhinoscopy
  p. rhizotomy
  p. sagittal diameter
  p. scleritis
  p. segment of eyeball
  p. spinocerebellar tract
  p. staphyloma
  superior labrum anterior and p.
    (SLAP)
  p. temporal branch
  p. tooth
  p. urethral valve
  p. vestibular branch
posterius
  cornu p.
posteroanterior (PA)
  p. projection
posteroexternal
posterointernal
posterolateral
  p. sclerosis
  p. sulcus
  p. thoracotomy
posteromedial
posteromedian
posterosuperior
postestrum
postestrus
postextrasystolic
  p. pause
  p. T wave
postganglionic
postgastrectomy syndrome
postglomerular arteriole
posthepatitic cirrhosis
posthioplasty
posthitis
posthypnotic suggestion
postictal automatism
postinfarction syndrome
postinfectious polyneuritis
postinfective bradycardia
postlumbar puncture syndrome
postmalaria neurologic syndrome
postmature infant
postmenopausal
postmortem
  p. delivery
  p. livedo
  p. lividity
  p. rigidity
  p. wart
postnasal drip
postnatal
postnecrotic cirrhosis
postoperative
  p. care
  p. course
  p. shock
postoral

postpartum
    p. atony
    p. blues
    p. depression
    p. hemorrhage
    p. psychosis
postpericardiotomy
    p. pericarditis
    p. syndrome
postpoliomyelitis syndrome
postpolio syndrome
postprandial
postpuberal
postpubertal
postpubescent
postrema
    camera p.
postremal chamber
postsphygmic
post–steady state
postsynaptic membrane
postterm infant
posttibial
posttransplant lymphoproliferative disease
posttraumatic
    p. amnesia
    p. delirium
    p. dementia
    p. epilepsy
    p. headache
    p. stress disorder
    p. syndrome
posttussive inspiratory rhonchi
postulate
    Ampère p.
    Avogadro p.
    Ehrlich p.
    Koch p.
postural
    p. alignment
    p. contraction
    p. drainage
    p. drainage system
    p. myoclonus
    p. resting position
    p. sway response
    p. syncope
    p. vertigo
posture
    p. sense
    Stern p.

posturography
    dynamic p.
postvaccinal encephalomyelitis
postvalvar
postvalvular
potable
Potain sign
potash
    caustic p.
potassium-39
potassium sparing diuretic
potency
potential
    action p.
    p. acuity meter
    average evoked p.
    bioelectric p.
    biotic p.
    brain p.
    brainstem auditory evoked p.
    chemical p.
    cochlear p.
    compound action p.
    demarcation p.
    early receptor p. (ERP)
    endocochlear p.
    p. energy
    evoked p.
    excitatory junction p. (EJP)
    excitatory postsynaptic p. (EPSP)
    generator p.
    inhibitory junction p. (IJP)
    inhibitory postsynaptic p. (IPSP)
    injury p.
    membrane p.
    oscillatory p.
    somatosensory evoked p. (SSEP)
    spike p.
    summating p.'s
    p. trauma
    visual evoked p.
    zoonotic p.
potentiation
Pott
    P. abscess
    P. aneurysm
    P. curvature
    P. disease
    P. fracture
    P. paraplegia

NOTES

P

potter
    p. phthisis
    P. syndrome
Potter-Bucky diaphragm
Potts
    P. clamp
    P. operation
pouch
    antral p.
    branchial p.
    Broca p.
    p. culture
    deep perineal p.
    Denis Browne p.
    Douglas p.
    endodermal p.
    Hartmann p.
    Heidenhain p.
    hepatorenal p.
    hypophysial p.
    ileoanal p.
    Kock p.
    laryngeal p.
    pararectal p.
    Physick p.
    Rathke p.
    rectouterine p.
    rectovesical p.
    uterovesical p.
poudrage
poultice
pourquoi
    folie du p.
Powassan encephalitis
powder
    bleaching p.
    p. burn
power
    aerobic p.
    anaerobic p.
    back vertex p.
    carbon dioxide combining p.
    equivalent p.
    muscular p.
    resolving p.
pox
    Kaffir p.
poxvirus
PPD
    purified protein derivative
PPO
    preferred provider organization
PQ interval
PR
    PR interval
    PR segment
practice
    evidence-based p.
    extramural p.

    family p.
    general p.
    group p.
    p. guideline
    intramural p.
practitioner
praecox
    dementia p.
    icterus p.
    lymphedema p.
    macrogenitosomia p.
pragmatism
Prague
    P. maneuver
    P. pelvis
prandial
pranobex
    inosine p.
praseodymium
Pratt symptom
praxis
PRCs
    packed red cells
preagonal
preanesthetic
preauricular
    p. pit
    p. sinus
preautomatic pause
preaxial
precancer
precancerous dermatosis
precapillary
precartilage
precava
precentral
    p. area
    p. gyrus
    p. sulcus
precipitable
precipitant
precipitate
    keratic p.'s
    p. labor
precipitation
    double antibody p.
    immune p.
precipitinogen
precipitin test
precision
preclinical
precocious puberty
precocity
precognition
precollagenous fiber
precommissure
preconceptual stage
preconscious
preconvulsive

precordia
precordial lead
precordium
precornu
precostal anastomosis
precuneate
precuneus
precursor
    angiotensin p.
    p. symptom
precursory cartilage
predecidual
predentin
pre-Descemet corneal dystrophy
prediabetes
prediastole
prediastolic
predictive value
predigestion
predispose
predisposition
preductal
preeclampsia
preepiglottic space
preexcitation syndrome
preference
    sexual p.
preferred provider organization (PPO)
prefrontal area
preganglionic
preglomerular arteriole
preglottic tonsillitis
pregnancy
    abdominal p.
    aborted ectopic p.
    ampullar p.
    cervical p.
    chemical p.
    combined p.
    compound p.
    cornual p.
    ectopic p.
    entopic p.
    extraamniotic p.
    extrachorial p.
    extramembranous p.
    extrauterine p.
    fallopian p.
    false p.
    p. gingivitis
    heterotopic p.
    higher order p.

    hydatid p.
    hysterical p.
    interstitial p.
    intraligamentary p.
    intramural p.
    intraperitoneal p.
    longitudinal p.
    mask of p.
    molar p.
    multiple p.
    ovarian p.
    placental p.
    postdate p.
    prolonged p.
    secondary abdominal p.
    tubal p.
    tuboabdominal p.
    tuboovarian p.
    vomiting of p.
pregnancy-induced hypertension
pregnane
pregnanediol
pregnanedione
pregnanetriol
pregnant
prehensile
prehension
prehormone
prehospital
    p. care
    p. care report
    p. provider
preictal
preinduction
preinfarction angina
prekallikrein
prelaminar branch
preleukemia
preload
    ventricular p.
prelogical thinking
premalignant
prematura
    alopecia p.
premature
    p. birth
    p. delivery
    p. ejaculation
    p. labor
    p. membrane rupture
    p. menopause

NOTES

premature *(continued)*
    p. ovarian failure
    p. systole
prematurity
    retinopathy of p.
premaxillary bone
premedication
premenstrual
    p. dysphoric disorder
    p. syndrome
    p. tension
premenstruum
premolar tooth
premonitory symptom
premonocyte
premorbid
premotor cortex
premunition
premunitive
premyeloblast
premyelocyte
prenaris
prenasal
prenatal diagnosis
preneoplastic
Prentice rule
preoperative
preosteoblast
preoxygenation
prepancreatic artery
preparation
    corrosion p.
    cytologic filter p.
    heart-lung p.
prepatellar
    p. bursa
    p. bursitis
prepatent period
preponderance
    directional p.
prepotential
prepped and draped
prepsychotic
prepuberal
prepubertal
prepubescent
prepuce
    hooded p.
    ventral apron p.
preputial
    p. calculus
    p. gland
preputiotomy
prepyloric vein
prerenal uremia
presacral
    p. fascia
    p. neurectomy
    p. sympathectomy

presbyacusis, presbyacusia
presbyastasis
presbyopia
presbyopic
prescribe
prescription
    exercise p.
presenile dementia
presenilis
    alopecia p.
    dementia p.
presenility
presentation
    acromion p.
    breech p.
    brow p.
    cephalic p.
    compound p.
    face p.
    foot p.
    footling p.
    frank breech p.
    head p.
    incomplete foot p.
    knee p.
    placental p.
    shoulder p.
    sincipital p.
    transverse p.
    vertex p.
presenting symptom
preseptal cellulitis
preservative
presomite
presphygmic
pressor
    p. amine
    p. base
    p. fiber
    p. nerve
pressoreceptive
pressoreceptor
pressosensitive
pressure
    abdominal p.
    absolute p.
    acoustic p.
    p. alopecia
    atmospheric p.
    back p.
    p. bandage
    barometric p.
    bilevel positive airway p.
    biting p.
    blood p. (BP)
    central venous p. (CVP)
    cerebrospinal p.
    continuous positive airway p.
     (CPAP)

p. controlled ventilation
coronary perfusion p.
critical p.
detrusor p.
diastolic p.
differential blood p.
Donders p.
p. dressing
effective osmotic p.
p. epiphysis
gauge p.
hydrostatic p.
inferior vena cava p. (IVCP)
intracranial p. (ICP)
intraocular p.
jugular venous p. (JVP)
leak point p.
left ventricular diastolic p.
left ventricular end-diastolic p.
left ventricular systolic p.
maximum expiratory p.
maximum inspiratory p.
mean pulmonary arterial p.
p. necrosis
negative end-expiratory p.
oncotic p.
osmotic p.
p. paralysis
partial p.
plateau p.
pleural p.
p. point
positive end-expiratory p. (PEEP)
pulmonary capillary wedge p.
pulse p.
p. pulse differentiation
p. reversal
p. sense
p. sore
standard p.
p. stasis
p. support ventilation
systemic arterial p. (SAP)
systolic p.
p. tapping
trans airway p.
transpulmonary p.
p. ulcer
p. ventilator
p. waveform
wedge p.
zero end-expiratory p.

pressure-volume index
pre-steady state
presumed ocular histoplasmosis
presuppurative
presynaptic membrane
presystole
presystolic
p. gallop
p. murmur
p. thrill
pretarsal
preterm
p. infant
p. membrane rupture
pretibial
p. fever
p. myxedema
prevalence
preventive
p. dentistry
p. medicine
p. treatment
prevertebral
p. ganglion
p. layer
previa
central placenta p.
placenta p.
vasa p.
Prevotella
P. bivia
P. denticola
P. heparinolytica
P. intermedia
P. melaninogenica
priapism
Price-Jones curve
prickle
p. cell
p. cell layer
prickly heat
prima
costa p.
primacy
genital p.
primal scene
primary
p. abscess
p. acquired cholesteatoma
p. adhesion
p. adrenocortical insufficiency
p. alcohol

NOTES

P

715

primary *(continued)*
    p. aldosteronism
    p. amenorrhea
    p. amine
    p. amyloidosis
    p. anesthetic
    p. atelectasis
    p. atypical pneumonia
    p. brain vesicle
    p. care
    p. care physician
    p. complex
    p. dementia
    p. dentin
    p. dentition
    p. deviation
    p. digestion
    p. disease
    p. dye test
    p. dysmenorrhea
    p. fissure
    p. gain
    p. hemochromatosis
    p. hemorrhage
    p. herpetic gingivostomatitis
    p. herpetic stomatitis
    p. immune response
    p. lateral sclerosis
    p. lysosome
    p. myopia
    p. nondisjunction
    p. nursing
    p. oocyte
    p. ovarian follicle
    p. pleurisy
    p. polycythemia
    p. process
    p. progressive aphasia
    p. pulmonary lobule
    p. senile dementia
    p. sex character
    p. spermatocyte
    p. splenic neutropenia
    p. sterility
    p. stuttering
    p. syphilis
    p. tooth
    p. tuberculosis
    p. union
primate
primigravida
    elderly p.
primipara
primiparity
primiparous
primitiva
    meninx p.
primitive
    p. groove

    p. gut
    p. knot
    p. node
    p. streak
primordia
primordial
    p. gut
    p. ovarian follicle
primordium
    genital p.
primum
    interatrial foramen p.
princeps pollicis artery
principal
    p. diagnosis
    p. optic axis
    p. point
principle
    active p.
    antianemic p.
    Bernoulli p.
    bitter p.
    closure p.
    consistency p.
    Fick p.
    follicle-stimulating p.
    founder p.
    hematinic p.
    Huygens p.
    Le Chatelier p.
    luteinizing p.
    mass action p.
    melanophore-expanding p.
    Mitrofanoff p.
    overload p.
    pain-pleasure p.
    Pauli exclusion p.
    pleasure p.
    reality p.
    reversibility p.
Prinzmetal angina
prion protein
prior
    p. to admission
    p. to arrival
prism
    p. bar
    p. diopter
    enamel p.
    Fresnel p.
    Risley rotary p.
proaccelerin
proacrosomal granule
proactivator
probability
    conditional p.
    joint p.
probacteriophage
    defective p.

proband
probe
    bipolar circumactive p. (BICAP)
    Bowman p.
    calibrated p.
    periodontal p.
    p. syringe
probiosis
probiotic
problem-oriented medical record
procapsid
procarboxypeptidase
procaryote
procaryotic
procedure
    back table p.
    Batista p.
    Belsey p.
    Buie p.
    Chamberlain p.
    Clagett p.
    Collis-Belsey p.
    commando p.
    Damus-Kaye-Stancel p.
    dideoxy p.
    Dor p.
    Eloesser p.
    endorectal pull-through p.
    Ewart p.
    Fontan p.
    Girdlestone p.
    Harada-Ito p.
    Hummelsheim p.
    Jatene p.
    Kestenbaum p.
    Konno p.
    Konno-Rastan p.
    lateral tarsal strip p.
    loop electrocautery excision p. (LEEP)
    loop electrosurgical excision p. (LEEP)
    McCall culdoplasty p.
    Mikulicz p.
    Mitchell p.
    Mohs p.
    Nick p.
    platelet neutralization p.
    Puestow p.
    Rashkind p.
    Reichel-Pólya stomach p.
    Ross p.
    sacrocolpopexy p.
    sacrospinous vaginal vault suspension p.
    Walsh p.
procelia
procentriole
procephalic
procerus muscle
process
    accessory p.
    acromial p.
    acromion p.
    agene p.
    alar p.
    alveolar p.
    anterior clinoid p.
    apical p.
    articular p.
    ascending p.
    auditory p.
    basilar p.
    binary p.
    Budde p.
    Burns falciform p.
    calcaneal p.
    caudate p.
    ciliary p.
    Civinini p.
    clinoid p.
    complex learning p.
    condylar p.
    condyloid p.
    conoid p.
    coracoid p.
    coronoid p.
    costal p.
    dendritic p.
    dental p.
    ensiform p.
    ethmoidal p.
    falciform p.
    Folli p.
    follian p.
    foot p.
    frontal p.
    frontonasal p.
    frontosphenoidal p.
    funicular p.
    globular p.
    hamular p.
    head p.
    inferior articular p.

NOTES

P

process *(continued)*
    Ingrassia p.
    intrajugular p.
    jugular p.
    lateral nasal p.
    Lenhossék p.
    lenticular p.
    malar p.
    mammillary p.
    mandibular p.
    Markov p.
    mastoid p.
    maxillary p.
    medial nasal p.
    mental p.
    middle clinoid p.
    odontoid p.
    orbital p.
    palatine p.
    primary p.
    pterygoid p.
    secondary p.
    spinous p.
    styloid p.
    supracondylar p.
    temporal p.
    transverse p.
    vocal p.
    xiphoid p.
    zygomatic p.
processing
    data p.
    perceptual p.
    sensory p.
processor
    speech p.
processus vaginalis
prochondral
prochymosin
procidentia
procoelia
procollagen
proconvertin
procreate
procreation
procreative
proctalgia
proctatresia
proctectomy
proctitis
    chronic ulcerative p.
    epidemic gangrenous p.
    idiopathic p.
proctocele
proctoclysis
proctococcypexy
proctocolectomy
proctocolonoscopy
proctocolpoplasty

proctocystoplasty
proctocystotomy
proctodaeum
proctodeal
proctodeum
proctodynia
proctologic
proctologist
proctology
proctoparalysis
proctopexy
proctoplasty
proctoplegia
proctoptosia
proctoptosis
proctorrhaphy
proctorrhea
proctoscope
    Tuttle p.
proctoscopy
proctosigmoidectomy
proctosigmoiditis
proctosigmoidoscopy
proctospasm
proctostenosis
proctostomy
proctotomy
    internal p.
proctotresia
proctovalvotomy
procursive epilepsy
prodromal
    p. labor
    p. myopia
    p. stage
    p. symptom
prodrome
prodromic
prodromous
prodrug
product
    cleavage p.
    double p.
    end p.
    fibrin/fibrinogen degradation p.
    fission p.
    orphan p.
    spallation p.
    substitution p.
production
    carbon dioxide p.
productive cough
proenzyme
proerythroblast
proerythrocyte
proestrogen
proestrus
professional
    allied health p.

Profeta law
profibrinolysin
proficiency
    p. sample
    p. testing
profile
    biochemical p.
    biophysical p.
    facial p.
    personality p.
    test p.
profiling
    DNA p.
profound
    p. anemia
    p. debility
    p. hematuria
profunda
    p. brachii artery
    p. femoris artery
    keratitis p.
    miliaria p.
profundus
    anulus inguinalis p.
    arcus palmaris p.
    lupus erythematosus p.
progastrin
progenia
progenitor
progeny
progeria
progestational hormone
progesterone
    p. challenge test
    p. receptor
progestin
progestogen
proglossis
proglottid
proglottis
prognathic
prognathism
    basilar p.
prognathous
prognosis, pl. **prognoses**
    denture p.
prognostic
prognosticate
prognostician
progonoma
    melanotic p.

program
    individualized education p.
programming
    neurolinguistic p.
progranulocyte
progressiva
    dysbasia lordotica p.
    fibrodysplasia ossificans p.
progressive
    p. bulbar paralysis
    p. cataract
    p. choroidal atrophy
    p. emphysematous necrosis
    p. hypertrophic polyneuropathy
    p. multifocal leukoencephalopathy
    p. muscular atrophy
    p. outer retinal necrosis
    p. staining
    p. tapetochoroidal dystrophy
progressive-resistance exercise
prohormone
proinsulin
projectile vomiting
projection
    p. angiogram
    anteroposterior p.
    AP p.
    apical lordotic p.
    axial p.
    base p.
    Caldwell p.
    cross-table lateral p.
    decubitus p.
    enamel p.
    erroneous p.
    false p.
    p. fiber
    Fischer p.
    frog-leg lateral p.
    Granger p.
    half-axial p.
    Haworth p.
    lateral p.
    maximum intensity p. (MIP)
    PA p.
    posteroanterior p.
    Rhese p.
    Waters p.
projective identification
prokaryote
prokaryotic
prolabium

NOTES

P

prolactin
prolactin-inhibiting
    p.-i. factor
    p.-i. hormone
prolactinoma
prolactin-producing adenoma
prolactin-releasing
    p.-r. factor
    p.-r. hormone
prolactoliberin
prolactostatin
prolapse
    first-degree p.
    iris p.
    mitral valve p.
    Morgagni p.
    second-degree p.
    third-degree p.
    p. of umbilical cord
    p. of uterus
prolapsed hemorrhoid
prolective
prolepsis
proleptic
prolidase
proliferans
    endarteritis p.
    retinitis p.
proliferate
proliferating
    p. cell nuclear antigen
    p. endarteritis
proliferation
    diffuse mesangial p.
    gingival p.
proliferative
    p. fasciitis
    p. inflammation
    p. retinopathy
proliferous
proligerous
prolinase
proline
    p. dipeptidase
    p. iminopeptidase
prolonged pregnancy
prolyl dipeptidase
promastigote
promegaloblast
prometaphase
promethium
prominence
    Ammon p.
    canine p.
    cardiac p.
    forebrain p.
    frontonasal p.
    hepatic p.
    hypothenar p.

    laryngeal p.
    lateral nasal p.
    mallear p.
    medial nasal p.
prominent heel
prominentia
promonocyte
promontory flush
promoter
promoting agent
promotion
    health p.
promyelocyte
pronasion
pronate
pronation
    rearfoot p.
pronator
    p. quadratus muscle
    p. teres muscle
    p. teres syndrome
pronephros
pronormoblast
pronucleus
prootic
prop
    mouth p.
propagate
propagation
propagative
proparathyroid hormone
propepsin
proper
    hepatic artery p.
properdin
    p. factor A, B, D, E
    p. system
properitoneal hernia
prophage
    defective p.
prophase
prophylactic treatment
prophylaxis
    active p.
    chemical p.
    dental p.
propionate
    calcium p.
    dromostanolone p.
    erythromycin p.
Propionibacterium
propionic acid
proportionate dwarfism
propositional speech
propositus
propria
    lamina p.
    tunica p.

proprietary
p. medicine
p. name
proprioception
proprioceptive
p. mechanism
p. neuromuscular facilitation
p. sensibility
proprioceptor
proprius
anterior fasciculus p.
lateral fasciculus p.
proptosis
proptotic
propulsion
propyl alcohol
propylene
pro re nata
prorennin
prorubricyte
prosecretin
prosect
prosector
prosencephalon
proserum prothrombin conversion accelerator
prosodemic
prosody
prosopagnosia
prosopalgia
prosopalgic
prosoplasia
prosopodiplegia
prosoponeuralgia
prosopoplegia
prosopoplegic
prosoposchisis
prosopospasm
prospective payment system
prostaglandin agonist
prostanoic acid
prostatae
apex p.
prostatalgia
prostate
female p.
p. gland
isthmus of p.
lobe of p.
transurethral resection of p. (TURP)

prostatectomy
perineal p.
radical retropubic p.
retropubic prevesical p.
suprapubic p.
prostate-specific antigen
prostatic
p. calculus
p. duct
p. ductule
p. fluid
p. intraepithelial neoplasia
p. massage
p. sinus
p. utricle
p. vesicle
prostatica
vesica p.
prostatism
prostatitis
prostatocystitis
prostatolithotomy
prostatomegaly
prostatorrhea
prostatotomy
prostatovesiculectomy
prostatovesiculitis
prosthesis, pl. **prostheses**
aortic p.
auditory p.
cardiac valve p.
cochlear p.
definitive p.
dental p.
discoid aortic p.
disc valve p.
feeding p.
heart valve p.
hybrid p.
knitted vascular p.
mandibular guide p.
maxillofacial p.
mitral p.
modular p.
ocular p.
penile p.
surgical p.
tilting disc valve p.
trileaflet aortic p.
prosthetic
dental p.
p. group

NOTES

prosthetic *(continued)*
    maxillofacial p.
    p. valve endocarditis
prosthetist
prosthion
prosthodontics
prosthodontist
prostration
    heat p.
protactinium
protamine
protanopia
protean
protease
    p. inhibitor
    Lon p.
    tricorn p.
protection test
protective laryngeal reflex
protector
    hearing p.
protein
    acute phase p.
    acyl carrier p.
    amyloid p.
    androgen binding p. (ABP)
    antitermination p.
    antitumor p.
    antiviral p.
    autologous p.
    basic p.
    Bence Jones p.
    cAMP receptor p.
    capping p.
    catabolite gene activator p.
    cholesterol ester transport p.
    circumsporozoite p.
    compound p.
    conjugated p.
    copper p.
    corticosteroid-binding p.
    C-reactive p.
    denatured p.
    derived p.
    docking p.
    encephalithogenic p.
    eosinophil cationic p.
    extrinsic p.
    fatty acid–binding p.
    fibrous p.
    foreign p.
    G p.
    glial fibrillary acidic p.
    globular p.
    heat shock p.
    heme p.
    heterologous p.
    homologous p.
    immune p.

    p. induced by vitamin K absence
    integral p.
    intrinsic p.
    iron-sulfur p.
    p. kinase C
    latent membrane p.
    low molecular weight p.
    M p.
    macrophage inflammatory p. (MIP)
    mannose-binding p.
    matrix Gla p.
    p. metabolism
    microtubule-associated p. (MAP)
    mild silver p.
    monocyte chemoattractant p.
    neutrophil-activating p.
    nonspecific p.
    p. p53
    pathologic p.
    plasma p.
    prion p.
    receptor p.
    p. S
    simple p.
    thrombospondin-related adhesive p.
    vitamin D–binding p.
proteinaceous
protein-losing enteropathy
proteinosis
    lipoid p.
    pulmonary alveolar p.
proteinuria
    Bence Jones p.
    gestational p.
    intrinsic p.
    isolated p.
    nonisolated p.
    residual p.
proteoglycan aggregate
proteolipid
proteolysis
proteolytic
proteometabolic
proteose
proteosome
protest
    masculine p.
Proteus
    P. morganii
    P. vulgaris
prothrombin
    p. accelerator
    p. test
    p. time
prothrombinase
protist
protocol
    Bruce p.
protocone

protoconid
protodiastolic gallop
protoduodenum
protoiodide
    mercury p.
proton
    p. pump
    p. pump inhibitor
protonymph
protooncogene
protopathic sensibility
protoplasm
protoplasmic
    p. astrocyte
    p. neuroglia
protoplast
protoporphyria
    erythropoietic p.
protoporphyrin
    iron p.
protostylid
prototroph
prototype
protovertebra
protozoal
protozoan
protozoiasis
protozoology
protozoon
protozoophage
protracted treatment
protraction
    mandibular p.
    maxillary p.
protractor
protruded disc
protruding ear
protrusion
    bimaxillary dentoalveolar p.
    double p.
protrusive
    p. excursion
    p. occlusion
protuberance
    Bichat p.
    external occipital p.
    internal occipital p.
    mental p.
protuberant abdomen
protuberantia
proud flesh
Proust space

provertebra
provider
    prehospital p.
provirus
provocation
    bronchial p.
provocative diagnosis
proximad
proximal
    p. deep inguinal lymph node
    p. incision
    p. latency
    p. myotonic myopathy
    p. splenorenal shunt
proximate
proximoataxia
proxy
    factitious illness by p.
prozone
prune belly
pruriginous
prurigo
    actinic p.
    Besnier p.
    Hebra p.
    p. mitis
    p. nodularis
    p. papule
    p. simplex
pruritic urticarial papule
pruritus
    p. ani
    aquagenic p.
    bath p.
    essential p.
    p. gravidarum
    senile p.
    p. senilis
    symptomatic p.
    p. vulvae
Prussian blue
psammoma
    p. body
    Virchow p.
psammomatous meningioma
psammous
pseudagraphia
pseudallescheriasis
pseudankylosis
pseudarthrosis
pseudesthesia
pseudoagraphia

NOTES

P

pseudoallelic
pseudoallelism
pseudoanemia
pseudoarthrosis
pseudobulbar
    p. palsy
    p. paralysis
pseudocartilage
pseudocast
pseudochancre
pseudochorea
pseudochromesthesia
pseudocoarctation
pseudocroup
pseudocryptorchism
pseudocyesis
pseudocylindroid
pseudocyst
    pancreatic p.
pseudodementia
pseudodiphtheria
pseudodiphtheriticum
    Corynebacterium p.
pseudodominance
pseudoedema
pseudoexfoliation syndrome
pseudoexfoliative glaucoma
pseudofolliculitis
pseudofracture
pseudoganglion
pseudogeusesthesia
pseudogeusia
pseudogout
pseudo-Graefe phenomenon
pseudohematuria
pseudohermaphrodite
pseudohermaphroditism
    female p.
    male p.
pseudohyperkalemia
pseudohyperparathyroidism
pseudohypertrophic
pseudohypertrophy
pseudohypoacusis
pseudohyponatremia
pseudohypoparathyroidism
pseudoicterus
pseudoisochromatic
pseudojaundice
pseudologia phantastica
pseudolymphoma
    cutaneous p.
pseudomalignancy
pseudomallei
    Burkholderia p.
pseudomania
pseudomembrane
pseudomembranous
    p. bronchitis

    p. colitis
    p. enteritis
    p. enterocolitis
    p. gastritis
    p. inflammation
pseudomilium
    colloid p.
pseudomonad
Pseudomonas
    cytochrome oxidase *P.*
pseudomonilethrix
pseudomucinous cystadenoma
pseudomyxoma peritonei
pseudoneoplasm
pseudoobstruction
    intestinal p.
pseudoosteomalacic pelvis
pseudopapilledema
pseudoparalysis
    arthritic general p.
    congenital atonic p.
pseudoparaplegia
    Basedow p.
pseudoparesis
pseudopelade
pseudoplatelet
pseudopod
pseudopodium
pseudopolyp
pseudopregnancy
pseudopterygium
pseudoptosis
pseudoreaction
pseudorickets
pseudorosette
pseudoscarlatina
pseudosmia
pseudospiralis
    Trichinella p.
pseudostrabismus
    pupillotonic p.
pseudostratified epithelium
pseudotortuosum
    Eubacterium p.
pseudotuberculosis
    Pasteurella p.
pseudotumor
    inflammatory p.
pseudotumour
pseudouridine
pseudoxanthoma elasticum
PSH
    past surgical history
psi phenomenon
psittaci
    Chlamydia p.
psittacosis

psoas
    p. abscess
    p. sign
psorelcosis
psoriasic
psoriasiform
psoriasis
    arthritis p.
    circinate p.
    diffused p.
    exfoliative p.
    flexural p.
    generalized pustular p.
    guttate p.
    nummular p.
    palmar p.
    pustular p.
    volar p.
psoriatica
    arthropathia p.
psoriatic arthritis
psoriaticum
    erythroderma p.
psychalgia
psychataxia
psyche
psychedelic
psychiatric rehabilitation
psychiatrist
psychiatry
    analytic p.
    biologic p.
    child p.
    contractual p.
    cross-cultural p.
    descriptive p.
    dynamic p.
    existential p.
    forensic p.
    industrial p.
    legal p.
    psychoanalytic p.
    social p.
psychic trauma
psychoactive substance abuse
psychoanalysis
    active p.
    adlerian p.
    freudian p.
    jungian p.
psychoanalyst

psychoanalytic
    p. psychiatry
    p. therapy
psychobiology
psychodiagnosis
psychodrama
psychodynamics
psychogenesis
psychogenetic
psychogenic
    p. deafness
    p. hearing impairment
    p. pain
    p. pain disorder
    p. vomiting
psychokinesia
psychokinesis
psycholinguistics
psychologic
psychological
psychologist
psychology
    abnormal p.
    adlerian p.
    analytical p.
    animal p.
    atomistic p.
    behavioral p.
    behavioristic p.
    child p.
    clinical p.
    cognitive p.
    constitutional p.
    counseling p.
    criminal p.
    depth p.
    developmental p.
    dynamic p.
    educational p.
    environmental p.
    existential p.
    experimental p.
    forensic p.
    genetic p.
    gestalt p.
    health p.
    holistic p.
    humanistic p.
    individual p.
    industrial p.
    medical p.
    social p.

NOTES

P

psychometrics
psychometry
psychomotor
    p. epilepsy
    p. seizure
psychoneurosis
psychoneurotic
psychopath
psychopathic
psychopathology
psychopharmaceuticals
psychopharmacology
psychophysical
psychophysics
psychophysiologic disorder
psychophysiology
psychosensorial
psychosensory
psychosexual
    p. development
    p. dysfunction
psychosis, pl. **psychoses**
    affective p.
    alcoholic p.
    bipolar p.
    Cheyne-Stokes p.
    depressive p.
    drug p.
    febrile p.
    functional p.
    hysterical p.
    ICU p.
    induced p.
    infection-exhaustion p.
    Korsakoff p.
    manic p.
    manic-depressive p.
    polyneuritic p.
    postpartum p.
    schizoaffective p.
    senile p.
    situational p.
    tardive p.
    toxic p.
psychosocial
psychosomatic
    p. disorder
    p. medicine
psychosomimetic
psychostimulant
psychosurgery
psychotherapeutics
psychotherapist
psychotherapy
    anaclitic p.
    autonomous p.
    brief p.
    contractual p.
    directive p.

    dyadic p.
    dynamic p.
    existential p.
    group p.
    heteronomous p.
    hypnotic p.
    intensive p.
    marathon group p.
psychotic disorder
psychotogenic
psychotomimetic
psychotropic
psychroalgia
psychrometry
psychrophil
psychrophile
psychrophilic
psychrophore
PTA
    percutaneous transluminal angioplasty
PTCA
    percutaneous transluminal coronary
      angioplasty
pteronyssinus
    Dermatophagoides p.
pterygium
pterygoid
    p. canal
    p. nerve
    p. process
pterygomandibular
pterygomaxillary
pterygomeningeal artery
pterygopalatine
    p. canal
    p. ganglion
ptomaine
ptosed
ptosis, pl. **ptoses**
    aponeurogenic p.
ptotic
PTT
    partial thromboplastin time
ptyalectasis
ptyalism
ptyalocele
pubarche
puberal
pubertal
puberty
    delayed p.
    precocious p.
    true precocious p.
pubescence
pubescent
pubic
    p. angle
    p. arch
    p. bone

p. crest
p. region
p. symphysis
pubiotomy
pubis
mons p.
osteitis p.
pecten p.
pediculosis p.
pubococcygeal muscle
pubococcygeus muscle
puboprostatic muscle
puborectalis muscle
puborectal muscle
pubovaginalis muscle
pubovaginal muscle
pubovesicalis muscle
pubovesical muscle
Puchtler-Sweat stain
pucker
macular p.
pudendal
p. canal
p. cleft
p. hernia
p. nerve
pudendum, pl. **pudenda**
pudic
puerpera, pl. **puerperae**
puerperal
p. eclampsia
p. fever
p. septicemia
p. tetanus
puerperant
puerperium
Puestow procedure
puff
chromosome p.
puffer poison
Pulfrich phenomenon
pulicicide
pulicide
pulley
anular p.
cruciform p.
p. suture
pulmoaortic
pulmonale
atrium p.
cor p.
P p.

pulmonalis
arteria p.
pulmonary
p. abscess
p. acinus
p. adcnomatosis
p. alveolar microlithiasis
p. alveolar proteinosis
p. alveolus
p. angiography
p. artery
p. artery atresia
p. artery catheter
p. bleb
p. capillary wedge pressure
p. circulation
p. collapse
p. dysmaturity syndrome
p. edema
p. embolism
p. emphysema
p. eosinophilia
p. fibrosis
p. function technician
p. function technologist
p. function test (PFT)
p. hamartoma
p. hypertension
p. insufficiency
p. intensive care unit (PIVU)
p. ligament
p. murmur
p. perfusion
p. phthisis
p. plexus
p. resection
p. stenosis
p. toilet
p. trunk
p. valve
p. vascular resistance
p. ventilation
pulmonic
p. atresia
p. murmur
p. stenosis
pulmonis
alveoli p.
apex p.
pulmonitis
pulp
p. amputation

NOTES

727

pulp (*continued*)
    p. canal
    p. cavity
    p. chamber
    coronal p.
    crown p.
    dead p.
    dental p.
    dentinal p.
    digital p.
    enamel p.
    exposed p.
    p. horn
    mummified p.
    necrotic p.
    nonvital p.
    radicular p.
    red p.
    root p.
    splenic p.
    p. stone
    p. test
    tooth p.
    vital p.
    white p.
pulpal
pulpectomy
pulpifaction
pulpitis
    hyperplastic p.
    hypertrophic p.
    irreversible p.
pulpotomy
pulpy
pulsate
pulsatile
pulsating empyema
pulsation
    balloon counter p.
pulse
    abdominal p.
    alternating p.
    amplitude of p.
    anacrotic p.
    anadicrotic p.
    apical p.
    bigeminal p.
    bisferious p.
    bulbar p.
    cannonball p.
    capillary p.
    carotid p.
    catacrotic p.
    catadicrotic p.
    cordy p.
    Corrigan p.
    coupled p.
    p. deficit
    dicrotic p.

    entoptic p.
    filiform p.
    gaseous p.
    p. generator
    guttural p.
    hard p.
    p. height analyzer
    intermittent p.
    irregular p.
    jerky p.
    jugular p.
    jugular venous p. (JVP)
    labile p.
    long p.
    p. oximeter
    p. oximetry
    oxygen p.
    paradoxic p.
    paradoxical p.
    plateau p.
    p. pressure
    Quincke p.
    p. rate
    Riegel p.
    p. sequence
    thready p.
    trigeminal p.
    undulating p.
    vagus p.
    venous p.
    vermicular p.
    water-hammer p.
    p. wave
    p. wave duration
    wiry p.
pulsed laser
pulse-field gel electrophoresis
pulseless
    p. disease
    p. electrical activity
pulsion
    p. diverticulum
    p. hernia
pulsus
    p. alternans
    p. bigeminus
    p. bisferiens
    p. celer
    p. differens
    p. paradoxus
    p. tardus
    p. trigeminus
pultaceous
pumilis
    Bacillus p.
pump
    breast p.
    calcium p.
    calf p.

Carrel-Lindbergh p.
constant infusion p.
dental p.
hydrogen p.
intraaortic balloon p.
ion p.
jet ejector p.
p. lung
proton p.
sodium p.
sodium-potassium p.
stomach p.
pumped laser
pump-oxygenator
punch
p. biopsy
p. graft
punchdrunk syndrome
puncta (*pl. of* punctum)
punctata
acne p.
dysplasia epiphysialis p.
keratitis p.
keratosis p.
rhizomelic chondrodysplasia p.
punctate
p. hemorrhage
p. hyalosis
punctiform
punctum, pl. puncta
p. cecum
p. fixa
kissing puncta
lacrimal p.
p. mobile
p. vasculosum
puncture
Bernard p.
cisternal p.
diabetic p.
lumbar p. (LP)
sternal p.
tracheoesophageal p.
transethmoidal p.
p. wound
pupil
Adie p.
amaurotic p.
Argyll Robertson p.
artificial p.
bounding p.
Bumke p.

catatonic p.
cat's-eye p.
p.'s equal, react to light (PERL)
p.'s equal, react to light and accommodation (PERLA)
p.'s equal, round, react to light and accommodation (PERRLA)
fixed p.
Gunn p.
Holmes-Adie p.
Horner p.
Hutchinson p.
keyhole p.
Marcus Gunn p.
pinhole p.
stiff p.
tonic p.
pupilla, pl. pupillae
sphincter pupillae
pupillary
p. block
p. distance
p. membrane
p. reflex
pupillary-skin reflex
pupillometer
pupillometry
pupillomotor
pupillostatometer
pupillotonic pseudostrabismus
pure
p. absence
p. autonomic failure
p. culture
p. flutter
p. tone
pure-tone
p.-t. audiogram
p.-t. average
purgation
purgative
purified protein derivative (PPD)
Purkinje
P. cell
P. cell layer
P. corpuscle
P. fiber
P. figure
P. network
P. phenomenon
Purkinje-Sanson image
Purmann method

NOTES

purple
    bromcresol p.
    Ruhemann p.
    visual p.
purpura
    allergic p.
    anaphylactoid p.
    factitious p.
    fibrinolytic p.
    p. fulminans
    p. hemorrhagica
    Henoch p.
    Henoch-Schönlein p.
    hyperglobulinemic p.
    idiopathic thrombocytopenic p.
     (ITP)
    immune thrombocytopenic p.
    nonthrombocytopenic p.
    orthostatic p.
    Schönlein p.
    senile p.
    p. senilis
    p. simplex
    thrombocytopenic p.
    thrombopenic p.
    thrombotic thrombocytopenic p.
purpuric
purpurin
    alizarin p.
purpurinuria
purse-string
    p.-s. instrument
    p.-s. suture
Purtscher retinopathy
purulence
purulency
purulent
    p. debris
    p. inflammation
    p. ophthalmia
    p. pachymeningitis
    p. pancreatitis
    p. pleurisy
    p. rhinitis
    p. salpingitis
    p. synovitis
puruloid
pus
    blue p.
    burrowing p.
    cheesy p.
    curdy p.
    green p.
    ichorous p.
    laudable p.
pustular
    p. eczema
    p. eruption
    p. psoriasis
    p. tonsillitis
pustulation
pustule
    malignant p.
pustulosa
    acne p.
pustulosis palmaris et plantaris
pustulosum
    eczema p.
Putnam-Dana syndrome
putrefaction
putrefactive
putrefy
putrescence
putrescent
putrescine
putrid
Putti-Platt operation
Puumala virus
pyarthrosis
pycnodysostosis
pyelectasia
pyelectasis
pyelitic
pyelitis
pyelocaliceal
pyelocystitis
pyelofluoroscopy
pyelogram
    dragon p.
    hydrated p.
    infusion p.
    intravenous p. (IVP)
    retrograde p.
pyelography
    antegrade p.
    intravenous p. (IVP)
    lateral p.
    retrograde p.
pyelolithotomy
pyelonephritis
    acute p.
    ascending p.
    asymptomatic p.
    chronic p.
pyeloplasty
    capsular flap p.
    Culp p.
    disjoined p.
    dismembered p.
    Foley Y-plasty p.
pyelorenal backflow
pyeloscopy
pyelostomy
pyelotomy
    extended p.
pyeloureterectasis
pyeloureterography

pyelovenous backflow
pyemesis
pyemia
    cryptogenic p.
pyemic
    p. abscess
    p. embolism
pyencephalus
pyesis
pygmy
pyknic
pyknodysostosis
pyknometer
pyknomorphous
pyknosis
pyknotic
pylephlebitis
pylethrombophlebitis
pylethrombosis
pylorectomy
pylori
    Campylobacter p.
    Helicobacter p.
pyloric
    p. antrum
    p. atresia
    p. canal
    p. cap
    p. constriction
    p. gland
    p. orifice
    p. sphincter
    p. stenosis
    p. vein
pyloristenosis
pyloroduodenitis
pylorogastrectomy
pyloromyotomy
pyloroplasty
    Finney p.
    Heineke-Mikulicz p.
    Jaboulay p.
    vagotomy and p.
pylorospasm
pylorostenosis
pylorostomy
pylorotomy
pylorus-preserving
  pancreaticoduodenectomy
pyocele
pyocephalus
    circumscribed p.

    external p.
    internal p.
pyochezia
pyococcus
pyocolpocele
pyocolpos
pyocyanic
pyocyanogenic
pyocyst
pyoderma gangrenosum
pyogenesis
pyogenetic
pyogenic granuloma
pyogenicum
    granuloma p.
pyohemothorax
pyoid
pyometra
pyometritis
pyomyositis
pyonephritis
pyonephrolithiasis
pyonephrosis
pyoovarium
pyopericarditis
pyopericardium
pyoperitoneum
pyoperitonitis
pyophysometra
pyopneumocholecystitis
pyopneumohepatitis
pyopneumopericardium
pyopneumoperitoneum
pyopneumoperitonitis
pyopneumothorax
pyopoiesis
pyopoietic
pyopyelectasis
pyorrhea
pyosalpingitis
pyosalpingo-oophoritis
pyosalpinx
pyosis
pyothorax
pyourachus
pyoureter
pyramid
    anterior p.
    cerebellar p.
    eating-right p.
    Ferrein p.
    Lallouette p.

NOTES

P

pyramid *(continued)*
    Malacarne p.
    malpighian p.
    medullary p.
    renal p.
    p. sign
    thyroid p.
pyramidal
    p. auricular muscle
    p. bone
    p. cataract
    p. cell
    p. decussation
    p. fracture
    p. lobe
    p. radiation
    p. tract
pyramidalis
    p. muscle
    radiatio p.
pyramidotomy
    medullary p.
pyramis renalis
pyranose
pyretic
pyrexia
pyrexial
pyridinium
pyridinoline
pyridoxamine
pyridoxine
pyriform thorax
pyrimidine

pyrin
pyrites
    iron p.
pyrogen
    endogenous p.
    exogenous p.
    leukocytic p.
pyrogenic
pyroglobulin
pyrolysis
pyromania
pyronin
pyrophobia
pyrophosphatase
    inorganic p.
pyrophosphate
    aneurine p.
    farnesyl p.
    geranyl p.
    geranylgeranyl p.
    lipothiamide p.
pyropoikilocytosis
    hereditary p.
pyrosis
pyrrole
pyrrolidine
pyruvate
    active p.
    enol p.
    p. kinase
pyruvic acid
pyuria

Q
    Q fever
    Q wave
Q-angle
Q-banding stain
QRB interval
QR interval
QRS
    QRS change
    QRS complex
    QRS deflection
QRST change
QS2 interval
Q-switched laser
QT interval
quadrangular lobule
quadrant
    left lower q. (LLQ)
    left outer q. (LOQ)
    left upper q. (LUQ)
    lower right q. (LRQ)
    outer upper right q. (OURQ)
    right lower q. (RLQ)
    upper left q. (ULQ)
    upper outer q. (UOQ)
quadrate lobe
quadratus
    q. femoris muscle
    q. labii superioris muscle
    q. lumborum muscle
    q. plantae muscle
quadribasic
quadriceps
    q. femoris muscle
    q. reflex
quadrigemina
    corpora q.
quadrigeminalis
    arteria q.
quadrigeminal rhythm
quadrigeminum
quadriparesis
quadripedal extensor reflex
quadriplegia
quadriplegic
quadrivalent
quadruplet
qualitative analysis
quality
    q. assurance
    q. control
    q. control chart
    q. of life
quantal effect
quantile

quantitative analysis
Quant sign
quantum
    q. theory
    q. yield
quarantine drain
quark
quartan
    double q.
    q. malaria
quartum
    Eubacterium q.
quasi-continuous wave laser
quasidominance
quasidominant
quaternary
Queckenstedt-Stookey test
quellung
    q. phenomenon
    q. reaction
    q. test
quenching
    fluorescence q.
questionnaire
    Holmes-Rahe q.
Queyrat
    erythroplasia of Q.
quickening
Quick test
quiescent
quiet lung
Quincke pulse
quinine
quinone
    dopa q.
quinsy
    lingual q.
quintan
quintana
    Bartonella q.
quintum
    Eubacterium q.
quintuplet
quit tam action
quodque
quotidian
    q. fever
    q. malaria
quotient
    achievement q.
    Ayala q.
    cognitive laterality q.
    extremal q.
    intelligence q. (IQ)
    Meyerhof oxidation q.

quotient *(continued)*
  respiratory q.

rabbeting
rabid
rabies
    dumb r.
    furious r.
    r. virus
raccoon eyes
racemase
    alanine r.
racemate
raceme
racemic
racemization
racemose
    r. aneurysm
    r. gland
rachial
rachicentesis
rachidial
rachigraph
rachilysis
rachiocentesis
rachiometer
rachiotomy
rachis
rachischisis
rachitic
    r. pelvis
    r. rosary
rachitis
rachitogenic
racket amputation
radectomy
radiability
radiable
radiad
radial
    r. collateral artery
    r. flexor muscle
    r. growth phase
    r. keratotomy
    r. nerve
    r. recurrent artery
    r. tunnel syndrome
    r. vein
radialis indicis artery
radian
radiant intensity
radiata
    corona r.
radiate
    r. crown
    r. ligament

radiatio
    r. optica
    r. pyramidalis
radiation
    acoustic r.
    afterloading r.
    alpha r.
    annihilation r.
    anterior thalamic r.
    background r.
    beta r.
    r. biology
    braking r.
    r. burn
    central thalamic r.
    Cerenkov r.
    characteristic r.
    corpuscular r.
    r. dermatitis
    r. dermatosis
    electromagnetic r.
    r. fibrosis
    gamma r.
    geniculocalcarine r.
    Gratiolet r.
    hemibody r.
    heterogeneous r.
    homogeneous r.
    hyperfractionated r.
    hypofractionated r.
    inferior thalamic r.
    interstitial r.
    ionizing r.
    monochromatic r.
    r. myelopathy
    r. necrosis
    r. oncology
    optic r.
    polychromatic r.
    pyramidal r.
    scattered r.
    secondary r.
    r. sickness
    r. syndrome
    r. therapy
radical
    acid r.
    color r.
    free r.
    r. hysterectomy
    r. mastectomy
    r. mastoidectomy
    r. neck dissection
    r. nephrectomy
    oxygen-derived free r.

R

radical *(continued)*
r. retropubic prostatectomy
r. surgery
radicle
radicotomy
radicula
radiculalgia
radicular
r. cyst
r. fila
r. pulp
radicularia
fila r.
radiculectomy
radiculitis
acute brachial r.
radiculoganglionitis
radiculomeningomyelitis
radiculomyelopathy
radiculoneuropathy
radiculopathy
diabetic thoracic r.
radiectomy
radii lentis
radioactive
r. constant
r. isotope
radioactivity
artificial r.
induced r.
radioallergosorbent test
radioautography
radiobicipital
radiobiology
radiocardiogram
radiocardiography
radiocarpal
r. joint
r. ligament
radiochemistry
radiocinematography
radiocurable
radiodense
radiodensity
radiodermatitis
radiodiagnosis
radiofrequency
radiograph
bitewing r.
cephalometric r.
decubitus r.
lateral decubitus r.
lateral oblique r.
lateral ramus r.
lateral skull r.
maxillary sinus r.
panoramic r.
periapical r.
radiographer

radiographic
r. artifact
r. contrast
r. density
radiography
advanced multiple-beam
equalization r. (AMBER)
air-gap r.
bedside r.
computed r. (CR)
digital r. (DR)
electron r.
filmless r.
magnification r.
mass r.
scanning equalization r.
serial r.
radioimmunity
radioimmunoassay
radioimmunodiffusion
radioimmunoelectrophoresis
radioimmunoprecipitation assay
radioimmunosorbent test
radioisotope
radiolesion
radioligand
radiologic
r. distortion
r. enteroclysis
r. sphincter
r. technologist
radiological anatomy
radiologist
radiology
cardiovascular r.
chest r.
diagnostic r.
interventional r.
therapeutic r.
radiolucency
radiolucent
radiometer
radiomimetic
radionecrosis
radioneuritis
radionuclide
r. angiocardiography
r. angiography
r. ejection fraction
r. generator
radiopacity
radiopaque
radiopathology
radiopelvimetry
radiopharmaceutical synovectomy
radioprotectant
radioreceptor
radioresistant
radiosensitive

radiosensitivity
radiotelemetry
radiotherapeutic
radiotherapeutics
radiotherapist
radiotherapy
    mantle r.
radiothermy
radiotoxaemia
radiotoxemia
radiotransparent
radiotropic
radisectomy
radium
radius
radon
Raeder paratrigeminal syndrome
Rainey corpuscle
Rainier
    hemoglobin R.
Raji cell assay
rale
    amphoric r.
    atelectatic r.
    bubbling r.
    cavernous r.
    clicking r.
    consonating r.
    crackling r.
    crepitant r.
    dry r.
    gurgling r.
    guttural r.
    laryngeal r.
    metallic r.
    moist r.
    sibilant r.
    sonorous r.
    whistling r.
raloxifene
ramal
rami (*pl. of* ramus)
ramification
ramify
ramisection
ramitis
Ramsay Hunt syndrome
Ramstedt operation
ramulus, pl. **ramuli**
ramus, pl. **rami**
    anterior r.
    communicating r.

    dental r.
    dorsal primary r.
    inferior dental r.
    inferior pubic r.
    internal r.
    ischial r.
    ischiopubic r.
    posterior r.
rancid
Randall plaque
random
    r. mating
    r. pattern flap
    r. sampling
randomization
range
    r. of accommodation
    r. of motion
    normal r.
    reference r.
    target heart rate r.
    therapeutic r.
ranine
Rankin clamp
Ransohoff sign
ranula
ranular
Ranvier
    node of R.
    R. node
Raoult law
raphe
    amnionic r.
    anogenital r.
    iliococcygeal r.
    lateral palpebral r.
    median longitudinal r.
    r. nucleus
    palatine r.
    penile r.
    perineal r.
    scrotal r.
rapid
    r. canities
    r. eye movements
    r. in-and-out surgery
    r. medical assessment
    r. trauma assessment
Rapoport-Leubering shunt
Rapoport test
rapport
rarefaction

R

NOTES

rare rhonchi
rash
    antitoxin r.
    black currant r.
    butterfly r.
    caterpillar r.
    crystal r.
    diaper r.
    drug r.
    heat r.
    hydatid r.
Rashkind
    R. operation
    R. procedure
Rasmussen
    R. aneurysm
    bundle of R.
    R. encephalitis
ras oncogene
raspatory
Rastelli operation
rat-bite fever
rate
    abortion r.
    age-specific r.
    attack r.
    average flow r.
    basal metabolic r. (BMR)
    baseline fetal heart r.
    birth r.
    case fatality r.
    concordance r.
    r. constants
    critical r.
    crude death r.
    death r.
    erythrocyte sedimentation r. (ESR)
    fatality r.
    fetal death r.
    fetal heart r.
    general fertility r.
    glomerular filtration r. (GFR)
    gross reproduction r.
    growth r.
    hazard r.
    heart r.
    inception r.
    incidence r.
    infant mortality r.
    initial r.
    lethality r.
    maternal death r.
    maximum expiratory flow r.
     (MEFR)
    metabolic clearance r. (MCR)
    mitotic r.
    morbidity r.
    mortality r.
    mucociliary clearance r.

    mutation r.
    neonatal mortality r.
    peak flow r. (PFR)
    pulse r.
    respiration r.
    respiratory r.
    sedimentation r.
    slew r.
    target heart r.
    5-year survival r.
ratellina
    Grisonella r.
Rathke
    R. cleft cyst
    R. pocket
    R. pouch
    R. pouch tumor
rathouisi
    Fasciolopsis r.
ratio
    absolute terminal innervation r.
    accommodative convergence-
     accommodation r.
    A/G r.
    albumin-globulin r.
    ALT:AST r.
    amylase-creatinine clearance r.
    body-weight r.
    cardiothoracic r.
    case fatality r.
    cup:disc r.
    extraction r.
    fertility r.
    flux r.
    functional terminal innervation r.
    grid r.
    gyromagnetic r.
    hand r.
    international normalized r. (INR)
    K:A r.
    ketogenic-antiketogenic r.
    lecithin/sphingomyelin r.
    magnetogyric r.
    mass-action r.
    maternal mortality r.
    M:E r.
    mendelian r.
    molecular weight r.
    nuclear:cytoplasmic r.
    respiratory exchange r.
    segregation r.
    sex r.
    signal-to-noise r.
    therapeutic r.
    ventilation/perfusion r.
    waist-to-hip r.
    zeta sedimentation r.
ration
    basal r.

rational
- r. formula
- r. symptom
- r. therapy

rationalization

ray
- actinic r.
- alpha r.
- anode r.
- Becquerel r.
- beta r.
- cathode r.
- chemical r.
- cosmic r.
- direct r.
- gamma r.
- glass r.
- grenz r.
- H r.
- hard r.
- incident r.
- indirect r.
- infrared r.
- intermediate r.
- marginal r.
- medullary r.
- roentgen r.

Raynaud
- R. phenomenon
- R. sign
- R. syndrome

razor
- Occam r.

R-banding stain

RCM
- right costal margin

RCU
- respiratory care unit

RDS
- respiratory distress syndrome

reactance

reactant
- acute phase r.

reaction
- accelerated r.
- acid r.
- acute phase r.
- acute situational r.
- acute stress r.
- adverse drug r. (ADR)
- alarm r.
- alkaline r.
- allergic r.
- amphoteric r.
- anamnestic r.
- anaphylactic r.
- anaplerotic r.
- antigen-antibody r. (AAR)
- anxiety r.
- Arias-Stella r.
- arousal r.
- Arthus r.
- Ascoli r.
- associative r.
- basic r.
- Bence Jones r.
- Berthelot r.
- bi bi r.
- Bittorf r.
- biuret r.
- Bloch r.
- Bordet and Gengou r.
- Brunn r.
- Burchard-Liebermann r.
- Cannizzaro r.
- capsular precipitation r.
- Carr-Price r.
- catalatic r.
- catastrophic r.
- cell-mediated r.
- chain r.
- Chantemesse r.
- chromaffin r.
- circular r.
- cocarde r.
- cockade r.
- colloidal gold r.
- complement-fixation r.
- consensual r.
- constitutional r.
- conversion r.
- cutaneous graft versus host r.
- cytotoxic r.
- Dale r.
- dark r.
- decidual r.
- delayed r.
- depot r.
- depressive r.
- dermotuberculin r.
- diazo r.
- digitonin r.
- Dische r.
- dissociative r.

NOTES

reaction *(continued)*
    dopa r.
    dystonic r.
    early r.
    echo r.
    Ehrlich benzaldehyde r.
    Ehrlich diazo r.
    eosinopenic r.
    error-prone polymerase chain r.
    eye-closure pupil r.
    false-negative r.
    false-positive r.
    Fenton r.
    Fernandez r.
    ferric chloride r.
    Feulgen r.
    fight or flight r.
    first-order r.
    fixation r.
    flocculation r.
    focal r.
    Folin r.
    foreign body r.
    r. formation
    Forssman antigen-antibody r.
    fragment r.
    Frei-Hoffmann r.
    fright r.
    fuchsinophil r.
    galvanic skin r.
    gel diffusion r.
    Gell and Coombs r.
    gemistocytic r.
    general adaptation r.
    Gerhardt r.
    graft versus host r. (GVHR)
    group r.
    Gruber r.
    Gruber-Widal r.
    Günning r.
    Haber-Weiss r.
    harlequin r.
    heel-tap r.
    hemoclastic r.
    Henle r.
    Herxheimer r.
    Hill r.
    homograft r.
    hunting r.
    hypersensitivity r.
    id r.
    immediate hypersensitivity r.
    immune r.
    incompatible blood transfusion r.
    indifference r.
    indirect pupillary r.
    intracutaneous r.
    intradermal r.
    iodate r.

    iodine r.
    irreversible r.
    Jaffe r.
    Jarisch-Herxheimer r.
    Jolly r.
    Kiliani-Fischer r.
    late r.
    lengthening r.
    lepromin r.
    leukemoid r.
    lid-closure r.
    Liebermann-Burchard r.
    ligase chain r.
    local anesthetic r.
    Loewenthal r.
    Lohmann r.
    lymphocytic leukemoid r.
    magnet r.
    Marchi r.
    Mazzotti r.
    Millon r.
    miostagmin r.
    Mitsuda r.
    mixed agglutination r.
    mixed lymphocyte culture r.
    near-point r.
    nested polymerase chain r.
    Neufeld r.
    ninhydrin r.
    polymerase chain r.
    quellung r.
    reverse transcriptase polymerase chain r.
    Schultz-Charlton r.
    serum r.
    specific r.
    startle r.
    stress r.
    symptomatic r.
    r. time
    transcription-based chain r.
    Weil-Felix r.
    Weinberg r.
    Wernicke r.
    wheal-and-erythema r.
    wheal-and-flare r.
    Yorke autolytic r.
reactivate
reactivator
    cholinesterase r.
reactive
    r. airways disease
    r. change
    r. depression
    r. hyperemia
reactivity
reading
    lip r.
    speech r.

R

reagent
Benedict-Hopkins-Cole r.
biuret r.
Cleland r.
diazo r.
Dische r.
Dische-Schwarz r.
Drabkin r.
Dragendorff r.
Edlefsen r.
Edman r.
Ehrlich diazo r.
Erdmann r.
Esbach r.
Exton r.
Fehling r.
Folin r.
Fouchet r.
Froehde r.
Frohn r.
Girard r.
Günzberg r.
Hahn oxine r.
Hammarsten r.
Ilosvay r.
Kasten fluorescent Schiff r.
Lloyd r.
Mandelin r.
Marme r.
Marquis r.
Mecke r.
Meyer r.
Millon r.
Schiff r.
reagin
atopic r.
reaginic antibody
REAL
Revised European-American
Classification of Lymphoid Neoplasms
REAL classification
reality
r. awareness
contact with r.
r. principle
retreat from r.
r. testing
real-time echocardiography
reamer
engine r.
intramedullary r.

rearfoot
r. pronation
r. supination
rearrangement
Amadori r.
reassignment
sex r.
rebound
r. nystagmus
r. phenomenon
r. tenderness
rebreathing
r. anesthesia
r. technique
r. volume
recalcification
recalcitrant
r. disease
r. hemorrhage
r. patient
recall bias
Récamier operation
recanalization
recapitulation theory
receptaculum
receptive aphasia
receptor
adrenergic r.
alpha-adrenergic r.
angiotensin r.
ANP clearance r.
asialoglycoprotein r.
B cell r.
beta-adrenergic r.
cholinergic r.
epidermal growth factor r. (EGFR)
estrogen r.
Fas r.
Fc r.
gustatory r.
kainate r.
laminin r.
low-density lipoprotein r.
metabotropic r.
olfactory r.
opiate r.
orphan r.
progesterone r.
r. protein
retinoic acid r.
retinoid X r.
ryanodine r.

NOTES

741

receptor *(continued)*
    scavenger r.
    stretch r.
    taste r.
    T-cell r.
    T-lymphocyte antigen r.
recess
    azygoesophageal r.
    cecal r.
    cerebellopontine r.
    cochlear r.
    costodiaphragmatic r.
    costomediastinal r.
    duodenojejunal r.
    elliptical r.
    epitympanic r.
    hepatoenteric r.
    hepatorenal r.
    Hyrtl epitympanic r.
    inferior duodenal r.
    inferior ileocecal r.
    inferior omental r.
    infundibular r.
    intersigmoid r.
    Jacquemet r.
    lateral r.
    mesentericoparietal r.
recession
    angle r.
    clitoral r.
    gingival r.
    tendon r.
recessive
    autosomal r.
    r. character
    r. inheritance
    r. trait
recidivation
recidivism
recidivist
reciprocal
    r. force
    r. gene
    r. transfusion
    r. translocation
Recklinghausen
    R. disease
    R. tumor
reclination
reclotting phenomenon
recognition factor
recombinant
    r. DNA
    r. human interleukin-11
    r. vector
recombination
    genetic r.
    homologous r.
    site-specific r.

recommended daily allowance
reconditum
    Dipetalonema r.
reconstruction
    ossicular r.
reconstructive
    r. mammaplasty
    r. rhinoplasty
    r. surgery
record
    anesthesia r.
    computer-based patient r.
    face-bow r.
    functional chew-in r.
    hospital r.
    interocclusal r.
    maxillomandibular r.
    medical r.
    problem-oriented medical r.
    unit r.
recorded detail
recording
    clinical r.
    depth r.
recovery
    active r.
    creep r.
    inversion r.
    r. room
recrudescence
recrudescent
    r. abscess
    r. pain
    r. typhus
recta (*pl. of* rectum)
rectal
    r. ampulla
    r. anesthesia
    r. column
    r. hernia
rectale
    Eubacterium r.
rectalgia
rectectomy
recti
    diastasis r.
rectify
rectitis
rectocele
rectococcygeal muscle
rectococcygeus muscle
rectococcypexy
rectocolic fossa
rectoischiadic excavation
rectolabial fistula
rectopexy
rectoplasty
rectoscope
rectosigmoid

rectostenosis
rectostomy
rectotomy
rectourethralis muscle
rectouterine
    r. excavation
    r. fold
    r. muscle
    r. pouch
rectovaginal septum
rectovesical
    r. excavation
    r. muscle
    r. pouch
    r. septum
rectovesicalis muscle
rectum, pl. recta, rectums
    per r.
    vasa recta
rectus
    r. abdominis muscle
    r. capitis anterior muscle
    r. capitis lateralis muscle
    r. capitis posterior major muscle
    r. capitis posterior minor muscle
    r. femoris muscle
recumbent incision
recuperate
recuperation
    rest and r. (R&R)
recurrence
    no evidence of r.
    r. risk
recurrens
    periadenitis mucosa necrotica r.
recurrent
    r. abortion
    r. aphthous ulcer
    r. aphthous ulcers
    r. herpetic stomatitis
    r. jaundice
    r. polyserositis
    r. respiratory papillomatosis
    r. ulcerative stomatitis
    r. ulnar artery
    r. upper respiratory tract infection
    r. vomiting
recurring digital fibroma
recurvation
recurvatum
    genu r.

red
    r. albinism
    aniline r.
    Biebrich scarlet r.
    r. blood cell
    Congo r.
    r. corpuscle
    cresol r.
    Darrow r.
    r. hepatization
    r. imported fire ant
    r. induration
    medicinal scarlet r.
    methyl r.
    r. muscle
    r. neuralgia
    r. nucleus
    r. oil
    r. pulp
    r. reflex
    r. tide
    vital r.
    r., white, and blue sign
redintegration
redox
reduce
reduced
    r. hematin
    r. hemoglobin
reducible hernia
reductant
reductase
    crotonyl-ACP r.
    cytochrome b5 r.
    cytochrome c r.
    cytochrome c2 r.
    dihydrobiopterin r.
    dihydrofolate r.
    enoyl-ACP r.
    enoyl-CoA r.
    ketose r.
5-reductase inhibitor
reduction
    afterload r.
    r. of chromosomes
    closed r.
    r. deformity
    r. left ventriculoplasty
    r. mammaplasty
    open r.
reduplication

NOTES

redux
    chancre r.
Reed-Frost model
Reed-Sternberg cell
reefing
reentrant
    r. mechanism
    r. pathway
reentry
    sinus nodal r.
reference
    biomechanical frame of r.
    delusion of r.
    idea of r.
    r. range
    r. value
referred
    r. pain
    r. sensation
reflectance spectrophotometry
reflected inguinal ligament
reflection coefficient
reflector
reflex
    abdominal r.
    abdominocardiac r.
    Abrams heart r.
    accommodation r.
    Achilles tendon r.
    acoustic r.
    acousticopalpebral r.
    acquired r.
    acromial r.
    adductor r.
    anal r.
    ankle r.
    antagonistic r.
    aortic r.
    aponeurotic r.
    r. arc
    Aschner r.
    Aschner-Dagnini r.
    attitudinal r.
    auditory oculogyric r.
    auricular r.
    auriculopalpebral r.
    auriculopressor r.
    auropalpebral r.
    axon r.
    Babinski r.
    Bainbridge r.
    Barkman r.
    basal joint r.
    Bechterew-Mendel r.
    behavior r.
    Benedek r.
    Bezold-Jarisch r.
    biceps femoris r.
    Bing r.

    bladder r.
    blink r.
    body righting r.
    brachioradial r.
    Brain r.
    bregmocardiac r.
    Brissaud r.
    bulbocavernosus r.
    bulbomimic r.
    Capps r.
    cardiac depressor r.
    carotid sinus r.
    celiac plexus r.
    cephalopalpebral r.
    Chaddock r.
    chain r.
    chin r.
    Chodzko r.
    ciliospinal r.
    clasping r.
    cochleo-orbicular r.
    cochleopalpebral r.
    cochleopupillary r.
    cochleostapedial r.
    conditioned r.
    conjunctival r.
    consensual light r.
    contralateral r.
    corneal r.
    costal arch r.
    costopectoral r.
    r. cough
    cough r.
    craniocardiac r.
    cremasteric r.
    crossed adductor r.
    crossed extension r.
    crossed knee r.
    crossed spino-adductor r.
    cuboidodigital r.
    cutaneous pupil r.
    cutaneous-pupillary r.
    darwinian r.
    deep abdominal r.
    deep tendon r. (DTR)
    defense r.
    deglutition r.
    Dejerine r.
    delayed r.
    depressor r.
    diffused r.
    digital r.
    diving r.
    dorsal r.
    dorsum pedis r.
    elbow r.
    enterogastric r.
    epigastric r.
    r. epilepsy

erector-spinal r.
esophagosalivary r.
exercise pressor r.
external oblique r.
eye r.
eyeball compression r.
eyeball-heart r.
eye-closure r.
facial r.
faucial r.
femoral r.
femoroabdominal r.
Ferguson r.
finger-thumb r.
flexor r.
forced grasping r.
front-tap r.
fundus r.
gag r.
gagging r.
Galant r.
galvanic skin r.
gastrocolic r.
gastroileac r.
Geigel r.
Gifford r.
gluteal r.
Gordon r.
grasp r.
grasping r.
great-toe r.
gripping r.
Guillain-Barré r.
gustatory-sudorific r.
H r.
hepatojugular r.
Hering-Breuer r.
Hoffmann r.
hypochondrial r.
hypogastric r.
inborn r.
r. inhibition
innate r.
interscapular r.
intrinsic r.
inverted radial r.
investigatory r.
ipsilateral r.
Jacobson r.
jaw r.
jaw-working r.
Joffroy r.

Kisch r.
knee r.
knee-jerk r.
labyrinthine righting r.
lacrimal r.
lacrimogustatory r.
laryngeal r.
laryngospastic r.
latent r.
laughter r.
let-down r.
lid r.
Liddell-Sherrington r.
light r.
lip r.
Lovén r.
lower abdominal periosteal r.
magnet r.
mandibular r.
mass r.
masseter r.
Mayer r.
McCarthy r.
mediopubic r.
Mendel-Bechterew r.
Mendel instep r.
metacarpohypothenar r.
metacarpothenar r.
metatarsal r.
micturition r.
milk-ejection r.
milk let-down r.
Moro r.
myopic r.
myotatic r.
nasal r.
neck-righting r.
r. neurogenic bladder
Oppenheim r.
orienting r.
palatal r.
palatine r.
parachute r.
paradoxical extensor r.
paradoxic pupillary r.
patellar r.
patelloadductor r.
Pavlov r.
pharyngeal r.
Phillipson r.
photic-sneeze r.
pilomotor r.

R

NOTES

reflex *(continued)*
plantar r.
protective laryngeal r.
pupillary r.
pupillary-skin r.
quadriceps r.
quadripedal extensor r.
red r.
Remak r.
righting r.
rooting r.
Rossolimo r.
Schäffer r.
snout r.
spinal r.
spinoadductor r.
stapedial r.
Starling r.
startle r.
statokinetic r.
stretch r.
Strümpell r.
superficial r.
swallowing r.
r. sympathetic dystrophy
r. symptom
tendon r.
tensor tympani r.
tonic neck r.
triceps surae r.
Trömner r.
unconditioned r.
vagus r.
vasopressor r.
vestibuloocular r.
vestibulospinal r.
vomiting r.
Westphal pupillary r.
wink r.
r. zone therapy
reflexa
decidua r.
placenta r.
tunica r.
reflexogenic
reflexograph
reflexology
reflexometer
reflexus
Argas r.
reflux
abdominojugular r.
esophageal r.
r. esophagitis
gastroesophageal r.
hepatojugular r.
intrarenal r.
r. otitis media
ureterorenal r.

vesicoureteral r.
vesicoureteric r.
refract
refraction
double r.
dynamic r.
refractionist
refractive
r. index
r. keratoplasty
r. keratotomy
refractivity
refractometer
refractometry
refractory
r. anemia
r. illness
r. period
r. state
refracture
refrigerant
refrigeration anesthesia
refringence
refringent
Refsum disease
refusion
Regaud fixative
regeneration
aberrant r.
guided tissue r.
regenerative polyp
regimen
region
abdominal r.
anal r.
ankle r.
anterior antebrachial r.
anterior brachial r.
anterior carpal r.
anterior cervical r.
anterior crural r.
anterior cubital r.
anterior hypothalamic r.
anterior knee r.
axillary r.
buccal r.
calcaneal r.
chromosomal r.
complementarity determining r.
constant r.
deltoid r.
dorsal hypothalamic r.
epigastric r.
face r.
femoral r.
framework r.
frontal r.
genitourinary r.
gluteal r.

R

heel r.
hinge r.
hypervariable r.
hypochondriac r.
hypogastric r.
I r.
iliac r.
inframammary r.
infraorbital r.
infrascapular r.
inguinal r.
r. of interest
intermediate hypothalamic r.
K r.
lateral abdominal r.
lateral cervical r.
lateral hypothalamic r.
lumbar r.
mammary r.
mental r.
pectoral r.
pelvic r.
pubic r.
sternocleidomastoid r.
submental r.
suprapubic r.
sural r.
temporal r.
umbilical r.
urogenital r.
vestibular r.
zygomatic r.
regional
r. anatomy
r. anesthesia
r. block
r. enteritis
r. enterocolitis
r. granulomatous lymphadenitis
r. hypothermia
r. ileitis
register
high risk r.
registration
maxillomandibular r.
sensory r.
regression analysis
regressive staining
regular astigmatism
regulation
enzyme r.
gene r.

regulator
r. gene
growth r.
humoral r.
regulatory
r. disorder
r. sequence
regulon
regurgitant murmur
regurgitate
regurgitation
aortic r.
ischemic mitral r.
r. jaundice
mitral r.
valvular r.
rehabilitation
aural r.
cardiac r.
r. medicine
physical medicine and r. (PMR)
psychiatric r.
rehearsal
rehydration
Reichel-Pólya stomach procedure
Reichert cartilage
Reid base line
Reifenstein syndrome
Reiki
Reil
island of R.
reimplantation
extravesical r.
ureteral r.
reinfection
reinforcement conditioning
reinforcer
Reinke space
reinnervation
reintegration
Reis-Bücklers corneal dystrophy
Reisseisen muscle
Reissner membrane
Reiter syndrome
rejection
accelerated r.
acute cellular r.
allograft r.
chronic allograft r.
first-set r.
hyperacute r.
relapse

NOTES

relapsing
r. febrile nodular nonsuppurative panniculitis
r. fever
r. polychondritis

relation
acquired centric r.
acquired eccentric r.
buccolingual r.
centric jaw r.
dynamic r.'s
eccentric r.
intermaxillary r.
maxillomandibular r.
median retruded r.
spatial r.
static r.

relationship
blood r.
coefficient of r.
dose-response r.
dual r.'s
Haldane r.
hypnotic r.
object r.

relative
r. accommodation
r. biologic effectiveness
blood r.
r. humidity
r. leukocytosis
r. molecular mass
r. polycythemia
r. scotoma
r. specificity
r. sterility

relaxant
depolarizing r.
muscular r.
r. reversal

relaxation
cardioesophageal r.
isometric r.
isovolumetric r.
isovolumic r.
longitudinal r.
r. suture
r. time
transverse r.

relearning

releasing
r. factor
r. hormone

reliability
equivalent form r.
interjudge r.

relief incision

relocation test

Remak
R. fiber
R. nuclear division
R. reflex
R. sign

remineralization

remission

remittence

remittent

remodeling
heart chamber r.

remote afterloading brachytherapy

removable
r. bridge
r. partial denture

renal
r. agenesis
r. amyloidosis
r. anuria
r. artery
r. calculus
r. column
r. corpuscle
r. cortex
r. fascia
r. ganglion
r. glycosuria
r. hematuria
r. hypertension
r. hypoplasia
r. labyrinth
r. medulla
r. osteodystrophy
r. papilla
r. pelvis
r. pyramid
r. retinopathy
r. rickets
r. scan
r. sinus
r. tubular acidosis
r. tubular osteomalacia
r. tubule
r. vein

renalis
cortex r.
medulla r.
pyramis r.

reniform

renin-angiotensin-aldosterone system

reniportal

renis
adeps r.
corpusculum r.

renninogen

rennogen

renogenic

renogram

renography

renomegaly
renoprival
renotrophic
renovascular hypertension
Renpenning syndrome
repalr
    chemical r.
    error-prone r.
    excision r.
    mismatch r.
reparative
    r. dentin
    r. granuloma
repeat
    inverted r.
repellent
repens
    dermatitis r.
repetition
    r. maximum
    r. time
repetition-compulsion
repetitive strain disorder
replacement
    cephalic r.
    r. therapy
replant
replantation
    intentional r.
repletion
replicase
replicate
replication
    bidirectional r.
    conservative r.
replicative form
replicator
replicon
repolarization
report
    prehospital care r.
reportable disease
reporting bias
repositioning
    gingival r.
    jaw r.
representation
    internal r.
repressible enzyme
repression
    catabolite r.

    end product r.
    enzyme r.
repressor
    active r.
    r. gene
    inactive r.
reproducibility
reproduction
    asexual r.
    cytogenic r.
    sexual r.
    somatic r.
reproductive cycle
reptilase
repulsion
requirement
    minimum protein r.
resectable
resection
    abdominoperineal r. (APR)
    gum r.
    loop r.
    pulmonary r.
    root r.
    septal r.
    transurethral r. (TUR)
    wedge r.
resectoscope electrode
reservatus
    coitus r.
reserve
    r. air
    alkali r.
    breathing r.
    cardiac r.
    r. force
    heart rate r.
    systolic r.
reservoir
    r. bag
    r. host
    r. of infection
    r. oxygen-conserving device
    r. sign
residual
    r. abscess
    r. air
    r. capacity
    r. proteinuria
    r. schizophrenia
    r. urine
    r. volume

R

NOTES

residue
    day r.
residuum
resin
    acrylic r.
    activated r.
    anion-exchange r.
    autopolymer r.
    autopolymerizing r.
    cation-exchange r.
    r. cement
    chemically cured r.
    cholestyramine r.
    cold cure r.
    cold-curing r.
    composite r.
    copolymer r.
    cross-linked r.
    direct filling r.
    dual-cure r.
    epoxy r.
    gum r.
    heat-curing r.
    Indian podophyllum r.
    ion-exchange r.
    ipomea r.
    jalap r.
    light-activated r.
    light-cured r.
    melamine r.
    methacrylate r.
resinous
resistance
    accommodating r.
    airway r.
    bacteriophage r.
    capillary r.
    dicumarol r.
    drug r.
    expiratory r.
    impact r.
    inductive r.
    insulin r.
    multidrug r.
    mutual r.
    natural r.
    peripheral r.
    r. plasmid
    pulmonary vascular r.
    systemic vascular r.
    r. thermometer
    vascular r.
resistance-transfer factor
resolution
resolving power
resonance
    amphoric r.
    bandbox r.
    bellmetal r.

    cavernous r.
    cough r.
    cracked-pot r.
    electron paramagnetic r. (EPR)
    electron spin r.
    hydatid r.
    nuclear magnetic r.
    skodaic r.
    tympanitic r.
    vesicular r.
    vesiculotympanitic r.
    vocal r.
    wooden r.
resonant frequency
resorb
resorption
    bone r.
    gingival r.
    horizontal r.
    internal r.
    r. lacunae
respirable
respiration
    abdominal r.
    aerobic r.
    amphoric r.
    anaerobic r.
    artificial r.
    assisted r.
    Biot r.
    bronchial r.
    bronchovesicular r.
    cavernous r.
    Cheyne-Stokes r.
    cogwheel r.
    controlled r.
    costal r.
    diffusion r.
    electrophrenic r.
    external r.
    forced r.
    internal r.
    interrupted r.
    jerky r.
    Kussmaul r.
    Kussmaul-Kien r.
    labored r.
    mouth-to-mouth r.
    paradoxical r.
    r. rate
    tissue r.
    vesicular r.
respirator
    cuirass r.
    Drinker r.
respiratory
    r. acidosis
    r. alkalosis
    r. bronchiole

r. burn
r. capacity
r. care
r. care unit (RCU)
r. center
r. compliance
r. distress syndrome (RDS)
r. enteric orphan virus
r. enzyme
r. exchange ratio
r. failure
r. frequency
r. gating
r. minute volume
r. pause
r. pigment
r. quotient
r. rate
r. scleroma
r. sounds
r. system compliance
r. therapist
r. therapy
r. tract
respirometer
Dräger r.
responder
first r.
response
acute phase r.
anamnestic r.
auditory brainstem r. (ABR)
automatic auditory brainstem r.
r. bias
biphasic r.
blink r.
booster r.
brainstem auditory evoked r. (BAER)
brainstem evoked r. (BSER)
conditioned r.
Cushing r.
depletion r.
early-phase r.
evoked r.
flight or fight r.
galvanic skin r. (GSR)
Henry-Gauer r.
hunting r.
immune r.
isomorphic r.
late auditory-evoked r.

late-phase r.
level-dependent frequency r.
middle latency r.
myotonic r.
orienting r.
postural sway r.
primary immune r.
secondary immune r.
target r.
triple r.
unconditioned r.
rest
adrenal r.
bed r.
Donath-Landsteiner r.
incisal r.
lingual r.
Malassez epithelial r.'s
Marchand r.
mesonephric r.
r. position
r. and recuperation (R&R)
r. of Serres
Walthard cell r.
wolffian r.
restenosis
restiform body
resting
r. energy expenditure
r. orthosis
r. tidal volume
r. tremor
restitope
restitution
Reston
Ebola virus R.
R. virus
restoration
acid-etched r.
combination r.
compound r.
direct acrylic r.
direct composite resin r.
silicate r.
restorative dentistry
restraint
restricted affect
restriction
asymmetric fetal growth r.
r. endonuclease
r. enzyme
fetal growth r.

NOTES

restriction *(continued)*
    r. fragment length polymorphism
    lactase r.
    r. site
    symmetric fetal growth r.
restriction-site polymorphism
restrictive ventilatory defect
restuans
    Culex r.
resuscitate
    do not r. (DNR)
resuscitation
    cardiopulmonary r. (CPR)
    mouth-to-mouth r.
retained
    r. foreign body
    r. menstruation
    r. products of conception
    r. testis
retainer
    continuous bar r.
    direct r.
    extracoronal r.
    Hawley r.
    indirect r.
    intracoronal r.
    matrix r.
retardation
    intrauterine growth r. (IUGR)
    mental r.
retarded dentition
retch
retching
rete
    r. cutaneum corii
    Haller r.
    malpighian r.
    r. ovarii
    r. ridge
    r. subpapillare
retention
    r. cyst
    denture r.
    direct r.
    indirect r.
    r. jaundice
    r. suture
    r. uremia
    r. vomiting
reticula (*pl. of* reticulum)
reticular
    r. activating system
    r. degeneration
    r. dystrophy
    r. fiber
    r. formation
    r. membrane
    r. substance
    r. tissue

reticulare
    magma r.
reticularis
    fetal r.
    livedo r.
    zona r.
reticulata
    folliculitis ulerythematosa r.
reticulated
    r. bone
    r. erythrocyte
reticulation
reticulatus
    Dermacentor r.
reticulin
reticulocyte production index
reticulocytopenia
reticulocytosis
reticuloendothelial
reticuloendothelium
reticulohistiocytoma
reticuloid
    actinic r.
reticulopenia
reticulosis
    benign inoculation r.
    leukemic r.
    malignant midline r.
reticulospinal tract
reticulum, pl. **reticula**
    agranular endoplasmic r.
    Ebner r.
    endoplasmic r.
    Golgi internal r.
    granular endoplasmic r.
    Kölliker r.
    sarcoplasmic r.
    stellate r.
    trabecular r.
    Wilder stain for r.
retiform tissue
retina
    detached r.
    detachment of r.
    fleck r.
    flecked r.
    hole in r.
    inferior nasal arteriole of r.
    inferior nasal venule of r.
    leopard r.
    physiologic r.
    shot-silk r.
retinaculum, pl. **retinacula**
    caudal r.
    extensor r.
    flexor r.
    inferior extensor r.
    inferior fibular r.
    inferior peroneal r.

R

lateral patellar r.
medial patellar r.
Morgagni r.
peroneal r.
superior extensor r.
retinae
dialysis r.
ischemia r.
ora serrata r.
retinal
r. adaptation
r. aplasia
r. astigmatism
r. cone
r. detachment
r. isomerase
r. migraine
r. tear
retinaldehyde
retinalis
lipemia r.
retinene
retinitis
albuminuric r.
apoplectic r.
circinate r.
diabetic r.
r. exudativa
exudative r.
leukemic r.
metastatic r.
r. pigmentosa
r. proliferans
serous r.
suppurative r.
retinoblastoma
retinochoroid
retinochoroiditis
bird shot r.
r. juxtapapillaris
retinoic
r. acid
r. acid receptor
retinoid X receptor
retinol dehydrogenase
retinopapillitis
retinopathy
arteriosclerotic r.
background r.
central angiospastic r.
central serous r.
circinate r.

compression r.
diabetic r.
dysproteinemic r.
electric r.
external exudative r.
hypertensive r.
Leber idiopathic stellate r.
leukemic r.
lipemic r.
macular r.
pigmentary r.
r. of prematurity
proliferative r.
Purtscher r.
renal r.
sickle cell r.
whiplash r.
retinopexy
fluid r.
gas r.
retinoschisis
juvenile r.
senile r.
retinoscope
luminous r.
retinoscopy
cylinder r.
fogging r.
retractile
retraction
gingival r.
mandibular r.
r. pocket
retractor
abdominal r.
contour r.
Desmarres r.
palate r.
retreat from reality
retrenchment
retrieval
retroauricular
r. fold
r. incision
r. lymph node
retrobulbar
r. anesthesia
r. neuritis
retrocalcaneal bursa
retrocalcaneobursitis
retrocardiac space
retrocession

NOTES

retroclusion
retrocochlear hearing loss
retrocursive
retrocuspid papilla
retrodeviation
retrodisplacement
retroflexion
retrognathic
retrognathism
retrograde
    r. amnesia
    r. beat
    r. block
    r. cystourethrogram
    r. ejaculation
    r. embolism
    r. hernia
    r. menstruation
    r. metastasis
    r. pyelogram
    r. pyelography
    r. urography
    r. VA conduction
retrogression
retrohyoid bursa
retroinguinalis
    lacuna musculorum r.
    lacuna vasorum r.
retrojection
retromandibular vein
retromolar pad
retroperitoneal
    r. fibrosis
    r. hematoma
    r. hernia
    r. space
retroperitonitis
    idiopathic fibrous r.
retropharynx
retroplasa
retroposed
retroposition
retroposon
retropubic
    r. prevesical prostatectomy
    r. space
retropulsion
retrosigmoid approach
retrospective falsification
retrospondylolisthesis
retrourethral catheterization
retroversioflexion
retroversion
retroverted
Retroviridae
retrovirus
retrusion

retrusive
    r. excursion
    r. occlusion
Rett syndrome
return
    r. extrasystole
    total anomalous pulmonary
     venous r.
    venous r.
Retzius
    foramen of R.
reuniens
    canaliculus r.
revascularization
reversal
    adrenaline r.
    epinephrine r.
    narcotic r.
    pressure r.
    relaxant r.
    sex r.
reverse
    r. Eck fistula
    r. osmosis
    r. passive hemagglutination
    r. pupillary block
    r. transcriptase
    r. transcriptase polymerase chain
     reaction
reversed
    r. coarctation
    r. peristalsis
reversibility principle
reversible calcinosis
reversion
revertant
review
    drug utilization r.
    peer r.
    r. of systems (ROS)
Revised European-American
  Classification of Lymphoid Neoplasms
  (REAL)
revivification
revulsion
Reye syndrome
Rh
    R. antigen incompatibility
    R. null syndrome
rhabdoid
rhabdomyoblast
rhabdomyolysis
    acute recurrent r.
    exertional r.
    familial paroxysmal r.
    idiopathic paroxysmal r.
rhabdomyoma
rhabdomyosarcoma
    embryonal r.

rhabdosarcoma
rhagades
rhegma
rhegmatogenous
rhenium
rheobase
rheobasic
rheology
rheometry
rheostosis
rheotaxis
rheotropism
Rhese projection
rhestocythemia
rheumatic
    r. arteritis
    r. endocarditis
    r. fever
    r. heart disease
    r. myocarditis
    r. pneumonia
    r. scoliosis
rheumatid
rheumatism
    articular r.
    cerebral r.
    chronic r.
    gonorrheal r.
    inflammatory r.
    lumbar r.
    Macleod r.
    nodose r.
rheumatoid
    r. arthritis
    r. factor
    r. nodule
    r. pocket
    r. spondylitis
    r. vasculitis
rheumatologist
rheumatology
Rh-immune globulin
rhinalgia
rhinal sulcus
rhinedema
rhinencephalic
rhinencephalon
rhinitis
    acute r.
    allergic r.
    atrophic r.
    caseous r.

    chronic r.
    fibrinous r.
    gangrenous r.
    hypertrophic r.
    membranous r.
    purulent r.
    tuberculous r.
    vasomotor r.
rhinocele
rhinocephalia
rhinocephaly
rhinocheiloplasty
rhinochiloplasty
rhinocleisis
rhinodynia
rhinogenous
rhinokyphosis
rhinolalia
rhinolith
rhinolithiasis
rhinologist
rhinology
rhinomanometer
rhinomanometry
rhinomycosis
rhinonecrosis
rhinopathy
rhinophonia
rhinophyma
rhinoplasty
    reconstructive r.
rhinorrhea
    cerebrospinal fluid r.
    gustatory r.
rhinorrhoea
rhinosalpingitis
rhinoscleroma
rhinoscleromatis
    Klebsiella r.
rhinoscope
rhinoscopic
rhinoscopy
    anterior r.
    median r.
    posterior r.
rhinosinusitis
rhinostenosis
rhinotomy
rhinovirus
    bovine r.
    equine r.
rhizoid

NOTES

rhizomelia
rhizomelic
    r. chondrodysplasia punctata
    r. dwarfism
rhizomeningomyelitis
rhizotomy
    anterior r.
    facet r.
    posterior r.
    trigeminal r.
Rhodesian trypanosomiasis
rhodium
rhodogenesis
rhodophylactic
rhodophylaxis
rhodopsin
rhombencephalic
    r. isthmus
    r. tegmentum
rhombencephalon
rhombic
rhombocele
rhomboid
    r. fossa
    r. ligament
    r. sinus
rhomboidal sinus
rhonchal fremitus
rhonchial
rhonchus, pl. **rhonchi**
    audible rhonchi
    bibasilar rhonchi
    bilateral rhonchi
    cavernous rhonchi
    coarse rhonchi
    diffuse rhonchi
    expiratory rhonchi
    faint rhonchi
    few rhonchi
    harsh rhonchi
    high-pitched rhonchi
    humming rhonchi
    inspiratory rhonchi
    low-pitched rhonchi
    marked rhonchi
    musical rhonchi
    occasional rhonchi
    posttussive inspiratory rhonchi
    rare rhonchi
    scattered rhonchi
    sibilant rhonchi
    sonorous rhonchi
    upper respiratory rhonchi
    whistling rhonchi
rhus dermatitis
rhusiopathiae
    Erysipelothrix r.
rhythm
    agonal r.

    alpha r.
    atrioventricular junctional r.
    AV junctional r.
    basic electrical r.
    Berger r.
    beta r.
    bigeminal r.
    cantering r.
    chaotic r.
    circadian r.
    circus r.
    coronary nodal r.
    coronary sinus r.
    coupled r.
    delta r.
    diurnal r.
    ectopic r.
    escape r.
    gallop r.
    idiojunctional r.
    idionodal r.
    idioventricular r.
    junctional escape r.
    r. method
    quadrigeminal r.
    scapulohumeral r.
    sinus r.
    theta r.
    trigeminal r.
    ventricular r.
rhytide
rhytidectomy
rhytidoplasty
rhytidosis
rib
    r. approximator
    beading of r.
    bicipital r.
    bifid r.
    cervical r.
    false r.
    first r.
    floating r.
    lumbar r.
    slipping r.
    spurious r.
    true r.
    vertebral r.
riboflavin
    methylol r.
ribonuclease
ribonucleic acid (RNA)
ribonucleoprotein
ribonucleoside
    cytosine r.
ribonucleotide
    glycineamide r.
    guanine r.
ribose

R

ribosomal RNA
ribosome
ribosuria
ribosyl
ribosylation
    ΛDP r.
ribothymidine
ribothymidylic acid
Ribot law of memory
Ricco law
rice starch
riches
    embarrassment of r.
Richter
    R. hernia
    R. syndrome
rickets
    acute r.
    adult r.
    celiac r.
    familial hypophosphatemic r.
    hemorrhagic r.
    hereditary hypophosphatemic r.
    late r.
    renal r.
    vitamin D-resistant r.
rickettsial
rickettsialpox
rickettsiosis
Riddoch phenomenon
Rideal-Walker coefficient
Ridell operation
rider's
    r. bone
    r. bursa
    r. sprain
ridge
    alveolar r.
    apical ectodermal r.
    basal r.
    bicipital r.
    buccocervical r.
    buccogingival r.
    bulbar r.
    bulboventricular r.
    cusp r.
    dental r.
    dermal r.
    epidermal r.
    epipericardial r.
    external oblique r.
    ganglion r.

    genital r.
    gluteal r.
    gonadal r.
    interpapillary r.
    key r.
    lateral epicondylar r.
    lateral supracondylar r.
    lateral supraepicondylar r.
    linguocervical r.
    linguogingival r.
    Mall r.
    mammary r.
    marginal r.
    medial epicondylar r.
    medial supracondylar r.
    medial supraepicondylar r.
    mesonephric r.
    milk r.
    oblique r.
    Passavant r.
    rete r.
    skin r.
    triangular r.
    urogenital r.
Riedel thyroiditis
Rieder
    R. cell
    R. cell leukemia
    R. lymphocyte
Riegel pulse
Rieger
    R. anomaly
    R. syndrome
Riehl melanosis
right
    r. atrium
    r. colic flexure
    r. costal margin (RCM)
    r. descending pulmonary artery
    deviation to the r.
    r. fibrous ring
    r. gastric artery
    r. gastric vein
    r. heart
    r. heart bypass
    r. hepatic duct
    r. lateral division
    r. liver
    r. lobe of liver
    r. lower extremity (RLE)
    r. lower quadrant (RLQ)
    r. lymphatic duct

NOTES

right *(continued)*
    r. medial division
    r. pulmonary artery
    shift to the r.
    r. upper extremity (RUE)
    r. ventricle
    r. ventricular failure
right-angle mattress suture
right-footed
right-handed
righting reflex
right-left discrimination
right-to-left shunt
rigid connector
rigidity
    cadaveric r.
    catatonic r.
    cerebellar r.
    clasp-knife r.
    cogwheel r.
    decerebrate r.
    decorticate r.
    hysterical r.
    lead-pipe r.
    muscular r.
    nuchal r.
    postmortem r.
    scleral r.
    spastic r.
rigidus
    hallux r.
rigor
    acid r.
    calcium r.
    heat r.
    r. mortis
rim
    bite r.
    r. incision
rimose
rimula
ring
    abdominal r.
    r. abscess
    amnion r.
    annuloplasty r.
    anterior limiting r.
    Balbani r.
    Bandl r.
    benzene r.
    Bickel r.
    Cannon r.
    cardiac lymphatic r.
    casting r.
    choroidal r.
    r. chromosome
    ciliary r.
    common tendinous r.
    conjunctival r.

    constriction r.
    crural r.
    deep inguinal r.
    external inguinal r.
    femoral r.
    fibrocartilaginous r.
    fibrous r.
    r. finger
    Fleischer r.
    Fleischer-Strümpell r.
    Flieringa r.
    gestational r.
    glaucomatous r.
    Graefenberg r.
    greater r.
    internal inguinal r.
    Kayser-Fleischer r.
    left fibrous r.
    Liesegang r.
    Lower r.
    lymphatic r.
    olive r.
    pathologic retraction r.
    physiologic retraction r.
    right fibrous r.
    Schwalbe r.
    r. scotoma
    superficial inguinal r.
    r. syringe
    tympanic r.
    umbilical r.
    vascular r.
    Vossius lenticular r.
Ringer
    lactated R. (LR)
    R. solution
ring-knife
ringlike corneal dystrophy
ringworm
    black-dot r.
    crusted r.
    honeycomb r.
Rinne test
Riolan anastomosis
Ripault sign
ripe cataract
Ripstein operation
risk
    assumption of r.
    attributable r.
    competing r.
    empiric r.
    recurrence r.
Risley rotary prism
risorius muscle
risticii
    Ehrlichia r.
Ritgen maneuver
Ritter opening tetanus

ritual
rituximab
rivalry
    binocular r.
    sibling r.
Rivers cocktail
Rivinus
    R. canal
    R. duct
riziform
RLE
    right lower extremity
RLQ
    right lower quadrant
RNA
    ribonucleic acid
      acceptor RNA
      antisense RNA
      chromosomal RNA
      heterogeneous nuclear RNA
      informational RNA
      messenger RNA
      messengerlike RNA
      nuclear RNA
      ribosomal RNA
      soluble RNA
      RNA splicing
      transfer RNA (tRNA)
      RNA tumor virus
RNase
    alkaline RNase
    RNase P
Roaf syndrome
Robertson
    Argyll R.
    R. sign
robertsonian translocation
Robinow syndrome
Robinson index
Robin syndrome
robotic
rocking microtome
Rocky Mountain spotted fever
rod
    analyzing r.
    Auer r.
    basal r.
    r. cell
    Corti r.
    enamel r.
    germinal r.
    r. granule

    Maddox r.
    surgical r.
rodenticide
rodent ulcer
roentgen-equivalent-man
roentgenogram
roentgenograph
roentgenography
roentgenologist
roentgenology
roentgen ray
Roesler-Dressler infarct
Roger
    R. Anderson pin fixation appliance
    R. bruit
    R. disease
    maladie de R.
    R. murmur
Rogers sphygmomanometer
Rokitansky
    R. disease
    R. hernia
    R. pelvis
rolandic
    r. epilepsy
    r. sleep
Rolando
    R. area
    fissure of R.
role
    complementary r.
    gender r.
    occupational r.
    sex r.
    sick r.
roll
    iliac r.
rollerball electrode
roller bandage
Rollet stroma
Romaña sign
Romanowsky blood stain
Romberg
    facial hemiatrophy of R.
    R. sign
rombergism
rongeur
Rónne nasal step
roof plate
room
    recovery r.
rooming-in

NOTES

759

root
  accessory r.
  r. amputation
  anatomical r.
  angelica r.
  aortic r.
  black r.
  buccal r.
  r. canal
  r. caries index
  clinical r.
  cochlear r.
  cranial r.
  Culver r.
  dorsal r.
  facial r.
  gentian r.
  hair r.
  inferior r.
  jaundice r.
  lateral r.
  marshmallow r.
  May apple r.
  medial r.
  r. pulp
  r. resection
  r. sheath
  ventral r.
root-form implant
rooting reflex
ROS
  review of systems
rosa
  mal de la r.
rosacea
  acne r.
  granulomatous r.
  hypertrophic r.
Rosai-Dorfman disease
rosary
  rachitic r.
rose
  attar of r.
  r. bengal
  essence of r.
  R. position
  r. spot
rosea
  pityriasis r.
Rosenbach
  R. law
  R. sign
Rosenmüller
  R. gland
  R. node
Rosenthal canal
roseola
  epidemic r.
  idiopathic r.

  r. infantilis
  r. infantum
  syphilitic r.
rosette
  EAC r.
  Homer-Wright r.'s
rosin
Ro spatula
Ross
  R. procedure
  R. River virus
rosso
  mal r.
Rossolimo
  R. reflex
  R. sign
Rostan asthma
rostellum
  armed r.
rostra (*pl. of* rostrum)
rostrad
rostral
rostrate pelvis
rostrum, pl. **rostra, rostrums**
rotamase
rotamer
rotary
  r. joint
  r. microtome
rotated tooth
rotating anode
rotation
  external r.
  r. flap
  internal r.
  intestinal r.
  lateral r.
  molecular r.
  off-vertical r.
  optic r.
  optical r.
  specific optic r.
rotational nystagmus
rotator
  r. cuff
  medial r.
rotatores muscle
rotatory
  r. joint
  r. nystagmus
Rotch sign
rote learning
Rothmund syndrome
Roth spot
Rotor syndrome
rotoscoliosis
rototome
Rouget bulb
roughage

R

rouleaux formation
round
    r. atelectasis
    r. heart
    r. ligament
    r., regular, and equal (RR&E)
    r. window
    r. window membrane
rounded atelectasis
roundworm
Rous-associated virus
Rous sarcoma virus
routing
    contralateral r.
Roux-en-Y
    R.-e.-Y anastomosis
    R.-e.-Y operation
Roux method
Roviralta
    Barraquer R.
Rovsing sign
R&R
    rest and recuperation
RR&E
    round, regular, and equal
rub
    friction r.
    pericardial r.
    pleural r.
    pleuritic r.
    pleuropericardial r.
rubber-bulb syringe
rubber dam clamp forceps
rubber-shod clamp
rubedo
rubefacient
rubefaction
rubella
    r. HI test
    measles, mumps, and r. (MMR)
    r. virus
rubeola virus
rubeosis iridis diabetica
rubescent
rubidium
rubidomycin
Rubivirus
rubor
rubra
    lochia r.
    miliaria r.

    pityriasis r.
    polycythemia r.
rubredoxins
rubriblast
rubricyte
rubrospinal decussation
Rubulavirus
rudiment
rudimentary
rudimentum
Rud syndrome
RUE
    right upper extremity
Ruffini corpuscle
rufous albinism
ruga, pl. **rugae**
    gastric r.
    vaginal rugae
rugal pattern
rugine
rugose
rugosity
rugous
Ruhemann purple
rule
    Abegg r.
    astigmatism against the r.
    astigmatism with the r.
    r. of bigeminy
    Chargaff r.
    Clark weight r.
    Cowling r.
    Durham r.
    Gibb phase r.
    Goriaew r.
    Haase r.
    Hückel r.
    Ingelfinger r.
    isoprene r.
    Jackson r.
    Le Bel-van't Hoff r.
    Liebermeister r.
    Meyer-Overton r.
    M'Naghten r.
    Nägele r.
    New Hampshire r.
    r. of nines
    Ogino-Knaus r.
    r. of outlet
    r. out myocardial infarction
    Prentice r.

NOTES

rule *(continued)*
>   stopping r.
>   Westgard r.

ruler
>   isometric r.

runaway pacemaker

runner's
>   r. bladder
>   r. knee

Runyon
>   R. classification
>   R. group I–IV mycobacteria

rupia

rupial

rupture
>   artificial membrane r.
>   intracapsular r.
>   membrane r.
>   premature membrane r.
>   preterm membrane r.

ruptured disc

Russell
>   R. body
>   hooked bundle of R.
>   R. Periodontal Index
>   R. sign
>   R. syndrome

Russell's
>   R. viper venom
>   R. viper venom clotting time

Rust phenomenon

rusty sputum

ruthenium

rutidosis

Ruysch
>   R. membrane
>   R. tube

R wave

ryanodine receptor

Ryan stain

Ryle tube

S-A
    sinuatrial
        S-A block
saber
    s. shin
    s. tibia
Sabia virus
sabot
    coeur en s.
Sabouraud dextrose agar
sabre
    coup de s.
sabulous
saburral colic
sac
    abdominal s.
    air s.
    allantoic s.
    alveolar s.
    amnionic s.
    aneurysmal s.
    aortic s.
    chorionic s.
    conjunctival s.
    cupular blind s.
    dental s.
    endolymphatic s.
    gestational s.
    heart s.
    hernial s.
    Hilton s.
    lacrimal s.
    lesser peritoneal s.
    lymph s.
    serous s.
    tear s.
saccadic
saccharate
    calcium s.
saccharide
sacchariferous
saccharolytic
saccharometabolic
saccharometabolism
saccharose
sacciform
saccular
    s. aneurysm
    s. gland
    s. nerve
sacculated
    s. aneurysm
    s. bladder
sacculation

saccule
    laryngeal s.
sacculocochlear
sacculus laryngis
saccus
sacra (*pl. of* sacrum)
sacrad
sacral
    s. canal
    s. crest
    s. flexure
    s. plexus
    s. splanchnic nerve
    s. vertebra
sacrales
    vertebra s.
sacralgia
sacralis
    hiatus s.
    kyphosis s.
sacrectomy
sacroanterior
    left s. (LSA)
    s. position
sacrococcygeal teratoma
sacrocolpopexy procedure
sacrodynia
sacroiliac
sacrolumbar
sacroposterior
    s. fetal position
    left s. (LSP)
sacrosciatic
sacrospinal
sacrospinous vaginal vault suspension procedure
sacrotransverse
    s. fetal position
    left s. (LST)
sacrouterine fold
sacrovertebral
sacrum, pl. **sacra**
    assimilation s.
saddle
    s. block anesthesia
    s. head
    s. joint
    s. nose
    s. thrombus
saddleback caterpillar
sadism
sadist
sadistic
sadomasochism

S

Saemisch
- S. section
- S. ulcer

Saenger
- S. operation
- S. sign

safety
- s. lens
- margin of s.

SAF fixative

sagittal
- s. axis
- s. fontanelle
- s. plane
- s. suture
- s. synostosis

sago spleen

saimiri
- Herpesvirus s.

Saint
- S. Anthony dance
- S. Anthony fire
- S. John dance
- S. triad
- S. Vitus dance

sakazakii
- *Enterobacter s.*

salad
- word s.

Salah sternal puncture needle

salicylate
- caffeine and sodium s.
- choline s.
- eserine s.
- menthyl s.
- mercuric s.
- methenamine s.
- methyl s.

salicylic acid

salicylism

salient findings

salinarius
- *Culex s.*

saline
- s. agglutinin
- normal s.
- physiologic s.
- s. solution

saliva
- ganglionic s.

salivant

salivarius
- *Lactobacillus s.*

salivary
- s. calculus
- s. digestion
- s. fistula
- s. gland
- s. gland disease

salivate

salivation

salivator

Salmonella
- *S. enterica choleraesuis*
- *S. enterica enteritidis*
- *S. enterica typhimurium*
- *S. typhi*
- *S. typhimurium*
- *S. typhosa*

salmonellosis

salpingectomy
- abdominal s.

salpingian

salpingitic

salpingitis
- chronic interstitial s.
- foreign body s.
- gonorrheal s.
- parenchymatous s.
- purulent s.

salpingocele

salpingography

salpingolysis

salpingoneostomy

salpingo-oophorectomy

salpingo-oophoritis

salpingo-oophorocele

salpingoperitonitis

salpingopexy

salpingopharyngeus muscle

salpingoplasty

salpingorrhaphy

salpingostomy

salpingotomy
- abdominal s.

salt
- acid s.
- artificial Carlsbad s.
- artificial Kissingen s.
- basic s.
- bile s.
- bone s.
- diazonium s.
- double s.
- effervescent s.
- Epsom s.
- Glauber s.
- hexazonium s.
- s. wasting

saltation

saltatory
- s. conduction
- s. evolution
- s. spasm

Salter incremental line

salting out

salt-losing nephritis

salubrious

saluresis
saluretic
salutary
salute
    allergic s.
salve
Salzmann nodular corneal degeneration
samarium
same-day surgery
sample
    cluster s.
    end-tidal s.
    Haldane-Priestley s.
    proficiency s.
sampling
    s. bias
    biological s.
    chemical s.
    continuous interleaved s.
    haphazard s.
    random s.
Samter syndrome
sanatorium
sanatory
sand
    brain s.
    hydatid s.
    intestinal s.
    urinary s.
Sandhoff disease
Sanfilippo syndrome
sanguifacient
sanguiferous
sanguification
sanguine
sanguineous
sanguinis
    fragilitas s.
sanguinolent
sanguinolenta
    lochia s.
sanguinolentis
    fetus s.
sanguinopurulent
sanguivorous
saniopurulent
sanioserous
sanious
sanitaire
    cordon s.
sanitarian
sanitarium

sanitary
sanitation
sanitization
Sansom sign
Sanson image
Santini booming sound
Santorini
    S. canal
    S. concha
    S. duct
    S. plexus
SAP
    systemic arterial pressure
sap
    cell s.
saphenous
    s. nerve
    s. opening
sapiens
    Homo s.
saponaceous
saponification
saponins
sapphism
saprobe
saprobic
saprogen
saprogenic
saprogenous
saprophyte
    facultative s.
saprophytic
saprozoic
saprozoonosis
sarcoblast
sarcoid
    Boeck s.
sarcoidal granuloma
sarcoidosis
    hypercalcemic s.
sarcolemma
sarcolemmal
sarcolemmic
sarcolemmous
sarcoma
    adipose s.
    alveolar soft part s.
    ameloblastic s.
    angiolithic s.
    avian s.
    botryoid s.
    endometrial stromal s.

S

NOTES

sarcoma *(continued)*
  Ewing s.
  fascial s.
  fascicular s.
  giant cell s.
  granulocytic s.
  immunoblastic s.
  Jensen s.
  juxtacortical osteogenic s.
  Kaposi s.
  leukocytic s.
  lymphatic s.
  medullary s.
  myeloid s.
  osteogenic s.
  telangiectatic osteogenic s.
sarcomatoid
sarcomatosis
sarcomatous
sarcomere
sarcopenia
sarcoplasm
sarcoplasmic reticulum
sarcopoietic
Sarcoptes scabiei
sarcoptic
sarcoptid
sarcosis
sarcostosis
sarcotic
sarcotubule
sarcous
sardonic grin
sargramostim
sartorius muscle
Sartwell incubation model
satellite
  s. abscess
  chromosome s.
  s. phenomenon
satellitosis
satiation
Sattler veil
saturate
saturated
  s. color
  s. fatty acid (SFA)
  s. solution
saturation
  s. index
  secondary s.
  s. sound pressure level
  transferrin s.
saturnina
  arthralgia s.
saturnine
satyri
  apex s.

satyriasis
saucerization
Savary bougie
saw
  crown s.
  Gigli s.
  hole s.
scabicidal
scabicide
scabiei
  Sarcoptes s.
scabies
  crusted s.
scala
  Löwenberg s.
scalded mouth syndrome
scale
  absolute s.
  activities of daily living s.
  adaptive behavior s.
  Allen cognitive level s.
  Ångström s.
  Baumé s.
  Binet s.
  Binet-Simon s.
  Borg s.
  Brazelton Neonatal Behavioral
    Assessment S.
  Cattell Infant Intelligence S.
  Celsius s.
  centigrade s.
  Charrière s.
  coma s.
  digital gray s.
  expanded disability status s.
  Fahrenheit s.
  French s.
  Gaffky s.
  Glasgow coma s.
  gray s.
  Guttman s.
  Hamilton anxiety rating s.
  Hamilton depression rating s.
  hardness s.
  homigrade s.
  interval s.
  Karnofsky s.
  Kelvin s.
  Kurtzke multiple sclerosis
    disability s.
  Likert s.
  Maryland coma s.
  masculinity-femininity s.
  Mohs s.
  Stanford-Binet intelligence s.
  Wechsler intelligence s.
scalenectomy
scalenotomy

scalenus
s. medius muscle
s. minimus muscle
scaler
hoe s.
scalloping
scalpel
plasma s.
scalp hair
scalprum
scaly
scan
bone s.
CT s.
duplex Doppler s.
HIDA s.
kidney s.
Meckel s.
multiple-gated acquisition s.
renal s.
sector s.
ventilation-perfusion s.
scandium
scanning
s. electron microscope
s. electron microscopy
s. equalization radiography
linker s.
s. speech
transvaginal s.
scanogram
Scanzoni maneuver
scaphocephalic
scaphocephalism
scaphocephaly
scaphoid
s. abdomen
s. bone
s. scapula
scaphoideum
os s.
scapula, pl. **scapulae**
s. alata
dorsum scapulae
scaphoid s.
spine of s.
winged s.
scapular
scapulectomy
scapuloclavicular
scapulocostal syndrome
scapulohumeral rhythm

scapulopexy
scapulothoracic joint
scar
s. carcinoma
cigarette-paper s.
hypertrophic s.
scarification
scarificator
scarlatina
s. anginosa
anginose s.
s. hemorrhagica
latent s.
scarlatinal
scarlatiniform
scarlet fever
Scarpa
S. fascia
S. method
S. operation
S. staphyloma
S. triangle
scarring alopecia
scatemia
scatologic
scatology
scatoscopy
scatter
Compton s.
scattered
s. radiation
s. rhonchi
scattering
Compton s.
scavenger receptor
scene
primal s.
SCFE
slipped capital femoral epiphysis
Schäffer reflex
Schapiro sign
Schaudinn fixative
Schede method
Scheibe hearing impairment
Scheie syndrome
Scheiner experiment
schema
body s.
scheme
body s.
Schenck disease
Scheuermann disease

S

NOTES

Schick test
Schiff reagent
Schilder disease
Schiller test
Schilling
    S. blood count
    S. test
schistocelia
schistocormia
schistocyte
schistocytosis
schistoglossia
Schistosoma
    S. haematobium
    S. japonicum
    S. mansoni
schistosomal dermatitis
schistosome
schistosomia
schistosomiasis
    Asiatic s.
    bladder s.
    ectopic s.
    s. haematobium
    intestinal s.
    Japanese s.
    s. japonica
    Manson s.
    s. mansoni
schistothorax
schizamnion
schizaxon
schizoaffective psychosis
schizogenesis
schizogony
schizogyria
schizoid
    s. personality
    s. personality disorder
    s. type
schizont
schizonychia
schizophasia
schizophrenia
    acute s.
    ambulatory s.
    catatonic s.
    childhood s.
    disorganized s.
    hebephrenic s.
    latent s.
    paranoid s.
    residual s.
    simple s.
    undifferentiated s.
schizophrenic
schizotrichia

schizotypal
    s. personality
    s. personality disorder
schizotypical personality
Schlatter
    S. disease
    S. operation
Schlatter-Osgood disease
Schlemm canal
Schlesinger sign
Schmidel anastomosis
Schmidt-Lanterman incisure
Schmidt syndrome
Schmorl
    S. ferric-ferricyanide reduction stain
    S. nodule
    S. picrothionin stain
Schneider
    S. carmine
    S. first rank symptoms
schneideri
    Elaeophora s.
Schnitzler syndrome
Schober test
Schönlein purpura
school
    biometrical s.
    dogmatic s.
    dynamic s.
    hippocratic s.
    iatromathematical s.
    mechanistic s.
    s. phobia
Schroeder operation
Schuchardt operation
Schüffner dot
Schüller
    S. phenomenon
    S. syndrome
Schultz-Charlton reaction
Schultze
    comma bundle of S.
    comma tract of S.
    S. mechanism
    S. phantom
    S. placenta
    S. sign
Schwalbe ring
Schwann
    S. cell
    sheath of S.
schwannoma
    acoustic s.
    vestibular s.
schwannosis
Schwartze sign
sciage
sciatic
    s. bursa

s. foramen
s. hernia
s. nerve
s. scoliosis
sciatica
science
behavioral s.
occupational s.
scientific theory
scientometrics
scimitar sign
scinticisternography
scintigram
scintigraphic
scintigraphy
scintillans
synchysis s.
scintillating scotoma
scintillation
s. camera
s. counter
scintillator
liquid s.
scintiphotography
scintiscan
scintiscanner
scirrhous carcinoma
scission
scissors
corneoscleral s.
craniotomy s.
de Wecker s.
s. gait
iris s.
scissura
scissure
sclera, pl. **sclerae**
blue s.
lamina cribrosa sclerae
sinus venosus sclerae
scleradenitis
scleral
s. buckle
s. crescent
s. icterus
s. plexus
s. rigidity
s. staphyloma
s. sulcus
s. vein
s. venous sinus
sclerectasia

sclerectomy
scleredema adultorum
sclerema neonatorum
scleritis
anterior s.
anular s.
brawny s.
deep s.
gelatinous s.
malignant s.
posterior s.
scleroblastema
sclerochoroiditis
scleroconjunctival
sclerocornea
sclerodactylia
sclerodactyly
scleroderma
linear s.
localized s.
systemic s.
sclerogenic
sclerogenous
scleroid
scleroiritis
sclerokeratitis
sclerokeratoiritis
scleroma
respiratory s.
scleromalacia
scleromere
scleronychia
sclero-oophoritis
sclerophthalmia
scleroprotein
sclerosal
sclerosant
sclerose
sclerosing
s. adenosis
s. hemangioma
s. keratitis
s. leukopenia
s. lymphosarcoma
s. osteitis
sclerosis, pl. **scleroses**
Alzheimer s.
amyotrophic lateral s. (ALS)
arterial s.
arteriocapillary s.
arteriolar s.
bone s.

S

NOTES

sclerosis *(continued)*
    Canavan s.
    central areolar choroidal s.
    cerebral s.
    combined s.
    diffuse infantile familial s.
    disseminated s.
    endocardial s.
    focal s.
    glomerular s.
    hippocampal s.
    idiopathic hypercalcemic s.
    insular s.
    laminar cortical s.
    lateral spinal s.
    lobar s.
    mantle s.
    menstrual s.
    Mönckeberg s.
    multiple s.
    posterolateral s.
    primary lateral s.
    valvular s.
    venous s.
sclerostenosis
sclerostomy
sclerotherapy
sclerotic
    s. body
    s. cemental mass
    s. dentin
sclerotica
sclerotome
sclerotomy
    anterior s.
sclerous
scolex
scoliokyphosis
scoliosis
    cicatricial s.
    coxitic s.
    empyemic s.
    habit s.
    myopathic s.
    rheumatic s.
    sciatic s.
    static s.
scoliotic pelvis
scombroid poisoning
scopophilia
scopophobia
scorbutic
scorbutigenic
scordinema
score
    Apgar s.
    Bishop s.
    discrimination s.
    Dubowitz s.

    Gleason s.
    Jarman s.
    outcome s.
    trauma s.
scoticum
    Diphyllobothrium s.
scotoma, pl. **scotomata**
    absolute s.
    anular s.
    arcuate s.
    Bjerrum s.
    cecocentral s.
    central s.
    color s.
    flittering s.
    glaucomatous nerve-fiber bundle s.
    hemianopic s.
    mental s.
    motile s.
    negative s.
    peripheral s.
    physiologic s.
    positive s.
    relative s.
    ring s.
    scintillating s.
    Seidel s.
    zonular s.
scotomatous
scotometer
scotometry
scotophilia
scotophobia
scotopia
scotopic
    s. adaptation
    s. eye
    s. vision
scotopsin
Scott operation
scotty dog
scout film
scratch test
screen
    Bjerrum s.
    fluorescent s.
    Hess s.
    intensifying s.
    s. memory
    multiple marker s.
    triple s.
    urine drug s.
screening
    carrier s.
    cytologic s.
    familial s.
    library s.
    mass s.
    s. test

screw
  afterloading s.
scriptorius
  calamus s.
scrobiculate
scrofulaceum
  Mycobacterium s.
scrofuloderma
scrofulosorum
  lichen s.
scrota (*pl. of* scrotum)
scrotal
  s. fat necrosis
  s. hemangioma
  s. hernia
  s. hydrocele
  s. hypospadias
  s. panniculitis
  s. raphe
  s. septum
scrotectomy
scroti
  elephantiasis s.
scrotitis
scrotoplasty
scrotum, pl. **scrota, scrotums**
  lymph s.
scrub
  s. nurse
  s. typhus
sculptatus
  hymen s.
Scultetus
  S. bandage
  S. position
scurf
scurvy
  Alpine s.
  hemorrhagic s.
  infantile s.
  land s.
scute
scutiform
scutular
scutulum
scutum
scybalous
scybalum
scyphoid
sea
  s. gull murmur
  s. louse
  s. nettle
  s. wasp
seabather's eruption
seal
  border s.
  golden s.
sealant
  dental s.
  fissure s.
seasickness
seasonal affective disorder
seat
  basal s.
seated massage
seatworm
sebaceous
  s. adenoma
  s. cyst
  s. epithelioma
  s. follicle
  s. gland
sebaceum
  adenoma s.
sebiferous
sebolith
seborrhea
  eczematoid s.
  s. faciei
  s. furfuracea
  s. sicca
seborrheic
  s. blepharitis
  s. dermatitis
  s. dermatosis
  s. keratosis
seborrheica
  corona s.
  dermatitis s.
  keratosis s.
sebum
second
  s. cranial nerve
  cycles per s. (cps)
  s. heart sound
  s. molar
  s. toe
  s. tooth
  s. wind
secondary
  s. abdominal pregnancy
  s. abscess
  s. acquired cholesteatoma

S

NOTES

secondary *(continued)*
s. adhesion
s. adrenocortical insufficiency
s. alcohol
s. aldosteronism
s. amenorrhea
s. amine
s. amyloidosis
s. anesthetic
s. atelectasis
s. axis
s. cataract
s. degeneration
s. dementia
s. dentin
s. dentition
s. deviation
s. digestion
s. disease
s. drive
s. dye test
s. dysmenorrhea
s. encephalitis
s. follicle
s. gain
s. glaucoma
s. gout
s. hemochromatosis
s. hemorrhage
s. hypertension
s. immune response
s. intention
s. lysosome
s. mucinosis
s. nondisjunction
s. oocyte
s. parkinsonism
s. polycythemia
s. process
s. radiation
s. saturation
s. sex character
s. spermatocyte
s. sterility
s. stuttering
s. syphilis
s. tuberculosis
s. tympanic membrane
s. union
second-degree
s.-d. AV block
s.-d. burn
s.-d. prolapse
second-look operation
second-set phenomenon
secretagogue
secretase
secrete
secretin test

secretion
cytocrine s.
external s.
secretoinhibitory
secretomotor
secretomotory
secretor
secretory
s. carcinoma
s. nerve
s. otitis media
section
abdominal s.
attached cranial s.
axial s.
cesarean s.
classical cesarean s.
coronal s.
cross s.
detached cranial s.
diagonal s.
frontal s.
frozen s.
Latzko cesarean s.
longitudinal s.
lower uterine segment cesarean s.
median s.
microscopic s.
midsagittal s.
oblique s.
perineal s.
Saemisch s.
serial s.
thin s.
transverse s.
trial of labor after cesarean s.
ultrathin s.
sector
s. echocardiography
s. scan
sectoranopia
sectorial tooth
secundigravida
secundines
secundipara
secundum
interatrial foramen s.
sedate
sedation
sedimentate
sedimentation
s. coefficient
s. constant
s. rate
s. test
sedimentator
sedimentometer
sedoxantrone trihydrochloride

seed
> celery s.
> millet s.
> s. wart

Seeligmüller sign
seesaw nystagmus
Seessel pocket
segment
> A1, A2 s.
> abnormal ST s.
> anterior basal s.
> anterior inferior renal s.
> anterior ocular s.
> anterior superior renal s.
> apical bronchopulmonary s.
> apicoposterior bronchopulmonary s.
> arterial s.
> bronchopulmonary s.
> cardiac s.
> cervical s.
> hepatic s.
> inferior lingular s.
> inferior lingular
> bronchopulmonary s.
> inferior renal s.
> interannular s.
> intermaxillary s.
> internodal s.
> Lanterman s.
> lateral basal bronchopulmonary s.
> lateral bronchopulmonary s.
> left anterior lateral hepatic s.
> left medial hepatic s.
> left posterior lateral hepatic s. III
> lower uterine s.
> lumbar s.
> M2 s.
> medial basal bronchopulmonary s.
> medial bronchopulmonary s.
> mesoblastic s.
> posterior hepatic s. I
> PR s.
> uterine s.

segmental
> s. anesthesia
> s. artery
> s. fracture
> s. neuritis

segmentation cavity
segmentectomy
segmented cell

segnis
> *Haemophilus s.*

segregation
> s. analysis
> s. ratio

Seidel
> S. scotoma
> S. sign

Seip syndrome
seizure
> absence s.
> akinetic s.
> anosognosic s.
> astatic s.
> atonic s.
> atypical absence s.
> audiogenic s.
> automotor s.
> autonomic s.
> clonic s.
> complex motor s.
> complex partial s.
> convulsive s.
> dileptic s.
> s. disorder
> early s.
> electrographic s.
> epileptic s.
> febrile s.
> focal motor s.
> gelastic s.
> generalized tonic-clonic s.
> grand mal s.
> hypermotor s.
> hypomotor s.
> jacksonian s.
> late s.
> lightning s.
> major motor s.
> minor motor s.
> myoclonic s.
> negative myoclonic s.
> neonatal s.
> partial s.
> psychomotor s.
> sylvian s.

Seldinger technique
selectin
> L s.
> P s.

selection
> artificial s.

NOTES

selection *(continued)*
    s. coefficient
    medical s.
    natural s.
    sexual s.
selective
    s. estrogen receptor modulator
    s. inhibition
    s. norepinephrine reuptake inhibitor
    s. serotonin reuptake inhibitor
    s. stain
selenium plate
self-awareness
self-concept
self concept
self-control
self-inflicted wound
selfish DNA
self-limited
self-love
self-obturation
    intermittent s.-o.
self-registering thermometer
self-retaining catheter
sella
    empty s.
    s. turcica
sellae
    diaphragm s.
    dorsum s.
sellar tumor
Sellick maneuver
Selye
    adaptation syndrome of S.
semantics
semen
semenuria
semialdehyde
    malonate s.
    methylmalonate s.
semicanal
semicanalis tubae auditoriae
Semichon acid carmine stain
semicircular
    s. canal
    s. duct
semiclosed anesthesia
semicoma
semicomatose
semiconscious
semi-Fowler position
semihorizontal heart
semilunar
    s. bone
    s. cartilage
    s. conjunctival fold
    s. fibrocartilage
    s. hiatus
    s. line

    s. notch
    s. valve
semimembranosus muscle
semimembranous bursa
seminal
    s. colliculus
    s. duct
    s. fluid
    s. gland
    s. granule
    s. lake
    s. vesicle
seminalis
    colliculus s.
    lacus s.
semination
seminiferous
    s. epithelium
    s. tubule
    s. tubule dysgenesis
seminoma
    spermacytic s.
seminuria
semiopen anesthesia
semiovale
    centrum s.
semipennate
semipermeable
semipolar bond
semispinalis
    s. capitis muscle
    s. cervicis muscle
    s. thoracis muscle
semisulcus
semisynthetic
semitendinosus muscle
semivertical heart
Semliki Forest virus
senescence
    dental s.
senescent
Sengstaken-Blakemore tube
senile
    s. amyloidosis
    s. arteriosclerosis
    s. cataract
    s. dementia
    s. hemangioma
    s. lentigo
    s. melanoderma
    s. neuritis
    s. osteomalacia
    s. plaque
    s. pruritus
    s. psychosis
    s. purpura
    s. retinoschisis
    s. tremor
    s. vaginitis

senilis
 alopecia s.
 arcus s.
 keratosis s.
 malum articulorum s.
 pruritus s.
 purpura s.
senility
sennetsu
 Ehrlichia s.
sensate
sensation
 delayed s.
 general s.
 girdle s.
 s. level
 objective s.
 perineal s.
 referred s.
 subjective s.
sense
 color s.
 s. of equilibrium
 geometric s.
 joint s.
 kinesthetic s.
 light s.
 muscular s.
 s. organ
 position s.
 posture s.
 pressure s.
 special s.
 visceral s.
sensibility
 articular s.
 bone s.
 cortical s.
 deep s.
 dissociation s.
 electromuscular s.
 epicritic s.
 proprioceptive s.
 protopathic s.
 splanchnesthetic s.
sensible perspiration
sensitive
sensitivity
 acquired s.
 analytical s.
 antibiotic s.
 clinical s.

 contrast s.
 culture and s. (C&S)
 diagnostic s.
 idiosyncratic s.
 induced s.
sensitization
 autoerythrocyte s.
 covert s.
 photodynamic s.
sensitize
sensitized
 s. antigen
 s. cell
sensor
sensorial
sensorimotor area
sensorineural
 s. deafness
 s. dysfunction
 s. hearing loss
sensorium
 general s.
sensory
 s. acuity level
 s. aphasia
 s. awareness
 s. cortex
 s. deprivation
 s. epilepsy
 s. ganglion
 s. hearing impairment
 s. image
 s. integration
 s. nerve
 s. neuronopathy
 s. paralysis
 s. phantom
 s. processing
 s. registration
 s. speech center
 s. urgency
sensu
 s. lato
 s. stricto
sensual
sentient
sentinel
 s. event
 s. gland
 s. lymph node
 s. node biopsy

S

NOTES

sentinel *(continued)*
    s. pile
    s. tag
Seoul virus
separation
    s. anxiety
    jaw s.
sepsis, pl. **sepses**
    intestinal s.
    s. syndrome
septa (*pl. of* septum)
septal
    s. defect
    s. resection
septate uterus
septectomy
septi
    falx s.
septic
    s. abortion
    s. fever
    s. infarct
    s. necrosis
    s. phlebitis
    s. pneumonia
    s. shock
    s. sore throat
    s. thrombus
    s. vasculitis
septica
    iridocyclitis s.
septicemia
    acute fulminating meningococcal s.
    anthrax s.
    cryptogenic s.
    metastasizing s.
    perinatal s.
    puerperal s.
septicemic abscess
septicopyemia
septicopyemic
septomarginal
septonasal
septooptic dysplasia
septoplasty
septorhinoplasty
septostomy
    atrial s.
    balloon s.
septulum
septum, pl. **septa**
    alveolar s.
    anteromedial intermuscular s.
    aortopulmonary s.
    atrioventricular s.
    Bigelow s.
    bony nasal s.
    bulbar s.
    cartilaginous s.

    Cloquet s.
    comblike s.
    crural s.
    deviated nasal s.
    distal spiral s.
    endovenous s.
    femoral s.
    gingival s.
    hanging s.
    interalveolar s.
    interatrial s.
    interdental s.
    interlobular s.
    intermediate cervical s.
    intermuscular s.
    interpulmonary s.
    interventricular s.
    intraalveolar s.
    lingual s.
    membranous s.
    nasal s.
    s. penis
    rectovaginal s.
    rectovesical s.
    scrotal s.
    transparent s.
sequela, pl. **sequelae**
sequence
    Alu s.
    chi s.
    coding s.
    insertion s.
    intervening s.
    s. ladder
    leader s.
    long terminal repeat s.'s
    pulse s.
    regulatory s.
    twin reversed arterial perfusion s.
sequencing
    dideoxy s.
    Maxim-Gilbert s.
sequential anastomosis
sequestral
sequestration
    bronchopulmonary s.
sequestrectomy
sequestrum
    eruption s.
sequoiosis
sera (*pl. of* serum)
seralbumin
serena
    gutta s.
Sergent white line
serial
    s. dilution
    s. extraction
    s. interval

s. radiography
s. section

series
acute abdominal s.
aromatic s.
erythrocytic s.
fatty s.
full-mouth s.
granulocytic s.
Hofmeister s.
homologous s.
lymphocytic s.
lymphoid s.
lyotropic s.
myeloid s.
thrombocytic s.
upper gastrointestinal s.

serocolitis
seroconversion
serodiagnosis
seroenteritis
seroepidemiology
serofibrinous pleurisy
serofibrous
serogroup
serologic test
serology
seroma
seromembranous
seromucoid
acid s.

seromucous gland
seronegative
seropositive
seropurulent
seropus
serosa
lochia s.
membrana s.

serosanguineous
seroserous
serositis
serosity
serosynovitis
serotherapy
serotina
decidua s.

serotonergic
serotonin
serotype
heterologous s.
homologous s.

serous
s. abscess
s. cell
s. cyst
s. cystadenoma
s. gland
s. inflammation
s. ligament
s. membrane
s. meningitis
s. otitis
s. otitis media
s. pleurisy
s. retinitis
s. sac
s. synovitis

serovaccination
serovar
serpiginosum
angioma s.

serpiginosus
lupus s.

serpiginous
serpigo
serrated
serrate suture
serration
serratus anterior muscle
serrefine
Serres
rest of S.

Sertoli
S. cell
S. cell tumor

Sertoli-cell-only syndrome
Sertoli-Leydig cell tumor
Sertoli-stromal cell tumor
serum, pl. **sera**
s. accelerator globulin
s. agglutinin
s. albumin
anticomplementary s.
antiepithelial s.
antilymphocyte s.
antirabies s.
antireticular cytotoxic s.
antitoxic s.
bacteriolytic s.
blood s.
convalescent s.
Coombs s.
s. disease

S

NOTES

777

serum (*continued*)
    dried human s.
    s. eruption
    foreign s.
    s. glutamic-oxaloacetic transaminase
    s. glutamic-pyruvic transaminase
    s. hepatitis virus
    hereditary erythroblastic
      multinuclearity associated with
      positive acidified s. (HEMPAS)
    human measles immune s.
    human pertussis immune s.
    human scarlet fever immune s.
    hyperimmune s.
    immune s.
    inactivated s.
    liquid human s.
    measles convalescent s.
    muscle s.
    s. nephritis
    nonimmune s.
    normal s.
    polyvalent s.
    s. prothrombin conversion
      accelerator
    s. reaction
    s. shock
    s. sickness
serumal
serum-fast
service
    ambulance s.
    ancillary s.'s
    denture s.
    emergency medical s. (EMS)
sesamoid
    s. bone
    s. cartilage
sesquihydrate
sessile
    s. lesion
    s. polyp
set
    haploid s.
    learning s.
    minimum data s.
setaceous
seton operation
setting sun sign
seventh cranial nerve
Sever disease
severity of illness
sex
    s. assignment
    s. cell
    s. chromatin
    s. chromosome
    s. determination
    s. hormone

    s. linkage
    s. ratio
    s. reassignment
    s. reversal
    s. role
sex-influenced inheritance
sex-limited inheritance
sex-linked
    s.-l. character
    s.-l. inheritance
sexology
sextant
sexual
    s. abuse
    s. asphyxia
    s. crisis
    s. dimorphism
    s. disorder
    s. dysfunction
    s. generation
    s. infantilism
    s. intercourse
    s. orientation
    s. preference
    s. reproduction
    s. selection
sexuality
    infantile s.
sexually transmitted disease
Sézary cell
SFA
    saturated fatty acid
shadow
    acoustic s.
    Gumprecht s.
    hilar s.
    Ponfick s.
    s. test
shaft
    hair s.
shagreen
    s. plaque
    s. skin
shaken baby syndrome
shallow breathing
shared epitope
sharp dissection
shave biopsy
shear
    Liston s.
    malleus s.
sheath
    anterior tarsal tendinous s.
    axillary s.
    carotid s.
    carpal tendinous s.
    caudal s.
    common flexor s.
    common peroneal tendon s.

crural s.
dentinal s.
dorsal carpal tendinous s.
dural s.
enamel rod s.
external root s.
fascial s.
femoral s.
fenestrated s.
fibrous digital s.
fibrous tendon s.
fibular tarsal tendinous s.
Henle s.
Hertwig s.
Huxley s.
infundibuliform s.
internal root s.
intertubercular tendon s.
Mauthner s.
medullary s.
microfilarial s.
mitochondrial s.
myelin s.
root s.
s. of Schwann
synovial s.
tendinous s.
tendon s.
Waldeyer s.
shedding
virus s.
Sheehan syndrome
sheet
beta s.
shelf
Blumer s.
dental s.
palatal s.
palatine s.
shell
cytotrophoblastic s.
diffusion s.
K s.
L s.
M s.
s. nail
O s.
s. shock
Shenton line
Shepherd fracture
Sherrington law
shiatsu

Shibley sign
shield
embryonic s.
nipple s.
shielding
stress s.
shift
antigenic s.
axis s.
chemical s.
chloride s.
Doppler s.
s. to the left
luteoplacental s.
permanent threshold s.
s. to the right
temporary threshold s.
Shiga-Kruse bacillus
Shigalike toxin
Shiga toxin
Shigella
S. boydii
S. dysenteriae
S. flexneri
S. sonnei
shigellosis
shin
s. bone
saber s.
shingles
ship
Fabricius s.
shipyard eye
shirt-stud abscess
shivering thermogenesis
shock
anaphylactic s.
anaphylactoid s.
anesthetic s.
break s.
burn s.
cardiac s.
cardiogenic s.
chronic s.
cultural s.
declamping s.
deferred s.
delayed s.
diastolic s.
electric s.
endotoxin s.
hemorrhagic s.

S

NOTES

shock *(continued)*
 histamine s.
 hypovolemic s.
 insulin s.
 irreversible s.
 s. lung
 postoperative s.
 septic s.
 serum s.
 shell s.
 s. therapy
 toxic s.
 s. treatment
shocklike appearance
Shone
 S. anomaly
 S. complex
 S. syndrome
short
 s. adductor muscle
 s. bone
 s. bowel syndrome
 s. extensor muscle
 s. flexor muscle
 s. gastric artery
 s. gastric vein
 s. gut syndrome
 s. gyrus
 s. increment sensitivity index
 s. leg cast
 s. radial extensor muscle
shortsightedness
short-term
 s.-t. exposure limit
 s.-t. memory
shot-silk retina
shotted suture
shotty node
shoulder
 s. apprehension sign
 s. blade
 s. complex
 s. dystocia
 frozen s.
 s. girdle
 s. joint
 Little League s.
 s. presentation
shoulder-girdle syndrome
shovel-shaped incisor
shudder
 carotid s.
shuffle
 exon s.
shunt
 aortopulmonary s.
 arteriovenous s.
 AV s.
 Blalock s.

Blalock-Taussig s.
cavopulmonary s.
Denver s.
dialysis s.
Dickens s.
distal splenorenal s.
Glenn s.
H s.
hexose monophosphate s.
jejunoileal s.
left-to-right s.
LeVeen s.
mesocaval s.
peritoneovenous s.
pleuroperitoneal s.
pleurovenous s.
portacaval s.
proximal splenorenal s.
Rapoport-Leubering s.
right-to-left s.
side-to-side s.
splenorenal s.
tracheoesophageal s.
transjugular intrahepatic
 portosystemic s.
ventriculoatrial s.
ventriculoperitoneal s.
shuttle
 glycerophosphate s.
 malate-aspartate s.
Shwartzman phenomenon
Shy-Drager syndrome
sialadenitis
sialagogue
sialectasis
sialemesis, sialemesia
sialic acid
sialidase
sialidosis
sialine
sialism
sialismus
sialoadenectomy
sialoadenitis
sialoadenotomy
sialoangiectasis
sialoangiitis
sialocele
sialodochitis
sialodochoplasty
sialogenous
sialogogue
sialogram
sialography
sialolith
sialolithiasis
sialolithotomy
sialorrhea
sialoschesis

sialosis
sialostenosis
Siamese twins
sibilant
  s. rale
  s. rhonchi
sibling rivalry
sibship
sicca
  s. complex
  hypophysis s.
  keratitis s.
  keratoconjunctivitis s.
  laryngitis s.
  seborrhea s.
  s. syndrome
  synovitis s.
siccant
siccative
siccus
  pannus s.
sick
  s. building syndrome
  s. headache
  s. role
sicklaemia
sickle
  s. cell
  s. cell anemia
  s. cell C disease
  s. cell crisis
  s. cell disease
  s. cell hemoglobin (Hb S)
  s. cell retinopathy
  s. cell trait
sicklemia
sickling test
sickness
  acute African sleeping s.
  aerial s.
  African sleeping s.
  air s.
  altitude s.
  balloon s.
  black s.
  caisson s.
  car s.
  cave s.
  chronic African sleeping s.
  chronic mountain s.
  decompression s.
  East African sleeping s.

  falling s.
  green tobacco s.
  Indian s.
  Jamaican vomiting s.
  milk s.
  morning s.
  motion s.
  mountain s.
  radiation s.
  serum s.
  sleeping s.
SICU
  surgical intensive care unit
side
  balancing s.
  s. chain
  s. effect
  working s.
side-chain theory
sideroachrestic anemia
sideroblast
sideroblastic anemia
siderocyte
siderofibrosis
sideropenia
sideropenic
siderophage
siderophil, siderophile
siderophilous
siderophore
siderosilicosis
siderosis
siderotic cataract
sidestream aerosol
side-to-end anastomosis
side-to-side
  s.-t.-s. anastomosis
  s.-t.-s. shunt
Siegert sign
Siegle otoscope
siemens
sieve
  molecular s.
sievert
sight
  day s.
  far s.
  long s.
sigmoid
  s. artery
  s. colon
  s. flexure

S

NOTES

sigmoid *(continued)*
    s. mesocolon
    s. sinus
    s. vein
sigmoidectomy
sigmoiditis
sigmoidopexy
sigmoidoproctostomy
sigmoidorectostomy
sigmoidoscope
    disposable s.
sigmoidoscopy
sigmoidostomy
sigmoidotomy
sign
    Aaron s.
    Abadie s.
    Abrahams s.
    accessory s.
    air cushion s.
    antecedent s.
    assident s.
    Auenbrugger s.
    Aufrecht s.
    auscultatory s.
    Auspitz s.
    Babinski s.
    Baccelli s.
    Balance s.
    Ballance s.
    Bamberger s.
    Bamberger-Pins-Ewart s.
    banana s.
    Bárány s.
    Barré s.
    barrel hoop s.
    Bassler s.
    Bastedo s.
    Battle s.
    B6 bronchus s.
    beak s.
    Bechterew s.
    Beevor s.
    Bergman s.
    Biederman s.
    Bielschowsky s.
    Biernacki s.
    Biot breathing s.
    Bird s.
    Bjerrum s.
    blue dot s.
    Blumberg s.
    Bonhoeffer s.
    Bozzolo s.
    Branham s.
    Braxton Hicks s.
    Broadbent s.
    Brockenbrough s.
    Brudzinski s.

burning drops s.
Burton s.
calcium s.
Calkins s.
Cantelli s.
Carman s.
Carnett s.
Carvallo s.
catheter coiling s.
Chaddock s.
Chadwick s.
chandelier s.
Chaussier s.
Chvostek s.
Claybrook s.
clenched fist s.
Collier tucked lid s.
colon cutoff s.
Comby s.
comet tail s.
commemorative s.
Comolli s.
contralateral s.
conventional s.
Cope s.
Corrigan s.
Courvoisier s.
crescent s.
Cruveilhier-Baumgarten s.
Cullen s.
Dalrymple s.
Dance s.
Danforth s.
Darier s.
Dejerine s.
Delbet s.
Demarquay s.
de Musset s.
D'Éspine s.
dimple s.
doll's eye s.
Dorendorf s.
double bubble s.
double ring s.
double track s.
drawer s.
drooping lily s.
Drummond s.
Duchenne s.
Dupuytren s.
Duroziez s.
Ebstein s.
echo s.
Epstein s.
Erb-Westphal s.
Ewart s.
Ewing s.
eyelash s.
Faget s.

fan s.
Federici s.
Fischer s.
fissure s.
flag s.
floating tooth s.
Forchheimer s.
Fothergill s.
Friedreich s.
Froment s.
Gaenslen s.
gauss s.
Glasgow s.
gloved-finger s.
Goggia s.
Goldstein toe s.
Goodell s.
Gordon s.
Gorlin s.
Gower s.
Graefe s.
Grasset s.
Grey Turner s.
Griesinger s.
Grocco s.
groove s.
Gubler s.
Gunn crossing s.
Guyon s.
halo s.
Hamman s.
Hawkins impingement s.
Hegar s.
Heim-Kreysig s.
Hennebert s.
Higoumenakia s.
Hill s.
Hoagland s.
Hoffmann s.
Homans s.
Hoover s.
Horn s.
iconic s.
impingement s.
indexical s.
inferior triangle s.
Jackson s.
Joffroy s.
Kehr s.
Kerandel s.
Kernig s.
Kestenbaum s.

Klemm s.
knuckle s.
Kocher s.
Kreysig s.
Kussmaul s.
Lancisi s.
Landolfi s.
Lasègue s.
Legendre s.
lemon s.
Leri s.
Leser-Trélat s.
Lhermitte s.
ligature s.
local s.
Lorenz s.
Lovibond profile s.
Macewen s.
Magendie-Hertwig s.
Magnan s.
Mannkopf s.
Marañón s.
Marcus Gunn s.
McBurney s.
meniscus s.
Metenier s.
Mirchamp s.
Möbius s.
Mosler s.
Müller s.
Munson s.
Murphy s.
Musset s.
Neer impingement s.
Néri s.
Nikolsky s.
objective s.
obturator s.
painful arc s.
Pastia s.
patellar apprehension s.
Payr s.
peroneal s.
physical s.
Pins s.
Pitres s.
pivot-shift s.
Potain s.
psoas s.
pyramid s.
Quant s.
Ransohoff s.

NOTES

S

sign *(continued)*
    Raynaud s.
    red, white, and blue s.
    Remak s.
    reservoir s.
    Ripault s.
    Robertson s.
    Romaña s.
    Romberg s.
    Rosenbach s.
    Rossolimo s.
    Rotch s.
    Rovsing s.
    Russell s.
    Saenger s.
    Sansom s.
    Schapiro s.
    Schlesinger s.
    Schultze s.
    Schwartze s.
    scimitar s.
    Seeligmüller s.
    Seidel s.
    setting sun s.
    Shibley s.
    shoulder apprehension s.
    Siegert s.
    silhouette s.
    Skoda s.
    soft s.
    Steinberg thumb s.
    Stellwag s.
    Stewart-Holmes s.
    Straus s.
    string s.
    subjective s.
    Sumner s.
    ten Horn s.
    Thomson s.
    Tinel s.
    Toma s.
    Topolanski s.
    Traube s.
    Trendelenburg s.
    Tresilian s.
    trough s.
    Trousseau s.
    Trunecek s.
    Vierra s.
    Vipond s.
    vital s.
    von Graefe s.
    Weiss s.
    Westermark s.
    Westphal s.
    Wilder s.
    Winterbottom s.
    wrist s.

signal
    arrest s.
    s. lymph node
    pause s.
    s. symptom
    termination s.
signal-processing circuit
signal-to-noise ratio
signature
    tumor s.
signet ring cell
significance
    atypical glandular cell of
      undetermined s. (AGUS)
    atypical squamous cell of
      undetermined s. (ASCUS)
    monoclonal gammopathy of
      unknown s. (MGUS)
silence
    electrocerebral s.
silent
    s. area
    s. aspiration
    s. gene
    s. myocardial infarction
silhouette sign
silica
silicate restoration
silicatosis
silicon
    amorphous s.
    s. dioxide
silicone
silicoproteinosis
silicosiderosis
silicosis
silicotuberculosis
silk
    floss s.
silo-filler's lung
silver
    s. impregnation
    s. protein stain
    s. stool
silver-ammoniac silver stain
silver-fork
    s.-f. deformity
    s.-f. fracture
Silverskiöld syndrome
simian virus
similar
    law of s.'s
    s. twins
similia similibus curantur
Simmonds disease
Simmons citrate medium
Simonart
    S. band
    S. ligament

Simon position
simple
    s. absence
    s. astigmatism
    s. dislocation
    s. endometrial hyperplasia
    s. fission
    s. fracture
    s. glaucoma
    s. goiter
    s. joint
    s. mastectomy
    s. mastoidectomy
    s. microscope
    s. necrosis
    s. nephrectomy
    s. obesity
    s. phobia
    s. protein
    s. schizophrenia
    s. squamous epithelium
    s. synovitis
simplex
    adiposis tuberosa s.
    glaucoma s.
    herpes s.
    ichthyosis s.
    lentigo s.
    prurigo s.
    purpura s.
Simplexvirus
Simplified Oral Hygiene Index (OHI-S)
Sims position
simulation
    computer s.
simultanagnosia
simultaneous communication
sincipital presentation
sinciput
Sindbis
    S. fever
    S. virus
Sinding-Larsen-Johansson syndrome
sinew
sine wave
singer's nodule
single
    s. bond
    s. microscope
    s. photon emission computed
    tomography
    s. vial fixative

single-armed suture
singleton
singultation
sinister
sinistra
    hemicardia s.
sinistrad
sinistral
sinistrality
sinistrocardia
sinistrocardiale
    P s.
sinistrocerebral
sinistrogyration
sinistromanual
sinistropedal
sinistrotorsion
sinistrum
    atrium cordis s.
Sin Nombre virus
sinoatrial
    s. block
    s. bradycardia
    s. node
sinopulmonary
sinuatrial (S-A)
    s. block
    s. node
sinus
    anal s.
    anterior s.
    aortic s.
    Arlt s.
    s. arrest
    s. arrhythmia
    barber pilonidal s.
    basilar s.
    s. block
    Breschet s.
    carotid s.
    cavernous s.
    cerebral s.
    cervical s.
    circular s.
    coccygeal s.
    confluence of s.
    coronary s.
    costomediastinal s.
    cranial s.
    dermal s.
    dural venous s.
    Englisch s.

S

NOTES

sinus *(continued)*
    ethmoidal s.
    frontal s.
    Guérin s.
    s. histiocytosis with massive
      lymphadenopathy
    Huguier s.
    inferior longitudinal s.
    inferior petrosal s.
    inferior sagittal s.
    intercavernous s.
    jugular s.
    lactiferous s.
    laryngeal s.
    lateral s.
    longitudinal vertebral venous s.
    Luschka s.
    lymph s.
    lymphatic s.
    Maier s.
    marginal s.
    mastoid s.
    maxillary s.
    Meyer s.
    middle ethmoidal s.
    Morgagni s.
    s. nodal reentry
    occipital s.
    paranasal s.
    s. pause
    pericardial s.
    pilonidal s.
    preauricular s.
    prostatic s.
    renal s.
    rhomboid s.
    rhomboidal s.
    s. rhythm
    scleral venous s.
    sigmoid s.
    sphenoidal s.
    sphenoparietal s.
    splenic s.
    straight s.
    tarsal s.
    tentorial s.
    terminal s.
    transverse pericardial s.
    tympanic s.
    uterine s.
    uteroplacental s.
    s. venosus
    s. venosus sclerae
    venous s.
sinusitis
sinusoid
sinusoidal
sinusotomy
siphon

siphonage
Sipple syndrome
sirenomelia
Sister Joseph nodule
site
    acceptor splicing s.
    active s.
    allosteric s.
    antibody-combining s.
    antigen-binding s.
    cleavage s.
    fragile s.
    immunologically privileged s.'s
    ligand-binding s.
    restriction s.
    switching s.
site-specific recombination
sitotaxis
sitotropism
situ
    adenocarcinoma in s.
    carcinoma in s. (CIS)
    in s.
    lobular carcinoma in s.
    malignant melanoma in s.
situational psychosis
situs inversus
sitz bath
sixth
    s. cranial nerve
    s. disease
sixth-year molar
size
    aerodynamic s.
    burst s.
    focal spot s.
Sjögren syndrome
skater's gait
skein
    choroid s.
skeletal
    s. age
    s. dysplasia
    s. extension
    s. muscle
    s. occlusion
    s. traction
skeleton
    appendicular s.
    articulated s.
    axial s.
    cardiac fibrous s.
    facial s.
    fibrous s.
    gill arch s.
    jaw s.
skeletonized
Skene tubule
skiascopy

skilled
    s. nursing care
    s. nursing facility (SNF)
skills validation
skimmed milk
skim milk
skin
    alligator s.
    bronzed s.
    citrine s.
    s. clip
    deciduous s.
    s. dose
    elastic s.
    farmer's s.
    fish s.
    glabrous s.
    glossy s.
    golfer's s.
    hidden nail s.
    loose s.
    marble s.
    nail s.
    piebald s.
    s. ridge
    shagreen s.
    s. tag
    s. test
    s. traction
skinfold measurement
Skoda
    S. sign
    S. tympany
skodaic resonance
skull
    s. base surgery
    cloverleaf s.
    inner table of s.
    maplike s.
    steeple s.
    tower s.
skullcap
slant culture
SLAP
    superior labrum anterior and posterior
        SLAP lesion
SLE
    systemic lupus erythematosus
sleep
    s. apnea
    s. deficit
    electric s.

electrotherapeutic s.
fast-wave s.
hypnotic s.
s. latency
light s.
paradoxical s.
s. paralysis
rolandic s.
slow-wave s.
sleeping sickness
sleeptalking
sleepwalking
slew rate
slide tracheoplasty
sliding
    s. flap
    s. hernia
    s. lock
    s. microtome
slip
    freudian s.
    s. joint
slipped
    s. capital femoral epiphysis (SCFE)
    s. hernia
slipping
    s. rib
    s. rib cartilage
slit
    Cheatle s.
    filtration s.
slitlamp
    Gullstrand s.
slope
    lower ridge s.
slough
slow
    s. channel-blocking agent
    s. virus
    s. virus disease
slow-reacting substance
slow-wave sleep
Sluder neuralgia
sludge
    activated s.
small
    s. calorie
    s. cardiac vein
    s. cell
    s. cell carcinoma
    s. increment sensitivity index

S

NOTES

small *(continued)*
    s. intestine
    s. pelvis
smaller posterior rectus muscle
smallpox
    confluent s.
    discrete s.
    fulminating s.
    hemorrhagic s.
    malignant s.
    modified s.
    s. virus
smear
    acid-fast s. (AFS)
    alimentary tract s.
    bronchoscopic s.
    buccal s.
    cervical s.
    colonic s.
    cul-de-sac s.
    s. culture
    cytologic s.
    duodenal s.
    ectocervical s.
    endocervical s.
    endometrial s.
    esophageal s.
    fast s.
    gastric s.
    lateral vaginal wall s.
    lower respiratory tract s.
    Pap s.
smegma
smegmalith
Smith
    S. fracture
    S. operation
Smith-Gibson operation
Smith-Indian operation
smoker's cancer
smoldering leukemia
smooth
    s. diet
    s. muscle
smudge cell
smut
    corn s.
snail track degeneration
snakeroot
    Canada s.
    European s.
snap
    closing s.
    mitral opening s.
    opening s.
snapping hip syndrome
snare
    cold s.

    galvanocaustic s.
    hot s.
Sneddon syndrome
Snellen test type
Snell law
SNF
    skilled nursing facility
sniff test
S-nitrosohemoglobin
snorting
snout reflex
snow
    s. blindness
    carbon dioxide s.
snuffbox
    anatomic s.
Snyder
    corneal dystrophy of S.
    S. test
soap
    animal s.
    Castile s.
    curd s.
    domestic s.
    green s.
    hard s.
    insoluble s.
    marine s.
    medicinal soft s.
Soave operation
social
    s. history
    s. phobia
    s. psychiatry
    s. psychology
socialization
socialized medicine
socioacusis
sociocentric
sociogenesis
sociopath
socket
    dry s.
    eye s.
    tooth s.
soda
    baking s.
    bicarbonate of s.
    caustic s.
sodium
    azlocillin s.
    s. bicarbonate
    s. borate
    cephapirin s.
    cilastatin s.
    colistimethate s.
    cromolyn s.
    dantrolene s.
    dextrothyroxine s.

dicloxacillin s.
divalproex s.
docusate s.
epoprostenol s.
estramustine phosphate s.
ethacrynate s.
fluorescein s.
fusidate s.
glucosulfone s.
glycocholate s.
heparin s.
iodohippurate s.
iodomethamate s.
iothiouracil s.
mercaptomerin s.
mercurophylline s.
methicillin s.
methiodal s.
methohexital s.
metrizoate s.
mezlocillin s.
s. phosphate 32P
s. pump
sulfobromophthalein s.

sodium-potassium pump
sodomist
sodomite
sodomy
soft

s. chancre
s. corn
s. diet
s. drusen
s. nevus
s. palate
s. sign
s. sore
s. tubercle
s. ulcer
s. wart

soil

night s.

solar

s. cheilitis
s. comedo
s. elastosis
s. urticaria

solation
soldering
soleus muscle

solid

color s.
s. teratoma

solis

ictus s.

solitary

s. bone cyst
s. lymphatic follicle
s. tract

sollicitans

Aedes s.

solubility test
soluble RNA
solute
solution

acetic s.
amaranth s.
aqueous s.
Benedict s.
Burow s.
chemical s.
colloidal s.
s. of contiguity
s. of continuity
Dakin s.
disclosing s.
Earle s.
ethereal s.
Fehling s.
Fonio s.
Gallego differentiating s.
Gey s.
Hanks s.
Hartman s.
Hartmann s.
Hayem s.
Krebs-Ringer s.
lactated Ringer s. (LRS)
Lange s.
Locke s.
Locke-Ringer s.
Lugol iodine s.
molecular dispersed s.
normal s.
ophthalmic s.
Ringer s.
saline s.
saturated s.
standard s.
standardized s.
supersaturated s.
test s.

S

NOTES

solution *(continued)*
    Tyrode s.
    volumetric s.
    Weigert iodine s.
solvent
    amphiprotic s.
    fat s.
soma
somasthenia
somatagnosia
somatalgia
somatasthenia
somatesthesia
somatesthetic
somatic
    s. antigen
    s. cell
    s. crossing-over
    s. death
    s. delusion
    s. motor nucleus
    s. mutation
    s. mutation theory
    s. nerve
    s. pain
    s. reproduction
    s. sensory cortex
    s. swallow
somatization disorder
somatochrome
somatocrinin
somatoform disorder
somatogenic
somatoliberin
somatomammotropin
    human chorionic s. (HCS)
somatomedin
somatopathic
somatopause
somatoplasm
somatopleure
somatopsychic
somatopsychosis
somatosensory
    s. aura
    s. cortex
    s. evoked potential (SSEP)
somatosexual
somatostatin
somatostatinoma
somatotherapy
somatotopagnosis
somatotopic
somatotopy
somatotropes
somatotroph
somatotropic, somatotrophic
    s. hormone
somatotropin release-inhibiting hormone

somatotropin-releasing
    s.-r. factor
    s.-r. hormone
somatotype
somatropin
somesthesia
somite
somnambulism
somnifacient
somniferous
somniloquence
somniloquism
somniloquy
somnipathy
somnocinematography
somnolence
somnolency
somnolent
somnolescent
Somogyi
    S. effect
    S. phenomenon
    S. unit
Sondermann canal
sonic
sonication
sonification
Sonne bacillus
sonnei
    Shigella s.
sonogram
sonograph
sonographer
sonography
sonorous
    s. rale
    s. rhonchi
sopor
soporific
sorbefacient
sordellii
    Clostridium s.
sordes
sore
    canker s.
    cold s.
    Delhi s.
    desert s.
    hard s.
    Lahore s.
    oriental s.
    pressure s.
    soft s.
    s. throat
    tropical s.
    venereal s.
soreness
    delayed onset muscle s.
Soret phenomenon

soroche
    chronic s.
sorption
Sorsby
    S. macular degeneration
    S. syndrome
sorter
    fluorescence-activated cell s.
Sotos syndrome
souffle
    cardiac s.
    fetal s.
    funic s.
    funicular s.
    mammary s.
    uterine s.
sound
    adventitious breath s.'s
    adventitious lung s.'s
    amphoric voice s.
    anvil s.
    atrial s.
    auscultatory s.
    bell s.
    bowel s.'s
    breath s.'s
    bronchial breath s.'s
    bronchovesicular breath s.'s
    Campbell s.
    cannon s.
    cardiac s.
    cavernous voice s.
    coconut s.
    complex s.
    cracked-pot s.
    Davis interlocking s.
    double-shock s.
    eddy s.
    ejection s.
    equal bilateral breath s.'s
    fetal heart s.
    s. field
    first heart s.
    flapping s.
    fourth heart s.
    friction s.
    gallop s.
    heart s.'s
    hippocratic succussion s.
    intensity of s.
    Jewett s.
    Korotkoff s.

    Le Fort s.
    McCrea s.
    Mercier s.
    percussion s.
    respiratory s.'s
    Santini booming s.
    second heart s.
    splitting of heart s.'s
    succussion s.
    third heart s.
    vesicular breath s.
    white s.
    Winternitz s.
source-to-image distance
South
    S. African tick-bite fever
    S. American blastomycosis
    S. American trypanosomiasis
Southern blot analysis
space
    alveolar dead s.
    anatomic dead s.
    antecubital s.
    anterior clear s.
    apical s.
    axillary s.
    Berger s.
    Bogros s.
    Böttcher s.
    Bowman s.
    Burns s.
    capsular s.
    cartilage s.
    cavernous s.
    central palmar s.
    Chassaignac s.
    Cloquet s.
    Colles s.
    corneal s.
    Cotunnius s.
    cranial extradural s.
    dead s.
    deep perineal s.
    denture s.
    disc s.
    Disse s.
    enclosed s.
    endolymphatic s.
    epidural s.
    episcleral s.
    epitympanic s.
    extradural s.

S

NOTES

space *(continued)*
    extraperitoneal s.
    filtration s.
    Fontana s.
    freeway s.
    gingival s.
    haversian s.
    Henke s.
    His perivascular s.
    infraglottic s.
    interalveolar s.
    intercostal s.
    interfascial s.
    interglobular s.
    intermembrane s.
    interocclusal rest s.
    interosseous metacarpal s.
    interosseous metatarsal s.
    interpleural s.
    interproximal s.
    interradicular s.
    interseptovalvular s.
    intersheath s.
    intervaginal subarachnoid s.
    intervillous s.
    intraretinal s.
    Kiernan s.
    Kretschmann s.
    Kuhnt s.
    lateral central palmar s.
    lateral midpalmar s.
    lateral pharyngeal s.
    leeway s.
    leptomeningeal s.
    lymph s.
    Magendie s.
    Malacarne s.
    masticator s.
    Meckel s.
    medial midpalmar s.
    mediastinal s.
    medullary s.
    middle palmar s.
    midpalmar s.
    Mohrenheim s.
    palmar s.
    paraglottic s.
    perilymphatic s.
    personal s.
    physiologic dead s.
    plantar s.
    pleural s.
    Poiseuille s.
    popliteal s.
    preepiglottic s.
    Proust s.
    Reinke s.
    retrocardiac s.
    retroperitoneal s.
    retropubic s.
    subarachnoid s.
    subchorial s.
    subdural s.
    thenar s.
    Westberg s.
    zonular s.

Spallanzani law
spallation product
span
    attention s.
    memory s.
Spanish influenza
sparing action
spasm
    accommodative s.
    affect s.
    anorectal s.
    arterial s.
    Bell s.
    cadaveric s.
    canine s.
    carpopedal s.
    clonic s.
    cynic s.
    diffuse esophageal s.
    epidemic transient diaphragmatic s.
    epileptic s.
    esophageal s.
    facial s.
    habit s.
    hemifacial s.
    infantile s.
    intention s.
    intentional s.
    masticatory s.
    mobile s.
    muscle s.
    nodding s.
    saltatory s.
    tonic s.
    tonoclonic s.
    torsion s.
    vascular s.
spasmodic
    s. dysmenorrhea
    s. dysphonia
spasmolysis
spasmolytic
spasmus nutans
spastic
    s. abasia
    s. aphonia
    s. colon
    s. diplegia
    s. dysarthria
    s. dysphonia
    s. gait
    s. hemiplegia

s. ileus
s. rigidity

spasticity
clasp-knife s.

spatial
s. agnosia
s. relation

spatula
iris s.
Ro s.

spatulate

spay

speaker's nodule

speaking tube

special
s. anatomy
s. sense

specialist

specialization

specialty referral center

speciation

species-specific antigen

specific
s. absorption coefficient
s. action
s. activity
s. building-related illnesses
s. dynamic action
s. extinction
s. gravity
s. immunity
s. opsonin
s. optic rotation
s. parasite
s. phobia
s. reaction

specificity
analytical s.
diagnostic s.
relative s.

specified
not otherwise s. (NOS)

specimen
cytologic s.

spectacles
bifocal s.
diver's s.
divided s.
Franklin s.
half-glass s.
hemianopic s.

lid crutch s.
Masselon s.

spectral

spectrin

spectrograph
mass s.

spectrometer

spectrometry
clinical s.

spectrophotometer

spectrophotometry
atomic absorption s.
flame emission s.
reflectance s.

spectroscope
direct vision s.

spectroscopic

spectroscopy
clinical s.
infrared s.
magnetic resonance s.
microabsorption s.

spectrum
absorption s.
antimicrobial s.
broad s.
chromatic s.
color s.
continuous s.
electromagnetic s.
excitation s.
fluorescence s.
fortification s.
frequency s.
infrared s.
invisible s.
line s.
visible s.
vocal s.

speculum, pl. **specula**
anal s.
bivalved s.
Cooke s.
duckbill s.
esophageal s.
eye s.
s. forceps
Kelly rectal s.
nasal s.
Pederson s.

Spee
curve of S.

S

NOTES

793

speech
- alaryngeal s.
- automatic s.
- s. awareness threshold
- s. bulb
- s. center
- cerebellar s.
- clipped s.
- cued s.
- s. detection threshold
- echo s.
- esophageal s.
- explosive s.
- s. frequency
- helium s.
- s. mechanism
- mirror s.
- nonpropositional s.
- s. pathology
- s. perception
- s. processor
- propositional s.
- s. reading
- s. reception threshold
- scanning s.
- spontaneous s.
- staccato s.
- subvocal s.
- telegraphic s.

speech-language
- s.-l. pathologist
- s.-l. pathology

speed
- film s.
- s. play

spelling
- finger s.

Spens syndrome
spermacytic seminoma
sperm-aster
spermatic
- s. cord
- s. duct

spermatid
spermatoblast
spermatocele
spermatocidal
spermatocide
spermatocytal
spermatocyte
- primary s.
- secondary s.

spermatocytogenesis
spermatogenesis
spermatogenic
spermatogonium
spermatoid
spermatolysis
spermatolytic

spermatopoietic
spermatorrhea
spermatozoal
spermatozoan
spermatozoon
spermaturia
spermicidal
spermicide
spermiduct
spermiogenesis
spermium
spermolith
sphacelate
sphacelation
sphacelism
sphaceloderma
sphacelous
sphacelus
sphaericus
- *Bacillus s.*

sphenion
sphenobasilar
sphenocephaly
sphenoethmoidectomy
sphenoid
- s. bone
- s. crest

sphenoidal
- s. conchae
- s. sinus
- s. spine

sphenoiditis
sphenoidotomy
sphenooccipital
sphenopalatine
- s. artery
- s. foramen
- s. neuralgia

sphenoparietal sinus
sphenorbital
sphenotic
sphere
- attraction s.

spherical
- s. aberration
- s. lens

spherocyte
spherocytic anemia
spherocytosis
- hereditary s.

spheroidal
spheroid joint
spherophakia
sphincter
- anal s.
- anatomic s.
- angular s.
- antral s.
- anular s.

artificial s.
basal s.
bicanalicular s.
Boyden s.
canalicular s.
cardiac s.
choledochal s.
colic s.
duodenal s.
duodenojejunal s.
external anal s.
external urethral s.
extrinsic s.
first duodenal s.
functional s.
Glisson s.
hepatopancreatic s.
hypertensive upper esophageal s.
Hyrtl s.
ileal s.
ileocecocolic s.
iliopelvic s.
inferior esophageal s.
internal anal s.
internal urethral s.
intrinsic s.
lower esophageal s. (LES)
macroscopic s.
marginal s.
mediocolic s.
microscopic s.
midgastric transverse s.
midsigmoid s.
s. muscle
s. of Oddi
s. of Oddi dysfunction
physiologic s.
s. pupillae
pyloric s.
radiologic s.
s. urethrae
s. vesicae
sphincteral
sphincteralgia
sphincterectomy
sphincterismus
sphincteritis
sphincterolysis
sphincteroplasty
sphincterotomy
external s.
internal s.

sphingolipid
sphingolipidosis
cerebral s.
sphingolipodystrophy
sphingomyelin phosphodiesterase
sphingomyelins
sphingosine
sphygmic interval
sphygmochronograph
sphygmogram
sphygmograph
sphygmographic
sphygmoid
sphygmomanometer
Mosso s.
Rogers s.
sphygmomanometry
sphygmometer
sphygmoscope
Bishop s.
sphygmoscopy
spica bandage
spicular
spicule
spider
s. angioma
arterial s.
s. belly
s. nevus
s. telangiectasia
vascular s.
spider-burst
Spiegelberg criteria
Spielmeyer acute swelling
spigelian
Spigelius lobe
spike
s. potential
s. and wave complex
spill
cellular s.
spilus
nevus s.
spin
s. density
s. echo
spina
s. bifida
s. bifida cystica
s. bifida occulta
spinal
s. akinesia

S

NOTES

spinal *(continued)*
    s. analgesia
    s. anesthesia
    s. arachnoid mater
    s. block
    s. branch
    s. canal
    s. column
    s. cord
    s. cord concussion
    s. curvature
    s. decompression
    s. dysraphism
    s. fusion
    s. ganglion
    s. gliosis
    s. headache
    s. instability
    s. muscle
    s. muscular atrophy
    s. mydriasis
    s. myoclonus
    s. nerve
    s. orthosis
    s. paralysis
    s. pia mater
    s. reflex
    s. stenosis
    s. tap
    s. vein

spinalis
    s. capitis muscle
    s. cervicis muscle
    dura mater s.
    funiculi medullae s.
    medulla s.
    s. thoracis muscle

spinalium
    ansae nervorum s.

spinate

spindle
    aortic s.
    s. cell
    s. cell carcinoma
    s. cell lipoma
    central s.
    cleavage s.
    His s.
    Krukenberg s.
    Kühne s.
    mitotic s.
    neuromuscular s.
    neurotendinous s.
    nuclear s.

spine
    alar s.
    angular s.
    anterior inferior iliac s.
    anterior nasal s.

    anterior superior iliac s.
    bamboo s.
    s. board
    cervical s.
    cleft s.
    dendritic s.
    dorsal s.
    s. fusion
    greater tympanic s.
    hemal s.
    Henle s.
    iliac s.
    ischiadic s.
    ischial s.
    kissing s.'s
    lesser tympanic s.
    lumbar s.
    meatal s.
    mental s.
    nasal s.
    neural s.
    palatine s.
    poker s.
    posterior nasal s.
    s. of scapula
    sphenoidal s.
    thoracic s.
    tibial s.
    trochanteric s.
    trochlear s.

spinnbarkeit

spinoadductor reflex

spinobulbar

spinocerebellar ataxia

spinocuneate fiber

spinogracile fiber

spinoolivary tract

spinous
    s. layer
    s. process

spinovestibular tract

spinulosa
    trichostasis s.

spinulosus
    lichen s.

spiradenoma
    eccrine s.

spiral
    s. bandage
    s. canal
    Curschmann s.
    s. fold
    s. fracture
    s. ganglion
    s. joint
    s. ligament
    s. organ
    s. vein

spirillar

spirillum
    Vincent s.
spirit
    ardent s.
    aromatic ammonia s.
    industrial methylated s.
    s. lamp
    methylated s.
spirochetemia
spirochetes
    Becker stain for s.
spirochetosis
    bronchopulmonary s.
spirogram
spirograph
spirometer
    chain-compensated s.
    incentive s.
    Krogh s.
spirometry
    closed-circuit s.
    forced s.
    open circuit s.
spissitude
spittle
Spitzer theory
Spitzka-Lissauer
    column of S.-L.
Spitz nevus
splanchnapophysial
splanchnapophysis
splanchnectopia
splanchnesthesia
splanchnesthetic sensibility
splanchnic
    s. anesthesia
    s. ganglion
    s. wall
splanchnicectomy
splanchnicotomy
splanchnicus
    Bacteroides s.
splanchnocele
splanchnography
splanchnolith
splanchnomegaly
splanchnopathy
splanchnopleure
splanchnoptosis, splanchnoptosia
splanchnosclerosis
splanchnoscopy
splanchnoskeletal

splanchnoskeleton
splanchnotomy
splanchnotribe
splay foot
spleen
    accessory s.
    diffuse waxy s.
    floating s.
    Gandy-Gamna s.
    gastric impression on s.
    kidneys, liver, s. (KLS)
    lardaceous s.
    movable s.
    sago s.
    waxy s.
splenectomize
splenectomy
    abdominal s.
splenectopia
splenectopy
splenic
    s. apoplexy
    s. artery
    s. flexure
    s. lymph follicle
    s. pulp
    s. sinus
    s. vein
splenitis
splenium
splenius
    s. capitis muscle
    s. cervicis muscle
splenocele
splenohepatomegalia
splenohepatomegaly
splenoid
splenoma
splenomalacia
splenomedullary
splenomegalia
splenomegaly
    congestive s.
    Egyptian s.
    hemolytic s.
    hyperreactive malarious s.
    Niemann s.
splenomyelogenous
splenomyelomalacia
splenopathy
splenopexy, splenopexia
splenoportography

NOTES

splenoptosia
splenoptosis
splenorenal
    s. ligament
    s. shunt
splenorrhagia
splenorrhaphy
splenosis
    thoracic s.
splenotomy
splenotoxin
splicing
    alternative s.
    gene s.
    RNA s.
splint
    acid etch cemented s.
    active s.
    air s.
    airplane s.
    anchor s.
    Anderson s.
    backboard s.
    Balkan s.
    cap s.
    coaptation s.
    contact s.
    Cramer wire s.
    Denis Browne s.
    dynamic s.
    Essig s.
    Frejka pillow s.
    functional s.
    Gunning s.
    inflatable s.
    interdental s.
    Kingsley s.
    labial s.
    ladder s.
    lingual s.
    pillow s.
    surgical s.
    Thomas s.
splinter hemorrhage
split
    s. hand
    s. pelvis
    s. products of fibrin
    s. uvula
split-thickness
    s.-t. flap
    s.-t. graft
splitting of heart sounds
spodogenous
spondylalgia
spondylarthritis
spondylitic
spondylitis
    ankylosing s.

    s. deformans
    rheumatoid s.
    tuberculous s.
spondyloepiphyseal
    s. dysplasia
    s. dysplasia congenita
    s. dysplasia tarda
spondylolisthesis
spondylolisthetic pelvis
spondylolysis
spondylopathy
spondylopyosis
spondyloschisis
spondylosis
    cervical s.
    hyperostotic s.
spondylosyndesis
sponge
    absorbable gelatin s.
    s. bath
    Bernays s.
    compressed s.
    contraceptive s.
    s. implant
spongiform encephalopathy
spongioblast
spongioblastoma
spongiocyte
spongioid
spongiosa
    decidua s.
    substantia s.
spongiose
spongiosis
spongiositis
spongiosum
    osteoma s.
    stratum s.
spongy
    s. bone
    s. iritis
    s. substance
spontaneous
    s. abortion
    s. amputation
    s. gangrene
    s. generation
    s. mutation
    s. nystagmus
    s. pneumothorax
    s. speech
    s. version
spoon
    cataract s.
    Daviel s.
    s. nail
    Volkmann s.
sporadic dysentery
sporangium

spore
    black s.
sporicidal
sporicide
sporidium
sporoagglutination
sporoblast
sporocyst
sporogenesis
sporogenous
sporogony, sporogeny
sporont
sporotrichosis
sporozoite
sports
    s. anemia
    s. massage
    s. medicine
sport-specific training
sporular
sporulation
sporule
spot
    acoustic s.
    Bitot s.
    blind s.
    blood s.
    blue s.
    Brushfield s.
    café au lait s.
    cherry-red s.
    corneal s.
    cotton-wool s.
    De Morgan s.
    Elschnig s.
    flame s.
    focal s.
    Fordyce s.
    Fuchs black s.
    hot s.
    hypnogenetic s.
    hypnogenic s.
    Koplik s.
    liver s.
    s. map
    Mariotte blind s.
    mental blind s.
    milk s.
    mongolian s.
    pain s.
    rose s.

    Roth s.
    Tardieu s.
    Tay cherry-red s.
    s. test
    Trousseau s.
    typhoid s.
    wet s.
spotted
    s. fever
    s. leprosy
spousal abuse
spouse abuse
sprain
    s. fracture
    rider's s.
spread
    common vehicle s.
spreader
    gutta-percha s.
Sprengel deformity
spring
    s. conjunctivitis
    hemoglobin Constant S.
springlike phenomenon
sprue
    celiac s.
    nontropical s.
    tropical s.
spun glass hair
spur
    bone s.
    calcaneal s.
    calcarine s.
    s. cell
    s. cell anemia
    Fuchs s.
    Grunert s.
    heel s.
    Michel s.
    occipital s.
    olecranon s.
spuria
    hemospermia s.
    melena s.
    placenta s.
spurious
    s. ankylosis
    s. labor
    s. parasite
    s. rib
Spurling test

S

NOTES

sputorum
>   *Campylobacter s.*

sputum, pl. **sputa**
>   globular s.
>   green s.
>   nummular s.
>   rusty s.

squalamine lactate
squama
>   frontal s.

squamate
squame
squamoparietal suture
squamosa
squamosal
squamous
>   s. cell
>   s. cell carcinoma
>   s. epithelium
>   s. metaplasia
>   s. odontogenic tumor
>   s. papilloma
>   s. suture

squamozygomatic
square
>   s. knot
>   Latin s.
>   least s.'s

squint
>   convergent s.
>   divergent s.
>   external s.
>   internal s.

squinting patella
SSEP
>   somatosensory evoked potential

St.
>   St. John's wort
>   St. Louis encephalitis virus

stab
>   s. cell
>   s. culture
>   s. drain

stabilate
stabile
stability
>   denture s.
>   detrusor s.
>   dimensional s.
>   endemic s.
>   enzootic s.

stabilization
stabilizer
>   endodontic s.

stable
>   s. isotope
>   vital signs s. (VSS)

staccato speech

staff
>   s. of Aesculapius
>   attending s.
>   s. cell
>   consulting s.
>   house s.
>   s. model HMO

stage
>   algid s.
>   Arneth s.
>   bell s.
>   bud s.
>   cap s.
>   cold s.
>   defervescent s.
>   end s.
>   eruptive s.
>   exoerythrocytic s.
>   genital s.
>   imperfect s.
>   incubative s.
>   intuitive s.
>   s. of labor
>   latent s.
>   perfect s.
>   preconceptual s.
>   prodromal s.
>   Tanner s.
>   tumor s.

staggered spondaic word test
staghorn calculus
staging
>   Jewett and Strong s.
>   TNM s.

stagnant anoxia
stagnation mastitis
Stahl ear
stain
>   Abbott s.
>   aceto-orcein s.
>   acid s.
>   Ag-AS s.
>   Albert diphtheria s.
>   Altmann anilin-acid fuchsin s.
>   Alzheimer s.
>   basic fuchsin-methylene blue s.
>   Bauer chromic acid leucofuchsin s.
>   Bennhold Congo red s.
>   Berg s.
>   Best carmine s.
>   Bielschowsky s.
>   Biondi-Heidenhain s.
>   Birch-Hirschfeld s.
>   Bodian copper-protargol s.
>   Borrel blue s.
>   Bowie s.
>   Brown-Brenn s.
>   Cajal astrocyte s.
>   carbol-thionin s.

C-banding s.
centromere banding s.
chromate s.
Ciaccio s.
contrast s.
Cresylecht violet s.
Da Fano s.
Dane s.
Dieterle s.
differential s.
double s.
Ehrlich acid hematoxylin s.
Ehrlich aniline crystal violet s.
Ehrlich triacid s.
Ehrlich triple s.
Einarson gallocyanin-chrome
 alum s.
Eranko fluorescence s.
Feulgen s.
Field rapid s.
Fink-Heimer s.
Flemming triple s.
fluorescence plus Giemsa s.
fluorescent s.
Fontana s.
Fontana-Masson silver s.
Foot reticulin impregnation s.
Fouchet s.
Fraser-Lendrum s.
Friedländer s.
G-banding s.
Giemsa chromosome banding s.
Glenner-Lillie s.
Golgi s.
Gomori aldehyde fuchsin s.
Gomori-Jones periodic acid-
 methenamine-silver s.
Goodpasture s.
Gordon and Sweet s.
Gram s.
Gram-chromotrope s.
green s.
Gridley s.
Grocott-Gomori methenamine-
 silver s.
Hale colloidal iron s.
Heidenhain azan s.
Heidenhain iron hematoxylin s.
hematoxylin and eosin s.
Hirsch-Peiffer s.
Hiss s.
Holmes s.

Hortega neuroglia s.
Hucker-Conn s.
immunofluorescent s.
India ink capsule s.
intravital s.
iodine s.
Jenner s.
Kasten fluorescent Feulgen s.
Kasten fluorescent PAS s.
Kinyoun s.
Kleihauer s.
Klinger-Ludwig acid-thionin s.
Klüver-Barrera Luxol fast blue s.
Kokoskin s.
Kossa s.
Kronecker s.
lacquer s.
lactophenol cotton blue s.
Laquer s.
lead hydroxide s.
Leishman s.
Lendrum phloxine-tartrazine s.
Lepehne-Pickworth s.
Levaditi s.
Lillie allochrome connective
 tissue s.
Lillie azure-eosin s.
Lillie ferrous iron s.
Lillie sulfuric acid Nile blue s.
Lison-Dunn s.
Loeffler caustic s.
Luna-Ishak s.
Macchiavello s.
MacNeal tetrachrome blood s.
malarial pigment s.
Maldonado-San Jose s.
Mallory aniline blue s.
Mallory collagen s.
Mallory iodine s.
Mallory phloxine s.
Mallory phosphotungstic acid
 hematoxylin s.
Mallory trichrome s.
Mallory triple s.
Mann methyl blue-eosin s.
Marchi s.
Masson argentaffin s.
Masson-Fontana ammoniac silver s.
Masson trichrome s.
Maximow s.
Mayer hemalum s.
Mayer mucicarmine s.

NOTES

stain *(continued)*
    Mayer mucihematein s.
    May-Grünwald s.
    metachromatic s.
    methenamine silver s.
    methyl green-pyronin s.
    modified acid-fast s.
    modified trichrome s.
    Mowry colloidal iron s.
    multiple s.
    Nair buffered methylene blue s.
    Nakanishi s.
    Nauta s.
    negative s.
    neutral s.
    Nicolle s.
    Nissl s.
    Noble s.
    nuclear s.
    Orth s.
    Papanicolaou s.
    picrocarmine s.
    port-wine s.
    positive s.
    Puchtler-Sweat s.
    Q-banding s.
    R-banding s.
    Romanowsky blood s.
    Ryan s.
    Schmorl ferric-ferricyanide
      reduction s.
    Schmorl picrothionin s.
    selective s.
    Semichon acid carmine s.
    silver-ammoniac silver s.
    silver protein s.
    supravital s.
    Taenzer s.
    Tizzoni s.
    Toison s.
    toluidine blue s.
    trichrome s.
    ultrafast Pap s.
    Unna s.
    van Ermengen s.
    van Gieson s.
    Verhoeff elastic tissue s.
    vital s.
    Weber s.
    Weigert iron hematoxylin s.
    Williams s.
    Wright s.
    Ziehl s.
staining
    progressive s.
    regressive s.
staircase phenomenon
stalagmometer
staleness

stalk
    allantoic s.
    body s.
    connecting s.
    infundibular s.
    pineal s.
    pituitary s.
    yolk s.
stammering bladder
stamping gait
stand
    Mayo s.
standard
    s. atmosphere
    s. bicarbonate
    s. deviation
    s. error of difference
    gold s.
    s. pressure
    s. solution
    s. temperature
    s. volume
standardization
standardized solution
standstill
    atrial s.
    auricular s.
    cardiac s.
Stanford-Binet intelligence scale
stannous
stannum
stapedectomy
stapedial reflex
stapediotenotomy
stapedius muscle
stapedotomy
stapes mobilization
staphylectomy
staphyledema
staphyline
staphylion
staphylococcal blepharitis
staphylococcemia
staphylococcosis
staphyloderma
staphylodermatitis
staphylodialysis
staphylokinase
staphylolysin
staphyloma
    anterior s.
    anular s.
    ciliary s.
    corneal s.
    equatorial s.
    intercalary s.
    posterior s.
    Scarpa s.
    scleral s.

staphylomatous
staphylopharyngorrhaphy
staphyloplasty
staphyloptosis
staphylorrhaphy
staphylotoxin
stapling
    gastric s.
star
    daughter s.
    lens s.'s
    polar s.
    venous s.
starch
    alant s.
    animal s.
    liver s.
    rice s.
Stargardt disease
Starling
    S. curve
    S. hypothesis
    S. reflex
startle
    s. disease
    s. epilepsy
    s. reaction
    s. reflex
starvation
    s. acidosis
    s. diabetes
stasis, pl. **stases**
    s. dermatitis
    s. dermatosis
    s. eczema
    intestinal s.
    papillary s.
    pressure s.
    s. syndrome
    urinary s.
state
    absent s.
    activated s.
    anxiety tension s.
    apallic s.
    carrier s.
    central excitatory s.
    clonic s.
    convulsive s.
    decerebrate s.
    decorticate s.
    dreamy s.

    eunuchoid s.
    excited s.
    gradient-recalled acquisition in the steady s. (GRASS)
    ground s.
    hypnoid s.
    hypnotic s.
    hypometabolic s.
    imperfect s.
    lacunar s.
    local excitatory s.
    multiple ego s.'s
    S. operation
    persistent vegetative s.
    post–steady s.
    pre-steady s.
    refractory s.
    steady s.
    tonic s.
    twilight s.
    vegetative s.
state-dependent learning
static
    s. compliance
    s. orthosis
    s. relation
    s. scoliosis
    s. symptom
statim
station
    base s.
statistics
    descriptive s.
    inferential s.
    vital s.
statoacoustic
statokinetic reflex
statolith
status
    s. asthmaticus
    s. epilepticus
    mental s.
    nonreassuring fetal s.
Stauffer syndrome
staurion
steady-rate exercise
steady state
steady-state exercise
steal
    coronary s.
    iliac s.

S

NOTES

steal (*continued*)
    subclavian s.
    s. syndrome
steapsin
stearate
    calcium s.
    erythromycin s.
stearic acid
Stearns alcoholic amentia
steatitis
steatocystoma
steatolysis
steatolytic
steatonecrosis
steatopyga, steatopygia
steatopygous
steatorrhea
    biliary s.
    intestinal s.
steatorrhoea
steatosis
    hepatic s.
Steell murmur
steeple skull
stegnosis
Steinberg thumb sign
steinstrasse
Stein test
stella, pl. **stellae**
stellate
    s. abscess
    s. block
    s. cataract
    s. cell
    s. fracture
    s. hair
    s. reticulum
    s. vein
    s. venule
stellula, pl. **stellulae**
Stellwag sign
stem
    brain s.
    s. cell
    s. cell factor
    s. cell leukemia
    infundibular s.
stenion
stenocardia
stenocephalic
stenocephalous
stenocephaly
stenochoria
Steno duct
stenopaic
stenopeic
stenosal murmur
stenosed

stenosing tenosynovitis
stenosis, pl. **stenoses**
    aortic s.
    bronchial s.
    buttonhole s.
    calcific nodular aortic s.
    congenital pyloric s.
    coronary ostial s.
    Dittrich s.
    double aortic s.
    fishmouth mitral s.
    hypertrophic pyloric s.
    idiopathic hypertrophic subaortic s.
    idiopathic subglottic s.
    infundibular s.
    laryngeal s.
    mitral s.
    pulmonary s.
    pulmonic s.
    pyloric s.
    spinal s.
    subaortic s.
    supravalvar s.
    tricuspid s.
stenostomia
stenothermal
stenothorax
stenotic
Stensen duct
stent
    s. dressing
    expandable s.
step
    Krönig s.
    Rønne nasal s.
step-down transformer
2-step exercise test
stephanial
stephanion
steppage gait
step-up transformer
stercobilin
stercolith
stercoraceous
    s. abscess
    s. vomiting
stercoral
    s. abscess
    s. colic
    s. ulcer
stercoroma
stercorous
stercus
stereoarthrolysis
stereocampimeter
stereochemical formula
stereochemistry
stereoelectroencephalography
stereoencephalometry

stereoencephalotomy
stereognosis
stereognostic
stereoisomer
stereoisomeric
stereoisomerism
stereometry
stereopathy
stereoradiography
stereoscopic
    s. microscope
    s. vision
stereoscopy
stereotactic, stereotaxic
    s. brachytherapy
    s. instrument
    s. surgery
stereotaxis
stereotaxy
stereotropic
stereotropism
stereotypy
steric
sterile cyst
sterility
    absolute s.
    aspermatogenic s.
    dysspermatogenic s.
    female s.
    male s.
    primary s.
    relative s.
    secondary s.
sterilization
    discontinuous s.
    fractional s.
    intermittent s.
sterilize
sterilizer
    glass bead s.
    hot salt s.
Stern
    S. position
    S. posture
sternal
    s. angle
    s. line
    s. muscle
    s. plane
    s. puncture
sternalgia
sternalis muscle

sternebra
sternoclavicular
    s. angle
    s. joint
sternocleidomastoid
    s. muscle
    s. region
    s. vein
sternocostal
sternodynia
sternoglossal
sternohyoid muscle
sternoid
sternomastoid muscle
sternopagia
sternopericardial
sternoschisis
sternothyroid muscle
sternotomy
    median s.
sternovertebral
sternutation
steroid
    s. acne
    anabolic s.
    androgenic s.
    s. cell tumor
    s. hormone
    s. myopathy
    s. ulcer
steroidal
steroidogenesis
sterol
stertor
    hen-cluck s.
stertorous
stethogoniometer
stethoscope
    binaural s.
    Bowles type s.
    differential s.
stethoscopic
stethoscopy
stethospasm
Stevens-Johnson syndrome
Stewart-Holmes sign
Stewart test
Stewart-Treves syndrome
sthenia
sthenic
stibialism
Stickler syndrome

S

NOTES

sticky-ended DNA
stiff
    s. man syndrome
    s. neck
    s. pupil
stiffness
    myocardial s.
stigma, pl. **stigmata**
    follicular s.
    malpighian s.
stigmal plate
stigmatic
stigmatism
stigmatization
stilbene
stilboestrol
still
    S. disease
    s. layer
    S. murmur
stillbirth
stillborn infant
stilus
stimulant
    diffusible s.
    general s.
    s. laxative
    local s.
stimulation
    caloric s.
    dorsal column s.
    fetal scalp s.
    Ganzfeld s.
    vagal nerve s.
    vagus s.
stimulator
    long-acting thyroid s.
stimulus, pl. **stimuli**
    adequate s.
    aversive s.
    conditioned s.
    s. control
    discriminant s.
    heterologous s.
    heterotopic s.
    homologous s.
    inadequate s.
    liminal s.
    maximal s.
    s. sensitive myoclonus
    threshold s.
    unconditioned s.
stinging caterpillar
stippling
    geographic s.
stirrup
stitch
    s. abscess
    lock s.

stock
    s. culture
    s. vaccine
Stocker line
Stockholm syndrome
stockinette dressing
stocking anesthesia
Stoffel operation
stoichiology
stoichiometric number
stoichiometry
Stokes
    S. amputation
    S. law
Stokes-Adams syndrome
stoma, pl. **stomas, stomata**
    s. blast
    s. button
    Fuchs s.
    loop s.
stomach
    s. ache
    bilocular s.
    cascade s.
    drain-trap s.
    dumping s.
    hourglass s.
    leather-bottle s.
    miniature s.
    s. pump
    s. tube
    water-trap s.
stomachal
stomal ulcer
stomas (*pl. of* stoma)
stomata (*pl. of* stoma)
stomatalgia
stomatitis
    allergic s.
    angular s.
    aphthous s.
    epidemic s.
    fusospirochetal s.
    gangrenous s.
    gonococcal s.
    infectious s.
    lead s.
    s. medicamentosa
    mercurial s.
    mycotic s.
    primary herpetic s.
    recurrent herpetic s.
    recurrent ulcerative s.
    ulcerative s.
    vesicular s.
stomatocytosis
stomatodynia
stomatognathic system
stomatomalacia

stomatomycosis
stomatonecrosis
stomatopathy
stomatoplastic
stomatoplasty
stomatorrhagia
stomodeal
stomodeum
stone
  artificial s.
  s. basket
  bladder s.
  s. heart
  kidney s.
  pulp s.
  tear s.
stonelike debris
Stookey-Scarff operation
stool
  butter s.
  currant jelly s.
  fatty s.
  mucous s.
  silver s.
  Trélat s.
stool-softening laxative
stop
  Krueger instrument s.
stopping rule
storage disease
storiform
storm
  thyroid s.
stove-in chest
strabismal
strabismus
  accommodative s.
  alternate day s.
  alternating s.
  A-pattern s.
  comitant s.
  concomitant s.
  convergent s.
  divergent s.
  incomitant s.
  kinetic s.
  manifest s.
  mechanical s.
  vertical s.
straight
  s. gyrus

  s. seminiferous tubule
  s. sinus
strain
  auxotrophic s.
  carrier s.
  cell s.
  congenic s.
  s. fracture
  hypothetical mean s.
  isogenic s.
  lysogenic s.
strain-counterstrain
straitjacket
straits
  dire s.
stramonium
  Datura s.
strand
  anticoding s.
  antiparallel s.
  antisense s.
  coding s.
  complementary s.
  minus s.
strangulated
  s. hemorrhoid
  s. hernia
strangulation
strangury
strap cell
strata (*pl. of* stratum)
stratification
stratified epithelium
stratigraphy
stratum, pl. **strata**
  s. basale
  s. basale epidermidis
  s. compactum
  s. corneum epidermidis
  s. functionale
  s. lucidum
  malpighian s.
  s. spinosum epidermidis
  s. spongiosum
Straus sign
straw-bed itch
strawberry
  s. cervix
  s. hemangioma
  s. mark
  s. nevus
  s. tongue

S

NOTES

straw itch
stray light
streak
    angioid s.
    s. culture
    germinal s.
    gonadal s.
    Knapp s.
    meningitic s.
    Moore lightning s.
    primitive s.
stream
    hair s.
streaming movement
street
    s. drug
    s. phobia
    s. virus
Streeter developmental horizon
strength
    associative s.
    biting s.
    compressive s.
    fatigue s.
    ionic s.
strephosymbolia
strepticemia
streptocerca
    Dipetalonema s.
streptococcal
    s. tonsillitis
    s. toxic shock syndrome
streptococcemia
streptococcic
streptococcus, pl. **streptococci**
    group A s. (GAS)
    group B s.
    hemolytic s.
    viridans s.
Streptococcus faecalis
streptokinase
streptolysin
streptosepticemia
streptozyme test
stress
    s. disorder
    s. fracture
    life s.
    s. reaction
    s. shielding
    s. test
    s. ulcer
    s. urinary incontinence
stress-broken
    s.-b. connector
    s.-b. joint

stretch
    s. receptor
    s. reflex
stria, pl. **striae**
    acoustic s.
    Amici s.
    anterior acoustic s.
    auditory s.
    Baillarger s.
    brown striae
    diagonalis s.
    Gennari s.
    intermediate acoustic s.
    Knapp s.
    Langhans s.
    lateral longitudinal s.
    malleolar s.
    medial longitudinal s.
    medullary s.
    Monakow s.
    Nitabuch s.
    terminal s.
    Wickham s.
striate
    s. body
    s. vein
striated
    s. border
    s. duct
    s. muscle
striation
    basal s.
striations
striatonigral
striatum
    Corynebacterium s.
    dorsal s.
striatus
    lichen s.
stricto
    sensu s.
stricture
    anastomotic s.
    anular s.
    bridle s.
    contractile s.
    functional s.
stricturotomy
stridor
    congenital s.
    expiratory s.
    inspiratory s.
    laryngeal s.
stridulosa
    laryngitis s.
stridulous
stridulus
    laryngismus s.

string
- auditory s.
- s. operation
- s. sign

striola

strip
- abrasive s.
- amalgam s.
- celluloid s.
- lightning s.

stripe
- Baillarger s.
- Hensen s.
- inner s.
- mallear s.
- Mees s.

stripper
- external s.
- internal s.
- intraluminal s.

stripping
- membrane s.

strobila

stroboscopic microscope

stroboscopy

stroke
- effective s.
- heart s.
- heat s.
- sun s.
- s. volume
- s. work index

stroking

stroma, pl. **stromata**
- lymphatic s.
- Rollet s.

stromal
- s. cell neoplasm
- s. corneal dystrophy
- s. keratitis

stromuhr
- Ludwig s.

strontium

strophulus

structural
- s. formula
- s. gene
- s. isomerism

structure
- accessory visual s.
- brush heap s.
- chi s.

- cointegrate s.
- complementary s.'s
- crystal s.
- denture-supporting s.
- fine s.
- gel s.
- Holliday s.
- tuboreticular s.

structured abstract

struma, pl. **strumae**
- Hashimoto s.
- ligneous s.
- s. ovarii

strumectomy

strumiform

strumipriva
- cachexia s.

strumitis

strumous abscess

Strümpell
- S. disease
- S. phenomenon
- S. reflex

struvite calculus

strychnine

strychninism

Stryker frame

ST-segment change

Stuart factor

Stuart-Prower factor

stuck-on appearance

study
- analytic s.
- blind s.
- case control s.
- cohort s.
- crossover s.
- cross-sectional s.
- diachronic s.
- double-blind s.
- ecologic s.
- flow-volume loop s.
- followup s.
- longitudinal s.
- synchronic s.

stump
- s. cancer
- s. hallucination

stupor
- benign s.
- catatonic s.
- depressive s.

S

NOTES

stupor *(continued)*
    epileptic s.
    lethargic s.
    malignant s.
stuporous melancholia
Sturm
    S. conoid
    S. interval
Sturmdorf operation
stuttering
    primary s.
    secondary s.
    urinary s.
sty
    meibomian s.
stylet
    endotracheal s.
styloglossus muscle
stylohyal
stylohyoid muscle
styloiditis
styloid process
stylomastoid
    s. artery
    s. foramen
    s. vein
stylopharyngeal muscle
stylopharyngeus muscle
stylus
styptic
subacetate
    aluminum s.
subacromial
    s. bursa
    s. bursitis
subacute
    s. bacterial endocarditis
    s. combined degeneration
    s. cystitis
    s. granulomatous thyroiditis
    s. inflammation
    s. migratory panniculitis
    s. necrotizing myelitis
    s. sclerosing panencephalitis
    s. spongiform encephalopathy
subaortic stenosis
subapical
subaponeurotic abscess
subarachnoid
    s. hemorrhage
    s. space
subarcuate fossa
subatomic
subaxial
subcallosal gyrus
subcapital fracture
subcapsular cataract
subcartilaginous

subchorial
    s. lake
    s. space
subclass
subclavian
    s. artery
    s. muscle
    s. nerve
    s. steal
    s. vein
subclavius muscle
subclinical
    s. coccidioidomycosis
    s. diabetes
subclinoid aneurysm
subconscious
subconsciousness
subcoracoid dislocation
subcortex
subcortical
subcostal
    s. artery
    s. muscle
    s. nerve
    s. plane
subcrepitant
subculture
subcutaneous
    s. emphysema
    s. flap
    s. mastectomy
    s. operation
    s. tenotomy
    s. tissue
    s. vein
subdeltoid bursa
subduce
subduct
subdural
    s. hematoma
    s. hemorrhage
    s. space
subendocardial
    s. branch
    s. layer
subendothelial layer
subendothelium
subependymoma
subfamily
subfertility
subgenus
subgingival curettage
subglenoid dislocation
subglossal
subgrundation
subhyoid pharyngotomy
subiculum
subiliac
subilium

subinfection
subinvolution
subitum
    exanthema s.
subjacent
subjective
    s. assessment data
    s. sensation
    s. sign
    s. symptom
subkingdom
sublation
sublethal
subleukemic leukemia
sublimate
    corrosive s.
sublimation
subliminal
sublingual
    s. artery
    s. cyst
    s. fossa
    s. gland
    s. nerve
    s. vein
subluxation
    arytenoid s.
submammary mastitis
submandibular
    s. duct
    s. fossa
    s. ganglion
    s. gland
    s. triangle
submaxilla
submaxillary
submental
    s. artery
    s. region
    s. vein
submentalis
    vena s.
submicroscopic
submucosa
submucosal plexus
submucous
    s. cleft palate
    s. cystitis
    s. laryngeal cleft
    s. ulcer
subnasion
subnucleus

suboccipital nerve
suboccipitobregmatic diameter
suborbital fossa
suborder
subpapillare
    rctc s.
subpapular
subparta
    ileus s.
subpectoral abscess
subperiosteal amputation
subperitoneal appendicitis
subphylum
subpleural edema
subpubic
    s. angle
    s. hernia
subsalicylate
    mercury s.
subscapular
    s. abscess
    s. artery
    s. muscle
subscapularis muscle
subscription
subsegmental atelectasis
subseptus
    hymen s.
subserosa
subsidence
subsidiary atrial pacemaker
subsigmoid fossa
substance
    s. abuse
    s. abuse disorder
    alpha s.
    anterior perforated s.
    autacoid s.
    bacteriotropic s.
    basophil s.
    basophilic s.
    blood group s.
    cementing s.
    central gray s.
    central and lateral intermediate s.'s
    chromidial s.
    chromophil s.
    compact s.
    controlled s.
    cortical s.
    s. dependence
    s. dependence disorder

S

NOTES

substance *(continued)*
    exophthalmos-producing s.
    filar s.
    gelatinous s.
    glandular s.
    gray s.
    ground s.
    H s.
    innominate s.
    Kendall s.
    medullary s.
    müllerian inhibiting s. (MIS)
    Nissl s.
    s. P
    reticular s.
    slow-reacting s.
    spongy s.
    threshold s.
    white s.
substantia, pl. substantiae
    basal s.
    s. medullaris
    s. nigra
    s. spongiosa
substantivity
substernal goiter
substitute
    blood s.
substitution
    generic s.
    s. product
    s. therapy
    s. transfusion
substrate
substrate-1
    insulin receptor s.-1
substructure
    implant denture s.
subtalar joint
subtendinous iliac bursa
subthalamic
subtraction
    s. angiography
    energy s.
subtrochanteric osteotomy
subtype
    tick-borne encephalitis Eastern s.
subungual
    s. abscess
    s. hematoma
    s. melanoma
subunguial
subunit vaccine
subvaginal
subvirion
subvocal speech
succedaneous tooth
succedaneum
    caput s.

succenturiate placenta
succinate
    active s.
    ferrous s.
succinyl-CoA
succinyl-coenzyme A
succorrhea
succubus
succussion
    hippocratic s.
    s. sound
sucking
    s. blister
    s. chest wound
sucrase
sucrose
sucrosemia
sucrosuria
suction
    s. catheter
    s. dilatation and curettage
    dilation and s.
    s. drainage
suctorial
sudamen
sudaminal
Sudan
    Ebola virus S.
    S. virus
    S. yellow
sudanophilic
sudanophobic
sudation
sudden
    s. deafness
    s. death
    s. exacerbation
    s. infant death syndrome
sudomotor
sudor
sudoral
sudoresis
sudoriferous
    s. abscess
    s. cyst
sudorific
sudoriparous abscess
suffocate
suffocation
suffocative goiter
suffusion
sugar
    amino s.
    blood s.
    brain s.
    corn s.
    deoxy s.
    desoxy s.
    fruit s.

gelatin s.
grape s.
invert s.
malt s.
manna s.
maple s.
milk s.
suggestibility
suggestible
suggestion
hypnotic s.
posthypnotic s.
suggillation
suicide
s. gene
physician-assisted s.
suis
Brucella s.
suit
anti-G s.
sulcal
sulcate
sulcatum
keratoderma plantare s.
keratolysis plantare s.
keratoma plantare s.
sulcus, pl. **sulci**
alveolobuccal s.
alveololabial s.
alveololingual s.
ampullary s.
anterior intermediate s.
anterior interventricular s.
anterior parolfactory s.
anterolateral s.
aortic s.
atrioventricular s.
basilar pontine s.
calcaneal s.
calcarine s.
callosal s.
callosomarginal s.
carotid s.
central s.
cerebellar s.
cerebral s.
s. chancre
chiasmatic s.
cingulate s.
circular s.
collateral s.
coronary s.

costophrenic s.
dorsal intermediate s.
dorsal median s.
dorsolateral s.
external spiral s.
fimbriodentate s.
gingival s.
gingivobuccal s.
gingivolabial s.
gingivolingual s.
habenular s.
hippocampal s.
hypothalamic s.
inferior frontal s.
inferior petrosal s.
inferior temporal s.
infrapalpebral s.
inner spiral s.
interatrial s.
internal spiral s.
interparietal s.
intertubercular s.
intragracile s.
intraparietal s.
labial s.
labiodental s.
lateral cerebral s.
lateral occipital s.
limiting s.
lip s.
longitudinal s.
lunate s.
malleolar s.
marginal s.
s. matricis unguis
medial s.
median s.
medullopontine s.
mentolabial s.
middle frontal s.
middle temporal s.
olfactory s.
parietooccipital s.
parolfactory sulci
postcentral s.
posterolateral s.
precentral s.
rhinal s.
scleral s.
superior temporal s.
s. test

NOTES

sulfatase
    iduronate s.
sulfate
    acid s.
    active s.
    atropine s.
    barium s.
    codeine s.
    copper s.
    cupric s.
    d-amphetamine s.
    debrisoquine s.
    dermatan s.
    dextran s.
    dextroamphetamine s.
    dodecyl s.
    dried ferrous s.
    effervescent magnesium s.
    ferric ammonium s.
    ferrous s.
    guanacline s.
    guanadrel s.
    guanochlor s.
    heparan s.
    heparitin s.
    hydroxychloroquine s.
    hyoscyamine s.
    iron s.
    isoprenaline s.
    isoproterenol s.
    keratan s.
    laminarin s.
    lobeline s.
    metaproterenol s.
    morphine s.
    s. salt of dehydroepiandrosterone (DHEAS)
sulfatidase
    cerebroside s.
sulfation
sulfhemoglobin
sulfhemoglobinemia
sulfhydryl
sulfide
    barium s.
    crude calcium s.
    hydrogen s.
    lead s.
sulfite
    exsiccated sodium s.
    s. oxidase
sulfmethemoglobin
sulfobromophthalein sodium
sulfonamide antibiotic
sulfonate
sulfone
sulfonic acid
sulfonylurea
sulfotransferase

sulfoxide
    dimethyl s.
sulfoximine
    buthionine s.
sulfur
    milk of s.
sulfur-35
sulfuric acid
sulfuryl
sulphate
    copper s.
summating potentials
summation gallop
summer
    s. acne
    s. diarrhea
Sumner sign
sump
    s. drain
    s. drainage system
    s. syndrome
sun
    s. protection factor
    s. stroke
sunburn
sundowning
sunscreen
sunstroke
superactivity
superacute
superciliary arch
supercompensation
    glycogen s.
superconducting magnet
superduct
superego
superexcitation
superficial
    s. brachial artery
    s. branch
    s. dorsal vein
    s. epigastric vein
    s. fascia
    s. flexor muscle
    s. inguinal ring
    s. investing fascia
    s. necrosis
    s. reflex
    s. transverse perineal muscle
superficialis
    anulus inguinalis s.
    arcus palmaris s.
superinduce
superinfection
superinvolution
superior
    s. alveolar nerve
    arcus dentalis s.
    arcus palpebralis s.

s. auricular muscle
s. basal vein
s. cerebellar artery
s. cerebellar peduncle
s. cerebral vein
s. constrictor muscle
s. dental arch
s. epigastric vein
s. extensor retinaculum
s. frontal gyrus
s. ganglion
s. gemellus muscle
s. labial vein
s. labrum anterior and posterior (SLAP)
s. laryngotomy
s. limbic keratoconjunctivitis
s. longitudinal fasciculus
s. macular arteriole
s. mediastinum
s. medullary velum
s. nasal concha
s. nasal retinal arteriole
s. oblique muscle
s. orbital fissure
s. pelvic aperture
s. rectus muscle
s. temporal line
s. temporal retinal arteriole
s. temporal sulcus
s. thalamostriate vein
s. vena cava
s. vena cava syndrome
s. vermian branch

superioris
musculus quadratus labii s.
superiority complex
superius
labrale s.
mediastinum s.
supermotility
supernumerary organ
superolateral
superoxide dismutase
supersaturate
supersaturated solution
superscription
supersonic
superstructure
implant denture s.
supinate

supination
rearfoot s.
supinator muscle
supplemental
s. air
s. groove
supplementary gene
support
advanced cardiac life s. (ACLS)
basic life s. (BLS)
supporting cusp
supportive therapy
suppository
glycerin s.
suppression
s. amblyopia
fixation s.
immune s.
intergenic s.
intragenic s.
missense s.
suppressive anuria
suppressor
amber s.
s. mutation
suppurate
suppurating mucocele
suppuration
suppurativa
hidradenitis s.
suppurative
s. appendicitis
s. arthritis
s. gingivitis
s. hyalitis
s. inflammation
s. mastitis
s. meningitis
s. nephritis
s. retinitis
suprabulge
supracervical hysterectomy
suprachoroid
supraciliaris
epicanthus s.
supraclavicular triangle
supraclinoid aneurysm
supracondylar process
supracostal
supracristal
supradiaphragmatic diverticulum
supraduction

NOTES

supraglottic
    s. laryngectomy
    s. swallow
supraglottitis
supraliminal
supramarginal gyrus
supramastoid crest
supramaxillary
suprameatal triangle
supranormal excitability
supranuclear paralysis
supraocclusion
supraomohyoid neck dissection
supraoptic commissure
supraorbital
    s. artery
    s. foramen
    s. margin
    s. nerve
    s. vein
supraorbitomeatal plane
suprapatellar bursa
suprapubic
    s. cystotomy
    s. prostatectomy
    s. region
suprarenal
    s. cortex
    s. gland
    s. medulla
suprarenalis
    macrogenitosomia praecox s.
suprascapular
    s. artery
    s. nerve
    s. vein
suprascleral
supraspinatus muscle
supraspinous muscle
supratrochlear
    s. artery
    s. nerve
    s. vein
supravaginal
    s. hysterectomy
    s. portion
supravalvar stenosis
supraventricular crest
supraversion
supravital stain
supreme nasal concha
sural
    s. artery
    s. nerve
    s. region
surface
    acromial articular s.
    s. anatomy
    anterior articular s.

anteroinferior s.
anterolateral s.
anterosuperior s.
approximal s.
articular s.
axial s.
balancing occlusal s.
basal s.
s. biopsy
buccal s.
cerebral s.
s. coil
colic s.
contact s.
costal s.
cuboidal articular s.
decayed, missing, and filled s.
  (DMFS)
denture basal s.
denture foundation s.
denture impression s.
denture occlusal s.
denture polished s.
diaphragmatic s.
dorsal s.
s. epithelium
external s.
facial s.
fibular articular s.
gastric s.
glenoid s.
gluteal s.
grinding s.
s. implant
incisal s.
inferior cerebral s.
inferolateral s.
infratemporal s.
interlobar s.
internal s.
interproximal s.
intestinal s.
lateral malleolar s.
lunate s.
malleolar articular s.
masticating s.
masticatory s.
maxillary s.
medial cerebral s.
mediastinal s.
mesial s.
s. microscopy
middle talar articular s.
Petzval s.
s. tension
s. thalamic vein
surfactant laxative
surgeon
    dental s.

genitourinary s.
s. knot
oral s.

surgery
ambulatory s.
aseptic s.
closed s.
conservative s.
cosmetic s.
craniofacial s.
day s.
elective s.
endolymphatic sac s.
esthetic s.
exploratory s.
functional endoscopic sinus s. (FESS)
general s.
in-and-out s.
keratorefractive s.
laparoscopic s.
laparoscopically assisted s.
left ventricular volume reduction s.
lung volume reduction s.
major s.
microscopically controlled s.
minimally invasive s.
minor s.
Mohs micrographic s.
open heart s.
oral s.
orthopedic s.
outpatient s.
palliative s.
plastic s.
radical s.
rapid in-and-out s.
reconstructive s.
same-day s.
skull base s.
stereotactic s.
ventricular reduction s.

surgical
s. abdomen
s. anatomy
s. anesthesia
s. diathermy
s. emphysema
s. intensive care unit (SICU)
s. microscope
s. pathology
s. prosthesis

s. rod
s. splint
s. vagotomy
surrogate mother
surround
acoustical s.
sursumduction
sursumversion
surveillance
immune s.
immunological s.
survey
field s.
survival
chain of s.
susceptibility cassette
suspended animation
suspension
amorphous insulin zinc s.
Coffey s.
crystalline insulin zinc s.
extended insulin zinc s.
insulin zinc s.
s. laryngoscopy
suspensoid
suspensory
s. bandage
s. ligament
s. muscle
sustained-action tablet
sustained-release tablet
sustentacular
sustentaculum
Sutton
S. disease
S. nevus
S. ulcer
sutural
s. bone
s. ligament
suture
s. abscess
absorbable surgical s.
Albert s.
alternating s.
angle s.
anterior palatine s.
apposition s.
approximation s.
atraumatic s.
back-and-forth s.
biparietal s.

S

NOTES

suture *(continued)*
black braided s.
blanket s.
braided s.
bridle s.
bunching s.
Bunnell s.
buried s.
button s.
cable wire s.
catgut s.
celluloid s.
chain s.
chromic catgut s.
circumcision s.
coaptation s.
cobbler's s.
collagen s.
compound s.
Connell s.
continuous s.
control release s.
coronal s.
cranial s.
cruciform s.
Cushing s.
cutaneous s.
cuticular s.
Czerny s.
Czerny-Lembert s.
delayed s.
dentate s.
double-button s.
doubly armed s.
Dupuytren s.
elastic s.
end-on mattress s.
epineural s.
ethmoidolacrimal s.
ethmoidomaxillary s.
Faden s.
false s.
far-and-near s.
figure-of-8 s.
fore-and-aft s.
free ligature s.
frontal s.
frontoethmoidal s.
frontolacrimal s.
frontomalar s.
frontomaxillary s.
frontonasal s.
frontozygomatic s.
Frost s.
Gély s.
glover s.
Gould s.
gridiron s.
groove s.

Gussenbauer s.
Halsted s.
harmonic s.
helical s.
horizontal mattress s.
imbricated s.
implanted s.
incisive s.
infraorbital s.
interlocking s.
intermaxillary s.
internasal s.
interpalatine s.
interparietal s.
interrupted s.
intradermal mattress s.
inverted s.
Jobert de Lamballe s.
kangaroo tendon s.
lacrimoconchal s.
lacrimomaxillary s.
lambdoid s.
Lembert s.
lens s.
s. ligature
locking s.
lock-stitch s.
malomaxillary s.
mammillary s.
mattress s.
median palatine s.
metopic s.
middle palatine s.
multifilament s.
multistrand s.
near-and-far s.
noose s.
over-and-over s.
overlapping s.'s
palatoethmoidal s.
palatomaxillary s.
Paré s.
peg-and-socket s.
pericostal s.
plane s.
plicating s.
posterior palatine s.
pulley s.
purse-string s.
relaxation s.
retention s.
right-angle mattress s.
sagittal s.
serrate s.
shotted s.
single-armed s.
squamoparietal s.
squamous s.
tendon s.

tension s.
tiger gut s.
transfixion s.
uninterrupted s.
vertical mattress s.
wedge-and-groove s.
whipstitch s.
white braided s.
zygomaticofrontal s.
zygomaticomaxillary s.
suturectomy
sutureless anastomosis
Svedberg
    S. of flotation
    S. unit
swallow
    barium s.
    Gastrografin s.
    Hypaque s.
    somatic s.
    supraglottic s.
    visceral s.
swallowing reflex
swamp fever
Swan-Ganz catheter
S wave
sweat
    s. gland
    s. gland carcinoma
    s. pore
Swedish massage
swelling
    albuminous s.
    arytenoid s.
    brain s.
    Calabar s.
    cloudy s.
    fugitive s.
    genital s.
    hunger s.
    labial s.
    labioscrotal s.
    lateral lingual s.
    levator s.
    Neufeld capsular s.
    Spielmeyer acute s.
Swift disease
swimmer's
    s. ear
    s. itch
swimming pool conjunctivitis

swing
    mood s.
swing-to gait
Swiss-cheese hyperplasia
switch
    class s.
switching
    class s.
    s. site
Swyer-James syndrome
Swyer syndrome
sycoma
sycosiform
sycosis
    lupoid s.
    tinea s.
Sydenham chorea
Sylvest disease
sylvian seizure
Sylvius
    fissure of S.
    fossa of S.
symballophone
symbion
symbiont
symbiosis
    dyadic s.
symbiote
symbiotic
symblepharon
symbolism
symbolization
symbrachydactyly
Syme
    S. amputation
    S. operation
symmetrical gangrene
symmetric fetal growth restriction
symmetry
    inverse s.
sympathectomy
    chemical s.
    periarterial s.
    presacral s.
sympathetic
    s. amine
    s. ganglion
    s. nerve
    s. nervous system
    s. ophthalmia
    s. symptom

NOTES

sympathetic *(continued)*
    s. trunk
    s. uveitis
sympathetoblast
sympathicoblast
sympathicolytic
sympathicomimetic
sympathicotonia
sympathicotonic
sympathicotripsy
sympathoadrenal
sympathoblast
sympathogonia
sympatholytic
sympathomimetic amine
symphalangism
symphalangy
symphyseotomy
symphyses (*pl. of* symphysis)
symphysial, symphyseal
symphysion
symphysiotomy
symphysis, pl. **symphyses**
    intervertebral s.
    mandibular s.
    manubriosternal s.
    mental s.
    pericardial s.
    pubic s.
sympodia
symport
symptom
    abstinence s.
    accessory s.
    accidental s.
    acute on chronic s.'s
    assident s.
    Baumès s.
    Bolognini s.
    cardinal s.
    characteristic s.
    s. complex
    concomitant s.
    consecutive s.
    constellation of s.'s
    constitutional s.
    conversion s.
    dearth of s.'s
    deficiency s.
    delayed s.
    direct s.
    Epstein s.
    equivocal s.
    factitious s.
    first rank s.'s (FRS)
    Fischer s.
    fundamental s.
    general s.
    Gordon s.

    guiding s.
    incarceration s.
    indirect s.
    induced s.
    local s.
    localizing s.
    Macewen s.
    negative s.
    objective s.
    pathognomonic s.
    positive s.
    Pratt s.
    precursor s.
    premonitory s.
    presenting s.
    prodromal s.
    rational s.
    reflex s.
    Schneider first rank s.'s
    signal s.
    static s.
    subjective s.
    sympathetic s.
    systemic s.
    Trendelenburg s.
    Wartenberg s.'s
    withdrawal s.'s
symptomatic
    s. porphyria
    s. pruritus
    s. reaction
    s. treatment
symptomatica
    alopecia s.
symptomatology
symptomatolytic
symptosis
sympus
    acephalus s.
synanamorph
synapse
    axoaxonic s.
    axodendritic s.
    axosomatic s.
    electrotonic s.
synapsis
synaptic
    s. cleft
    s. conduction
    s. vesicle
synaptinemal complex
synaptosome
synarthrodia
synarthrodial joint
synarthrophysis
synarthrosis
syncanthus
syncephalus
syncephaly

syncheiria
synchondrodial joint
synchondroseotomy
synchondrosis
    anterior intraoccipital s.
    arycorniculate s.
    cranial s.
synchondrotomy
synchronia
synchronic study
synchronism
synchronized intermittent mandatory
  ventilation
synchronous
synchrony
    bilateral s.
synchysis scintillans
synclitic
synclitism
synclonus
syncopal
syncope
    Adams-Stokes s.
    cardiac s.
    carotid sinus s.
    deglutition s.
    hysterical s.
    laryngeal s.
    local s.
    micturition s.
    postural s.
    tussive s.
    vasodepressor s.
    vasovagal s.
syncopic
syncytial knot
syncytiotrophoblast
syncytium
syndactylia, syndactylism, syndactyly
syndactylous
syndesis
syndesmectomy
syndesmectopia
syndesmitis
syndesmodial
syndesmopexy
syndesmophyte
syndesmoplasty
syndesmorrhaphy
syndesmosis
syndesmotic
syndesmotomy

syndrome
    Aagenaes s.
    Aarskog-Scott s.
    abdominal muscle deficiency s.
    abstinence s.
    Achard s.
    Achard-Thiers s.
    Achenbach s.
    acquired immunodeficiency s.
    (AIDS)
    acrofacial s.
    acroparesthesia s.
    acute organic brain s.
    acute radiation s.
    acute respiratory distress s.
    (ARDS)
    Adams-Stokes s.
    addisonian s.
    adherence s.
    Adie s.
    adiposogenital s.
    adrenal cortical s.
    adrenal virilizing s.
    adrenogenital s.
    adult respiratory distress s. (ARDS)
    afferent loop s.
    aglossia-adactylia s.
    Ahumada-del Castillo s.
    Aicardi s.
    Alagille s.
    Albright s.
    alcohol amnestic s.
    Aldrich s.
    Alice in Wonderland s.
    Allen-Masters s.
    Allgrove s.
    Alport s.
    Alström s.
    amenorrhea-galactorrhea s.
    amnesic s.
    amnionic band s.
    amnionic fluid s.
    Amsterdam s.
    androgen insensitivity s.
    androgen resistance s.
    Angelman s.
    Angelucci s.
    angioosteohypertrophy s.
    ankyloglossia superior s.
    anorectal s.
    anterior chamber cleavage s.
    anterior tibial compartment s.

NOTES

S

syndrome *(continued)*

antibody deficiency s.
antiphospholipid antibody s.
Anton s.
anxiety s.
aortic arch s.
apallic s.
Apert s.
Arnold-Chiari s.
arterial thoracic outlet s.
Ascher s.
Asherman s.
asplenia s.
ataxia telangiectasia s.
auriculotemporal nerve s.
autoerythrocyte sensitization s.
Avellis s.
AV strabismus s.
Ayerza s.
Babinski s.
baby bottle s.
bacterial overgrowth s.
Balint s.
Bamberger-Marie s.
Bannwarth s.
Banti s.
Bardet-Biedl s.
bare lymphocyte s.
Barlow s.
Barrett s.
Bart s.
Barth s.
Bartter s.
basal cell nevus s.
Bassen-Kornzweig s.
battered child s.
battered spouse s.
Bauer s.
Bazex s.
Beckwith-Wiedemann s.
Behçet s.
Behr s.
Benedikt s.
Beradinelli s.
Berardinelli s.
Bernard-Horner s.
Bernard-Sergent s.
Bernard-Soulier s.
Bernhardt-Roth s.
Bernheim s.
Besnier-Boeck-Schaumann s.
Beuren s.
Biemond s.
billowing mitral valve s.
Björnstad s.
Blatin s.
blind loop s.
Bloch-Sulzberger s.
Bloom s.

blue diaper s.
blue toe s.
Boerhaave s.
Bonnet-Dechaume-Blanc s.
Bonnier s.
Böök s.
Börjeson-Forssman-Lehmann s.
bowel bypass s.
Bradbury-Eggleston s.
bradytachycardia s.
branchiootorenal s.
Briquet s.
Brissaud-Marie s.
Brock s.
bronze baby s.
Brown s.
Brown-Séquard s.
Budd s.
Budd-Chiari s.
Bürger-Grütz s.
burner s.
Burnett s.
burning foot s.
burning mouth s.
burning tongue s.
burning vulva s.
Buschke-Ollendorf s.
Caffey s.
Caffey-Kempe s.
Caffey-Silverman s.
camptomelic s.
Capgras s.
Caplan s.
carbonic anhydrase II deficiency s.
carcinoid s.
cardiofacial s.
Caroli s.
carotid sinus s.
carpal tunnel s.
Carpenter s.
cataract-oligophrenia s.
cat-cry s., cat's cry s.
cat's-eye s.
cauda equina s.
cavernous sinus s.
Ceelen-Gellerstedt s.
celiac s.
cellular immunity deficiency s.
central cord s.
cerebellar s.
cerebellomedullary malformation s.
cerebellopontine angle s.
cerebrohepatorenal s.
cervical compression s.
cervical disc s.
cervical fusion s.
cervical rib s.
cervical tension s.
cervicooculoacoustic s.

Cestan-Chenais s.
chancriform s.
Chandler s.
Charcot s.
Charcot-Weiss-Baker s.
Chauffard s.
Chédiak-Higashi s.
Chédiak-Steinbrinck-Higashi s.
Cheney s.
cherry-red spot myoclonus s.
Chiari-Budd s.
Chiari-Frommel s.
Chiari II s.
chiasma s.
Chilaiditi s.
CHILD s.
Chinese restaurant s.
Chotzen s.
Christian s.
chromosomal breakage s.
chromosomal instability s.
chronic brain s.
chronic fatigue s.
chronic hyperventilation s.
Churg-Strauss s.
Cianca s.
Clarke-Hadfield s.
classic cervical rib s.
Claude s.
click s.
climacteric s.
clitoral engorgement s.
cloverleaf skull s.
Cobb s.
Cockayne s.
Coffin-Lowry s.
Coffin-Siris s.
Cogan s.
Cogan-Reese s.
cold agglutinin s.
Collet-Sicard s.
combined immunodeficiency s.
compartment s.
complete androgen insensitivity s.
compression s.
congenital rubella s.
Conn s.
Conradi-Hünermann s.
Cornelia de Lange s.
Costen s.
costochondral s.
costoclavicular s.

Cotard s.
Crandall s.
CREST s.
cri-du-chat s., cri du chat syndrome
Crigler-Najjar s.
crocodile tears s.
Cronkhite-Canada s.
Crouzon s.
Crow-Fukase s.
crush s.
Cruveilhier-Baumgarten s.
cryptophthalmus s.
cubital tunnel s.
Cushing s.
cutaneomucouveal s.
Dandy-Walker s.
dead arm s.
dead fetus s.
dead-in-bed s.
Debré-Sémélaigne s.
de Clerambault s.
Degos s.
Dejerine-Klumpke s.
Dejerine-Roussy s.
de Lange s.
Del Castillo s.
de Morsier s.
dengue shock s.
Denys-Drash s.
depersonalization s.
depressive s.
dermatitis-arthritis-tenosynovitis s.
De Sanctis-Cacchione s.
dialysis disequilibrium s.
dialysis encephalopathy s.
Diamond-Blackfan s.
diencephalic s.
Di Ferrante s.
DiGeorge s.
Di Guglielmo s.
disc s.
disconnection s.
disputed neurogenic thoracic
  outlet s.
distal intestinal obstructive s.
Donath-Landsteiner s.
Donohue s.
Doose s.
Dorfman-Chanarin s.
dorsal midbrain s.
Down s.
Dressler s.

S

NOTES

syndrome *(continued)*

dry eye s.
Duane s.
Dubin-Johnson s.
Dubreuil-Chambardel s.
dumping s.
Duncan s.
Dyggve-Melchior-Clausen s.
dysarthria–clumsy hand s.
dyskinesia s.
dysmnesic s.
dysplastic nevus s.
Eagle-Barrett s.
early dumping s.
Eaton-Lambert s.
ectopic ACTH s.
ectrodactyly–ectodermal
  dysplasia–clefting s.
Edwards s.
egg-white s.
Ehlers-Danlos s. (EDS)
Eisenmenger s.
Ekbom s.
elfin facies s.
Ellis-van Creveld s.
E-M s.
EMG s.
encephalotrigeminal vascular s.
eosinophilia-myalgia s.
episodic dyscontrol s.
erythrodysesthesia s.
euthyroid sick s.
Evans s.
exfoliation s.
extrapyramidal s.
Faber s.
false memory s.
familial aortic ectasia s.
familial chylomicronemia s.
Fanconi s.
FAPA s.
Farber s.
Favre-Racouchot s.
Felty s.
fetal alcohol s.
fetal aspiration s.
fetal face s.
fetal hydantoin s.
fetal trimethadione s.
fetal warfarin s.
fibrinogen-fibrin conversion s.
fibromyalgia s.
Fiessinger-Leroy-Reiter s.
fifth digit s.
first arch s.
Fisher s.
Fitz-Hugh and Curtis s.
flashing pain s.
flecked retina s.

floppy valve s.
Flynn-Aird s.
Foix-Alajouanine s.
Foix-Cavany-Marie s.
folded-lung s.
Forbes-Albright s.
Foster Kennedy s.
Foville s.
fragile X s.
Fraley s.
Franceschetti s.
Franceschetti-Jadassohn s.
Fraser s.
Freeman-Sheldon s.
Frey s.
Friderichsen-Waterhouse s.
Fröhlich s.
Froin s.
Fuchs s.
functional prepubertal castration s.
G s.
Gaisböck s.
Ganser s.
Gardner s.
Gardner-Diamond s.
gastrocardiac s.
gastrojejunal loop obstruction s.
gay bowel s.
Gélineau s.
gender dysphoria s.
general adaptation s.
Gerstmann s.
Gerstmann-Sträussler-Scheinker s.
Gianotti-Crosti s.
Gilbert s.
Gilles de la Tourette s.
Gillespie s.
Gitelman s.
glucagonoma s.
Goldenhar s.
Goldmann-Favre s.
gold-myokymia s.
Goltz s.
Goodpasture s.
Gopalan s.
Gorham s.
Gorlin s.
Gorlin-Chaudhry-Moss s.
Gougerot-Carteaud s.
Gowers s.
gracilis s.
Gradenigo s.
gray baby s.
Greig cephalopolysyndactyly s.
Grönblad-Strandberg s.
Gubler s.
Guillain-Barré s.
Gulf War s.
Gunn s.

gustatory sweating s.
Guyon tunnel s.
Haber s.
Hallermann-Streiff s.
Hallermann-Streiff-François s.
Hallervorden s.
Hallervorden-Spatz s.
Hallgren s.
Hamman s.
Hamman-Rich s.
hand-and-foot s.
hand-foot s.
Hanhart s.
hantavirus pulmonary s.
happy puppet s.
Harada s.
Harris s.
Hartnup s.
Hayem-Widal s.
head-bobbing doll s.
Hegglin s.
HELLP s.
Helweg-Larssen s.
hemolytic uremic s.
Henoch-Schönlein s.
hepatonephoric s.
hepatonephric s.
hepatorenal s.
Herlitz s.
Hermansky-Pudlak s.
heroin overdose s.
Herrmann s.
Hinman s.
HIV wasting s.
holiday heart s.
Holmes-Adie s.
Holt-Oram s.
Horner s.
Houssay s.
Houston-Harris s.
Hughes-Stovin s.
Hunt s.
Hunter s.
Hurler s.
Hurler-Scheie s.
Hutchinson-Gilford s.
Hutchison s.
hyaline membrane s.
hydralazine s.
hyperabduction s.
hyperactive child s.
hypereosinophilic s.

hyper-IgM s.
hyperimmunoglobulin E s.
hyperkinetic heart s.
hypersensitive xiphoid s.
hyperventilation s.
hyperviscosity s.
hypometabolic s.
hypoparathyroidism s.
hypophysial s.
hypophysiosphenoidal s.
hypoplastic left heart s.
iliotibial band friction s.
Imerslünd-Grasbeck s.
immotile cilia s.
immune dysfunction s.
immunodeficiency s.
impingement s.
indifference to pain s.
infection-associated
  hemophagocytic s. (IAHS)
infertile male s.
inspissated bile s.
internal capsule s.
inversed jaw-winking s.
iridocorneal endothelial s.
iris-nevus s.
irritable bowel s.
Irvine-Gass s.
Isaac s.
Isaac-Merton s.
Ivemark s.
Jadassohn-Lewandowski s.
Jahnke s.
jaw-winking s.
Jeghers-Peutz s.
Jervell and Lange-Nielsen s.
Jeune s.
Job s.
Johanson-Blizzard s.
Joubert s.
jugular foramen s.
Kallmann s.
Kanner s.
Kartagener s.
Kasabach-Merritt s.
Kast s.
Katayama s.
Kawasaki s.
Kearns-Sayre s.
Kennedy s.
Kenny-Caffey s.
Kimmelstiel-Wilson s.

S

NOTES

syndrome *(continued)*

Kleine-Levin s.
Klinefelter s.
Klippel-Feil s.
Klippel-Trenaunay-Weber s.
Klüver-Bucy s.
Kniest s.
Kobberling-Dunnigan s.
Kocher-Debré-Sémélaigne s.
Koenig s.
Koerber-Salus-Elschnig s.
Kohlmeier-Degos s.
Korsakoff s.
Kostmann s.
Kuskokwim s.
Laband s.
Lady Windemere's s.
Lambert s.
Lambert-Eaton s.
Landau-Kleffner s.
Landry s.
Landry-Guillain-Barré s.
Langer-Saldino s.
Larsen s.
Lasègue s.
late dumping s.
lateral medullary s.
Launois-Bensaude s.
Launois-Cléret s.
Laurence-Moon s.
Lawrence-Seip s.
Lejeune s.
Lenègre s.
Lennox s.
Lennox-Gastaut s.
LEOPARD s.
Leriche s.
Leri-Weill s.
Lermoyez s.
Lesch-Nyhan s.
Lev s.
Libman-Sacks s.
Li-Fraumeni cancer s.
liver kidney s.
locked-in s.
loculation s.
Loeffler s. I, II
Löffler s.
long QT s.
Lorain-Lévi s.
Louis-Bar s.
Lowe s.
Lowe-Terrey-MacLachlan s.
Lown-Ganong-Levine s.
low salt s.
low sodium s.
lupus-like s.
Lutembacher s.
Lyell s.

lymphoproliferative s.
Lynch s.
Macleod s.
Mad Hatter s.
Maffucci s.
Magendie-Hertwig s.
malabsorption s.
malignant carcinoid s.
malignant mole s.
Mallory-Weiss s.
mandibulofacial dysotosis s.
mandibulo-oculofacial s.
Marchiafava-Micheli s.
Marcus Gunn s.
Marfan s.
Marie-Robinson s.
Marine-Lenhart s.
Marinesco-Garland s.
Marinesco-Sjögren s.
marker X s.
Maroteaux-Lamy s.
Marshall s.
Martin-Bell s.
Martorell s.
MASS s.
massive bowel resection s.
maternal deprivation s.
Mauriac s.
Mayer-Rokitansky-Küster-Hauser s.
May-White s.
McArdle s.
McCune-Albright s.
Meadows s.
Meckel s.
Meckel-Gruber s.
meconium aspiration s.
meconium blockage s.
megacystic s.
megacystitis-megaureter s.
megacystitis-microcolon-intestinal
    hypoperistalsis s.
Meigs s.
Meischer s.
Melkersson-Rosenthal s.
Melnick-Needles s.
Ménétrier s.
Ménière s.
Menkes s.
menopausal s.
Meretoja s.
metastatic carcinoid s.
Meyenburg-Altherr-Uehlinger s.
Meyer-Betz s.
middle lobe s.
Mikulicz s.
milk-alkali s.
Milkman s.
Millard-Gubler s.
minimal-change nephrotic s.

Mirizzi s.
mitral valve prolapse s.
Möbius s.
Mohr s.
Monakow s.
monofixation s.
Morgagni s.
Morton s.
mucocutaneous lymph node s.
multiple endocrine deficiency s.
multiple mucosal neuroma s.
myasthenic s.
myelodysplastic s.
myeloproliferative s.
Naegeli s.
Nance-Insley s.
Nelson s.
nephritic s.
nephrotic s.
Netherton s.
neural crest s.
neuroleptic malignant s.
Noack s.
Noonan s.
Nothnagel s.
numb chin s.
Ogilvie s.
Oldfield s.
Olmsted s.
Omenn s.
Opitz BBB s.
Opitz G s.
organic brain s.
overtraining s.
overuse s.
Pancoast s.
pancreatorenal s.
paraneoplastic s.
Parenti-Fraccaro s.
Parinaud oculoglandular s.
Parkes Weber s.
patellofemoral stress s.
Pendred s.
Pfeiffer s.
Picchini s.
pickwickian s.
Pierre Robin s.
pigment dispersion s.
Pins s.
placental transfusion s.
Plummer-Vinson s.
Poland s.

polycystic ovary s.
postadrenalectomy s.
postcommissurotomy s.
postconcussion s.
posterior leukoencephalopathy s.
postgastrectomy s.
postinfarction s.
postlumbar puncture s.
postmalaria neurologic s.
postpericardiotomy s.
postpolio s.
postpoliomyelitis s.
posttraumatic s.
Potter s.
preexcitation s.
premenstrual s.
pronator teres s.
pseudoexfoliation s.
pulmonary dysmaturity s.
punchdrunk s.
Putnam-Dana s.
radial tunnel s.
radiation s.
Raeder paratrigeminal s.
Ramsay Hunt s.
Raynaud s.
Reifenstein s.
Reiter s.
Renpenning s.
respiratory distress s. (RDS)
Rett s.
Reye s.
Rh null s.
Richter s.
Rieger s.
Roaf s.
Robin s.
Robinow s.
Rothmund s.
Rotor s.
Rud s.
Russell s.
Samter s.
Sanfilippo s.
scalded mouth s.
scapulocostal s.
Scheie s.
Schmidt s.
Schnitzler s.
Schüller s.
Seip s.
sepsis s.

S

NOTES

syndrome *(continued)*
    Sertoli-cell-only s.
    shaken baby s.
    Sheehan s.
    Shone s.
    short bowel s.
    short gut s.
    shoulder-girdle s.
    Shy-Drager s.
    sicca s.
    sick building s.
    Silverskiöld s.
    Sinding-Larsen-Johansson s.
    Sipple s.
    Sjögren s.
    snapping hip s.
    Sneddon s.
    Sorsby s.
    Sotos s.
    Spens s.
    stasis s.
    Stauffer s.
    steal s.
    Stevens-Johnson s.
    Stewart-Treves s.
    Stickler s.
    stiff man s.
    Stockholm s.
    Stokes-Adams s.
    streptococcal toxic shock s.
    sudden infant death s.
    sump s.
    superior vena cava s.
    Swyer s.
    Swyer-James s.
    systemic capillary leak s.
    tachycardia-bradycardia s.
    Tapia s.
    Taussig-Bing s.
    tegmental s.
    temporomandibular joint pain-dysfunction s.
    Terry s.
    Terson s.
    testicular feminization s.
    Thiemann s.
    thoracic outlet s.
    Thorn s.
    thrombocytopenia-absent radius s.
    Tietz s.
    Tietze s.
    TMJ s.
    Tolosa-Hunt s.
    Tornwaldt s.
    Torre s.
    Tourette s.
    toxic shock s.
    transfusion s.
    Treacher Collins s.
    trisomy 21 s.
    trophic s.
    tropical splenomegaly s.
    Trousseau s.
    Turner s.
    Ullmann s.
    ulnar nerve compression s.
    ulnar tunnel s.
    uncombable hair s.
    Usher s.
    uveoencephalitic s.
    VACTERL s.
    van Buchem s.
    van der Hoeve s.
    vanishing lung s.
    Van Lohuizen s.
    Vernet s.
    voice fatigue s.
    wasting s.
    Waterhouse-Friderichsen s.
    Weber s.
    Wermer s.
    Werner s.
    Wernicke s.
    Wernicke-Korsakoff s.
    West s.
    Williams s.
    Williams-Beuren s.
    Wissler s.
    withdrawal s.
    Wolff-Parkinson-White s.
    Wolfram s.
    Wright s.
    Wyburn-Mason s.
    X-linked lymphoproliferative s.
    XO s.
    XXY s.
    XYY s.
    Zollinger-Ellison s.

syndromic
synechia, pl. **synechiae**
    anular s.
synechiotomy
synencephalocele
syneresis
synergism
synergist
synergistic muscle
synergy
synesthesia
synesthesialgia
syngamy
syngeneic
syngenesis
syngenetic
syngraft
synizesis
synkaryon
synkinesis

synkinetic
synonychia
synophthalmia
synorchidism
synorchism
synoscheos
synostosis
    sagittal s.
synostotic
synotia
synovectomy
    radiopharmaceutical s.
synovial
    s. bursa
    s. cavity
    s. crypt
    s. cyst
    s. fluid
    s. hernia
    s. joint
    s. ligament
    s. membrane
    s. sheath
synovioma
synovitis
    bursal s.
    chronic hemorrhagic villous s.
    dry s.
    filarial s.
    pigmented villonodular s.
    purulent s.
    serous s.
    s. sicca
    simple s.
    tendinous s.
    transient s.
synovium
syntenic
synteny
synthase
    glutamate s.
    glycine s.
    glycogen s.
    glycogen starch s.
    holo-ACP s.
    lactose s.
    malate s.
synthesis, pl. **syntheses**
    activity s.
    enzymatic s.
    Kiliani-Fischer s.

    Merrifield s.
    s. period
synthesize
synthetase
    acetyl-CoA s.
    acyl-CoA s.
    butyryl-CoA s.
    cholyl-coenzyme A s.
    dodecanoyl-CoA s.
    holocarboxylase s.
synthetic sentence identification
syntonic
syntrophoblast
syntropic
syntropy
    inverse s.
syphilid
syphilis
    cardiovascular s.
    congenital s.
    early latent s.
    endemic s.
    hereditary s.
    late benign s.
    late latent s.
    latent s.
    meningovascular s.
    primary s.
    secondary s.
    tertiary s.
syphilitic
    s. aneurysm
    s. endocarditis
    s. laryngitis
    s. leukoderma
    s. neuritis
    s. roseola
syphilitica
    alopecia s.
syphiloma
syringadenoma
syringe
    air s.
    chip s.
    control s.
    Davidson s.
    dental s.
    fountain s.
    hypodermic s.
    Luer s.
    Luer-Lok s.
    probe s.

S

NOTES

syringe *(continued)*
    ring s.
    rubber-bulb s.
syringectomy
syringes (*pl. of* syrinx)
syringitis
syringoadenoma
syringobulbia
syringocarcinoma
syringocele
syringocystadenoma
syringocystoma
syringoma
    chondroid s.
syringomeningocele
syringomyelia
syringomyelocele
syringotomy
syrinx, pl. **syringes**
syrup
    ipecac s.
system
    absorbent s.
    aerobic s.
    alimentary s.
    anterolateral s.
    arch-loop-whorl s.
    association s.
    autonomic nervous s.
    Bethesda s.
    blood group s.'s
    blood-vascular s.
    2-bottle drainage s.
    3-bottle drainage s.
    bulbosacral s.
    cardiovascular s.
    caudal neurosecretory s.
    centimeter-gram-second s.
    central auditory nervous s.
    central nervous s. (CNS)
    cerebrospinal s.
    chromaffin s.
    circulatory s.
    closed water-seal drainage s.
    collecting s.
    colloid s.
    complement s.
    continuous suction drainage s.
    craniosacral nervous s.
    cytochrome P-450 s.
    digestive s.
    ecological s.
    electron-transport s.
    EMS s.
    endocrine s.
    endomembrane s.
    esthesiodic s.
    exterofective s.
    extrapyramidal motor s.

    feedback s.
    foot-pound-second s.
    French-American-British
      classification s.
    Galton s.
    gamma motor s.
    gated s.
    genital s.
    genitourinary s.
    geographic information s.
    glandular s.
    haversian s.
    health information s.
    hematopoietic s.
    hepatic portal s.
    heterogeneous s.
    hexaxial reference s.
    His-Tawara s.
    homogeneous s.
    hypophyseoportal s.
    hypophysial portal s.
    hypophysioportal s.
    hypothalamohypophysial portal s.
    hypoxia warning s.
    immediate energy s.
    immune s.
    incident command s.
    incident management s.
    indicator s.
    information s.
    integumentary s.
    intermediary s.
    interofective s.
    involuntary nervous s.
    kallikrein s.
    kinetic s.
    limbic s.
    lymphatic s.
    lymphoid s.
    masticatory s.
    metameric nervous s.
    meter-kilogram-second s.
    metric s.
    mononuclear phagocyte s.
    movement s.
    nervous s.
    ossicular s.
    peripheral nervous s.
    Pinel s.
    portal s.
    postural drainage s.
    properdin s.
    prospective payment s.
    renin-angiotensin-aldosterone s.
    reticular activating s.
    review of s.'s (ROS)
    stomatognathic s.
    sump drainage s.
    sympathetic nervous s.

tidal drainage s.
trauma care s.
urogenital s.
vacuum drainage s.
vascular s.
water seal drainage s.

systematized delusion
systemic
s. anaphylaxis
s. arterial pressure (SAP)
s. capillary leak syndrome
s. circulation
s. death
s. lesion
s. lupus erythematosus (SLE)
s. scleroderma

s. symptom
s. vascular resistance

systole
aborted s.
atrial s.
auricular s.
electrical s.
electromechanical s.
late s.
premature s.

systolic
s. murmur
s. pressure
s. reserve
s. thrill
s. time interval

NOTES

S

θ (*var. of* theta)
τ (*var. of* tau)
T
    T antigen
    T cytotoxic cell
    T helper subset 1, 2 cell
    T lymphocyte
    Ortho-Kung T (OKT)
    T tubule
    T wave
tabanid
tabes
    t. dorsalis
    t. mesenterica
tabescent
tabetic
    t. arthropathy
    t. neurosyphilis
tabetiform
tablature
table
    Aub-DuBois t.
    contingency t.
    examining t.
    Gaffky t.
    internal t.
    life t.
tablespoon
tablet
    buccal t.
    compressed t.
    dispensing t.
    enteric coated t.
    hypodermic t.
    sustained-action t.
    sustained-release t.
taboparesis
tabular
tache
tachetic
tachometer
tachyarrhythmia
tachycardia
    atrial chaotic t.
    atrioventricular junctional t.
    auricular t.
    AV junctional t.
    bidirectional ventricular t.
    Coumel t.
    double t.
    ectopic t.
    essential t.
    fetal t.
    junctional t.
    multifocal atrial t. (MAT)

    nodal t.
    orthostatic t.
    paroxysmal t.
    t. window
tachycardia-bradycardia syndrome
tachycardiac
tachycrotic
tachypnea
tachyrhythmia
tachysterol
tachysystole
tackler's exostosis
tactile
    t. agnosia
    t. anesthesia
    t. corpuscle
    t. defensiveness
    t. fremitus
    t. hallucination
    t. hypoesthesia
    t. image
    t. meniscus
    t. papilla
tactometer
tactual
tactus
    meniscus t.
taeniorhynchus
    Aedes t.
Taenzer stain
tag
    anal skin t.
    epiploic t.
    sentinel t.
    skin t.
    triage t.
tail
    t. bud
    t. fold
    t. of pancreas
4-tailed
    4-t. bandage
    4-t. dressing
Taiwan Dobrava-Belgrade virus
Takayasu arteritis
talar
talc operation
talcosis
talipedic
talipes
    t. calcaneovalgus
    t. calcaneovarus
    t. calcaneus
    t. cavus
    t. equinovalgus

T

talipes *(continued)*
    t. equinovarus
    t. equinus
    t. planus
    t. valgus
    t. varus
talocalcaneal joint
talocalcaneonavicular joint
talocrural joint
talofibular ligament
talon
talonavicular articulation
talonid
tambour
    bruit de t.
Tamm-Horsfall mucoprotein
tampon
    Corner t.
    nasal t.
tamponade
    balloon t.
    cardiac t.
    chronic t.
    heart t.
tamponage
tandem gait
tangentiality
tangible body macrophage
tank
    Hubbard t.
Tanner
    T. growth chart
    T. operation
    T. stage
tannic acid
Tansini operation
tantalum
tantrum
tap
    heel t.
    mitral t.
    pleural t.
    spinal t.
tape
    adhesive t.
tapering-off
tapetum
tapeworm
Tapia syndrome
tapir mouth
tapotement
tapping
    pressure t.
tar
    birch t.
    coal t.
    juniper t.
tarantula
    American t.

    black t.
    European t.
tarda
    osteogenesis imperfecta t.
    porphyria cutanea t.
    spondyloepiphyseal dysplasia t.
Tardieu
    T. ecchymosis
    T. petechia
    T. spot
tardive
    cyanose t.
    t. cyanosis
    t. psychosis
tardus
    pulsus t.
target
    t. cell
    t. gland
    t. heart rate
    t. heart rate range
    t. lesion
    t. organ
    t. response
Tarlov cyst
Tarnier forceps
tarry cyst
tarsal
    t. bone
    t. cyst
    t. gland
    t. joint
    t. sinus
tarsalgia
tarsalis
    epicanthus t.
tarsectomy
tarsitis
tarsoclasia
tarsoclasis
tarsomalacia
tarsomegaly
tarsometatarsal
    t. joint
    t. ligament
tarsophalangeal
tarsorrhaphy
tarsotomy
tarsus
    inferior t.
tartar
    cream of t.
tart cell
tartrate
    acid t.
    dihydrocodeine t.
    levallorphan t.
    levorphanol t.
    metoprolol t.

tastant
taste
    t. bud
    t. cell
    color t.
    franklinic t.
    t. hair
    t. receptor
tattoo
    amalgam t.
tau, τ
    interferon t.
taurocholic acid
Taussig-Bing syndrome
Taussig-Morton operation
Taussig operation
tautomeric fiber
tautomerism
taxane
taxonomic
taxonomy
    chemical t.
Tay cherry-red spot
Taylor disease
Tay-Sachs disease
T-binder
T-cell receptor
T-cell–rich, B-cell lymphoma
tea
    Hottentot t.
    Jesuit t.
    Mexican t.
teaching hospital
Teale amputation
tear
    artificial t.'s
    bucket-handle .t.
    crocodile t.'s
    t. gas
    horizontal t.
    longitudinal t.
    Mallory-Weiss t.
    parrot's beak t.
    retinal t.
    t. sac
    t. stone
teardrop cell
technetium
technetium-99m
technician
    cardiac care t.
    cardiac rescue t.

    emergency medical t. (EMT)
    pulmonary function t.
technique
    airbrasive t.
    air-gap t.
    atrial-well t.
    ballpoint pen t.
    Barcroft-Warburg t.
    Begg light wire differential
      force t.
    cellulose tape t.
    direct t.
    enzyme-multiplied immunoassay t.
      (EMIT)
    Ficoll-Hypaque t.
    flicker fusion frequency t.
    fluorescent antibody t.
    flush t.
    Hampton t.
    Hartel t.
    high-kV t.
    Ilizarov t.
    immunoperoxidase t.
    indirect t.
    Jerne t.
    Judkins t.
    Kleihauer-Betke t.
    Knott t.
    long cone t.
    McGoon t.
    Merendino t.
    microetching t.
    Mohs fresh tissue chemosurgery t.
    muscle energy t.
    Ouchterlony t.
    PAP t.
    rebreathing t.
    Seldinger t.
    vacuum pack t.
technologist
    nuclear medicine t.
    pulmonary function t.
    radiologic t.
technology
    assisted reproductive t.
tecta
    zona t.
tectal
tectocephaly
tectonic keratoplasty
tectorial membrane
tectorium

T

NOTES

tectospinal tract
tectum of midbrain
TED
    thromboembolic disease
      TED hose
teeth (*pl. of* tooth)
teething
tegmen mastoideum
tegmental
    t. decussation
    t. nucleus
    t. syndrome
tegmentum, pl. tegmenta
    mesencephalic t.
    midbrain t.
    rhombencephalic t.
tegument
tegumental
tegumentary
Teichmann crystal
teichoic acid
teichopsia
telangiectasia
    ataxia t.
    calcinosis, Raynaud phenomenon,
      esophageal motility disorder,
      sclerodactyly, and t. (CREST)
    cephalooculocutaneous t.
    essential t.
    hereditary benign t.
    hereditary hemorrhagic t.
    spider t.
telangiectasis
telangiectatic
    t. angioma
    t. fibroma
    t. granuloma
    t. osteogenic sarcoma
    t. wart
telangiectatica
    livedo t.
telangiectodes
    elephantiasis t.
    neuroma t.
telangiosis
telecanthus
telediagnosis
telegraphic speech
telemetry
    cardiac t.
telencephalic flexure
teleomitosis
teleopsia
teleorganic
telepathy
telephone ear
teleradiography
teleradiology
telergy

teleroentgenography
telescope
    Hopkins rod-lens t.
teletherapy
television microscopy
telluric
tellurium
telodendron
telogen effluvium
telolecithal
telomere
telophase
temperament
temperance
temperate bacteriophage
temperature
    absolute t.
    basal body t.
    body t.
    core t.
    critical t.
    effective t.
    equivalent t.
    eutectic t.
    maximum t.
    mean t.
    melting t.
    t. midpoint
    minimum t.
    normal t.
    standard t.
tempolabile
temporal
    t. arteritis
    t. bone
    t. fossa
    t. hemianopia
    t. lobe
    t. lobe epilepsy
    t. muscle
    t. plane
    t. pole
    t. process
    t. region
temporalis
    fossa t.
    t. muscle
temporary
    t. cartilage
    t. denture
    t. parasite
    t. threshold shift
    t. tooth
temporomandibular
    t. disorder
    t. joint (TMJ)
    t. joint dysfunction
    t. joint pain-dysfunction syndrome
    t. nerve

temporomaxillary
temporoparietalis muscle
temporoparietal muscle
temporopontine
  t. fiber
  t. tract
tempostabile
tempostable
tenacious
tenacity
  cellular t.
tenaculum forceps
tenalgia
tenant
  locum t.
tenax
  Trichomonas t.
tenderness
  costovertebral angle t. (CVAT)
  rebound t.
tender point
tendinea
  inscriptio t.
tendineae
  chordae t.
  false chordae t.
tendineus
  arcus t.
tendinis
tendinitis
tendinoplasty
tendinosuture
tendinous
  t. arch
  t. cord
  t. sheath
  t. synovitis
tendolysis
tendon
  Achilles t.
  calcaneal t.
  t. cell
  central t.
  conjoined t.
  conjoint t.
  coronary t.
  cricoesophageal t.
  Gerlach annular t.
  hamstring t.
  heel t.
  t. recession
  t. reflex

  t. sheath
  t. suture
  t. tucker
tendonitis
  calcific t.
tendoplasty
tendosynovitis
tendotomy
tendovaginal
tendovaginitis
tenectomy
tenens
  locum t.
tenesmic
tenesmus
ten Horn sign
tenia, pl. teniae
  colic teniae
  free t.
  medullary teniae
  mesocolic t.
teniacide
tenial
teniasis
tennis
  t. elbow
  t. thumb
tenodynia
tenolysis
tenomyoplasty
tenomyotomy
Tenon capsule
tenonectomy
tenonitis
tenontitis
tenontodynia
tenontomyoplasty
tenontoplasty
tenophyte
tenoplasty
tenoreceptor
tenorrhaphy
tenositis
tenostosis
tenosuspension
tenosuture
tenosynovectomy
tenosynovitis
  adhesive t.
  de Quervain t.
  localized nodular t.
  pigmented villonodular t.

T

NOTES

tenosynovitis *(continued)*
    stenosing t.
    villous t.
tenotomy
    curb t.
    fenestrated t.
    graduated t.
    open t.
    subcutaneous t.
tenovaginitis
tension
    arterial t.
    t. curve
    t. headache
    interfacial surface t.
    myocardial t.
    ocular t.
    t. pneumopericardium
    t. pneumothorax
    premenstrual t.
    surface t.
    t. suture
    tissue t.
tension-type headache
tensor
    t. fasciae latae muscle
    t. tympani muscle
    t. tympani reflex
    t. veli palati muscle
tentacle
tenth cranial nerve
tentorial
    t. basal branch
    t. sinus
tentorium
    cerebellar t.
tenue
    Eubacterium t.
tenuis
    meninx t.
    pannus t.
teratic
teratism
teratoblastoma
teratocarcinoma
teratogen
teratogenesis
teratogenetic
teratogenic
teratogenicity
teratoid tumor
teratologic
teratology
teratoma
    adult t.
    anaplastic malignant t.
    benign cystic t.
    cystic t.
    differentiated t.

    immature t.
    malignant t.
    mature t.
    sacrococcygeal t.
    solid t.
    trophoblastic malignant t.
    undifferentiated malignant t.
teratomatous
teratosis
    atresic t.
    ceasmic t.
    ectogenic t.
    ectopic t.
    hypergenic t.
teratozoospermia
terbium
teres
    t. major muscle
    t. minor muscle
terminal
    t. artery
    axon t.
    t. bar
    t. boutons
    t. bronchiole
    carboxy t.
    t. dementia
    t. deoxynucleotidyl transferase
    t. disinfection
    t. duct carcinoma
    t. filum
    t. hair
    t. hinge position
    t. ileitis
    t. infection
    t. latency
    t. line
    t. nerve
    t. nucleus
    t. sinus
    t. stria
terminale
    filum t.
terminalis
    bronchiolus t.
termination
    t. codon
    t. signal
terminaux
    bouton t.
terminoterminal anastomosis
terminus
    C t.
    N t.
terms
    hierarchy of t.
ternary
terreus
    Aspergillus t.

Terrien marginal degeneration
territoriality
territorial matrix
terrors
    night t.
Terry syndrome
Terson syndrome
tertian
    double t.
tertiary
    t. alcohol
    t. amine
    t. care
    t. dentin
    t. syphilis
    t. vitreous
tessellated fundus
test
    acetone t.
    achievement t.
    acidified serum t.
    acid perfusion t.
    acid reflux t.
    acoustic stimulation t.
    ACTH stimulation t.
    Addis t.
    adhesion t.
    Adler t.
    Adson t.
    agglutination t.
    Albarran t.
    alkali denaturation t.
    Allen t.
    Allen-Doisy t.
    Alpha t.
    alternate binaural loudness
     balance t.
    alternate cover t.
    alternating light t.
    Ames t.
    Amsler t.
    Anderson-Collip t.
    Anderson and Goldberger t.
    anoxemia t.
    anterior apprehension t.
    antibiotic sensitivity t.
    antiglobulin t.
    antihuman globulin t.
    antithrombin t.
    Apt t.
    aptitude t.
    Army alpha t.

    Army beta t.
    Ascoli t.
    ascorbate-cyanide t.
    association t.
    Astwood t.
    atropine t.
    augmented histamine t.
    aussage t.
    autohemolysis t.
    Bachman t.
    Bachman-Pettit t.
    Bagolini t.
    Bárány caloric t.
    Barlow t.
    Bauer-Kirby t.
    belt t.
    Bender Visual Motor Gestalt t.
    Benedict t.
    bentiromide t.
    bentonite flocculation t.
    benzidine t.
    Bernstein t.
    Berson t.
    Beta t.
    Betke-Kleihauer t.
    Bettendorff t.
    Bial t.
    bile acid tolerance t.
    bile esculin t.
    bile solubility t.
    binaural alternate loudness
     balance t.
    Binet t.
    bithermal caloric t.
    biuret t.
    blind t.
    block design t.
    Bonney t.
    breath t.
    breath-holding t.
    Brigg t.
    bromphenol t.
    bromsulphalein t.
    BSP t.
    butanol-extractable iodine t.
    California psychological inventory t.
    Calmette t.
    caloric t.
    cancer antigen 125 t.
    capillary fragility t.
    capillary resistance t.
    carbohydrate utilization t.

T

NOTES

test *(continued)*

carotid sinus t.
Carr-Price t.
Casoni intradermal t.
Casoni skin t.
Chick-Martin t.
chi-square t.
Clauberg t.
clonidine growth hormone
  stimulation t.
coccidioidin t.
coin t.
cold bend t.
cold pressor t.
colloidal gold t.
complement-fixation t.
contraction stress t.
Coombs t.
Corner-Allen t.
cover t.
cover-uncover t.
CO2-withdrawal seizure t.
Crampton t.
crank t.
cutaneous tuberculin t.
cyanide-nitroprusside t.
cytotropic antibody t.
DA pregnancy t.
Day t.
D-dimer t.
Dehio t.
dehydrocholate t.
Denver Developmental Screening T.
dexamethasone suppression t.
Dick t.
differential renal function t.
differential ureteral catheterization t.
dilute Russell's viper venom t.
dinitrophenylhydrazine t.
direct Coombs t.
direct fluorescent antibody t.
discontinuation t.
Doerfler-Stewart t.
double-blind t.
Dragendorff t.
drawer t.
Ducrey t.
Dugas t.
Duke bleeding time t.
dye disappearance t.
dye exclusion t.
Ebbinghaus t.
Ellsworth-Howard t.
E-rosette t.
erythrocyte adherence t.
erythrocyte fragility t.
exercise stress t.
FANA t.
Farnsworth-Munsell color t.

fern t.
ferric chloride t.
Finckh t.
finger-nose t.
finger-to-finger t.
Finkelstein t.
Fishberg concentration t.
Fisher exact t.
fistula t.
FIT t.
Fleitmann t.
flocculation t.
fluorescein instillation t.
fluorescein string t.
fluorescent antinuclear antibody t.
fluorescent treponemal antibody-
  absorption t.
foam stability t.
Folin t.
Folin-Looney t.
formol-gel t.
Fosdick-Hansen-Epple t.
Foshay t.
fragility t.
Frei t.
FTA-ABS t.
functional t.
fusion-inferred threshold t.
Gaddum and Schild t.
galactose tolerance t.
gel diffusion precipitin t.
Gellé t.
Gerhardt t.
germ tube t.
2-glass t.
3-glass t.
glucose oxidase paper strip t.
glucose tolerance t.
glycerol dehydration t.
Gmelin t.
Gofman t.
Goldscheider t.
Goodenough draw-a-man t.
goodness of fit t.
Göthlin t.
graded exercise t.
Graham-Cole t.
group t.
guaiac t.
Günzberg t.
Guthrie t.
Gutzeit t.
Ham t.
Hardy-Rand-Ritter t.
Harrington-Flocks t.
Harris and Ray t.
head-dropping t.
heat coagulation t.
heat instability t.

heel-tap t.
heel-to-knee-to-toe t.
heel-to-shin t.
Heinz body t.
hemadsorption virus t.
hemagglutination t.
Hemoccult t.
Hering t.
Hershberg t.
Hines-Brown t.
Hinton t.
Hirschberg t.
Histalog t.
histamine t.
histoplasmin-latex t.
Hollander t.
Holmgren wool t.
homovanillic acid t.
Howard t.
Huhner t.
hyperventilation t.
hypoxemia t.
immune adhesion t.
immunologic pregnancy t.
impingement t.
indirect Coombs t.
indirect fluorescent antibody t.
indirect hemagglutination t.
indole t.
inkblot t.
insulin hypoglycemia t.
intelligence t.
intradermal t.
iodine t.
Ishihara t.
131I uptake t.
Ivy bleeding time t.
Jacquemin t.
Jaffe t.
Janet t.
Jolles t.
Jones t.
Jones I, II t.
Katayama t.
ketogenic corticoids t.
Knoop hardness t.
Kober t.
Kolmer t.
Korotkoff t.
Krimsky t.
Kurzrok-Ratner t.
Kveim t.

Kveim-Siltzbach t.
Lachman t.
Lancaster red green t.
Landsteiner-Donath t.
Lange t.
latex agglutination t.
latex fixation t.
LE cell t.
Legal t.
leishmanin t.
lepromin t.
leukocyte adherence assay t.
leukocyte bactericidal assay t.
leukocyte esterase t.
Liebermann-Burchard t.
line t.
lipase t.
Lombard voice-reflex t.
Lücke t.
lupus band t.
lupus erythematosus cell t.
Machado-Guerreiro t.
Maclagan thymol turbidity t.
macrophage migration inhibition t.
Mantel-Haenszel t.
Mantoux t.
Marshall t.
Marshall-Marchetti t.
Master 2-step exercise t.
maximal Histalog t.
Mazzotti t.
McMurray t.
McNemar t.
McPhail t.
t. meal
Meinicke t.
Meltzer-Lyon t.
metabisulfite t.
methacholine challenge t.
methylene blue t.
metrotrophic t.
MHA-TP t.
microhemagglutination-*Treponema pallidum* t.
microprecipitation t.
migration inhibition t.
migration inhibitory factor t.
milk-ring t.
Millon-Nasse t.
Minnesota Multiphasic Personality Inventory t.
mixed agglutination t.

T

NOTES

test *(continued)*
    mixed lymphocyte culture t.
    Molisch t.
    Moloney t.
    monocyte function t.
    Mörner t.
    multiple puncture tuberculin t.
    Nagel t.
    neutralization t.
    nitroprusside t.
    nonstress t.
    Ober t.
    oxytocin challenge t.
    Pachon t.
    Pap t.
    parallax t.
    patch t.
    Patrick t.
    Perthes t.
    photo-patch t.
    Pirquet t.
    plasmacrit t.
    postcoital t.
    precipitin t.
    primary dye t.
    t. profile
    progesterone challenge t.
    protection t.
    prothrombin t.
    pulmonary function t. (PFT)
    pulp t.
    Queckenstedt-Stookey t.
    quellung t.
    Quick t.
    radioallergosorbent t.
    radioimmunosorbent t.
    Rapoport t.
    relocation t.
    Rinne t.
    rubella HI t.
    Schick t.
    Schiller t.
    Schilling t.
    Schober t.
    scratch t.
    screening t.
    secondary dye t.
    secretin t.
    sedimentation t.
    serologic t.
    shadow t.
    sickling t.
    skin t.
    sniff t.
    Snyder t.
    solubility t.
    t. solution
    spot t.
    Spurling t.
    staggered spondaic word t.
    Stein t.
    2-step exercise t.
    Stewart t.
    streptozyme t.
    stress t.
    sulcus t.
    thematic apperception t.
    Thompson t.
    Thormählen t.
    thyrotropin-releasing hormone
      stimulation t.
    tilt t.
    tine t.
    tolbutamide t.
    Trendelenburg t.
    TRH stimulation t.
    t. tube
    tuberculin t.
    t. type
    vitality t.
    Weil-Felix t.
    Western blot t.
    whiff t.
    Whitaker t.
testalgia
testectomy
testes (*pl. of* testis)
testicle
testicular
    t. artery
    t. cord
    t. feminization syndrome
    t. tubule
testing
    bedside t.
    bench t.
    competence t.
    contrast sensitivity t.
    genetic t.
    histocompatibility t.
    limit t.
    proficiency t.
    reality t.
testis, pl. **testes**
    abdominal t.
    cryptorchid t.
    ectopia t.
    ectopic t.
    mediastinum t.
    obstructed t.
    peeping t.
    perineal t.
    retained t.
    tunica vaginalis t.
    undescended t.
testitis
testosterone
testotoxicosis

test-tube baby
tetani
    Clostridium t.
tetanic
tetaniform
tetanigenous
tetanism
tetanization
tetanize
tetanode
tetanoid
tetanospasmin
tetanus
    acoustic t.
    benign t.
    cathodal opening t. (COTe)
    cephalic t.
    cerebral t.
    complete t.
    drug t.
    generalized t.
    incomplete t.
    intermittent t.
    local t.
    t. neonatorum
    puerperal t.
    Ritter opening t.
    toxic t.
    t. toxin
    traumatic t.
tetany
    duration t.
    gastric t.
    hyperventilation t.
    hypoparathyroid t.
    infantile t.
    manifest t.
    neonatal t.
    parathyroid t.
tetrachloride
    carbon t.
tetracrotic
tetracycline antibiotic
tetrad
    Fallot t.
tetradactyl
tetraethyl
    lead t.
tetralogy
    Eisenmenger t.
    t. of Fallot
tetrameric

tetramerous
tetranitrate
    erythrityl t.
    erythrol t.
tetraparesis
tetrapeptide
tetraphosphate
    adenosine t.
tetraplegia
tetraploid
tetrasaccharide
tetrasomic
tetravalent
tetrose
tetroxide
    lead t.
text blindness
textiform
textural
texture
thalamencephalon
thalami (*pl. of* thalamus)
thalamic peduncle
thalamocortical
thalamostriate vein
thalamotomy
    parafascicular t.
thalamus, pl. thalami
    dorsal t.
thalassemia, thallasanemia
    A2 t.
    F t.
    Lepore t.
    t. major
    t. minor
thallic
thallium
thanatobiologic
thanatognomonic
thanatoid
thanatology
Thayer-Martin agar
theca
    t. cordis
    t. folliculi
thecal
thecitis
thecoma
Theden method
Theile canal
Theiler mouse encephalomyelitis virus
thelarche

NOTES

theleplasty
thelium
thelorrhagia
thematic apperception test
thenar
t. eminence
t. space
theophyllinate
choline t.
theophylline
mersalyl t.
theorem
Bernoulli t.
central limit t.
Gibbs t.
theory
adsorption t.
aerodynamic t.
Altmann t.
Arrhenius-Madsen t.
atomic t.
Baeyer t.
balance t.
beta-oxidation-condensation t.
Bohr t.
Brønsted t.
Burn and Rand t.
Cannon t.
Cannon-Bard t.
catastrophe t.
cellular immune t.
chaos t.
chemiosmotic t.
cloacal t.
clonal deletion t.
clonal selection t.
cognitive dissonance t.
darwinian t.
decay t.
dipole t.
Ehrlich t.
5-element t.
emergency t.
Flourens t.
Frerichs t.
Freud t.
game t.
gastrea t.
gate-control t.
germ layer t.
gestalt t.
Haeckel gastrea t.
Helmholtz-Gibbs t.
Hering t.
humoral t.
hydrate microcrystal t.
incasement t.
information t.
instructive t.

kern-plasma relation t.
Knoop t.
Ladd-Franklin t.
lamarckian t.
learning t.
libido t.
Liebig t.
lipoid t.
mass action t.
membrane expansion t.
Metchnikoff t.
Meyer-Overton t.
miasma t.
Miller chemicoparasitic t.
mnemic t.
molecular dissociation t.
Ollier t.
omega-oxidation t.
Planck t.
quantum t.
recapitulation t.
scientific t.
side-chain t.
somatic mutation t.
Spitzer t.
traveling wave t.
van't Hoff t.
Warburg t.
Young-Helmholtz t.
therapeutic
t. abortion
t. crisis
t. drug
t. index
t. malaria
t. orthosis
t. radiology
t. range
t. ratio
t. ultrasound
therapist
athletic t.
physical t.
respiratory t.
therapy
adjuvant t.
aerosol t.
alimentary t.
alkali t.
analytic t.
anticoagulant t.
antisense t.
autoserum t.
aversion t.
behavior t.
client-centered t.
cognitive t.
cold t.
compression t.

conditioning t.
conjoint t.
convulsive t.
craniosacral t.
cytoreductive t.
depot t.
diathermic t.
directly observed t.
electroconvulsive t. (ECT)
electroshock t.
electrotherapeutic sleep t.
estrogen replacement t.
extended family t.
family t.
fast-neutron radiation t.
fever t.
foreign protein t.
functional orthodontic t.
gene t.
geriatric t.
gestalt t.
helium t.
heterovaccine t.
hormone replacement t. (HRT)
hyperbaric oxygen t.
implosive t.
individual t.
inhalation t.
insulin coma t.
interstitial t.
intralesional t.
light t.
maintenance drug t.
marital t.
marriage t.
massage t.
microwave t.
milieu t.
myofunctional t.
neoadjuvant t.
occupational t. (OT)
osteopathic manipulative t.
photodynamic t.
photoradiation t.
physical t.
play t.
polarity t.
psychoanalytic t.
radiation t.
rational t.
reflex zone t.
replacement t.

respiratory t.
shock t.
substitution t.
supportive t.
thrombolytic t.
Time-Line t.
tongue thrust t.
transtracheal oxygen t.
thermal
    t. anesthesia
    t. artifact
    t. burn
    t. capacity
thermalgesia
thermalgia
thermanalgesia
thermanesthesia
thermesthesia
thermesthesiometer
thermic anesthesia
thermionic emission
thermoanalgesia
thermoanesthesia
thermochemistry
thermocoagulation
thermocouple
thermodiffusion
thermoduric
thermodynamics
thermoesthesia
thermoesthesiometer
thermoexcitory
thermogenesis
    nonshivering t.
    shivering t.
thermogenetic
thermogenic
thermogram
thermograph
thermography
    infrared t.
    liquid crystal t.
thermoinhibitory
thermolabile
thermoluminescent dosimeter
thermolysis
thermolytic
thermomassage
thermometer
    air t.
    axilla t.
    axillary t.

NOTES

T

thermometer *(continued)*
>black globe t.
>bulb t.
>clinical t.
>differential t.
>gas t.
>resistance t.
>self-registering t.
>wet-bulb t.

thermometric
thermometry
thermophil, thermophile
thermophilic
thermophore
thermoreceptor
thermoregulation
thermostabile
thermostable
thermosteresis
thermotactic, thermotaxic
thermotaxis
thermotherapy
thermotonometer
thermotropism
theta, θ
>t. rhythm
>t. wave

thetaiotamicron
>*Bacteroides* t.

thiamin
thiazide
thiazin dye
thick-layer autoradiography
thickness
>Breslow t.

Thiemann syndrome
thienylalanine
Thiersch canaliculus
thigh
>Heilbronner t.

thigmesthesia
thigmotaxis
thigmotropism
thinking
>abstract t.
>archaic-paralogical t.
>concrete t.
>creative t.
>magical t.
>prelogical t.
>t. through

thin-layer chromatography
thin section
thiocyanoacetate
>isobornyl t.

thioglucose
>gold t.

thiokinase
>acetate t.
>fatty acid t.

thiolase
>acetoacetyl-CoA t.
>acetyl-CoA t.

thiosulfuric acid
third
>t. cranial nerve
>t. disease
>t. heart sound
>t. molar
>t. peroneal muscle
>t. toe
>t. ventricle
>t. ventriculostomy

third-degree
>t.-d. burn
>t.-d. prolapse

third-party payer
thirst
>false t.
>insensible t.

Thiry fistula
thixolabile
thixotropic
thixotropy
Thoma
>T. ampulla
>T. fixative
>T. law

Thomas
>T. operation
>T. splint

Thompson test
Thomsen disease
Thomson sign
thoracalgia
thoracentesis
thoraces (*pl. of* thorax)
thoracic
>t. aorta
>t. cage
>t. cardiac nerve
>t. cavity
>t. duct
>t. kyphosis
>t. longissimus muscle
>t. outlet syndrome
>t. spinal nerve
>t. spine
>t. splenosis
>t. vertebra
>t. wall

thoracica
>kyphosis t.

thoracici
>arcus ductus t.

thoracoabdominal incision

thoracoacromial
  t. artery
  t. vein
thoracoceloschisis
thoracocentesis
thoracocyllosis
thoracocyrtosis
thoracodorsal
  t. artery
  t. nerve
thoracodynia
thoracoepigastric vein
thoracogastroschisis
thoracolumbar fascia
thoracolumbosacral orthosis
thoracolysis
thoracometer
thoracomyodynia
thoracoplasty
  conventional t.
thoracoschisis
thoracoscope
thoracoscopy
thoracostenosis
thoracosternotomy
  transverse t.
thoracostomy
thoracotomy
  anterior t.
  axillary t.
  clamshell t.
  t. incision
  muscle-sparing t.
  posterolateral t.
thorax, pl. **thoraces**
  amazon t.
  barrel-shaped t.
  Peyrot t.
  pyriform t.
thorium
Thormählen test
thorn
  dendritic t.
  T. syndrome
thought
  t. disorder
  trend of t.
threaded implant
threadworm
thready pulse
threatened abortion
threonine

threshold
  absolute t.
  achromatic t.
  acoustic reflex t.
  auditory t.
  brightness difference t.
  convulsant t.
  differential t.
  displacement t.
  double-point t.
  fibrillation t.
  fusion-inferred t. (FIT)
  galvanic t.
  lactate t.
  light differential t.
  t. limit value
  minimum light t.
  speech awareness t.
  speech detection t.
  speech reception t.
  t. stimulus
  t. substance
  t. trait
  ventilatory t.
thrill
  aneurysmal t.
  aortic t.
  diastolic t.
  hydatid t.
  presystolic t.
  systolic t.
thrive
  failure to t.
throat
  clergyman's sore t.
  ears, nose, and t. (ENT)
  eye, ear, nose, and t. (EENT)
  hospital sore t.
  septic sore t.
  sore t.
  ulcerated sore t.
thrombasthenia
  Glanzmann t.
  hereditary hemorrhagic t.
thrombectomy
thrombi (*pl. of* thrombus)
thrombin
  human t.
thromboangiitis obliterans
thromboarteritis
thromboasthenia
thromboclastic

T

NOTES

thrombocyst
thrombocystis
thrombocyte
thrombocythemia
thrombocytic series
thrombocytopathy
thrombocytopenia
  autoimmune neonatal t.
  essential t.
  immune t.
  isoimmune neonatal t.
thrombocytopenia-absent radius syndrome
thrombocytopenic purpura
thrombocytopoiesis
thrombocytosis
thromboelastogram
thromboelastograph
thromboembolic disease (TED)
thromboembolism
thromboendarterectomy
thrombogenic
thromboid
thrombokinase
thrombolymphangitis
thrombolysis
thrombolytic therapy
thrombon
thrombopathy
  constitutional t.
thrombopenia
thrombopenic purpura
thrombophilia
thrombophlebitis
thromboplastid
thromboplastin
thrombopoiesis
thrombopoietin
thrombosed hemorrhoid
thrombosis, pl. thromboses
  agonal t.
  arterial t.
  atrophic t.
  cerebral t.
  compression t.
  coronary t.
  creeping t.
  deep venous t.
  dilation t.
  effort-induced t.
  intracardiac t.
  marantic t.
  marasmic t.
  mesenteric t.
  mural t.
  traumatic t.
thrombospondin-related adhesive protein
thrombostasis
thrombotic thrombocytopenic purpura

thromboxane
thrombus, pl. thrombi
  agglutinative t.
  agonal t.
  antemortem t.
  ball t.
  ball-valve t.
  bile t.
  currant jelly t.
  fibrin t.
  globular t.
  hyaline t.
  infective t.
  laminated t.
  marantic t.
  marasmic t.
  mixed t.
  mural t.
  obstructive t.
  organized t.
  parietal t.
  saddle t.
  septic t.
  traumatic t.
  valvular t.
through
  t. drainage
  thinking t.
  working t.
throughput
thrush esophagitis
thrust
  tongue t.
thumb
  bifid t.
  bowler's t.
  t. forceps
  gamekeeper's t.
  hitchhiker t.
  tennis t.
  trigger t.
thunderclap headache
thymectomy
  extended t.
  maximal t.
  transcervical t.
thymi (*pl. of* thymus)
thymic
  t. alymphoplasia
  t. aplasia
  t. corpuscle
  t. vein
thymicolymphatic
thymidine
thymine
thyminuria
  hyperuracil t.
thymitis
thymocyte

thymogenic
thymokinetic
thymoma
thymoprival
thymoprivic
thymoprivous
thymus, pl. thymi
    cortex thymi
    t. gland
thyroaplasia
thyroarytenoid muscle
thyrocardiac disease
thyrocele
thyrocervical trunk
thyroepiglottic muscle
thyroepiglottidean muscle
thyrogenic
thyrogenous
thyroglobulin
thyroglossal
thyrohyal
thyrohyoideus
    musculus t.
thyrohyoid muscle
thyroid
    t. bruit
    t. cartilage
    t. crisis
    t. follicle
    t. gland
    t. pyramid
    t. storm
thyroidal hernia
thyroidectomy
thyroiditis
    autoimmune t.
    chronic atrophic t.
    chronic fibrous t.
    chronic lymphadenoid t.
    chronic lymphocytic t.
    de Quervain t.
    focal lymphocytic t.
    giant cell t.
    giant follicular t.
    Hashimoto t.
    ligneous t.
    lymphocytic t.
    Riedel t.
    subacute granulomatous t.
thyroid-stimulating
    t.-s. hormone
    t.-s. immunoglobulin

thyroliberin
thyromegaly
thyronine
thyroparathyroidectomy
thyropriva
    cachexia t.
thyroprival
thyroptosis
thyrotomy
thyrotoxic crisis
thyrotoxicosis
    apathetic t.
thyrotroph
thyrotrophin
thyrotropic, thyrotrophic
thyrotropin
thyrotropin-releasing
    t.-r. hormone (TRH)
    t.-r. hormone stimulation test
thyroxin
thyroxine
    labeled t.
thyrse
    en t.
TIA
    transient ischemic attack
tibia, pl. tibiae
    saber t.
    t. valga
    t. vara
tibial
    t. collateral ligament
    t. malleolus
    t. nerve
    t. spine
tibialis
    t. anterior muscle
    t. posterior muscle
tic
    blinking t.
    bowing t.
    convulsive t.
    degenerative t.
    t. douloureux
    facial t.
    glossopharyngeal t.
    habit t.
    local t.
tick
    t. fever
    t. paralysis
    t. typhus

T

NOTES

tick-borne
    t.-b. encephalitis Eastern subtype
    t.-b. encephalitis virus
tidal
    t. air
    t. drainage
    t. drainage system
    t. volume
tide
    acid t.
    alkaline t.
    fat t.
    red t.
Tietze syndrome
Tietz syndrome
tiger gut suture
tight junction
tilt
    pantoscopic t.
    t. test
tilting
    t. disc valve
    t. disc valve prosthesis
time
    activated clotting t. (ACT)
    activated partial thromboplastin t.
      (aPTT)
    t. agnosia
    AH conduction t.
    association t.
    biologic t.
    bleeding t.
    circulation t.
    clot retraction t.
    clotting t.
    coagulation t.
    doubling t.
    euglobulin clot lysis t.
    fading t.
    filter bleeding t.
    forced expiratory t. (FET)
    HR conduction t.
    HV conduction t.
    inertia t.
    interatrial conduction t.
    intraatrial conduction t.
    kaolin clotting t.
    left ventricular ejection t. (LVET)
    PA conduction t.
    partial thromboplastin t. (PTT)
    PH conduction t.
    prothrombin t.
    reaction t.
    relaxation t.
    repetition t.
    Russell's viper venom clotting t.
    tissue thromboplastin inhibition t.
    total breathing cycle t.
    turnaround t.

Time-Line therapy
tinctorial
tincture
    alcoholic t.
    ammoniated t.
    belladonna t.
    digitalis t.
    ethereal t.
    glycerinated t.
    green soap t.
    hydroalcoholic t.
    iodine t.
tinea
    t. barbae
    t. capitis
    t. circinata
    t. corporis
    t. cruris
    t. imbricata
    t. kerion
    t. pedis
    t. sycosis
    t. unguium
    t. versicolor
Tinel sign
tine test
tinnitus
    clicking t.
    Leudet t.
    nervous t.
    objective t.
    vibratory t.
tip pinch
tissue
    adenoid t.
    adipose t.
    areolar t.
    bone t.
    bronchus-associated lymphoid t.
      (BALT)
    brown adipose t.
    cancellous t.
    cardiac muscle t.
    cartilaginous t.
    cavernous t.
    chondroid t.
    chromaffin t.
    connective t.
    t. culture
    dartoic t.
    elastic t.
    epithelial t.
    erectile t.
    fatty t.
    fibrohyaline t.
    fibrous t.
    Gamgee t.
    gelatinous t.
    gingival t.

granulation t.
gut-associated lymphoid t. (GALT)
Haller vascular t.
hard t.
hemopoietic t.
indifferent t.
interstitial t.
investing t.
islet t.
t. lymph
lymphatic t.
lymphoid t.
mesenchymal t.
mesonephric t.
metanephrogenic t.
mucosa-associated lymphoid t.
  (MALT)
mucous connective t.
muscular t.
myeloid t.
osseous t.
t. plasminogen activator (TPA, t-
  PA, tPA)
t. respiration
reticular t.
retiform t.
subcutaneous t.
t. tension
t. thromboplastin inhibition time
tissue-specific antigen
titration
colorimetric t.
formol t.
titubating tremor
titubation
Tizzoni stain
T-lymphocyte antigen receptor
TMJ
temporomandibular joint
  TMJ syndrome
TNM
tumor node metastasis
  TNM staging
toast
bananas, rice cereal, applesauce, t.
  (BRAT)
tobacco
t. abuse
t. heart
tobacco-alcohol amblyopia
tocainide hydrochloride
tocodynagraph

tocodynamometer
tocography
tocolytic
tocopherol
Todd postepileptic paralysis
toe
t. drop brace
fourth t.
great t.
hammer t.
little t.
Morton t.
second t.
third t.
turf t.
toe-drop
toenail
ingrowing t.
togavirus
toilet
pulmonary t.
Toison stain
Toker cell
tolbutamide test
Toldt membrane
tolerance
acoustic t.
cross t.
t. dose
frustration t.
high dose t.
immunologic high dose t.
impaired glucose t.
individual t.
t. limit
tolerant
tolerize
tolerogenic
Tolosa-Hunt syndrome
toluidine blue stain
Toma sign
tomentum cerebri
Tommaselli disease
tomogram
tomograph
tomography
computed t. (CT)
computerized axial t. (CAT)
conventional t.
dynamic computed t.
electron beam t. (EBT)
helical computed t.

NOTES

T

tomography *(continued)*
    high-resolution computed t. (HRCT)
    hypocycloidal t.
    panoramic t.
    positron emission t.
    single photon emission computed t.
    ultrasonic t.
    wide-angle t.

tone
    affective t.
    emotional t.
    feeling t.
    fetal heart t.
    fundamental t.
    heart t.'s
    muscle t.
    pure t.
    Traube double t.

tongue
    amyloid t.
    baked t.
    bald t.
    bifid t.
    black hairy t.
    burning t.
    cleft t.
    coated t.
    t. crib
    dotted t.
    fissured t.
    furred t.
    geographic t.
    grooved t.
    hairy t.
    hobnail t.
    lobulated t.
    magenta t.
    mandibular t.
    strawberry t.
    t. thrust
    t. thrust therapy

tongue-swallowing
tongue-tie
tonic
    bitter t.
    t. contraction
    t. convulsion
    t. epilepsy
    t. neck reflex
    t. pupil
    t. spasm
    t. state

tonicity
tonicoclonic
tonoclonic spasm
tonofibril
tonofilament
tonograph
tonography

tonometer
    applanation t.
    Gärtner t.
    Goldmann applanation t.
    Mackay-Marg t.
    Mueller electronic t.
    pneumatic t.

tonometry
tonoplast
tonotopic
tonotropic
tonsil
    cerebellar t.
    eustachian t.
    faucial t.
    Gerlach t.
    laryngeal t.
    lingual t.
    Luschka t.
    palatine t.
    pharyngeal t.

tonsillar
    t. crypt
    t. fossa
    t. hernia

tonsillary
tonsillectomy
tonsillitis
    lacunar t.
    preglottic t.
    pustular t.
    streptococcal t.
    Vincent t.

tonsillolith
tonsillotomy
tonsilolith
tonus
    baseline t.

tooth, pl. **teeth**
    acoustic t.
    acrylic resin t.
    anatomic t.
    ankylosed t.
    anterior t.
    auditory teeth
    baby t.
    back t.
    bicuspid t.
    buck t.
    t. bud
    canine t.
    carnassial t.
    cheek t.
    Corti auditory teeth
    crossbite t.
    cuspid t.
    cuspidate t.
    cutting teeth
    dead t.

deciduous t.
devitalized t.
distal surface of t.
embedded t.
extruded teeth
eye t.
fluoridated t.
fused teeth
geminated teeth
t. germ
ghost t.
green t.
Horner teeth
Huschke auditory teeth
Hutchinson teeth
impacted t.
incisor t.
lingual surface of t.
metal insert teeth
migrating teeth
milk t.
molar t.
pegged t.
permanent t.
posterior t.
premolar t.
primary t.
t. pulp
rotated t.
second t.
sectorial t.
t. socket
succedaneous t.
temporary t.
tube t.
Turner t.
wandering t.
wisdom t.
toothache
topagnosis
topalgia
topesthesia
tophaceous gout
tophus, pl. **tophi**
gouty t.
topical
t. anesthesia
t. antibiotic
topoanesthesia
Topografov virus
topographical orientation
topographic anatomy

topography
Topolanski sign
toponarcosis
tori (*pl. of* torus)
Tornwaldt
T. abscess
T. cyst
T. syndrome
Torovirus
torpid
torpor
torque
Torre syndrome
torsade de pointes
torsion
extravaginal t.
t. fracture
intravaginal t.
t. spasm
torsional deformity
torsiversion
torso
torsoclusion
torti
pili t.
torticollar
torticollis
benign paroxysmal t.
congenital t.
dermatogenic t.
dystonic t.
fixed t.
hysterical t.
infantile t.
labyrinthine t.
myogenic t.
neurogenic t.
tortuosum
Eubacterium t.
tortuous
toruloidea
Hendersonula t.
torulopsosis
torulus
torus, pl. **tori**
t. fracture
mandibular t.
t. mandibularis
t. palatinus
tosylate
itramin t.

T

NOTES

total
- t. anomalous pulmonary venous return
- t. aphasia
- t. body hypothermia
- t. body surface area
- t. breathing cycle time
- t. communication
- t. cricoid cleft
- t. daily energy expenditure
- t. end-diastolic diameter
- t. end-systolic diameter
- t. hip arthroplasty
- t. hyperopia
- t. iron binding capacity
- t. joint arthroplasty
- t. knee arthroplasty
- t. laryngectomy
- t. lesion
- t. lung capacity
- t. necrosis
- t. ophthalmoplegia
- t. parenteral hyperalimentation
- t. parenteral nutrition (TPN)
- t. transfusion

totalis
- alopecia t.
- alopecia capitis t.

totipotence
totipotency
totipotent
totipotential
Toupet fundoplication
Tourette
- T. disease
- T. syndrome

tourniquet
- Dupuytren t.
- Esmarch t.
- t. paralysis

Touton giant cell
Tovell tube
towel
- t. clamp
- t. clip

tower skull
toxemia
toxemic
toxic
- t. appearance
- t. cirrhosis
- t. deafness
- t. epidermal necrolysis
- t. goiter
- t. hemoglobinuria
- t. megacolon
- t. nephrosis
- t. neuritis
- t. paraplegia
- t. psychosis
- t. shock
- t. shock syndrome
- t. tetanus
- t. unit

toxica
- alopecia t.

toxicity
- oxygen t.

toxicogenic
toxicologic
toxicologist
toxicology
toxicosis
- endogenic t.
- exogenic t.

toxicum
- erythema t.

toxigenic
toxin
- animal t.
- anthrax t.
- bacterial t.
- bee t.
- botulinus t.
- cholera t.
- cobra t.
- Crotalus t.
- diagnostic diphtheria t.
- Dick test t.
- dinoflagellate t.
- diphtheria t.
- erythrogenic t.
- extracellular t.
- intracellular t.
- Shiga t.
- Shigalike t.
- tetanus t.
- t. unit

toxinic
toxinogenic
toxocariasis
toxoid
toxophore
toxophorous
toxoplasmosis
- acquired t.
- congenital t.

toxopyrimidine
Toynbee
- T. maneuver
- T. tube

TPA, t-PA, tPA
- tissue plasminogen activator

TPN
- total parenteral nutrition

trabecula, pl. **trabeculae**
- anterior chamber t.

trabecular
  t. bone
  t. meshwork
  t. reticulum
trabeculoplasty
  laser t.
trabeculotomy
trace element
tracer
trachea
  bifurcation of t.
tracheal
  t. cartilage
  t. tube
  t. vein
trachealis muscle
tracheitis
trachelectomy
trachelism
trachelismus
trachelitis
trachelobregmatic diameter
trachelodynia
trachelorrhaphy
trachelotomy
tracheoaerocele
tracheobronchial
tracheobronchitis
tracheobronchoscopy
tracheocele
tracheoesophageal
  t. fistula
  t. puncture
  t. shunt
tracheolaryngeal
tracheomalacia
tracheomegaly
tracheopathia
tracheopathy
tracheopharyngeal
tracheophony
tracheoplasty
  slide t.
tracheorrhagia
tracheoschisis
tracheoscopic
tracheoscopy
tracheostenosis
tracheostome
  end t.

tracheostomy
  t. mask
  t. tube
tracheotomy tube
trachitis
trachoma
  t. body
  follicular t.
  granular t.
trachomatis
  Chlamydia t.
trachomatous
  t. conjunctivitis
  t. keratitis
tracing
  arrow point t.
  cephalometric t.
  Gothic arch t.
tract
  alimentary t.
  anterior corticospinal t.
  anterior raphespinal t.
  anterior spinocerebellar t.
  anterior spinothalamic t.
  anterior trigeminothalamic t.
  anterolateral t.
  Arnold t.
  association t.
  auditory t.
  bulboreticulospinal t.
  Burdach t.
  caerulospinal t.
  central tegmental t.
  cerebellorubral t.
  cerebellothalamic t.
  Collier t.
  corticobulbar t.
  corticopontine t.
  corticospinal t.
  crossed pyramidal t.
  cuneocerebellar t.
  dead t.
  deiterospinal t.
  dentatothalamic t.
  descending t.
  digestive t.
  direct pyramidal t.
  dorsal spinocerebellar t.
  dorsal trigeminothalamic t.
  dorsolateral t.
  fastigiobulbar t.
  fastigiospinal t.

T

NOTES

tract *(continued)*
    Flechsig t.
    frontopontine t.
    frontotemporal t.
    gastrointestinal t.
    geniculocalcarine t.
    genital t.
    GI t.
    Gowers t.
    habenulointerpeduncular t.
    habenulopeduncular t.
    Hoche t.
    hypothalamohypophysial t.
    iliopubic t.
    iliotibial t.
    interpositospinal t.
    interstitiospinal t.
    James t.
    lateral corticospinal t.
    lateral pyramidal t.
    lateral raphespinal t.
    lateral reticulospinal t.
    lateral spinothalamic t.
    lateral vestibulospinal t.
    Lissauer t.
    Loewenthal t.
    mamillothalamic t.
    Marchi t.
    medial reticulospinal t.
    medial vestibulospinal t.
    medullary reticulospinal t.
    mesencephalic t.
    Monakow t.
    nucleus of solitary t.
    optic t.
    posterior spinocerebellar t.
    pyramidal t.
    respiratory t.
    reticulospinal t.
    solitary t.
    spinoolivary t.
    spinovestibular t.
    tectospinal t.
    temporopontine t.
    urinary t.
    vocal t.
traction
    t. alopecia
    axis t.
    Bryant t.
    Buck t.
    t. diverticulum
    elastic t.
    t. epiphysis
    external t.
    halo t.
    halter t.
    intermaxillary t.
    internal t.

    isometric t.
    isotonic t.
    maxillomandibular t.
    skeletal t.
    skin t.
tractor
    Lowsley t.
tractotomy
    anterolateral t.
    intramedullary t.
tractus
tragal lamina
tragicus muscle
tragus, pl. **tragi**
    accessory t.
trainer
    athletic t.
training
    assertive t.
    athletic t.
    aversive t.
    avoidance t.
    circuit resistance t.
    circuit weight t.
    continuous t.
    dynamic constant external
      resistance t.
    escape t.
    t. group
    interval t.
    long slow distance t.
    plyometric t.
    sport-specific t.
    variable resistance t.
training-sensitive zone
trait
    Bombay t.
    categorical t.
    chromosomal t.
    codominant t.
    dominance of t.'s
    dominant lethal t.
    galtonian t.
    intermediate t.
    liminal t.
    marker t.
    mendelian t.
    nonpenetrant t.
    recessive t.
    sickle cell t.
    threshold t.
trance
    death t.
    induced t.
tranquilizer
    major t.
    minor t.
transacetylase
    glyoxylate t.

transacetylation
transactional analysis
transacylase
trans airway pressure
transaldolation
transamidinase
    glycine t.
transamidination
transaminase
    alanine t.
    glutamic-oxaloacetic t.
    glutamic-pyruvic t.
    serum glutamic-oxaloacetic t.
    serum glutamic-pyruvic t.
transamination
transcalent
transcarbamoylase
transcarboxylase
transcellular fluid
transcervical thymectomy
transcobalamins
transcochlear approach
transcortical aphasia
transcortin
transcriptase
    reverse t.
transcription
transcription-based chain reaction
transcriptionist
    medical t.
transcutaneous blood gas monitor
transcytosis
transducer cell
transduction
    abortive t.
    complete t.
    general t.
    high-frequency t.
    low-frequency t.
    mechanoelectric t.
transection incision
transesophageal echocardiography
transethmoidal puncture
transfection
transfer
    t. board
    embryo t.
    t. factor
    Fourier t.
    gamete intrafallopian t. (GIFT)
    group t.
    Jones t.

    linear energy t.
    t. RNA (tRNA)
transferase
    chloramphenicol acetyl t.
    CoA t.
    dipeptidyl t.
    lecithin-cholesterol t.
    terminal deoxynucleotidyl t.
transference
    counter t.
    extrasensory thought t.
    t. neurosis
transferrin saturation
transfixion suture
transform
    Fourier t.
transformation
    blast t.
    cavernous t.
    cell t.
    Haldane t.
    Lobry de Bruyn-van Ekenstein t.
    logit t.
    lymphocyte t.
transformer
    step-down t.
    step-up t.
transforming factor
transfuse
transfusion
    direct t.
    drip t.
    exchange t.
    exsanguination t.
    fetomaternal t.
    immediate t.
    indirect t.
    intramedullary t.
    intrauterine t.
    t. jaundice
    mediate t.
    t. nephritis
    reciprocal t.
    substitution t.
    t. syndrome
    total t.
    twin-twin t.
transgenesis
transglottic
transglycosylase
    dextrin t.
transhiatal esophagectomy

NOTES

857

transient
- t. acantholytic dermatosis
- t. cerebral ischemic episode
- t. evoked otoacoustic emission
- t. global amnesia
- t. hypogammaglobulinemia
- t. ischemic attack (TIA)
- t. synovitis

transilient

transition
- cervicothoracic t.
- isomeric t.
- t. mutation

transitional
- t. cell carcinoma
- t. dentition
- t. denture
- t. epithelium
- t. gyrus
- t. object
- t. zone

transjugular intrahepatic portosystemic shunt

transketolation

translabyrinthine approach

translation

translocation
- bacterial t.
- balanced t.
- group t.
- t. mongolism
- reciprocal t.
- robertsonian t.
- unbalanced t.

transmeatal incision

transmethylase

transmethylation

transmigration

transmissible

transmission
- duplex t.
- horizontal t.
- iatrogenic t.
- vertical t.

transmural necrosis

transmutation

transnasal
- t. approach
- t. fiberoptic laryngoscopy

transparent
- t. dentin
- t. septum

transpeptidase

transpeptidation

transphosphorylation

transpiration

transplant
- Gallie t.
- hair t.

transplantation
- bone marrow t.
- cardiopulmonary t.
- corneal t.
- heart t.
- heart-lung t.

transport
- active t.
- air medical t.
- axoplasmic t.
- facilitated t.
- hydrogen t.
- t. maximum
- t. medium
- mucociliary t.
- vesicular t.

transposable element

transposase

transpose

transposition of the great vessels

transposon

transpulmonary pressure

transrectus incision

transsection

transseptal approach

transsexual

transsexualism

transsynaptic degeneration

transthoracic esophagectomy

transtracheal oxygen therapy

transudate

transudation

transureteroureterostomy

transurethral
- t. resection (TUR)
- t. resection of bladder (TURB)
- t. resection of prostate (TURP)

transvaginal scanning

transvalensis
- Nocardia t.

transvector

transversalis fascia

transverse
- t. amputation
- t. carpal ligament
- t. cervical artery
- t. cervical nerve
- t. cervical vein
- t. colon
- t. diameter
- t. facial artery
- t. facial vein
- t. fissure
- t. foramen
- t. fracture
- t. hermaphroditism
- t. horizontal axis
- t. lie
- t. mesocolon

t. muscle
t. pericardial sinus
t. perineal ligament
t. plane
t. presentation
t. process
t. rectal fold
t. relaxation
t. rhombencephalic flexure
t. scapular artery
t. section
t. tarsal joint
t. temporal gyrus
t. thoracosternotomy
transversectomy
transversion mutation
transversospinalis muscle
transversospinal muscle
transversus

t. abdominis muscle
t. menti muscle
t. nuchae muscle
t. thoracis muscle
transvestism
transvestite
transvestitism
Trantas dot
trapezial
trapeziform
trapezium bone
trapezius muscle
trapezoid

t. bone
t. ligament
t. line
Traube

T. bruit
T. corpuscle
T. double tone
T. sign
Traube-Hering

T.-H. curve
T.-H. wave
trauma

acoustic t.
birth t.
t. care system
t. center
occlusion t.
periodontal t.
potential t.

psychic t.
t. score
traumasthenia
traumatic

t. amenorrhea
t. amnesia
t. amputation
t. anemia
t. anesthesia
t. asphyxia
t. atrophy
t. convulsion
t. discopathy
t. encephalopathy
t. glaucoma
t. headache
t. myoglobinuria
t. neuritis
t. neuroma
t. neurosis
t. occlusion
t. pneumothorax
t. tetanus
t. thrombosis
t. thrombus
traumatism
traumatogenic occlusion
traumatopnea
traveler's diarrhea
traveling wave theory
Travel operation
traverse
tray

acrylic resin t.
annealing t.
impression t.
Treacher Collins syndrome
treatment

active t.
aggressive t.
Carrel t.
causal t.
conservative t.
Dakin-Carrel t.
dietetic t.
empiric t.
endodontic t.
Goeckerman t.
heat t.
insulin coma t.
insulin shock t.
isoserum t.

NOTES

T

859

treatment *(continued)*
    Kenny t.
    light t.
    medical t.
    Mitchell t.
    neurodevelopmental t.
    palliative t.
    preventive t.
    prophylactic t.
    protracted t.
    shock t.
    symptomatic t.
treble increase at low levels
tree
    cabbage t.
    decision t.
    maidenhair t.
Treitz hernia
Trélat stool
tremacamra
trematoid
trembling abasia
tremens
    delirium t. (DT, DTs)
tremor
    action t.
    alcoholic withdrawal t.
    alternating t.
    alternative t.
    benign essential t.
    coarse t.
    continuous t.
    essential t.
    familial t.
    fine t.
    flapping t.
    head t.
    heredofamilial t.
    hysterical t.
    intention t.
    kinetic t.
    pill-rolling t.
    resting t.
    senile t.
    titubating t.
    volitional t.
    wing-beating t.
tremulous
trench
    t. fever
    t. lung
    t. mouth
Trendelenburg
    T. gait
    T. operation
    T. position
    T. sign
    T. symptom
    T. test

trend of thought
trepan
trepanation
    corneal t.
trephination
trephine
trepidans
    abasia t.
trepidant
trepidatio cordis
trepidation
Treponema
    T. pallidum
    T. pertenue
treponematosis
treponeme
treponemiasis
treponemicidal
treppe
Tresilian sign
tresis
Treves operation
TRH
    thyrotropin-releasing hormone
    TRH stimulation test
triacetic acid
triacylglycerol lipase
triad
    acute compression t.
    Beck t.
    Charcot t.
    Fallot t.
    female athlete t.
    hepatic t.
    Hull t.
    Hutchinson t.
    Kartagener t.
    portal t.
    Saint t.
triage tag
trial
    Bernoulli t.
    clinical t.
    t. denture
    double-blind clinical t.
    t. frame
    t. of labor after cesarean section
    t. lenses
triangle
    anal t.
    Assézat t.
    auricular t.
    47auscultatory t.
    t. of auscultation
    axillary t.
    Béclard t.
    Bonwill t.
    Bryant t.
    Burger t.

Burow t.
Calot t.
cardiohepatic t.
carotid t.
cephalic t.
cervical t.
clavipectoral t.
Codman t.
color t.
crural t.
cystohepatic t.
deltoideopectoral t.
deltopectoral t.
digastric t.
Einthoven t.
Elaut t.
facial t.
Farabeuf t.
femoral t.
frontal t.
Garland t.
Gombault t.
Grocco t.
Grynfeltt t.
Hesselbach t.
iliofemoral t.
inferior carotid t.
inferior lumbar t.
inferior occipital t.
infraclavicular t.
inguinal t.
interscalene t.
Killian t.
Koch t.
Labbé t.
Langenbeck t.
lateral pelvic wall t.
Lesser t.
Lesshaft t.
Lieutaud t.
lumbar t.
lumbocostal t.
lumbocostoabdominal t.
Macewen t.
Malgaigne t.
Marcille t.
muscular t.
Petit lumbar t.
Scarpa t.
submandibular t.
supraclavicular t.
suprameatal t.

vesical t.
Ward t.
Weber t.
Wilde t.
triangular
   t. area
   t. bandage
   t. bone
   t. muscle
   t. ridge
triangularis
   alopecia t.
triatriatum
   cor t.
tribasic
tribrachia
tricarboxylic acid cycle
triceps
   t. brachii muscle
   t. surae muscle
   t. surae reflex
trichiasis
trichilemmoma
trichina
Trichinella pseudospiralis
trichinosis granuloma
trichinous
trichitis
trichloride
   ethinyl t.
   indium-111 t.
trichloroacetic acid
trichobezoar
trichoclasia
trichoclasis
trichodes
   Lactobacillus t.
trichodiscoma
trichoepithelioma
   desmoplastic t.
   hereditary multiple t.
trichoglossia
trichoid
tricholith
trichologia
trichomegaly
trichomonacide
trichomonad
trichomonal vaginitis
Trichomonas
   T. tenax
   T. vaginalis

NOTES

trichomoniasis
trichomycosis axillaris
trichonocardiosis
trichonodosis
trichonosis
trichopathic
trichopathy
trichophagy
trichophytic
trichophytid
trichophytobezoar
trichophytosis
trichoptilosis
trichorrhexis
    t. invaginata
    t. nodosa
trichoschisis
trichosis
trichostasis spinulosa
trichotillomania
trichromatic
trichromatism
    anomalous t.
trichromatopsia
trichrome stain
trichromic
trichuriasis
tricipital
triconodont
tricorn protease
tricornute
tricrotic
tricuspid
    t. atresia
    t. insufficiency
    t. murmur
    t. orifice
    t. stenosis
    t. valve
tricuspidal
tricuspidate
tridentate
tridermic
triethiodide
    gallamine t.
trifacial neuralgia
trifid
trifocal lens
trifurcation
trigastric
trigeminal
    t. cave
    t. ganglion
    t. nerve
    t. neuralgia
    t. neurolysis
    t. pulse
    t. rhizotomy
    t. rhythm

trigeminus
    pulsus t.
trigeminy
trigger
    t. area
    ECG t.
    EKG t.
    t. finger
    t. point
    t. thumb
    t. zone
triggered activity
triglyceride
trigonal
trigone
    t. of bladder
    cerebral t.
    collateral t.
    deltoideopectoral t.
    fibrous t.
    habenular t.
    hypoglossal t.
    inguinal t.
    left fibrous t.
    lemniscal t.
    Lieutaud t.
    vertebrocostal t.
trigonid
trigonitis
trigonocephalic
trigonocephaly
trigonum
    t. lumbale
    os t.
trihydric alcohol
trihydride
    arsenic t.
trihydrochloride
    sedoxantrone t.
trilabe
trilaminar
trileaflet aortic prosthesis
trilobate
trilobed
trilocular
triloculare
    cor t.
trilogy of Fallot
trimester
trimethylamine
trimethylaminuria
trinucleotide
triose
triosephosphate isomerase
trioxide
    arsenic t.
    chromium t.
triphosphatase
    adenosine t.

triphosphate
    adenosine t.
triphosphopyridine nucleotide
Tripier amputation
triple
    t. bond
    t. repeat disorder
    t. response
    t. screen
    t. vision
triplegia
triplet
    nonsense t.
triploid
triploidy
triplopia
tripod
    t. fracture
    Haller t.
triquetral bone
triquetrum
triseriatus
    Aedes t.
trismus
trisomic
trisomy 21 syndrome
trisplanchnic
tristichia
trisulcate
tritanomaly
tritanopia
tritici
    farina t.
tritium
triton tumor
tritubercular
triturable
triturate
trituration
trivalence
trivalency
trivalent
trivial name
trivittatus
    Aedes t.
tRNA
    transfer RNA
        initiation tRNA
        isoacceptor tRNA
trocar
    t. catheter
    Hasson t.

trochanter
    greater t.
    lesser t.
trochanterian
trochanteric spine
trochc
trochlea, pl. **trochleae**
    fibular t.
trochlear
    t. nerve
    t. notch
    t. spine
trochleiform
trochoid joint
Troisier ganglion
trombiculiasis
tromethamine
    carboprost t.
Trömner reflex
trophectoderm
trophesic
trophesy
trophic
    t. lesion
    t. syndrome
    t. ulcer
trophoblastic
    t. lacuna
    t. malignant teratoma
    t. neoplasm
trophoblastin
trophoblast interferon
trophodermatoneurosis
trophoneurosis
trophoneurotic leprosy
trophoplast
trophotaxis
trophotropic
trophotropism
trophozoite
tropica
    frambesia t.
tropical
    t. abscess
    t. acne
    t. anemia
    t. bubo
    t. diarrhea
    t. disease
    t. eosinophilia
    t. lichen
    t. medicine

T

NOTES

tropical *(continued)*
    t. sore
    t. splenomegaly syndrome
    t. sprue
    t. typhus
    t. ulcer
tropicalis
    Candida t.
tropicum
    granuloma t.
tropicus
    lichen t.
tropism
    viral t.
tropocollagen
tropomyosin
troponin
trough
    gingival t.
    Langmuir t.
    t. sign
trousers
    military antishock t. (MAST)
Trousseau
    T. point
    T. sign
    T. spot
    T. syndrome
true
    t. ankylosis
    t. diverticulum
    t. lumen
    t. pelvis
    t. precocious puberty
    t. rib
    t. twins
    t. vocal cord
truncal vagotomy
truncate
truncus, pl. **trunci**
Trunecek sign
trunk
    accessory nerve t.
    brachiocephalic arterial t.
    bronchomediastinal lymphatic t.
    celiac arterial t.
    costocervical arterial t.
    inferior t.
    intestinal lymphatic t.
    jugular lymphatic t.
    linguofacial arterial t.
    lumbar lymphatic t.
    lumbosacral nerve t.
    middle t.
    pulmonary t.
    sympathetic t.
    thyrocervical t.
    vagal t.

Trusler rule for pulmonary artery banding
truss
trypanocidal
trypanocide
trypanosome
trypanosomiasis
    acute t.
    African t.
    American t.
    chronic t.
    Cruz t.
    East African t.
    Gambian t.
    Rhodesian t.
    South American t.
trypanosomic
trypanosomid
trypanosomosis
trypsin
    crystallized t.
trypsinogen
trypsogen
tryptic
tryptophan
tryptophanase
tryptophanuria
tsetse
tsutsugamushi disease
tuba auditoria
tubaeforme
    Ancylostoma t.
tubal
    t. abortion
    t. air cell
    t. ligation
    t. pregnancy
tubam
    per t.
tube
    Abbott t.
    air t.
    auditory t.
    Babcock t.
    Bouchut t.
    bronchial t.
    Cantor t.
    cardiac t.
    Carlen t.
    cathode ray t. (CRT)
    Celestin t.
    chest t.
    Coolidge t.
    Crookes-Hittorf t.
    digestive t.
    drainage t.
    Durham t.
    empyema t.
    endobronchial t.

endocardial t.
endotracheal t.
esophageal t.
eustachian t.
fallopian t.
feeding t.
Ferrein t.
field emission t.
Geiger-Müller t.
germ t.
Haldane t.
intestinal t.
intratracheal t.
intubation t.
Levin t.
Martin t.
medullary t.
Miescher t.
Miller-Abbott t.
molybdenum target t.
Moss t.
nasogastric t.
nasotracheal t.
nephrostomy t.
orotracheal t.
pharyngotympanic auditory t.
Ruysch t.
Ryle t.
Sengstaken-Blakemore t.
speaking t.
stomach t.
test t.
t. tooth
Tovell t.
Toynbee t.
tracheal t.
tracheostomy t.
tracheotomy t.
tympanostomy t.
uterine t.

tubectomy
tubed flap
tuber

ashen t.
calcaneal t.
eustachian t.
frontal t.
gray t.

tubercle

accessory t.
acoustic t.
adductor t.

amygdaloid t.
anatomic t.
anterior thalamic t.
areolar t.
ashen t.
auricular t.
Babès t.
t. bacillus
calcaneal t.
Carabelli t.
carotid t.
caseous t.
Chassaignac t.
conoid t.
corniculate t.
crown t.
cuneate t.
cuneiform t.
darwinian t.
deltoid t.
dental t.
dissection t.
dorsal t.
epiglottic t.
fibrous t.
genial t.
genital t.
Gerdy t.
Ghon t.
gracile t.
gray t.
greater t.
hard t.
hyaline t.
iliac t.
inferior thyroid t.
infraglenoid t.
intercolumnar t.
intercondylar t.
intervenous t.
jugular t.
labial t.
lesser t.
Lisfranc t.
Lister t.
Lower t.
mammillary t.
marginal t.
medial t.
mental t.
molar t.
Montgomery t.

T

NOTES

tubercle *(continued)*
    Müller t.
    soft t.
tubercular eruption
tuberculate
tuberculated
tuberculid
    papular t.
    papulonecrotic t.
tuberculin
    Koch old t.
    t. test
tuberculitis
tuberculocele
tuberculofibroid
tuberculoid
    t. leprosy
    t. myocarditis
tuberculoma
tuberculosis
    abdominal t.
    acute t.
    adult t.
    aerogenic t.
    anthracotic t.
    arrested t.
    attenuated t.
    basal t.
    cerebral t.
    childhood type t.
    cutaneous t.
    t. cutis verrucosa
    disseminated t.
    endothelial t.
    enteric t.
    esophageal t.
    exudative t.
    generalized t.
    genital t.
    healed t.
    ileocecal t.
    inactive t.
    miliary t.
    Mycobacterium t.
    open t.
    primary t.
    secondary t.
    warty t.
tuberculostatic
tuberculous
    t. abscess
    t. enteritis
    t. laryngitis
    t. meningitis
    t. myocarditis
    t. peritonitis
    t. rhinitis
    t. spondylitis
    t. wart

tuberculum arthriticum
tuberositas
tuberosity
    bicipital t.
    calcaneal t.
    coracoid t.
    costal t.
    deltoid t.
    gluteal t.
    greater t.
    iliac t.
    infraglenoid t.
    ischial t.
    lateral femoral t.
    lesser t.
    malar t.
    masseteric t.
    maxillary t.
    medial femoral t.
tuberosum
    xanthoma t.
tuberous
tuboabdominal pregnancy
tuboovarian
    t. abscess
    t. pregnancy
tuboplasty
tuboreticular structure
tubotorsion
tubotympanal
tubotympanic cleft
tubouterine
tubular
    t. atrophy
    t. carcinoma
    t. cyst
    t. diuresis
    t. forceps
    t. gland
    t. necrosis
    t. vision
tubule
    connecting t.
    convoluted seminiferous t.
    dental t.
    dentinal t.
    discharging t.
    Henle t.
    Kobelt t.
    malpighian t.
    mesonephric t.
    metanephric t.
    renal t.
    seminiferous t.
    Skene t.
    straight seminiferous t.
    T t.
    testicular t.
tubuli *(pl. of tubulus)*

tubulin
tubuloacinar gland
tubulocyst
tubuloglomerular feedback
tubulointerstitial nephritis
tubulorrhexis
tubulus, pl. **tubuli**
tubus
tucker
    tendon t.
tuft
    enamel t.
    malpighian t.
tufted cell
tularemia
    glandular t.
tularemic chancre
tularensis
    Francisella t.
Tullio phenomenon
tumefaction
tumefy
tumescence
tumescent liposuction
tumid
tumor
    acinar cell t.
    acoustic t.
    acute splenic t.
    adenoid t.
    adenomatoid odontogenic t.
    adipose t.
    ameloblastic adenomatoid t.
    amyloid t.
    t. angiogenic factor
    t. antigen
    aortic body t.
    Bednar t.
    benign t.
    blood t.
    t. blush
    borderline ovarian t.
    Brenner t.
    Brooke t.
    brown t.
    t. burden
    calcifying epithelial odontogenic t.
    carcinoid t.
    carotid body t.
    cellular t.
    cerebellopontine angle t.
    chromaffin t.

Codman t.
collision t.
connective t.
dermal duct t.
dermoid t.
desmoid t.
desmoplastic small cell t.
dysembryoplastic neuroepithelial t.
eighth nerve t.
embryonal t.
embryonic t.
endocervical sinus t.
endodermal sinus t.
endometrioid t.
epidermoid t.
Erdheim t.
Ewing t.
exuberant t.
fecal t.
fibroid t.
gastrointestinal autonomic nerve t.
gastrointestinal stromal t.
giant cell t.
glomus jugulare t.
glomus tympanicum t.
Godwin t.
granular cell t.
granulosa cell t.
Grawitz t.
heterologous t.
hilar cell t.
histoid t.
homologous t.
Hürthle cell t.
innocent t.
interstitial cell t.
islet cell t.
juxtaglomerular cell t.
Klatskin t.
Krukenberg t.
Landschutz t.
Leydig cell t.
Lindau t.
low malignant potential t.
malignant mixed mesodermal t.
  (MMMT)
malignant mixed müllerian t.
  (MMMT)
t. marker
melanotic neuroectodermal t.
Merkel cell t.
mesonephroid t.

T

NOTES

tumor *(continued)*
    mixed mesodermal t.
    t. necrosis factor
    neurogenic t.
    t. node metastasis (TNM)
    nonresponsive t.
    oncocytic hepatocellular t.
    organoid t.
    papillary t.
    phantom t.
    pilar t.
    Rathke pouch t.
    Recklinghausen t.
    sellar t.
    Sertoli cell t.
    Sertoli-Leydig cell t.
    Sertoli-stromal cell t.
    t. signature
    squamous odontogenic t.
    t. stage
    steroid cell t.
    t. suppressor gene
    teratoid t.
    triton t.
    vascular t.
    t. virus
    Wilms t.
tumoricidal
tumorigenesis
    foreign body t.
tumorigenic
tumor-specific transplantation antigen
tungstate
    lithium t.
tungsten
tunic
    Bichat t.
    Brücke t.
    fibrous t.
    mucous t.
    muscular t.
    vascular t.
tunica
    t. albuginea
    t. media
    t. propria
    t. reflexa
    t. vaginalis testis
    t. vasculosa
tunicary hernia
tuning
    t. curve
    t. fork
tunnel
    t. anemia
    carpal t.
    Corti t.
    t. infection
    t. vision

tunneled implant
TUR
    transurethral resection
TURB
    transurethral resection of bladder
turbid
turbidimetry
turbidity
turbinate
    nasal t.
turbinated
turbinectomy
turbinotomy
turbulence
    heart rate t.
turbulent flow
turcica
    sella t.
Türck degeneration
turf toe
turgescence
turgescent
turgid
turgor
turista
turnaround time
Turner
    T. syndrome
    T. tooth
turnover number
TURP
    transurethral resection of prostate
turpentine
    Canada t.
    larch t.
tussal
tussis
tussive
    t. fremitus
    t. syncope
Tuttle proctoscope
T-wave change
twelfth cranial nerve
twelfth-year molar
twilight state
twin
    allantoidoangiopagous t.
    binovular t.
    conjoined t.'s
    conjoined asymmetric t.'s
    conjoined equal t.'s
    conjoined symmetric t.'s
    conjoined unequal t.'s
    dichorial t.
    diovular t.'s
    dissimilar t.
    dizygotic t.
    enzygotic t.
    fraternal t.

heterologous t.
identical t.
incomplete conjoined t.'s
locked t.'s
monoamniotic t.
monozygotic t.'s
t. placenta
t. poles
t. reversed arterial perfusion
  sequence
Siamese t.'s
similar t.'s
true t.'s
uniovular t.'s
unlike t.'s

twinge
twinning
twin-twin transfusion
twisted hairs
tying forceps
tylectomy
tyloma
tylosis
tylotic
tyloticum

eczema t.

tympanal
tympanectomy
tympani

canaliculus chordae t.
cavum t.
chorda t.

tympanic

t. antrum
t. bone
t. canaliculus
t. cavity
t. ganglion
t. membrane
t. nerve
t. opening
t. plexus
t. ring
t. sinus
t. vein

tympanica

pars t.

tympanicus

anulus t.
canaliculus t.

tympanism
tympanites

tympanitic

t. abscess
t. resonance

tympanitis
tympanocentesis
tympanogram
tympanomastoid fissure
tympanometry
tympanoplasty
tympanosclerosis
tympanostomy tube
tympanotomy
tympanous
tympany

Skoda t.

Tyndall phenomenon
type

t. A, B behavior
t. A, B personality
basic personality t.
blood t.
Bombay blood t.
buffalo t.
t. culture
t. 1, 2 diabetes
t. 1–6 glycogenosis
t. I, II diabetes
t. I–V familial hyperlipoproteinemia
Jaeger test t.
schizoid t.
Snellen test t.
test t.

typhi

Salmonella t.

typhimurium

Salmonella t.
Salmonella enterica t.

typhlectasis
typhlectomy
typhlenteritis
typhlitis
typhlodicliditis
typhloenteritis
typhlolithiasis
typhlopexia
typhlopexy
typhlorrhaphy
typhlosis
typhlostomy
typhlotomy
typhoid

abdominal t.

T

NOTES

869

typhoid *(continued)*
    ambulatory t.
    apyretic t.
    t. bacillus
    t. fever
    fowl t.
    latent t.
    t. meningitis
    t. spot
typhoidal
typhosa
    Salmonella t.
typhous
typhus
    Australian tick t.
    endemic t.
    epidemic t.
    European t.
    exanthematous t.
    flea-borne t.
    Indian tick t.

    louse-borne t.
    Manchurian t.
    Mexican t.
    mite t.
    mite-born t.
    murine t.
    recrudescent t.
    scrub t.
    tick t.
    tropical t.
typical drusen
typing
    bacteriophage t.
    DNA t.
    HLA t.
Tyrode solution
tyroketonuria
tyroma
tyrosine
tyrosinuria
tyrosyluria

UA
> urinalysis

ubiquinol
ubiquinone
ubiquitin
ubiquitin-protease pathway
ulcer
> acute decubitus u.
> Allingham u.
> anastomotic u.
> Buruli u.
> chronic u.
> cold u.
> contact u.
> Cruveilhier u.
> Curling u.
> Cushing u.
> decubitus u.
> dendritic corneal u.
> dental u.
> Dieulafoy u.
> diphtheritic u.
> distention u.
> elusive u.
> fascicular u.
> Fenwick-Hunner u.
> fever, adenitis, pharyngitis, and aphthous u.'s (FAPA)
> follicular u.
> Gaboon u.
> gastric u.
> gastroduodenal u.
> gastrojejunal u.
> gravitational u.
> gummatous u.
> hard u.
> healed u.
> herpetic u.
> Hunner u.
> hypopyon u.
> indolent u.
> inflamed u.
> Kocher u.
> Mann-Williamson u.
> marginal ring u.
> Marjolin u.
> Meleney u.
> Mooren u.
> peptic u.
> perforated u.
> perforating u.
> phagedenic u.
> pressure u.
> recurrent aphthous u.
> rodent u.
> Saemisch u.
> soft u.
> stercoral u.
> steroid u.
> stomal u.
> stress u.
> submucous u.
> Sutton u.
> trophic u.
> tropical u.
> varicose u.
> venereal u.
> venous u.

ulcerate
ulcerated
> u. cancer
> u. sore throat

ulcerating granuloma
ulceration
ulcerative
> u. colitis
> u. stomatitis
> u. vulvitis

ulceromembranous gingivitis
ulcerous
ulerythema
Ullmann
> U. line
> U. syndrome

ULN
> upper limit of normal

ulnad
ulnar
> u. artery
> u. drift
> u. drift deformity
> u. extensor muscle
> u. flexor muscle
> u. malleolus
> u. nerve
> u. nerve compression syndrome
> u. palsy
> u. tunnel syndrome
> u. vein

ulodermatitis
uloid
ULQ
> upper left quadrant

ultracentrifuge
ultradian
ultrafast Pap stain
ultrafiltration
ultraligation
ultramicroscopic
ultramicroscopy

U

ultramicrotome
ultrashortwave diathermy
ultrasonic
    u. lithotripsy
    u. nebulizer
    u. tomography
ultrasonics
ultrasonogram
ultrasonograph
ultrasonographer
ultrasonography
    Doppler u.
    duplex u.
    endovaginal u.
    gray-scale u.
ultrasound
    u. cardiography
    diagnostic u.
    therapeutic u.
ultrastructural anatomy
ultrathin section
ultraviolet
    extravital u.
    u. index
    intravital u.
    u. keratoconjunctivitis
    u. microscope
ultravirus
umbilical
    u. artery
    u. catheter
    u. cord
    u. hernia
    u. region
    u. ring
    u. vein
umbilicalis
    anulus u.
umbilicate
umbilicated
umbilication
umbilicus, pl. **umbilici**
    areola u.
    areola umbilici
umbrella iris
unbalanced translocation
uncal herniation
unci (*pl. of* uncus)
unciform
    u. bone
    u. fasciculus
uncinate
    u. fasciculus
    u. gyrus
uncombable hair syndrome
uncomfortable level
uncompensated alkalosis
uncompetitive inhibitor

unconditioned
    u. reflex
    u. response
    u. stimulus
unconscious
    collective u.
unconsciousness
uncovertebral
unction
unctuous
uncus, pl. **unci**
undecylate
    estradiol u.
underbite
underdrive pacing
underlying cause of death
undershoot
underwater weighing
undescended testis
undetermined nitrogen
undifferentiated
    u. malignant teratoma
    u. schizophrenia
    u. type fever
undulant fever
undulate
undulating
    u. membrane
    u. pulse
undulatory membrane
undulipodium
ungual
unguent
unguinal
unguis
    matrix u.
    sulcus matricis u.
unguium
    dystrophia u.
    tinea u.
uniaxial joint
unicameral bone cyst
unicamerate
unicellular gland
unicollis
    uterus bicornis u.
unicornous
unicorn uterus
unigerminal
uniglandular
unilateral
    u. amelia
    u. anesthesia
    u. hemianopia
    u. hermaphroditism
    u. hyperlucent lung
    u. lobar emphysema
    u. nystagmus
unilobar

unilocal
unilocular
    u. cyst
    u. joint
unimolecular
uninhibited neurogenic bladder
uninterrupted suture
union
    autogenous u.
    faulty u.
    fibrous u.
    primary u.
    secondary u.
    vicious u.
uniovular twins
unipennate
unipolar
    u. lead
    u. neuron
unit
    absolute u.
    alexin u.
    Allen-Doisy u.
    alpha u.
    amboceptor u.
    androgen u.
    Ångström u.
    Ansbacher u.
    antigen u.
    antitoxic u.
    antitoxin u.
    antivenene u.
    atomic mass u.
    base u.
    Bethesda u.
    biological standard u.
    bird u.
    Bodansky u.
    British thermal u. (BTU)
    burn u.
    capon u.
    capon-comb u.
    cardiac intensive care u. (CICU)
    cardiology intensive care u. (CICU)
    centimeter-gram-second u.
    CGS u.
    chlorophyll u.
    chorionic gonadotropin u.
    Clauberg u.
    colony-forming u.
    complement u.
    Corner-Allen u.

    coronary care u. (CCU)
    coronary intensive care u. (CICU)
    critical care u. (CCU)
    CT u.
    Dam u.
    digitalis u.
    diphtheria antitoxin u.
    dog u.
    electromagnetic u.
    electrostatic u.
    epidermal-melanin u.
    equine gonadotropin u.
    equivalent normal child u. (encu)
    equivalent normal son u. (ensu)
    estradiol benzoate u.
    estrone u.
    Fishman-Lerner u.
    Florey u.
    foot-pound-second u.
    FPS u.
    G u.
    gravitational u.
    hemolysin u.
    hemolytic u.
    heparin u.
    Holzknecht u.
    Hounsfield u.
    Howell u.
    insulin u.
    intensive care u. (ICU)
    international u. (IU)
    Jenner-Kay u.
    Karmen u.
    Kienböck u.
    King u.
    King-Armstrong u.
    lung u.
    u. membrane
    meter-kilogram-second u.
    MKS u.
    Montevideo u.
    motor u.
    neonatal intensive care u. (NICU)
    neurological intensive care u. (NICU)
    pediatric intensive care u. (PICU)
    physiologic u.
    pulmonary intensive care u. (PIVU)
    u. record
    respiratory care u. (RCU)
    Somogyi u.
    surgical intensive care u. (SICU)

NOTES

U

unit *(continued)*
    Svedberg u.
    toxic u.
    toxin u.
    workload u.
univalence
univalency
univalent antibody
universal
    u. dental nomenclature
    u. donor
universale
    melasma u.
universalis
    adiposis u.
    alopecia u.
    calcinosis u.
unlike twins
unmyelinated
    u. fiber
Unna
    U. disease
    U. nevus
    U. stain
unofficial
unphysiologic
unsanitary
unsaturated fatty acid
unsharpness
    geometric u.
unspecified
    peripheral T-cell lymphoma, u.
unstable
    u. angina
    u. lie
unstriated
unsystematized delusion
Unverricht disease
UOQ
    upper outer quadrant
upbeat nystagmus
upper
    u. airway
    u. extremity
    u. gastrointestinal series
    u. left quadrant (ULQ)
    u. limb
    u. limit of normal (ULN)
    u. outer quadrant (UOQ)
    u. respiratory disease
    u. respiratory infection (URI)
    u. respiratory rhonchi
    u. respiratory tract infection
      (URTI)
upregulation
upregulation/downregulation hypothesis
upsilon, Ψ

uptake
    131I u. test
    maximal oxygen u.
urachal
urachus
uracil
uranium
uranoplasty
uranorrhaphy
uranoschisis
uranostaphyloschisis
uranyl
urarthritis
urate
    u. calculus
    u. oxidase
uratemia
uratosis
uraturia
Urban operation
urea
    u. clearance
    u. cycle
    u. frost
    u. nitrogen
ureagenesis
ureapoiesis
urease
uredema
ureidosuccinic acid
urelcosis
uremia
    hypercalcemic u.
    prerenal u.
    retention u.
uremic
    u. acidosis
    u. coma
    u. convulsion
    u. frost
uremigenic
uresiesthesia
uresis
ureter
    aberrant u.
    curlicue u.
    double u.
    ectopic u.
    ileal u.
ureteral
    u. catheter
    u. ectopia
    u. reimplantation
ureteralgia
uretercystoscope
ureterectasia
ureterectomy
ureteric orifice
ureteritis

ureterocele
    ectopic u.
    orthotopic u.
ureterocelorraphy
ureterocolostomy
ureterocystoplasty
ureterocystoscope
ureterocystostomy
ureteroenterostomy
ureterography
ureteroileal anastomosis
ureteroileoneocystostomy
ureteroileostomy
ureterolithiasis
ureterolithotomy
ureterolysis
ureteroneocystostomy
ureteronephrectomy
ureteropelvic
    u. junction
    u. junction obstruction
ureteroplasty
ureteropyelitis
ureteropyelography
ureteropyeloplasty
ureteropyelostomy
ureteropyosis
ureterorenal reflux
ureterorrhagia
ureterorrhaphy
ureterosigmoidostomy
ureterostomy
    cutaneous loop u.
ureterotomy
ureteroureterostomy
ureterovesical
    u. angle (UVA)
    u. junction (UVJ)
ureterovesicostomy
urethra
    anterior u.
    female u.
    male u.
    membranous u.
urethrae
    labium u.
    sphincter u.
urethral
    u. artery
    u. caruncle
    u. crest
    u. gland

    u. groove
    u. hematuria
    u. papilla
    u. valve
urethralgia
urethralis
    anulus u.
    colliculus u.
    lacuna u.
    papilla u.
urethrectomy
urethremorrhagia
urethrism
urethrismus
urethritis
    anterior u.
    follicular u.
    gonorrheal u.
    granular u.
    u. petrificans
urethrobulbar
urethrocele
urethrocutaneous fistula
urethrocystometry
urethrodynia
urethroperineoscrotal
urethroplasty
    Cecil u.
urethrorrhagia
urethrorrhaphy
urethrorrhea
urethroscope
urethroscopic
urethroscopy
urethrospasm
urethrostaxis
urethrostenosis
urethrostomy
urethrotomy
    external u.
    internal u.
urethrovaginal fistula
urethrovesical angle
urethrovesicopexy
urge incontinence
urgency
    u. incontinence
    motor u.
    sensory u.
urhidrosis
URI
    upper respiratory infection

NOTES

urica
    cornea u.
uric acid
uricase
uricolysis
uricolytic
uricosuria
uridine
uridrosis
uridylic acid
uriesthesia
urinal
urinalysis (UA)
urinariae
    fundus vesicae u.
urinarius
    meatus u.
urinary
    u. bladder
    u. calculus
    u. fistula
    u. meatus
    u. nitrogen
    u. sand
    u. stasis
    u. stuttering
    u. tract
    u. tract infection
urinate
urination
urine
    ammoniacal u.
    anemic u.
    black u.
    chylous u.
    cloudy u.
    crude u.
    u. drug panel
    u. drug screen
    febrile u.
    feverish u.
    gouty u.
    honey u.
    incontinence of u.
    maple syrup u.
    milky u.
    residual u.
urinogenous
urinoma
urinometry
urinoscopy
urobilin
urobilinemia
urobilinogen
urobilinuria
urocanate hydratase
urocanic acid
urocele
urochesia

urochrome
urodynia
uroflavin
urofollitropin
urogastrone
urogenital
    u. canal
    u. diaphragm
    u. peritoneum
    u. region
    u. ridge
    u. sinus anomaly
    u. system
urogenitale
    peritoneum u.
urogenous
urogram
    intravenous u. (IVU)
urography
    antegrade u.
    cystoscopic u.
    descending u.
    excretory u.
    intravenous u.
    retrograde u.
urohaematin
urohematin
urokinase
urolithiasis
urolithic
urologic
urological
urologist
urology
uroncus
uronephrosis
uropathy
    obstructive u.
urophanic
uropoiesis
uropoietic
uroporphyrin
uroporphyrinogen
uroradiology
uroschesis
uroscopic
uroscopy
urosepsis
urothelial
    u. carcinoma
    u. papilloma
urothelium
urothorax
URTI
    upper respiratory tract infection
urticant
urticaria
    acute u.
    allergic u.

aquagenic u.
cholinergic u.
chronic u.
cold u.
endemic u.
u. endemica
u. epidemica
exercise-induced u.
factitious u.
febrile u.
giant u.
heat u.
hemorrhagic u.
u. medicamentosa
papular u.
u. pigmentosa
solar u.
urticarial vasculitis
urticarious
urticate
urtication
urticatus
lichen u.
Usher syndrome
usual interstitial pneumonia
uteri (*pl. of* uterus)
uterine
u. artery
u. atony
u. calculus
u. cavity
u. contraction
u. gland
u. hernia
u. ostium
u. segment
u. sinus
u. souffle
u. tube
u. vein
uterinus
vagitus u.
utero
in u.
uterocystostomy
uterofixation
uteroglobin
uteroglobin-adducin
uterometer
uteropexy
uteroplacental sinus
uteroplasty

uterosalpingography
uteroscope
uteroscopy
uterotomy
uterotonic
uterotubography
uterovaginal canal
uterovesical
u. ligament
u. pouch
uterus, pl. **uteri**
adenomyosis uteri
adnexa uteri
anomalous u.
arcuate u.
bicornate u.
u. bicornis bicollis
u. bicornis unicollis
bifid u.
biforate u.
bipartite u.
cavum uteri
cervix uteri
cordiform u.
Couvelaire u.
u. didelphys
double-mouthed u.
duplex u.
gliosis uteri
gravid u.
heart-shaped u.
horn of u.
incudiform u.
isthmus of u.
labia uteri
masculine u.
prolapse of u.
septate u.
unicorn u.
utricle
prostatic u.
utricular nerve
utriculitis
utriculoampullar nerve
utriculosaccular
UVA
ureterovesical angle
uveae
ectropion u.
uveal
uveitic
uveitis, pl. **uveitides**

U

NOTES

uveitis *(continued)*
    anterior u.
    Förster u.
    Fuchs u.
    heterochromic u.
    intermediate u.
    lens-induced u.
    peripheral u.
    sympathetic u.
uveoencephalitic syndrome
uveoparotid fever
uveoscleritis
uviform
UVJ
    ureterovesical junction
uvula, pl. **uvuli**

    bifid u.
    u. cerebelli
    cleft u.
    Lieutaud u.
    palatine u.
    split u.
    u. vermis
uvular muscle
uvulectomy
uvuli (*pl. of* uvula)
uvulitis
uvuloptosis
uvulotomy
U wave

V, v
volt
V wave
vaccae
Mycobacterium v.
vaccinal
vaccinate
vaccination
vaccine
adjuvant v.
aqueous v.
attenuated v.
autogenous v.
bacillus Calmette-Guérin v.
BCG v.
brucella strain 19 v.
Calmette-Guérin v.
cholera v.
crystal violet v.
diphtheria toxoid, tetanus toxoid,
and pertussis v. (DTP)
duck embryo origin v.
Flury strain v.
foot-and-mouth disease virus v.
Haemophilus influenzae type B v.
Haffkine v.
hepatitis B v.
heterogenous v.
Hib v.
high-egg-passage v.
hog cholera v.
human diploid cell v. (HDCV)
human diploid cell rabies v.
inactivated poliovirus v. (IPV)
influenza virus v.
live oral poliovirus v.
low-egg-passage v.
v. lymph
measles, mumps, and rubella v.
measles virus v.
multivalent v.
oral poliovirus v.
poliovirus v.
polysaccharide conjugated v.
polyvalent v.
stock v.
subunit v.
vital v.
vaccinia
generalized v.
v. lymph
VACTERL syndrome
vacuo
hydrocephalus ex v.
in v.

vacuolar
vacuolate
vacuolated
vacuolation
vacuole
autophagic v.
contractile v.
digestive v.
vacuolization
vacutome
vacuum
v. drainage system
v. pack technique
vagabond's disease
vagal
v. nerve stimulation
v. trunk
vagi (*pl. of* vagus)
vagina, pl. **vaginae**
bipartite v.
fossa of vestibule of v.
vaginal
v. agenesis
v. artery
v. atresia
v. celiotomy
v. cuff
v. gland
v. hernia
v. hysterectomy
v. intraepithelial neoplasia
v. nerve
v. orifice
v. portion
v. rugae
v. vault
vaginalis
flatus v.
Gardnerella v.
processus v.
Trichomonas v.
vaginate
vaginectomy
vaginismus
vaginitis
adhesive v.
amebic v.
atrophic v.
desquamative inflammatory v.
Gardnerella v.
papulous v.
senile v.
trichomonal v.
vaginocele
vaginodynia

V

vaginofixation
vaginolabial hernia
vaginomycosis
vaginopathy
vaginoperineoplasty
vaginoperineorrhaphy
vaginoperineotomy
vaginopexy
vaginoplasty
vaginoscopy
vaginosis
    bacterial v.
vaginotomy
vagitus uterinus
vagolysis
vagolytic
vagomimetic
vagotomy
    bilateral v.
    v. and pyloroplasty
    surgical v.
    truncal v.
vagotropic
vagovagal
vagrant's disease
vagus, pl. vagi
    v. nerve
    v. pulse
    v. reflex
    v. stimulation
valence
valency
Valentine position
valerate
    amyl v.
    estradiol v.
valga
    coxa v.
    tibia v.
valgum
    genu v.
valgus
    cubitus v.
    v. deformity
    hallux v.
    hindfoot v.
    v. laxity
    talipes v.
validation
    consensual v.
    skills v.
validity
    concurrent v.
    construct v.
    content v.
    criterion-related v.
    face v.
valine

vallate papilla
vallecula, pl. valleculae
    epiglottic v.
Valleix point
Valsalva maneuver
value
    acetyl v.
    buffer v.
    C v.
    caloric v.
    Hehner v.
    homing v.
    iodine v.
    maturation v.
    normal v.
    phenotypic v.
    predictive v.
    reference v.
    threshold limit v.
valve
    Amussat v.
    anal v.
    anterior urethral v.
    aortic v.
    atrioventricular v.
    AV v.
    ball v.
    Bauhin v.
    Béraud v.
    bicuspid aortic v.
    bi-leaflet v.
    biologic v.
    Björk-Shiley v.
    Blom-Singer v.
    Bochdalek v.
    Braune v.
    Carpentier-Edwards v.
    caval v.
    congenital v.
    coronary v.
    eustachian v.
    flail mitral v.
    Gerlach v.
    Guérin v.
    Heister v.
    Heyer-Pudenz v.
    Hoboken v.
    Huschke v.
    ileocecal v.
    ileocolic v.
    Kerckring v.
    Krause v.
    left atrioventricular v.
    Mercier v.
    mitral v.
    parachute mitral v.
    posterior urethral v.
    pulmonary v.
    semilunar v.

tilting disc v.
tricuspid v.
urethral v.
vesicoureteral v.

valvoplasty

valvotomy
mitral v.

valvula, pl. **valvulae**
Amussat v.
Gerlach v.

valvular
v. endocarditis
v. insufficiency
v. pneumothorax
v. regurgitation
v. sclerosis
v. thrombus

valvule
Foltz v.
lymphatic v.

valvulitis
mitral v.

valvuloplasty
mitral v.

valvulotomy

van
v. Buchem syndrome
v. Buren operation
v. der Hoeve syndrome
v. der Waals force
v. Ermengen stain
v. Gieson stain
V. Lohuizen syndrome

vanadium group

vanbreuseghemi
Microsporum v.

vanillism

vanillylmandelic acid

vanishing lung syndrome

van't
v. Hoff equation
v. Hoff law
v. Hoff theory

vapor
anesthetic v.

vaporization

vaporize

vaporizer
flow-over v.

Vaquez disease

vara
coxa v.

false coxa v.
tibia v.

variabilis
Dermacentor v.
erythrokeratodermia v.

variability
baseline v.
beat-to-beat v.

variable
continuous random v.
dependent v.
discrete random v.
independent v.
intermediate v.
intervening v.
mixed discrete-continuous
random v.
moderator v.
v. resistance training

variance
analysis of v. (ANOVA)
ball v.

varians
Micrococcus v.

variant
v. angina
v. angina pectoris
inherited albumin v.
L-phase v.

variation
antigenic v.
coefficient of v. (CV)
continuous v.

varication

variceal

varicella encephalitis

varicella-zoster virus

varicelliform

varicellosus
herpes zoster v.

varices (*pl. of* varix)

variciform

varicoblepharon

varicocele

varicocelectomy

varicography

varicomphalus

varicophlebitis

varicose
v. aneurysm
v. placenta

V

NOTES

varicose *(continued)*
    v. ulcer
    v. vein
varicosis
varicosity
varicotomy
varicula
varicule
variegate porphyria
variegatum
       Amblyomma v.
variegatus
       Aedes v.
variolar
variolate
variola virus
varioliform
varioliformis
    acne v.
varioloid
variolous
varix, pl. **varices**
    aneurysmal v.
    cirsoid v.
    conjunctival v.
    esophageal v.
    gelatinous v.
    lymph v.
varum
    genu v.
varus
    cubitus v.
    v. deformity
    hallux v.
    hindfoot v.
    v. laxity
    metatarsus v.
    talipes v.
vas, pl. **vasa**
    v. deferens
    vasa lymphatica
    vasa previa
    vasa recta
    vasa vasorum
vasal
vascular
    v. cataract
    v. circle
    v. dementia
    v. endothelium
    v. headache
    v. lacuna
    v. lamina
    v. leiomyoma
    v. malformation
    v. neoplasm
    v. nerve
    v. parkinsonism
    v. polyp

    v. resistance
    v. ring
    v. spasm
    v. spider
    v. system
    v. tumor
    v. tunic
vascularis
    nevus v.
vascularity
vascularization
vascularized graft
vasculature
vasculitis
    cutaneous v.
    granulomatous v.
    hypersensitivity v.
    hypocomplementemic v.
    leukocytoclastic v.
    livedo v.
    lymphomatoid v.
    necrotizing v.
    nodular v.
    rheumatoid v.
    septic v.
    urticarial v.
vasculomyelinopathy
vasculopathy
vasculosa
    meninx v.
    tunica v.
vasculosum
    punctum v.
vasculosus
    nevus v.
vasectomy
vasifaction
vasifactive
vasiform
vasitis
vasoactive
    v. amine
    v. intestinal polypeptide
vasoconstriction
    active v.
vasoconstrictive
vasoconstrictor
vasodepression
vasodepressor syncope
vasodilatation
vasodilation
    active v.
vasodilative
vasodilator
vasoepididymostomy
vasoformation
vasoformative cell
vasoganglion
vasography

vasohypertonic
vasohypotonic
vasoinhibitor
vasoinhibitory
vasoligation
vasomotion
vasomotor
    v. imbalance
    v. nerve
    v. paralysis
    v. rhinitis
    v. wave
vasoneuropathy
vaso-orchidostomy
vasoparalysis
vasoparesis
vasopressin
    arginine v.
vasopressor reflex
vasopuncture
vasoreflex
vasorelaxation
vasorum
    lacuna v.
    vasa v.
vasosection
vasosensory
vasospasm
vasospastic
vasostimulant
vasostomy
vasotomy
vasotonia
vasotonic
vasotrophic
vasotropic
vasovagal syncope
vasovasostomy
vasovesiculectomy
vastomy
vastus
    v. intermedius muscle
    v. lateralis muscle
    v. medialis muscle
Vater
    ampulla of V.
vault
    cranial v.
    vaginal v.
vector
    biologic v.
    biological v.

    cloning v.
    expression v.
    instantaneous v.
    manifest v.
    mean manifest v.
    mechanical v.
    recombinant v.
vector-borne infection
vectorcardiogram
vectorcardiography
vectorial
vegan
vegetal pole
vegetation
    bacterial v.
vegetative
    v. bacteriophage
    v. endocarditis
    v. pole
    v. state
veil
    aqueduct v.
    Jackson v.
    Sattler v.
vein
    accessory cephalic v.
    accessory hemiazygos v.
    accessory saphenous v.
    accessory vertebral v.
    accompanying v.
    anastomotic v.
    angular v.
    anonymous v.
    anterior auricular v.
    anterior basal v.
    anterior cardiac v.
    anterior cardinal v.
    anterior cerebral v.
    anterior ciliary v.
    anterior circumflex humeral v.
    anterior facial v.
    anterior intercostal v.
    anterior jugular v.
    anterior labial v.
    anterior pontomesencephalic v.
    anterior scrotal v.
    anterior tibial v.
    anterior vertebral v.
    apical v.
    apicoposterior v.
    appendicular v.
    aqueous v.

V

NOTES

vein *(continued)*
    arciform v.
    arcuate v.
    arterial v.
    ascending lumbar v.
    auricular v.
    axillary v.
    azygos v.
    basal v.
    basilic v.
    basivertebral v.
    Baumgarten v.
    Boyd communicating perforation v.
    brachial v.
    brachiocephalic v.
    Breschet v.
    bronchial v.
    Browning v.
    Burow v.
    capillary v.
    cardiac v.
    cardinal v.
    cavernous v.
    central retinal v.
    cephalic v.
    cerebellar v.
    cerebral v.
    cervical v.
    choroid v.
    ciliary v.
    circumflex scapular v.
    Cockett communicating
     perforating v.
    colic v.
    common basal v.
    common cardinal v.
    common facial v.
    common iliac v.
    common modiolar v.
    companion v.
    condylar emissary v.
    conjunctival v.
    coronary v.
    costoaxillary v.
    cutaneous v.
    Cuvier v.
    cystic v.
    deep cervical v.
    deep circumflex iliac v.
    deep dorsal v.
    deep epigastric v.
    deep facial v.
    deep femoral v.
    deep lingual v.
    deep middle cerebral v.
    deep temporal v.
    digital v.
    diploic v.
    direct lateral v.

dorsal callosal v.
dorsal digital v.
dorsal lingual v.
dorsal metacarpal v.
dorsal metatarsal v.
dorsal scapular v.
dorsispinal v.
emissary v.
epigastric v.
episcleral v.
esophageal v.
ethmoidal v.
external iliac v.
external jugular v.
external nasal v.
external palatine v.
external pudendal v.
facial v.
femoral v.
fibular v.
frontal v.
gastric v.
gastroepiploic v.
genicular v.
gluteal v.
great cardiac v.
great cerebral v.
great saphenous v.
hemiazygos v.
hemorrhoidal v.
hepatic portal v.
highest intercostal v.
hypogastric v.
ileal v.
ileocolic v.
iliac v.
iliolumbar v.
inferior anastomotic v.
inferior basal v.
inferior cardiac v.
inferior cerebral v.
inferior choroid v.
inferior epigastric v.
inferior gluteal v.
inferior hemiazygos v.
inferior hemorrhoidal v.
inferior labial v.
inferior laryngeal v.
inferior mesenteric v.
inferior ophthalmic v.
inferior palpebral v.
inferior phrenic v.
inferior rectal v.
inferior thalamostriate v.
inferior thyroid v.
inferior ventricular v.
infrasegmental v.
innominate cardiac v.
insular v.

intercapitular v.
intercostal v.
interlobar v.
interlobular v.
intermediate antebrachial v.
intermediate basilic v.
intermediate cephalic v.
intermediate cubital v.
intermediate hepatic v.
internal auditory v.
internal cerebral v.
internal iliac v.
internal jugular v.
internal pudendal v.
internal thoracic v.
intersegmental v.
intervertebral v.
intrasegmental v.
jugular v.
key v.
Krukenberg v.
Labbé v.
labial v.
labyrinthine v.
lacrimal v.
large saphenous v.
laryngeal v.
Latarget v.
lateral atrial v.
lateral circumflex femoral v.
lateral direct v.
lateral sacral v.
lateral thoracic v.
left colic v.
left coronary v.
left gastric v.
left gastroepiploic v.
left gastroomental v.
left hepatic v.
left inferior pulmonary v.
left ovarian v.
left superior intercostal v.
left superior pulmonary v.
left suprarenal v.
left testicular v.
left umbilical v.
levoatrio-cardinal v.
lingual v.
lingular v.
long saphenous v.
long thoracic v.
lumbar v.

Marshall oblique v.
masseteric v.
mastoid emissary v.
maxillary v.
Mayo v.
medial atrial v.
medial circumflex femoral v.
median antebrachial v.
median basilic v.
median cephalic v.
median cubital v.
median sacral v.
mediastinal v.
medium v.
meningeal v.
mesencephalic v.
mesenteric v.
metacarpal v.
middle cardiac v.
middle colic v.
middle hemorrhoidal v.
middle hepatic v.
middle lobe v.
middle meningeal v.
middle rectal v.
middle temporal v.
middle thyroid v.
musculophrenic v.
nasofrontal v.
oblique v.
obturator v.
occipital cerebral v.
palatine v.
palpebral v.
pancreatic v.
pancreaticoduodenal v.
paraumbilical v.
parotid v.
pectoral v.
perforating v.
pericardiacophrenic v.
pericardial v.
peroneal v.
pharyngeal v.
popliteal v.
portal v.
posterior intercostal v.
posterior labial v.
prepyloric v.
pyloric v.
radial v.
renal v.

V

NOTES

vein *(continued)*
   retromandibular v.
   right gastric v.
   scleral v.
   short gastric v.
   sigmoid v.
   small cardiac v.
   spinal v.
   spiral v.
   splenic v.
   stellate v.
   sternocleidomastoid v.
   striate v.
   stylomastoid v.
   subclavian v.
   subcutaneous v.
   sublingual v.
   submental v.
   superficial dorsal v.
   superficial epigastric v.
   superior basal v.
   superior cerebral v.
   superior epigastric v.
   superior labial v.
   superior thalamostriate v.
   supraorbital v.
   suprascapular v.
   supratrochlear v.
   surface thalamic v.
   thalamostriate v.
   thoracoacromial v.
   thoracoepigastric v.
   thymic v.
   tracheal v.
   transverse cervical v.
   transverse facial v.
   tympanic v.
   ulnar v.
   umbilical v.
   uterine v.
   varicose v.
   vertebral v.
   vesical v.
   vestibular v.
   vortex v.
   vorticose v.
vela *(pl. of* velum)
velamen, pl. **velamina**
velamentous
velocity
   initial v.
   maximum v.
velopharyngeal insufficiency
Velpeau
   V. bandage
   V. hernia
velum, pl. **vela**
   anterior medullary v.
   inferior medullary v.
   v. palatinum
   superior medullary v.
vena, pl. **venae**
   agger valvae venae
   venae comitantes
   v. epigastrica
   v. submentalis
venacavography
   inferior v.
venectasia
venectomy
venenata
   acne v.
venenation
venerea
   lues v.
venereal
   v. bubo
   v. disease
   v. lymphogranuloma
   v. sore
   v. ulcer
   v. wart
venereum
   granuloma v.
   lymphogranuloma v.
   malum v.
veneris
   corona v.
venesection
Venezuelan hemorrhagic fever
venipuncture
venogram
venography
   peripheral v.
venom
   kokoi v.
   Russell's viper v.
venomotor
venoocclusive disease
venosclerosis
venosity
venostasis
venostomy
venosus
   ductus v.
   sinus v.
venotomy
venous
   v. admixture
   v. angioma
   v. angle
   v. blood
   v. capillary
   v. catheter
   v. claudication
   v. embolism
   v. hum
   v. hyperemia

v. insufficiency
v. malformation
v. murmur
v. pulse
v. return
v. sclerosis
v. sinus
v. star
v. ulcer
venovenostomy
venovenous access
ventilate
ventilation
airway pressure release v.
alveolar v.
artificial v.
assist-control v.
assisted v.
bag v.
continuous positive pressure v.
  (CPPV)
controlled mechanical v. (CMV)
high-frequency v.
intermittent mandatory v. (IMV)
intermittent positive pressure v.
  (IPPV)
inverse-ratio v.
liquid v.
mandatory minute v.
manual v.
maximum voluntary v.
mechanical v.
minute v.
negative pressure v.
positive pressure v.
pressure controlled v.
pressure support v.
pulmonary v.
synchronized intermittent
  mandatory v.
volume controlled v.
ventilation/perfusion ratio
ventilation-perfusion scan
ventilator
automatic transport v.
cuirass v.
flow-controlled v.
pressure v.
volume v.
ventilatory threshold
ventrad

ventral
v. apron prepuce
v. celiotomy
v. hernia
v. horn
v. plate
v. root
v. thalamic peduncle
ventricle
Arantius v.
cerebral v.
double outlet right v.
Duncan v.
fifth v.
fourth v.
laryngeal v.
lateral v.
left v.
right v.
third v.
ventricular
v. afterload
v. artery
v. assist device
v. band
v. complex
v. conduction
v. contour
v. escape
v. extrasystole
v. fibrillation
v. flutter
v. fold
v. fusion beat
v. hypertrophy
v. pacing
v. preload
v. reduction surgery
v. rhythm
v. septal defect
ventriculectomy
partial left v.
ventriculi
anadenia v.
filtrum v.
fundus v.
Merkel filtrum v.
ventriculitis
ventriculoatrial shunt
ventriculoatriostomy
ventriculocisternostomy
ventriculography

V

NOTES

ventriculomastoidostomy
ventriculonector
ventriculoperitoneal shunt
ventriculoplasty
    reduction left v.
ventriculopuncture
ventriculoscopy
ventriculostomy
    third v.
ventriculosubarachnoid
ventriculotomy
ventriculus
ventriduction
ventroscopy
ventrotomy
venular
venule
    high endothelial postcapillary v.
    inferior macular v.
    inferior nasal retinal v.
    inferior temporal retinal v.
    medial v.
    pericytic v.
    postcapillary v.
    stellate v.
vera
    cutis v.
    decidua v.
    hemospermia v.
    melena v.
    polycythemia v.
verbal
    v. apraxia
    v. autopsy
    v. dyspraxia
verbigeration
verge
    anal v.
vergence
Verhoeff elastic tissue stain
Vermale operation
vermicidal
vermicide
vermicular
    v. movement
    v. pulse
vermiculation
vermiculose
vermiculous
vermiform appendix
vermiformis
    appendix v.
vermilion border
vermilionectomy
vermin
vermination
verminous
    v. abscess

    v. appendicitis
    v. colic
vermis
    uvula v.
vernal conjunctivitis
Vernet syndrome
Verneuil operation
vernix caseosa
vero cytotoxin
verruca, pl. **verrucae**
    v. necrogenica
    v. peruana
    v. peruviana
    v. plana
    v. plantaris
verruciform
verrucosa
    tuberculosis cutis v.
verrucose
verrucosis
    lymphostatic v.
verrucosum
    eczema v.
verrucosus
    lichen planus v.
verrucous
    v. endocarditis
    v. hemangioma
    v. nevus
    v. xanthoma
verruga peruana
versicolor
    pityriasis v.
    tinea v.
version
    bimanual v.
    bipolar v.
    cephalic v.
    combined v.
    external cephalic v.
    internal cephalic v.
    internal podalic v.
    pelvic v.
    podalic v.
    spontaneous v.
    Wright v.
vertebra, pl. **vertebrae**
    basilar v.
    block v.
    butterfly v.
    v. C1
    v. C2
    cervical v.
    coccygeal v.
    codfish v.
    cranial v.
    v. dentata
    dorsal v.
    false v.

first cervical v.
hourglass v.
H-shape v.
ivory v.
v. lumbales
lumbar v.
v. plana
sacral v.
v. sacrales
thoracic v.
vertebral
v. arch
v. artery
v. canal
v. column
v. foramen
v. formula
v. nerve
v. notch
v. rib
v. vein
vertebrate
vertebrated catheter
vertebrectomy
vertebroarterial foramen
vertebrochondral
vertebrocostal trigone
vertebrosternal
vertex, pl. **vertices**
corneal v.
v. presentation
vertical
v. banded gastroplasty
v. growth phase
v. heart
v. mattress suture
v. muscle
v. nystagmus
v. overlap
v. strabismus
v. transmission
verticillata
cornea v.
verticillate
vertiginous
vertigo
arteriosclerotic v.
auditory v.
aural v.
benign paroxysmal positional v.
Charcot v.
chronic v.

endemic paralytic v.
epidemic v.
essential v.
gastric v.
height v.
horizontal v.
hysterical v.
labyrinthine v.
laryngeal v.
lateral v.
mechanical v.
ocular v.
organic v.
positional v.
postural v.
visual v.
vesicae
apex v.
bullous edema v.
sphincter v.
vesical
v. calculus
v. diverticulum
v. hematuria
v. triangle
v. vein
vesicalis
anus v.
vesicans
collodion v.
vesicant
vesica prostatica
vesication
vesicle
acoustic v.
acrosomal v.
air v.
allantoic v.
amniocardiac v.
auditory v.
blastodermic v.
cerebral v.
cervical v.
coated v.
encephalic v.
forebrain v.
germinal v.
v. hernia
hindbrain v.
lens v.
lenticular v.
malpighian v.

V

NOTES

vesicle *(continued)*
    matrix v.
    midbrain v.
    ophthalmic v.
    otic v.
    primary brain v.
    prostatic v.
    seminal v.
    synaptic v.
vesicocele
vesicoclysis
vesicocolonic fistula
vesicointestinal fistula
vesicopustular
vesicorectal fistula
vesicorectostomy
vesicosigmoidostomy
vesicospinal
vesicostomy
    cutaneous v.
vesicotomy
vesicoumbilical fistula
vesicoureteral
    v. reflux
    v. valve
vesicoureteric reflux
vesicourethral canal
vesicouterine
    v. excavation
    v. fistula
    v. fold
vesicovaginal fistula
vesicula, pl. **vesiculae**
vesicular
    v. appendage
    v. breath sound
    v. emphysema
    v. eruption
    v. keratitis
    v. murmur
    v. ovarian follicle
    v. resonance
    v. respiration
    v. stomatitis
    v. transport
vesiculate
vesiculation
vesiculectomy
vesiculiform
vesiculitis
vesiculocavernous
vesiculography
vesiculopapular
vesiculoprostatitis
vesiculopustular
vesiculosum
    eczema v.
vesiculotomy
vesiculotubular

vesiculotympanitic resonance
vesiculous
vessel
    absorbent v.
    afferent v.
    anastomosing v.
    anastomotic v.
    blood v.
    capillary v.
    choroid blood v.
    chyle v.
    collateral v.
    corkscrew v.
    deep lymph v.
    efferent v.
    hairpin v.
    intrapulmonary blood v.
    lacteal v.
    lymph v.
    lymphatic v.
    nutrient v.
    transposition of the great v.'s
vestibula (*pl. of* vestibulum)
vestibular
    v. canal
    v. crest
    v. fold
    v. ganglion
    v. membrane
    v. nerve
    v. neurectomy
    v. neuronitis
    v. nucleus
    v. nystagmus
    v. organ
    v. region
    v. schwannoma
    v. vein
vestibule
    aortic v.
    buccal v.
    esophagogastric v.
    gastroesophageal v.
    labial v.
    nasal v.
    oral v.
vestibuli
    fenestra v.
vestibulocochlear
    v. nerve
    v. nucleus
vestibuloocular reflex
vestibulopathy
    idiopathic bilateral v.
    migraine-related v.
vestibuloplasty
vestibulospinal reflex
vestibulotomy
vestibulum, pl. **vestibula**

vestige
vestigial organ
veterinarian
vexans
    Aedes v.
viable birth
vibrating line
vibratory tinnitus
vibrio
    V. alginolyticus
    V. cholerae
    El Tor v.
    V. fetus
    V. fluvialis
    V. furnissii
    V. mimicus
    V. parahaemolyticus
    V. vulnificus
vibriosis
vibrissa
vibrocardiogram
vicarious
    v. hypertrophy
    v. menstruation
vicious
    v. circle
    v. union
videoendoscope
videoendoscopy
vidian
Vierra sign
Vieth-Müller circle
view
    axial v.
    base v.
    Caldwell v.
    half axial v.
    Judet v.
    long axis v.
vigil
    coma v.
vigilambulism
villi (*pl. of* villus)
villoma
villose
villositis
villosity
villous
    v. adenoma
    v. carcinoma
    v. tenosynovitis
villus, pl. villi

    anchoring v.
    arachnoid v.
    chorionic v.
    floating v.
    free v.
    intestinal v.
villusectomy
vimentin
Vincent
    V. angina
    V. bacillus
    V. disease
    V. infection
    V. spirillum
    V. tonsillitis
vincula
vinculum
    long v.
vinegar eel
violence
    domestic v.
violet
    aniline gentian v.
    crystal v.
    gentian v.
    Hoffman v.
    Lauth v.
    methyl v.
    visual v.
vipoma
Vipond sign
viral
    v. conjunctivitis
    v. dysentery
    v. envelope
    v. hemagglutination
    v. hepatitis
    v. hepatitis type A, B, D
    v. load
    v. pharyngitis
    v. spongiform encephalopathy
    v. tropism
Virchow
    V. node
    V. psammoma
viremia
viridans streptococcus
viridis
    Euglena v.
virile
virilescence

V

NOTES

virilis
>   mamma v.

virilism
>   adrenal v.

virility

virilization

virilizing

virion

virologist

virology

virtual endoscopy

virucidal

virucide

virulence

virulent bacteriophage

viruliferous

viruria

virus
>   Abelson murine leukemia v.
>   adeno-associated v. (AAV)
>   adenoidal-pharyngeal-conjunctival v.
>   adenosatellite v.
>   AIDS-related v.
>   amphotropic v.
>   Andes v.
>   A-P-C v.
>   Argentine hemorrhagic fever v.
>   attenuated v.
>   Aujeszky disease v.
>   Australian X disease v.
>   avian encephalomyelitis v.
>   avian influenza v.
>   avian leukosis-sarcoma v.
>   avian lymphomatosis v.
>   avian neurolymphomatosis v.
>   avian pneumoencephalitis v.
>   avian viral arthritis v.
>   B v.
>   B19 v.
>   bacterial v.
>   Barmah Forest v.
>   Bayou v.
>   Bittner v.
>   BK v.
>   Black Creek Canal v.
>   bluetongue v.
>   Bolivian hemorrhagic fever v.
>   Borna disease v.
>   Bornholm disease v.
>   bovine leukemia v.
>   bovine leukosis v.
>   bovine papular stomatitis v.
>   bovine virus diarrhea v.
>   Bunyamwera v.
>   Bwamba v.
>   CA v.
>   California v.
>   canine distemper v.
>   Capim v.

Caraparu v.
Catu v.
CELO v.
Central European tick-borne
  encephalitis v.
C group v.
Chagres v.
chickenpox v.
Coe v.
cold v.
Colorado tick fever v.
common cold v.
Côte-d'Ivoire v.
cowpox v.
coxsackie v.
Crimean-Congo hemorrhagic
  fever v.
croup-associated v.
cytopathogenic v.
defective v.
delta v.
dengue v.
distemper v.
DNA v.
dog distemper v.
duck hepatitis v.
duck influenza v.
duck plague v.
Duvenhage v.
eastern equine encephalomyelitis v.
EB v.
Ebola v.
ecotropic v.
ectromelia v.
EEE v.
emerging v.
encephalitis v.
encephalomyocarditis v.
enteric cytopathogenic human
  orphan v.
enteric cytopathogenic monkey
  orphan v.
enteric cytopathogenic swine
  orphan v.
enzootic encephalomyelitis v.
ephemeral fever v.
epidemic gastroenteritis v.
epidemic keratoconjunctivitis v.
epidemic myalgia v.
epidemic parotitis v.
epidemic pleurodynia v.
Epstein-Barr v. (EBV)
FA v.
fibrous bacterial v.
filamentous bacterial v.
filtrable v.
fixed v.
Flury strain rabies v.
FMD v.

foamy v.
foot-and-mouth disease v.
Four Corners v.
Friend leukemia v.
GAL v.
gallus adenolike v.
gastroenteritis v. type A, B
GB v.
German measles v.
Germiston v.
goatpox v.
Graffi v.
green monkey v.
Gross leukemia v.
Guama v.
Guanarito v.
Guaroa v.
HA1 v.
HA2 v.
hand-foot-and-mouth disease v.
Hantaan v.
helper v.
Hendra v.
hepatitis A v. (HAV)
hepatitis B v. (HBV)
hepatitis C v. (HCV)
hepatitis D v.
hepatitis delta v. (HDV)
hepatitis E v. (HEV)
hepatitis G v. (HGV)
herpes simplex v. (HSV)
herpes zoster v.
hog cholera v.
horsepox v.
human immunodeficiency v. (HIV)
human papilloma v.
human T-cell
  lymphoma/leukemia v. (HTLV)
human T-cell lymphotropic v.
human T-cell lymphotropic v., type
  1 (HTLV-I)
human T-cell lymphotropic v., type
  2 (HTLV-II)
human T-cell lymphotropic v., type
  3 (HTLV-III)
human T lymphotrophic v.
Ilhéus v.
inclusion conjunctivitis v.
infantile gastroenteritis v.
infectious ectromelia v.
infectious hepatitis v.
infectious papilloma v.

infectious porcine
  encephalomyelitis v.
influenza v.
insect v.
iridescent v.
Jamestown Canyon v.
Japanese B encephalitis v.
JC v.
JH v.
Junin v.
K v.
Kasokero v.
Kelev strain rabies v.
v. keratoconjunctivitis
Kilham rat v.
Koongol v.
Korean hemorrhagic fever v.
Kyasanur Forest disease v.
La Crosse v.
lactate dehydrogenase v.
Lassa v.
latent rat v.
louping-ill v.
Lucké v.
Lunyo v.
lymphadenopathy-associated v.
  (LAV)
lymphocytic choriomeningitis v.
lymphogranuloma venereum v.
Machupo v.
malignant catarrhal fever v.
Marburg v.
Marek disease v.
marmoset v.
masked v.
Mason-Pfizer v.
Mayaro v.
measles v.
Menangle v.
Mengo v.
milkers' nodule v.
mink enteritis v.
MM v.
Mokola v.
molluscum contagiosum v.
Moloney v.
mumps v.
naked v.
New York v.
Nipah v.
Norwalk v.
oncogenic v.

NOTES

V

virus *(continued)*
    orphan v.
    Pacheco parrot disease v.
    parainfluenza v.
    poliomyelitis v.
    Puumala v.
    rabies v.
    respiratory enteric orphan v.
    Reston v.
    RNA tumor v.
    Ross River v.
    Rous-associated v.
    Rous sarcoma v.
    rubella v.
    rubeola v.
    Sabia v.
    Semliki Forest v.
    Seoul v.
    serum hepatitis v.
    v. shedding
    simian v.
    Sindbis v.
    Sin Nombre v.
    slow v.
    smallpox v.
    St. Louis encephalitis v.
    street v.
    Sudan v.
    Taiwan Dobrava-Belgrade v.
    Theiler mouse encephalomyelitis v.
    tick-borne encephalitis v.
    Topografov v.
    tumor v.
    varicella-zoster v.
    variola v.
    xenotropic v.
    Zaire v.

virus-1
    human immunodeficiency v.-1 (HIV-1)

virus-2
    human immunodeficiency v. (HIV-2)

virusoid

virus-transformed cell

viscerad

visceral
    v. anesthesia
    v. cleft
    v. fascia
    v. layer
    v. leishmaniasis
    v. lymph node
    v. pain
    v. pleurisy
    v. sense
    v. swallow

viscerale
    cranium v.

visceralgia

viscerocranium
    membranous v.

viscerogenic

visceroinhibitory

visceromegaly

visceromotor

visceropleural

visceroptosia

visceroptosis

viscerosensory

visceroskeletal

visceroskeleton

viscerosomatic

viscerotrophic

viscerotropic

viscid

viscidity

viscosity
    absolute v.
    anomalous v.
    apparent v.
    coefficient of v.
    dynamic v.
    kinematic v.

viscosus
    Actinomyces v.

viscous

viscus

visible spectrum

vision
    achromatic v.
    binocular v.
    blue v.
    central v.
    chromatic v.
    colored v.
    cone v.
    direct v.
    double v.
    duplicity theory of v.
    facial v.
    green v.
    halo v.
    haploscopic v.
    indirect v.
    multiple v.
    night v.
    oscillating v.
    peripheral v.
    photopic v.
    scotopic v.
    stereoscopic v.
    triple v.
    tubular v.
    tunnel v.

visual
    v. agnosia
    v. angle

v. aphasia
v. area
v. aura
v. axis
v. closure
v. cortex
v. evoked potential
v. field
v. hallucination
v. inspection
v. memory
v. neglect
v. orientation
v. pigment
v. purple
v. receptor cell
v. vertigo
v. violet

visual-kinetic dissociation
visuognosis
visuomotor
visuosensory
visuospatial
vital

v. capacity
v. index
v. pulp
v. red
v. sign
v. signs stable (VSS)
v. stain
v. statistics
v. vaccine

vitality test
vitalometer
vitam

intra v.

vitamin

v. A
v. A1 acid
antiberiberi v.
antihemorrhagic v.
antineuritic v.
antirachitic v.
antiscorbutic v.
antisterility v.
v. B
v. B1
v. B6
v. B12
v. B complex
v. B12 neuropathy

v. C
coagulation v.
v. D
v. D2
v. D3
v. D–binding protein
v. D milk
v. D-resistant rickets
v. E
fat-soluble v.
fertility v.
v. K
v. K1
v. K2
microbial v.

vitelliform retinal dystrophy
vitellina

membrana v.

vitelline pole
vitellointestinal cyst
vitellus
vitiation
vitiliginous choroiditis
vitiligo
vitrea

camera v.

vitrectomy

anterior v.

vitreitis
vitreodentin
vitreoretinal
vitreoretinopathy

exudative v.

vitreotapetoretinal dystrophy
vitreous

v. body
v. chamber
v. detachment
v. hernia
v. humor
v. lamella
v. membrane
v. opacity
persistent anterior hyperplastic
  primary v.
persistent posterior hyperplastic
  primary v.
tertiary v.

vitreum
vitreus

humor v.

vitrification

V

NOTES

vitro
    in v.
vitronectin
Vittaforma
vivax
    v. malaria
    Plasmodium v.
vivification
viviparous
vivisection
vivisectionist
vivisector
vivo
    ex v.
    in v.
vocal
    v. fold
    v. fremitus
    v. fry
    v. ligament
    v. muscle
    v. nodule
    v. process
    v. resonance
    v. spectrum
    v. tract
vocalis
    glottis v.
    v. muscle
vogeli
    Echinococcus v.
Vogel law
voice
    amphoric v.
    bronchial v.
    cavernous v.
    epigastric v.
    eunuchoid v.
    v. fatigue syndrome
    gravel v.
void
    flow v.
voiding
    v. cystogram
    v. cystourethrogram
volar psoriasis
volatile oil
volatilization
volitantes
    muscae v.
volition
volitional tremor
Volkmann
    V. cheilitis
    V. contracture
    V. spoon
volt (V, v)
    kiloelectron v. (keV)
voltage

voltampere
Voltolini disease
volume
    atomic v.
    closing v.
    compressible v.
    v. controlled ventilation
    distribution v.
    end-diastolic v.
    end-systolic v.
    expiratory reserve v. (ERV)
    extracellular fluid v. (ECFV)
    forced expiratory v. (FEV)
    v. index
    inspiratory reserve v. (IRV)
    maximum expiratory flow v. (MEFV)
    mean corpuscular v. (MCV)
    minute v.
    partial v.
    rebreathing v.
    residual v.
    respiratory minute v.
    resting tidal v.
    standard v.
    stroke v.
    tidal v.
    v. ventilator
volumetric
    v. analysis
    v. solution
voluminous hernia
voluntary
    v. muscle
    v. nystagmus
volute
volvulus
    cecal v.
    gastric v.
    mesenteroaxial v.
vomerine cartilage
vomeronasal cartilage
vomit
    Barcoo v.
    bilious v.
    black v.
    coffee-ground v.
vomiting
    cerebral v.
    cyclic v.
    dry v.
    epidemic v.
    explosive v.
    fecal v.
    hysterical v.
    nausea and v. (N&V)
    pernicious v.
    v. of pregnancy
    projectile v.

psychogenic v.
recurrent v.
v. reflex
retention v.
stercoraceous v.

vomiturition
vomitus
von

V. Bergman hernia
v. Gierke disease
v. Graefe sign
v. Spee curve
v. Willebrand disease

vortex, pl. **vortices**

v. corneal dystrophy
Fleischer v.
v. lentis
v. vein

vorticose vein
Vossius lenticular ring
voulu

déjà v.

voyeur
voyeurism
V-pattern

V-p. esotropia
V-p. exotropia

VSS

vital signs stable

vu

déjà v.

vulgaris

acne v.
ichthyosis v.
impetigo v.
lupus v.
pemphigus v.
Proteus v.

vulnerable phase
vulnificus

Vibrio v.

Vulpian atrophy
vulsella forceps, vulsellum forceps
vulvae

elephantiasis v.
kraurosis v.
leukoplakia v.
pruritus v.

vulvar

v. intraepithelial neoplasia
v. nevus

vulvectomy
vulvitis

chronic atrophic v.
chronic hypertrophic v.
follicular v.
ulcerative v.

vulvovaginitis

NOTES

V

Wachendorf membrane
waddling gait
wadsworthii
    Legionella w.
waist-to-hip ratio
Waldenström macroglobulinemia
Waldeyer sheath
Walker chart
walking
    chromosome w.
walk-through angina
wall
    cavity w.
    cell w.
    chest w.
    enamel w.
    hitting the w.
    inferior w.
    jugular w.
    labyrinthine w.
    lateral w.
    mastoid w.
    medial w.
    membranous w.
    parietal w.
    splanchnic w.
    thoracic w.
wallerian degeneration
wall-eye
wall-eyed bilateral internuclear
  ophthalmoplegia
Walsh procedure
Walthard cell rest
Walther
    W. dilator
    W. duct
    W. ganglion
waltzed flap
wandering
    w. abscess
    w. cell
    w. goiter
    w. kidney
    w. pacemaker
    w. tooth
Warburg
    W. apparatus
    W. theory
Wardrop method
Ward triangle
warming
    global w.
warm-up phenomenon
war neurosis

wart
    anatomic w.
    anatomical w.
    asbestos w.
    common w.
    digitate w.
    filiform w.
    flat w.
    fugitive w.
    genital w.
    Henle w.
    infectious w.
    mosaic w.
    necrogenic w.
    Peruvian w.
    pitch w.
    plantar w.
    postmortem w.
    seed w.
    soft w.
    telangiectatic w.
    tuberculous w.
    venereal w.
Wartenberg symptom
warty tuberculosis
wash-out
    open-circuit nitrogen w.-o.
wasp
    sea w.
wastage
    fetal w.
wasting
    w. palsy
    w. paralysis
    salt w.
    w. syndrome
water
    alkaline w.
    aromatic w.
    bag of w.'s
    baryta w.
    bitter w.
    bound w.
    w. brash
    bromine w.
    calcic w.
    carbonated w.
    carbon dioxide-free w.
    carbonic w.
    chalybeate w.
    chlorine w.
    deionized w.
    distilled w.
    w. diuresis
    earthy w.

W

water *(continued)*
    false w.'s
    free w.
    gentian aniline w.
    hard w.
    heavy w.
    indifferent w.
    intracellular w.
    w. itch
    lime w.
    mineral w.
water-hammer pulse
Waterhouse-Friderichsen syndrome
Waters
    W. operation
    W. projection
water-seal drainage system
watershed infarction
water-trap stomach
Watson-Crick helix
Watson operation
wave
    A w.
    acid w.
    alkaline w.
    alpha w.
    arterial w.
    B w.
    beta w.
    brain w.
    C w.
    cannon w.
    D w.
    delta w.
    dicrotic w.
    electrocardiographic w.
    epsilon w.
    excitation w.
    F w.
    f w.
    fibrillary w.
    fibrillatory w.
    flat top w.
    fluid w.
    flutter-fibrillation w.
    microelectric w.
    mucosal w.
    oscillation w.
    overflow w.
    P w.
    percussion w.
    postextrasystolic T w.
    pulse w.
    Q w.
    R w.
    S w.
    sine w.
    T w.

    theta w.
    Traube-Hering w.
    U w.
    V w.
    vasomotor w.
waveform
    pressure w.
wavelength
wax
    animal w.
    baseplate w.
    bleached w.
    bone w.
    boxing w.
    Brazil w.
    carnauba w.
    casting w.
    Chinese w.
    ear w., earwax
    earth w.
    emulsifying w.
    grave w.
    Horsley bone w.
    inlay w.
    Japan w.
    mineral w.
waxing
waxing-up
waxy
    w. degeneration
    w. kidney
    w. spleen
2-way catheter
weakness
    directional w.
wear-and-tear pigment
web
    esophageal w.
    laryngeal w.
webbed
    w. finger
    w. neck
webbing
Weber
    W. law
    W. paradox
    W. stain
    W. syndrome
    W. test for hearing
    W. triangle
Weber-Fechner law
Wechsler intelligence scale
wedge
    w. bone
    dental w.
    w. fracture
    w. pressure
    w. resection

wedge-and-groove
    w.-a.-g. joint
    w.-a.-g. suture
weed
    Jamestown w.
    jimson w.
Weeks bacillus
Weeksella zoohelcum
Wegener granulomatosis
Weigert
    W. iodine solution
    W. iron hematoxylin stain
    W. law
    W. stain for actinomyces
    W. stain for elastin
    W. stain for fibrin
    W. stain for myelin
    W. stain for neuroglia
weighing
    hydrostatic w.
    underwater w.
weight
    apothecaries w.
    atomic w. (AW)
    avoirdupois w.
    birth w.
    combining w.
    dry w.
    equivalent w.
    gram-atomic w.
    gram-molecular w.
    molecular w.
weight-supported exercise
Weil disease
Weil-Felix
    W.-F. reaction
    W.-F. test
Weinberg reaction
Weiss sign
Welch bacillus
welchii
    Clostridium w.
well-differentiated lymphocytic lymphoma
Wenckebach
    W. block
    W. period
Werlhof disease
Wermer syndrome
werneckii
    Exophiala w.
Werner syndrome

Wernicke
    W. aphasia
    W. center
    W. reaction
    W. syndrome
Wernicke-Korsakoff
    W.-K. encephalopathy
    W.-K. syndrome
Wertheim operation
Westberg space
Westergren method
Westermark sign
western
    W. blot
    W. blot analysis
    W. blot test
    W. blotting
    w. equine encephalomyelitis
Westgard rule
Westphal
    W. pupillary reflex
    W. sign
Westphal-Strümpell disease
West syndrome
wet
    w. gangrene
    w. lung
    w. mount
    w. pleurisy
    w. spot
wet-bulb thermometer
wet-technique liposuction
wet-to-dry dressing
Wharton
    W. duct
    W. jelly
wheal
wheal-and-erythema reaction
wheal-and-flare reaction
Wheatstone bridge
wheel
    Burlew w.
wheeze
    asthmatoid w.
whey
    alum w.
whiff test
whiplash
    w. injury
    w. retinopathy
Whipple
    W. disease

W

NOTES

Whipple *(continued)*
  W. incision
  W. operation
whipstitch suture
whispered bronchophony
whistle
  Galton w.
whistling
  w. rale
  w. rhonchi
Whitaker test
white
  w. blood cell
  w. braided suture
  w. corpuscle
  w. fiber
  w. gangrene
  w. graft
  w. infarct
  w. limbal girdle
  w. line
  w. lung
  w. matter
  w. matter disease
  w. muscle
  w. noise
  w. piedra
  w. pulp
  w. sound
  w. substance
Whitehead operation
whitlow
  herpes w.
  herpetic w.
Whitman frame
whole blood
whole-body counter
whooping cough
whorl
  coccygeal w.
  digital w.
  hair w.
Wickham stria
wide-angle
  w.-a. glaucoma
  w.-a. tomography
wideband
wide dynamic range compression
Wilbrand knee
Wilder
  W. sign
  W. stain for reticulum
Wildermuth ear
Wilde triangle
Wilkie artery
will
  living w.

Williams
  W. stain
  W. syndrome
Williams-Beuren syndrome
Willis
  circle of W.
  W. cord
Williston law
Wilms tumor
Wilson
  W. block
  curve of W.
  W. disease
  W. method
wind
  second w.
windburn
windchill index
window
  aortic w.
  aorticopulmonary w.
  aortic-pulmonic w.
  aortopulmonary w.
  cochlear w.
  lung w.
  mediastinal w.
  oval w.
  round w.
  tachycardia w.
windpipe
wind-sucking
wine
  high w.
  low w.
wing
  angel w.
  ashen w.
  gray w.
  greater w.
  lesser w.
wing-beating tremor
winged
  w. catheter
  w. scapula
winking
  jaw w.
wink reflex
Winslow
  foramen of W.
Winterbottom sign
Winternitz sound
winthemi
  Margaropus w.
wire
  arch w.
  guide w.
  Kirschner w.
  ligature w.

w. mesh implant
olive w.
wiring
circumferential w.
circumzygomatic w.
continuous loop w.
craniofacial suspension w.
Gilmer w.
Ivy loop w.
Wirsung
W. canal
W. duct
wiry pulse
wisdom tooth
Wise operation
Wissler syndrome
witch's milk
withdrawal
w. symptoms
w. syndrome
withering cancer
within normal limits (WNL)
Witzel operation
WNL
within normal limits
Wolfe graft
wolffian
w. body
w. cyst
w. duct
w. rest
Wolff law
Wolff-Parkinson-White syndrome
wolframium
Wolfram syndrome
Wollaston doublet
Wolman
W. disease
W. xanthomatosis
womb
falling of the w.
wood
W. glass
W. lamp
W. light
orange w.
wooden resonance
word
w. blindness
w. deafness
w. salad
workaholic

work of breathing
working
w. occlusion
w. out
w. side
w. through
workload unit
worm
caddis w.
Manson eye w.
meal w.
wormian bone
wort
St. John's w.
Worth amblyoscope
Woulfe bottle
wound
abraded w.
avulsed w.
w. biopsy
w. clip
crease w.
glancing w.
gunshot w.
gutter w.
incised w.
lacerating w. (LW)
nonpenetrating w.
open w.
penetrating w.
perforating w.
puncture w.
self-inflicted w.
sucking chest w.
woven bone
W-plasty
wrap
cardiac muscle w.
wreath
ciliary w.
Wright
W. stain
W. syndrome
W. version
wrinkle
glabellar w.
wrist
w. joint
w. sign
wrist-drop
wrist-hand orthosis
writhing in pain

NOTES

W

903

writing hand
wuchereriasis

Wyburn-Mason syndrome

xanthelasma
  generalized x.
  x. palpebrarum
xanthemia
xanthene dye
xanthic
xanthine
xanthism
xanthochromatic
xanthochromia
xanthochromic
xanthoderma
xanthogranuloma
  juvenile x.
xanthoma
  x. disseminatum
  eruptive x.
  fibrous x.
  x. multiplex
  x. planum
  x. tuberosum
  verrucous x.
xanthomatosis
  biliary x.
  x. bulbi
  cerebrotendinous x.
  chronic idiopathic x.
  familial hypercholesteremic x.
  generalized plane x.
  Wolman x.
xanthomatous
xanthophyll
xanthopsia
xanthosine
xanthosis
X chromosome
xenic culture
xenobiotic
xenodiagnosis
xenogeneic
xenogenic
xenogenous
xenograft
xenon

xenon-133
xenoparasite
xenophobia
xenotropic virus
xerochilia
xeroderma pigmentosum
xerogram
xerography
xeroma
xerophthalmia
xeroradiograph
xeroradiography
xerosis
  Corynebacterium x.
xerostomia
xerotic
X-inactivation
xiphisternal
xiphisternum
xiphoid
  x. cartilage
  x. process
xiphoiditis
X-linked
  X-l. gene
  X-l. infantile
    hypogammaglobulinemia
  X-l. lymphoproliferative syndrome
  X-l. recessive bulbospinal
    neuronopathy
XO syndrome
X-pattern
  X-p. esotropia
  X-p. exotropia
x-ray
  x-r. alopecia
  x-r. microscope
XXY syndrome
xylidine
  ponceau de x.
xylose
xylulose
xysma
XYY syndrome

X

Y
Y cartilage
Y chromosome
Yakima
hemoglobin Y.
yaw
bosch y.
foot y.
mother y.
year
disability-adjusted life y. (DALY)
5-year survival rate
yeast
brewers' y.
compressed y.
cultivated y.
dried y.
yellow
acridine y.
butter y.
y. cartilage
y. fever
y. fiber
y. hepatization
hydrazine y.
indicator y.
lead oxide y.
Leipzig y.

lemon y.
martius y.
metanil y.
methyl y.
Sudan y.
yellowish
eosin y.
light green SF y.
yersiniosis
yield
quantum y.
Y-linkage
Y-linked gene
yoke
alveolar y.
yolk
y. membrane
y. stalk
Yorke autolytic reaction
Young-Helmholtz theory
Young modulus
yo-yo dieting
Y-shaped
Y-s. cartilage
Y-s. ligament
ytterbium
yttrium

Y

Z

Z band
Z filament
Z line

Zahn

Z. infarct
line of Z.

Zaire

Ebola virus Z.
Z. virus

Zarit burden interview
Zavanelli maneuver
Zeis gland
Zenker

Z. degeneration
Z. diverticulum
Z. fixative
Z. paralysis

zero

absolute z.
z. end-expiratory pressure

zetacrit
zeta sedimentation ratio
Z-flap incision
Ziehl stain
Ziemann dot
zigzag

z. incision
z. laceration

Zimmerlin atrophy
Zimmerman operation
zinc-65
zinc sulfate flotation concentration
Zinn

anulus of Z.
Z. zonule

zirconium
zoacanthosis
zoanthropic
zoanthropy
Zollinger-Ellison syndrome
Zöllner line
zona, pl. **zonae**

z. arcuata
z. fasciculata
z. glomerulosa
z. ophthalmica
z. orbicularis
z. pectinata
z. pellucida
z. reticularis
z. tecta

zonal necrosis
zone

abdominal z.
anal transitional z.
androgenic z.
arcuate z.
Barnes z.
cervical z.
ciliary z.
comfort z.
contact area z.
dentofacial z.
dolorogenic z.
entry z.
ependymal z.
epigastric z.
epileptogenic z.
equivalence z.
erogenous z.
erotogenic z.
fetal z.
gingival z.
Golgi z.
grenz z.
Head z.
hemorrhoidal z.
inner z.
intermediate z.
interpalpebral z.
intertubular z.
isoelectric z.
isopycnic z.
language z.
large loop excision of
    transformation z. (LLETZ)
latent z.
lateral z.
Lissauer marginal z.
Looser z.
mantle z.
Marchant z.
marginal z.
medial z.
mesogastric z.
pectinate z.
pellucid z.
training-sensitive z.
transitional z.
trigger z.

zonesthesia
zonifugal
zoning
zonipetal
zonography
zonula, pl. **zonulae**
zonular

z. cataract

Z

zonular *(continued)*
  z. scotoma
  z. space
zonule
  ciliary z.
  Zinn z.
zonulitis
zonulolysis
zonulysis
zoo blot analysis
zooerastia
zoograft
zoografting
zoohelcum
  Weeksella z.
zooid
zoolagnia
zoonosis
  direct z.
zoonotic
  z. cutaneous leishmaniasis
  z. potential
zooparasite
zoophilism
  erotic z.
zoophobia
zooplasty
zootoxin
zoster
  geniculate z.
  herpes z.
zosteroid
Z-plasty
Z-protein
Zsigmondy dental nomenclature
Zuckerkandl body
Zülch
  giant cell monstrocellular sarcoma
  of Z.

zwitter hypothesis
zwitterions
zygal
zygapophysis
zygoma
zygomatic
  z. arch
  z. bone
  z. nerve
  z. process
  z. region
zygomaticofacial foramen
zygomaticofrontal suture
zygomaticomaxillary suture
zygomaticoorbital
  z. artery
  z. foramen
zygomaticotemporal foramen
zygomaticus
  arcus z.
  z. major muscle
zygomaxillary point
zygomycosis
zygon
zygonema
zygosis
zygosity
zygote
zygotene
zygotic
zymodeme
zymogen
zymogenesis
zymogenic cell

Common Prefixes, Suffixes, and Combining Forms

a-	not, without, less	-ary	pertaining to
ab-, abs-	away from	-ase	an enzyme
-ac	pertaining to	-asthenia	weakness
acou-	hearing	-ate	a salt or ester of an
acr(o)-	extremity, topmost		"-ic" acid
acu-	hearing; needle	athero-	pasty, fatty
-acusis	hearing condition	-ation	process
ad-	increase, adherence, motion toward, very	audi(o)-	hearing
		aur(i)-, auro-	ear
-ad	toward, in the direction of	aut(o)-	self, same
		bacteri(o)-	bacteria
aden(o)-	gland	balan(o)-	glans penis
adip(o)-	fat	bi-	twice, double
adren(o)-	gland	bio-	life
aer(o)-	air, gas	blasto-	germ or bud
-agog, -agogue	promoter, stimulator	blephar(o)-	eyelid
-al	pertaining to	brachio(o)-	arm
alge-, algesi-	pain	brady-	slow
-algia, algio-, algo-	pain	bronch(i)o-	bronchus
		bucc(o)-	cheek
allo-	other, different	carcin(o)-	cancer
ambi-	around, on all sides, both	cardi(o)-	heart; esophageal opening of stomach
ambly(o)-	dull	carpo-	wrist
amyl(o)-	starch, polysaccharide	cata-	down
an-	not, without	caud(o)-	tail, lower part of body
ana-	up, toward, apart	-cele	hernia, swelling
ankylo-	crooked, stiff	-centesis	surgical puncture
ante-	before	centi-	one-hundredth
anthraco-	coal, carbon	cephal(o)-	the head
anti-	against, opposed to; curative; antibody	chem(o)-	chemistry, drug
		chir(o)-	hand
apo-	separated from, derived from	chlor(o)-	green; chlorine
		chol(e)-	bile
aque(o)-	water	chondrio-, chondr(o)-	cartilage; granular; gritty
-ar	pertaining to		
arteri(o)-	artery	chrom-, chromat-, chromo-	color
arthr(o)-	joint, articulation		
articul(o)-	joint		

chron(o)-	time	**-desis**	binding
-cidal, -cide	killing, destroying	**dextr(o)-**	right, toward or on the right side
circum-	around		
cis-	on this side, on the near side	**di-**	separation, taking apart, reversal, not, un-
-clast	breaker		
-clysis	washing	**dif-**	separation, taking apart, reversal, not, un-
co-, col-	with, together, in association, very, complete		
		dipso-	thirst
colo-	colon	**dir-, dis-**	separation, taking apart, reversal, not, un-
colp(o)-	vagina		
com-, con-	with, together, in association, very, complete		
		duo-	two
		duodeno-	duodenum
conio-	dust	**dynamo-**	force, energy
cor-	with, together, in association, very, complete	**-dynia**	pain
		dys-	bad, difficult
		-eal	pertaining to
coreo-	pupil	**ec-**	out, away
cost(o)-	rib	**ect-**	outer, on the outside
crani(o)-	cranium	**-ectasia, -ectasis**	dilation, stretching
-crine	secretion		
cry(o)-	cold	**ecto-**	outer, on the outside
crypt(o)-	hidden	**-ectomy**	excision
culdo-	cul-de-sac	**-emia**	blood condition
cyan(o)-	blue; cyanide	**-emphraxis**	obstruction
cycl-	circle, cycle; ciliary body	**encephal(o)-**	brain
		end(o)-	within, inner
cyst(i), cysto-	bladder; cyst; cystic duct	**enter(o)-**	intestine
cyt-, cyte-, cyt(o)-	cell	**ent(o)-**	inner, within
		ep-, epi-	upon, following, subsequent to
-cyte	cell		
dacry(o)-	tears	**ergo-**	work
dactyl(o)-	finger, toe	**erythr(o)-**	red, redness
de-	away from; cessation	**eso-**	inward
deca-	ten	**esthesio-**	sensation, perception
deci-	one-tenth	**eu-**	good, well
deka-	ten	**ex-**	out of, from, away from
dent(i)-	tooth	**exo-**	exterior, external, outward
derm-, derma-	skin		
dermat(o)-, dermo-		**extra-**	without, outside of
		ferro-	metallic iron; ferrous ion

fibr(o)-	fiber	-ic	pertaining to
-form	in the form or shape of	-icle	small
galact(o)-	milk	-ics	organized knowledge,
gastr(o)-	stomach; belly		practice, treatment
gen-, -gen	producing, coming to	ileo-	ileum
	be; precursor	ilio-	ilium
giga-	one billion	in-	in; not
gingiv(o)-	gums	infra-	below
gloss(o)-	tongue	inguino-	groin
gluco-	glucose	inter-	between, among
glyco-	sugars	intra-, intro-	within
gnath(o)-	jaw	irid(o)-	iris
gonio-	angle	ischi(o)-	ischium
gon(o)-	seed, semen, angle	-ism	condition, disease;
-gram	writing, recording		practice, doctrine
granul(o)-	granular, granule	-ismus	spasm; contraction
-graph	recording instrument	iso-	equal, like; isomer;
gyn(e),	woman		sameness
gyneco-,		-ist	one who specializes in
gyno-		-ite	of the nature of,
hecto-	one hundred		resembling
hem(a),	blood	-ites	-y, -like
hemat(o)-		-itides	plural of -itis
hemi-	one-half	-itis	inflammation
hemo-	blood	-ium	structure, tissue
hepat-,	liver	kal(i)-	potassium
hepatico-,		kary(o)-	nucleus
hepato-		kerat(o)-	cornea, cornified
hept(a)-	seven		epithelium
hidr(o)-	sweat	kilo-	one thousand
hist-, histio-,	tissue	kin(e)-,	movement
histo-		kinesi(o)-	
homeo-	same, constant	kineso-,	
hydr(o)-	water; hydrogen	kino-	
hyper-	above, excessive	kyph(o)-	humped
hypo-	below, deficient	labio-	lip
hyster(o)-	uterus; hysteria; late,	lacrim(o)-	tears
	following	lact(i), lacto-	milk
-ia	condition	laparo-	abdomen, abdominal
-iasis	condition, infestation,		wall
	infection	laryng(o)-	larynx
-iatrics	treatment	lateri-, latero-	lateral, to one side, side
-iatry	treatment	lei(o)-	smooth

-lepsis, -lepsy	seizure	**micro-**	small, microscopic, one-millionth
lepto-	light, slender, thin, frail	**milli-**	one-thousandth
leuk(o)-	white	**mon(o)-**	single
lien(o)-	spleen	**morph(o)-**	form, shape, structure
linguo-	tongue	**musculi(o)-**	muscle
lip(o)-	fat, lipid	**my(o)-**	muscle
lith(o)-	stone, calculus, calcification	**myc(o)-**	fungus
-log, log(o)-	speech, words	**myel(o)-**	bone marrow; spinal cord
-logist	one who specializes in study or treatment of	**myring(o)-**	tympanic membrane
-logy	study of; collecting	**myx(o)-**	mucus
lymph(o)-	lymph; lymphocyte	**nano-**	dwarf; one-billionth
lys(o)-, -lysis, -lytic	dissolution, disintegration; release	**nas(o)-**	nose
		natr(i)-	sodium
macr(o)-	large; long	**necr(o)-**	death, necrosis
mal-	bad, deficient	**neo-**	new
-malacia	softening	**nephr(o)-**	kidney
mamm-, mamm(a)-, mammo-, mast(o)-	breast	**neur(i), neuro-**	nerve, nervous system
		norm(o)-	normal
		octo-	eight
		oculo-	eye
meg-	large, oversize	**odont(o)-**	tooth
mega-	large, oversize; one million	**odyn(o)-, -odynia**	pain
megal(o)-	large	**-oid**	resemblance to
-megaly	enlargement	**olig(o)-**	few, little
melan(o)-	black	**-oma**	tumor, neoplasm
men-	menstruation	**-omata**	plural of –oma
mening(o)-	meninges	**oncho-, onco-**	tumor, bulk, volume
meno-	menstruation	**-one**	ketone
ment(o)-	chin	**onych(o)-, -onychia**	fingernail, toenail
-mer	member of a series		
mes(o)-	middle, mean, intermediate; attaching membrane	**oo-**	egg, ovary
		oophor(o)-	ovary
		ophthalm(o)-	eye
meta-	after, behind; joint action, sharing	**-opia, -opsia, -opsis**	vision
-meter	measurement, measuring device	**or-**	mouth
		orchi-, orchido-, orchio-	testis
metr(o)-	uterus		
-metry	process of measuring		
micr-	small, microscopic	**ori-, oro-**	mouth

orth(o)-	straight, normal, in proper order
-ose	sugar
-oses	plural of -osis
-osis	process, condition, state
osseo-	bony
ossi-	bone
ost(e)-, osteo-	bone
ot(o)-	ear
-ous	pertaining to
ovari(o)-	ovary
ov(i)-, ovo-	egg
ox(a)-, oxo-	oxygen
oxy-	sharp, acid; acute, shrill, quick; oxygen
pachy-	thick
pan-, pant(o)-	all, entire
para-	beside, near; similar; subordinate; abnormal
pari-	equal
path(o)-	disease, abnormality
-pathy	disease, abnormality
ped(i)-, pedo-	child; foot
pelvi-, pelvio-, pelvo-	the pelvis
-penia	deficiency
penta-	five
per-	through, thoroughly, intensely
peri-	around, about
-pexy	fixation, usually surgical
phaco-	lens
-phage, -phagia, phago-, -phagy	eating, devouring
phako-	lens
phanero-	visible, evident
pharmaco-	drug, medicine
pharyng(o)-	pharynx
phil-, -philia, philo-	attraction; chemical affinity
phleb(o)-	vein
-phobe, -phobia	fear; chemical repulsion
phon(o)-	sound, speech
phor(o)-	carrying, bearing
phos-, phot(o)-	light
phren(i)-, phrenico-, phreno-	diaphragm; mind; phrenic
-phrenia	mind
-phyaxis	protection
phyll(o)-	leaf
physi(o)-	physical; natural
physo-	swelling, inflation; air, gas
phyt(o)-	plants
pico-	one-trillionth
plan(i)-, plan(o)-	flat
-plasia	formation
plasm(a)-, plasmat(o)-, plasmo-	plasma
-plasty	surgical repair, reconstruction
platy-	wide, flat
-plegia	paralysis
pleo-	more
plesio-	near, similar
pleur(a)-, pleuro-	rib, side, pleura
pluri-	several, more
-pnea, -pneo	breath, respiration
pneum/ pneuma-	air, lung
pneum(a)-, pneumat(o)-	air, gas; lung; breathing
pod(o)-	foot, foot-shaped
-poiesis, -poietic	production
poikilo-	irregular, variable

polio-	gray	**scot(o)-**	shadow, darkness
poly-	many, multiple; polymer	**semi-**	one-half; partly
post-	after, behind, posterior	**sept-, septo-**	seven; septum; sepsis, infection
pre-	anterior, before		
presby-	old	**septi-**	seven
pro-	before, forward; precursor	**sial(o)-**	saliva, salivary gland
		sider(o)-	iron
proct(o)-	anus, rectum	**sigmoid(o)-**	S-shaped; sigmoid colon
prot(o)-	first		
pseud(o)-	false	**sin-, sin(o)-, sinu-**	sinus
psych(e)-, psycho-	mind		
		sinistr(o)-	left, toward the left
-ptosis	sagging, falling	**sito-**	food, grain
pyel(o)-	(renal) pelvis	**somat-, somato- somatico-**	body, bodily
pykn(o)-	dense, compact		
pyo-	suppuration, pus		
pyreto-	fever	**somno-**	sleep
pyro-	fire, heat, fever	**son(o)-**	sound; ultrasound
quadr(i)-	four	**spasmo-**	spasm
rachi(o)-	spinal column	**sperm(a)-, spermat(o)- spermo-**	semen, spermatozoa
radio-	radiation, x-ray; radius		
re-	again, back, backward		
rect(i)-	straight	**sphygmo-**	pulse
rect(o)-	rectum	**spir(o)-**	breathing
ren(o)-	kidney	**splanchn(i)-, splanchno-**	viscera
reticul(o)-	reticulum; reticular		
retro-	backward, behind	**splen(o)-**	spleen
rhabd(o)-	rod; rod-shaped	**spondyl(o)-**	vertebra
rhin(o)-	nose	**staphyle(o)-**	grape, bunch of grapes; staphylococci
-rrhagia	discharge, bleeding		
-rrhaphy	surgical suturing	**-stasis**	stopping
-rrhea	flow	**-stat**	arresting change or movement
-rrhexis	rupture		
salping(o)-	tube	**steno-**	narrowness, constriction
sarco-	flesh, muscle		
schisto-, schiz(o)-	split, cleft, division	**stereo-**	solid
		stheno-	strength, force, power
scler(o)-	hardness, sclerosis; ocular sclera	**stom(a)-, stomat(o)-**	mouth
scoli(o)-	crooked	**-stomy**	artificial or surgical opening
-scope	instrument for viewing		
		sub-	beneath, less than normal, inferior
-scopy	viewing		

super-	above, in excess, superior	**tri-**	three
supra-	above	**trich(i)-,** **-trichia,** **tricho-**	hair
sy-, syl-, sym-, **syn-, sys-**	together		
tachy-	rapid	**tris-**	three
tel(e)-	distant	**-trophic,** **tropho-,** **-trophy**	food, nutrition
ten-, tendin- **teno-,** **tenont(o)-**	tendon		
		-tropia, **-tropic,** **-tropy**	turning, tendency, affinity
tera-	one quadrillion		
tetra-	four	**tympan(o)-**	tympanum
thel(o)-	nipple	**ule-, ulo-**	scar, scarring; the gums; curly
therm(o)-	heat		
thora-, **thorac(i)-** **thoracico-,** **thoraco-**	chest, thorax	**ultra-**	beyond
		uni-	one, single
		ure-	urine
		uri-	uric acid
thromb(o)-	blood clot	**-uria**	urine, urination
thyre(o)-, **thyr(o)-**	thyroid gland	**uric(o)-**	uric acid
		urin-, uro-	urine
toco-, toko-	childbirth	**varico-**	varix, varicose, varicosity
-tome	cutting instrument; segment, section		
		vas-	duct, blood vessel
-tomy	cutting operation	**vasculo-**	blood vessel
tono-	tone, tension, pressure	**vaso-**	duct, blood vessel
top(o)-	place, topical	**vesic(o)-**	urinary bladder, vesicle
tox(i)-, **toxico-,** **toxo-**	toxin, poison		
		xanth(o)-	yellow
		xero-	dry
trache(o)-	trachea	**zo(o)-**	animal; life
trans-	across, through, beyond	**zym(o)-**	fermentation, enzyme

Appendix 2
Ligaments

Shoulder/upper arm
acromioclavicular
collateral ulnar
conoid
coracoacromial
coracoclavicular
coracohumeral
costoclavicular
glenohumeral
inferior transverse
interclavicular
superior transverse
trapezoid

Hand/forearm
anular ligament of radius
collateral ligament of interphalangeal
   articulation
collateral ligament of
   metacarpophalangeal articulation
collateral radial
deep transverse metacarpal
dorsal carpometacarpal
dorsal intercarpal
dorsal metacarpal
dorsal radiocarpal
interosseous intercarpal
interosseous metacarpal
palmar carpometacarpal
palmar intercarpal
palmar ligament of interphalangeal
   articulation
palmar metacarpal
palmar radiocarpal
palmar ulnocarpal
pisohamate
pisometacarpal
quadrate

radial carpal
radiate ligament of wrist
superficial transverse metacarpal
transverse carpal
ulnar carpal

Spine
alar
anterior longitudinal
anterior sacrococcygeal
anterior sacroiliac
apical dental
caudal retinaculum
cruciform ligament of atlas
costotransverse
deep posterior sacrococcygeal
iliofemoral
iliolumbar
interarticular
interspinal
intertransverse
lateral atlantooccipital
lateral costotransverse
lateral sacrococcygeal
lumbocostal
nuchal
posterior longitudinal
sacrospinal
superficial posterior sacrococcygeal
supraspinal
transverse ligament of atlas

Hip/thigh
inguinal
ischiofemoral
ligament of head of femur
round ligament of femur
transverse ligament of acetabulum

Knee/calf

anterior cruciate ligament of knee
anterior ligament of head of fibula
anterior meniscofemoral
anterior tibiofibular
arcuate popliteal
collateral fibular
collateral tibial
cruciate ligament of knee
oblique popliteal
patellar
posterior cruciate of knee
posterior ligament of head of fibula
posterior meniscofemoral
posterior tibiofibular
transverse ligament of knee

Foot/ankle

anterior talofibular
bifurcate
calcaneocuboid
calcaneofibular
calcaneonavicular
calcaneotibial
collateral of metatarsophalangeal
  articulation
deep transverse metatarsal
dorsal calcaneonavicular
dorsal cuboideonavicular
dorsal cuneocuboid
dorsal intercuneiform
dorsal ligament of tarsus
dorsal metatarsal
dorsal tarsometatarsal
inferior extensor of foot
interosseous cuneocuboid
interosseous cuneometatarsal
interosseous intercuneiform
interosseous ligament of tarsus
interosseous metatarsal
interosseous talocalcaneal
lateral ligament of ankle
lateral talocalcaneal
long plantar
medial ligament of ankle
medial talocalcaneal
plantar calcaneocuboid
plantar calcaneonavicular
plantar cuboideonavicular
plantar cuneocuboid
plantar ligament of metatarsophalangeal
  articulation
plantar ligament of tarsus
plantar metatarsal
plantar tarsometatarsal
superficial transverse metatarsal
superior extensor retinaculum
talonavicular

Appendix 3

Muscles

Shoulder
deltoid
infraspinatus
latissimus dorsi
subscapularis
supraspinatus
teres major
teres minor

Arm
anconeus
biceps brachii
brachialis
coracobrachialis
triceps

Anterior forearm
flexor carpi radialis
flexor carpi ulnaris
flexor digitorum profundus
flexor digitorum superficialis
flexor pollicis longus
palmaris longus
pronator quadratus
pronator teres

Posterior forearm
abductor pollicis longus
brachioradialis
extensor carpi radialis brevis
extensor carpi radialis longus
extensor carpi ulnaris
extensor digiti minimi
extensor digitorum
extensor indicis
extensor pollicis brevis
extensor pollicis longus
supinator

Hand
abductor digiti minimi
abductor pollicis
abductor pollicis brevis
adductor pollicis
dorsal interosseous
flexor digiti minimi brevis
flexor pollicis brevis
lumbrical
opponens digiti minimi
opponens pollicis
palmar interosseus
palmaris brevis

Anterior thigh
iliacus
rectus femoris
sartorius
vastus intermedius
vastus lateralis
vastus medialis

Medial thigh
adductor brevis
adductor longus
adductor magnus
adductor minimus
gracilis
obturator externus
pectineus

Gluteal region
gluteus maximus
gluteus medius
gluteus minimus
inferior gemellus
obturator internus
piriformis

quadratus femoris
superior gemellus
tensor fasciae latae

Posterior thigh
biceps femoris
semimembranosus
semitendinosus

Anterior leg
extensor digitorum longus
extensor hallucis longus
peroneus tertius
tibialis anterior

Lateral leg
peroneus brevis
peroneus longus

Posterior leg
flexor digitorum longus
flexor hallucis longus
gastrocnemius
plantaris
popliteus
soleus
tibialis posterior

Foot
abductor digiti minimi
abductor hallucis
dorsal interosseus
extensor digitorum brevis
extensor hallucis brevis
flexor digiti minimi brevis
flexor digitorum brevis
flexor hallucis brevis
lumbrical
quadratus plantae
plantar interosseus

Thoracic wall
external intercostal
innermost intercostal
internal intercostal
levator costarum
subcostalis
transverse thoracic

Anterior abdominal wall
cremaster
external oblique
internal oblique
pyramidalis
rectus abdominis
transversus abdominis

Posterior abdominal wall
psoas major
psoas minor
quadratus lumborum

Superficial back
latissimus dorsi
levator scapulae
rhomboid major
rhomboid minor
serratus posterior-inferior
serratus posterior-superior
trapezius

Suboccipital region
obliquus capitis inferior
obliquus capitis superior
rectus capitis posterior major
rectus capitis posterior minor

Neck
digastric
geniohyoid
mylohyoid
omohyoid

platysma
sternocleidomastoid
sternohyoid
sternothyroid
stylohyoid
thyrohyoid

Prevertebral region
anterior scalene
longus capitis
longus colli
middle scalene
posterior scalene
rectus capitis anterior
rectus capitis lateralis

Facial expression
auricularis anterior
auricularis posterior
auricularis superior
buccinator
corrugator supercilii
depressor anguli oris
depressor labii inferioris
depressor septi
levator anguli oris
levator labii superioris alaeque nasi
mentalis
nasalis
occipitofrontalis
orbicularis oculi
orbicularis oris
procerus
risorius
zygomaticus major
zygomaticus minor

Mastication
lateral pterygoid
masseter
medial pterygoid
temporalis

Eye movement
ciliary
inferior oblique
inferior rectus
lateral rectus
levator palpebrae superioris
medial rectus
superior oblique
superior rectus

Palate
levator veli palatini
musculus uvulae
palatoglossus
palatopharyngeus
tensor veli palatini

Tongue
genioglossus
hyoglossus
palatoglossus
styloglossus

Pharynx
inferior constrictor
middle constrictor
palatopharyngeus
salpingopharyngeus
stylopharyngeus
superior constrictor

Larynx
aryepiglottic
cricothyroid
lateral cricoarytenoid
oblique arytenoid
posterior cricoarytenoid
thyroarytenoid
thyroepiglottic
transverse arytenoid
vocalis

Common Professional Titles and Degrees

AA Anesthesiologist's Assistant
ADN Associate Degree in Nursing
AHN Army Head Nurse
    Assistant Head Nurse
AHP Assistant House Physician
AHS Assistant House Surgeon
AMO Assistant Medical Officer
ANP Adult Nurse Practitioner
    Advanced Nurse Practitioner
ARNP Advanced Registered Nurse
    Practitioner
ART Accredited Record Technician
ATh Associate in Therapy
ATR Activities Therapist, Registered
AuD Doctorate of Audiology
BAMS Bachelor of Ayurvedic Medicine
    and Surgery
BAO Bachelor of the Art of Obstetrics
BCh Bachelor of Surgery, Baccalaureus
    Chirurgiae
BChD Bachelor of Dentistry
BCNP Board Certified Nuclear Pharmacist
BDent Bachelor of Dentistry
BdentSci, BDSc Bachelor of Dental
    Science
BDS Bachelor of Dental Surgery
BHyg Bachelor of Hygiene
BM, BMed Bachelor of Medicine
BMedBiol Bachelor of Medical Biology
BMedSci, BMS Bachelor of Medical
    Science
BMET Biomedical Equipment Technician
BMic Bachelor of Microbiology
BMT Bachelor of Medical Technology
BNEd Bachelor of Nursing Education
BNSc Bachelor of Nursing Science
BO Bachelor of Osteopathy
BP, BPharm Bachelor of Pharmacy
BPH Bachelor of Public Health
BPHEng Bachelor of Public Health
    Engineering
BPHN Bachelor of Public Health Nursing
BS Bachelor of Science
    Bachelor of Surgery

BSc Bachelor of Science
BSM Bachelor of Science in Medicine
BSN Bachelor of Science in Nursing
BSOT Bachelor of Science in Occupational
    Therapy
BSPh Bachelor of Science in Pharmacy
BSS Bachelor of Sanitary Science
BVMS Bachelor of Veterinary Medicine
    and Surgery
BVSc Bachelor of Veterinary Science
CA Certified Acupuncturist
CAC Certified Addictions Counselor
CAP College of American Pathologists
CARN Certified Addictions Registered
    Nurse
CCDN Certified Chemical Dependency
    Nurse
CCM Certified Case Manager
CCRN Critical Care Registered Nurse
CDA Certified Dental Assistant
CDE Certified Diabetes Educator
CDT Certified Dental Technician
CEN Certificate for Emergency Nursing
CEO Chief Executive Officer
CFO Chief Financial Officer
CFP Clinical Fellowship Program
CGC Certified Gastrointestinal Clinician
ChB Bachelor of Surgery; Chirurgiae
    Baccalaureus
ChD, Chir. Doct. Doctor of Surgery;
    Chirurgiae Doctor
ChM Master of Surgery; Chirurgiae
    Magister
CHN Certified Hemodialysis Nurse
    Community Health Nurse
CHP Coordinating Hospital Physician
CIC Certified Infection Control
CIH Certificate in Industrial Health
CLA Certified Laboratory Assistant
CLA (ASCP) Clinical Laboratory Assistant
    (American Society of Clinical
    Pathologists)
CLSp(MB) Certified Laboratory Specialist
    in Molecular Biology

CLS(NCA) Clinical Laboratory Scientist certified by National Credentialing Agency
CLSP Clinical Laboratory Specialist
CLT Certified Laboratory Technician
Clinical Laboratory Technician
Clinical Laboratory Technologist
CLT(NCA) Clinical Laboratory Technician certified by National Credentialing Agency
CM Master in Surgery; Chirurgiae Magister
CMA Certified Medical Assistant
CMHN Community Mental Health Nurse
CMO Chief Medical Officer
CMT Certified Medical Transcriptionist
CNM Certified Nurse-Midwife
CNMT Certified Nuclear Medicine Technologist
CNOR Certified Nurse, Operating Room
CNP Community Nurse Practitioner
CNRN Certified Neuroscience Registered Nurse
CNS Chief, Nursing Services
Clinical Nurse Specialist
CNSN Certified Nutrition Support Nurse
CO Certified Orthotist
COMA Certified Ophthalmic Medical Assistant
CORD Commissioned Officer Residency Deferment
CORT Certified Operating Room Technician
COS Chief of Staff
COTA Certified Occupational Therapy Assistant
CP Certified Prosthetist
CPAN Certified Post-Anesthesia Nurse
CPed Certified Pedorthist
CPH Certificate in Public Health
CPNP/A Certified Pediatric Nurse Practitioner/Associate
CPO Certified Prosthetist and Orthotist
CR Chief Resident
CRL Certified Record Librarian
CRNA Certified Registered Nurse Anesthetist
CRNI Certified Registered Nurse Intravenous

CRNP Certified Registered Nurse Practitioner
CRT Certified Respiratory Therapist
CRTT Certified Respiratory Therapy Technician
CS Chief of Staff
CST Certified Surgical Technician
CSW Certified Social Worker
CT Cardiovascular Technologist
Cytotechnologist
CT(ASCP) Cytotechnologist (American Society of Clinical Pathologists)
CVO Chief Veterinary Officer
D, Dip Diplomate
DA Dental Assistant
Diploma in Anesthetics
DBIR Director of Biotechnology Information Resources
DC Doctor of Chiropractic
DCH Diploma in Child Health
DCh Doctor of Surgery; Doctor Chirurgiae
DchO Doctor of Ophthalmic Surgery
DCM Doctor of Comparative Medicine
DCO Diploma of the College of Optics
DCP Diploma in Clinical Pathology
Diploma in Clinical Psychology
District Community Physician
DD Doctor of Divinity
DDH Diploma in Dental Health
DDM Diploma in Dermatological Medicine
Doctor of Dental Medicine
DDO Diploma in Dental Orthopaedics
DDR Diploma in Diagnostic Radiology
DDS Director of Dental Services
Doctor of Dental Surgery
DDSc Doctor of Dental Science
DGO Diploma in Gynaecology and Obstetrics
DH Dental Hygienist
DHg, DHy, DHyg, Dhyg, DrHyg Doctor of Hygiene
DHMSA Diploma of History of Medicine, Society of Apothecaries
Diet. Tech. Dietetic Technician
Dip Diplomate
DipBact Diploma in Bacteriology
DipChem Diploma in Chemistry
DipClinPath Diploma in Clinical Pathology

DipMicrobiol Diploma in Microbiology
DipSocMed Diploma in Social Medicine
DLO Diploma in Laryngology and Otology
DM Doctor of Medicine; Doctor Medicinae
DMA Director of Medical Affairs
DMD Doctor of Dental Medicine
DME Director of Medical Education
DMJ Diploma in Medical Jurisprudence
DMR Diploma in Medical Radiology
　　Directorate of Medical Research
DMRE Diploma in Medical Radiology and
　　Electrology
DMS, DMSc Doctor of Medical Science
DMT Doctor of Medical Technology
DMV Doctor of Veterinary Medicine
DN Diploma in Nursing
　　Diploma in Nutrition
　　District Nurse
　　Doctor of Nursing
DNB Diplomate of the National Board (of
　　Medical Examiners)
DNE Director of Nursing Education
　　Doctor of Nursing Education
DNO District Nursing Officer
DNS Director of Nursing Services
　　Doctor of Nursing Services
DO Diploma in Ophthalmology
　　Diploma in Osteopathy
　　Doctor of Ophthalmology
　　Doctor of Osteopathy
DOHyg Diploma in Occupational Hygiene
DOM Doctor of Oriental Medicine
DOMS Diploma in Ophthalmic Medicine
　　and Surgery
　　Doctor of Orthopedic Medicine and
　　Surgery
DON Director of Nursing
Doph Doctor of Ophthalmology
DOPS Director of Pharmacy Service(s)
Dorth Diploma in Orthodontics
　　Diploma in Orthoptics
DOS Doctor of Ocular Science
　　Doctor of Optical Science
DP Doctor of Pharmacy
　　Doctor of Podiatry
DPD Diploma in Public Dentistry
DPH Diploma in Public Health
　　Doctor of Public Health/Hygiene

DPharm Doctor of Pharmacy
DPhC Doctor of Pharmaceutical Chemistry
DPhc Doctor of Pharmacology
DPHN Doctor of Public Health Nursing
Dphys Diploma in Physiotherapy
DphysMed Diploma in Physical Medicine
DPM Diploma in Psychological Medicine
　　Doctor of Physical Medicine
　　Doctor of Podiatric Medicine
　　Doctor of Preventative Medicine
　　Doctor of Psychiatric Medicine
DPR Department of Professional
　　Regulation
DPsy Doctor of Psychology
Dr, DR Doctor
DrHyg Doctor of Hygiene
Dr Med Doctor of Medicine
DrMT Doctor of Mechanotherapy
DrPH Doctor of Public Health
　　Doctor of Public Health/Hygiene
DS, DSc Doctor of Science
DSC Doctor of Surgical Chiropody
DSE Doctor of Sanitary Engineering
DSIM Doctor of Science in Industrial
　　Medicine
DSM Diploma in Social Medicine
DSSc Diploma in Sanitary Science
DSur Doctor of Surgery
DSW Doctor of Social Work
DTCD Diploma in Tuberculosis and Chest
　　Diseases
DVM Doctor of Veterinary Medicine
DVMS Doctor of Veterinary Medicine and
　　Surgery
DVR Diploma in Vocational Rehabilitation
　　Doctor of Veterinary Radiology
DVS Doctor of Veterinary Science
　　Doctor of Veterinary Surgery
DVSc Doctor of Veterinary Science
EEG T Electroencephalographic
　　Technologist
EMT Emergency Medical Technician
EMT-A Emergency Medical Technician,
　　Advanced
　　Emergency Medical Technician,
　　Ambulance
EMT-B Emergency Medical Technician,
　　Basic

EMT-D Emergency Medical Technician, Defibrillation
EMT-I Emergency Medical Technician, Intermediate
EMT-M Emergency Medical Technician, Military
EMT-P Emergency Medical Technician, Paramedic
EN Enrolled Nurse
FAAAI Fellow of the American Academy of Allergy and Immunology
FAAAAI Fellow of the American Academy of Allergy, Asthma and Immunology
FAAFP Fellow of the American Academy of Family Physicians
FAAN Fellow of the American Academy of Nursing
FAAO Fellow of the American Academy of Osteopathy
FAAOS Fellow of the American Academy of Orthopedic Surgeons
FAAP Fellow of the American Academy of Pediatrics
FACA Fellow of the American College of Anesthesiology
FACAG Fellow of the American College of Angiology
FACAI Fellow of the American College of Allergy and Immunology
FACAL Fellow of the American College of Allergy
FACAN Fellow of the American College of Anesthesiologists
FACAS Fellow of the American College of Abdominal Surgeons
FACC Fellow of the American College of Cardiologists
FACCP Fellow of the American College of Chest Physicians
FACCPC Fellow of the American College of Pharmacology and Chemotherapy
FACD Fellow of the American College of Dentists
FACE Fellow of the American College of Endocrinology
FACEM Fellow of the American College of Emergency Medicine

FACEP Fellow of the American College of Emergency Physicians
FACFP Fellow of the American College of Family Physicians
FACFS Fellow of the American College of Foot Surgeons
FACG Fellow of the American College of Gastroenterology
FACHA Fellow of the American College of Hospital Administrators
FACLM Fellow of the American College of Legal Medicine
FACN Fellow of the American College of Nutrition
FACNM Fellow of the American College of Nuclear Medicine
FACNP Fellow of the American College of Neuropsychopharmacology
Fellow of the American College of Nuclear Physicians
FACO Fellow of the American College of Otolaryngology
FACOG Fellow of the American College of Obstetricians and Gynecologists
FACOS Fellow of the American College of Orthopedic Surgeons
FACP Fellow of the American College of Physicians
Fellow of the American College of Prosthodontists
FACPM Fellow of the American College of Preventative Medicine
FACR Fellow of the American College of Radiology
FACS Fellow of the American College of Surgeons
FACSM Fellow of the American College of Sports Medicine
FAMA Fellow of the American Medical Association
FANS Fellow of the American Neurological Society
FAOTA Fellow of the American Occupational Therapy Association
FAPA Fellow of the American Psychiatric Association
FAPHA Fellow of the American Public Health Association

FASHP Fellow of the American Society of Health-System Pharmacists

FCAP Fellow of the College of American Pathologists

FCCP Fellow of the College of Chest Physicians

FCGP Fellow of the College of General Practitioners

FChS Fellow of the Society of Chiropodists

FCMS Fellow of the College of Medicine and Surgery

FCO Fellow of the College of Osteopathy

FCPS Fellow of the College of Physicians and Surgeons

FCSP Fellow of the Chartered Society of Physiotherapy

FCST Fellow of the College of Speech Therapists

FDS Fellow in Dental Surgery

FFA Fellow of the Faculty of Anaesthetists

FFARCS Fellow of the Faculty of Anaesthetists of the Royal College of Surgeons

FFCM Fellow of the Faculty of Community Medicine

FFD Fellow in the Faculty of Dentistry

FFHom Fellow of the Faculty of Homeopathy

FFOM Fellow of the Faculty of Occupational Medicine

FFR Fellow of the Faculty of Radiologists

FHA Fellow of the Institute of Hospital Administrators

FIAC Fellow of the International Academy of Cytology

FIB Fellow of the Institute of Biology

FIC Fellow of the Institute of Chemistry

FICC Fellow of the International College of Chiropractors

FICD Fellow of the International College of Dentists

FICS Fellow of the International College of Surgeons

FIMLT Fellow of the Institute of Medical Laboratory Technology

FMCA Forensic Medicine Consultant Advisor

FMS Fellow of the Medical Society

FNAAOM Fellow of the National Academy of Acupuncture and Oriental Medicine

FNP Family Nurse Practitioner

FPS Fellow of the Pathological Society Fellow of the Pharmaceutical Society

FRCGP Fellow of the Royal College of General Practitioners

FRCOG Fellow of the Royal College of Obstetricians and Gynaecologists

FRCP Fellow of the Royal College of Physicians (England)

FRCPC Fellow of the Royal College of Physicians of Canada

FRCPE Fellow of the Royal College of Physicians of Edinburgh

FRCPI Fellow of the Royal College of Physicians of Ireland

FRCR Fellow of the Royal College of Radiologists

FRCS Fellow of the Royal College of Surgeons

FRCSC Fellow of the Royal College of Surgeons of Canada

FRCSE Fellow of the Royal College of Surgeons of England

FRCSI Fellow of the Royal College of Surgeons of Ireland

FRS Fellow of the Royal Society

FRSC Fellow of the Royal Society of Canada Fellow of the Royal Society of Chemistry

FSR Fellow of the Society of Radiographers

GDMO General Duties Medical Officer

GMO General Medical Officer

GN Graduate Nurse

GNP Geriatric Nurse Practitioner Gerontological Nurse Practitioner

GNS Gerontological Nurse Specialist

GNT Graduate Nurse Technician

GNTP Graduate Nurse Transition Program

GPN Graduate Practical Nurse

GRT Graduate Respiratory Therapist

GRTT Graduate Respiratory Therapist Technician

HAD Hospital Administrator

HHA Home Health Aid

HHD Doctor of Holistic Health
HNC Holistic Nurse Certified
HOC Health Officer Certificate
HP House Physician
HT Histologic Technician
HT(ASCP) Histologic Technician (American Society of Clinical Pathologists)
HTL(ASCP) Histotechnologist (American Society of Clinical Pathologists)
ICN Infection Control Nurse
ICP Infection Control Practitioner
IEMT Intermediate Emergency Medical Technician
IG Inspector General
IME Independent Medical Examiner
IMP Individual Medicaid Practitioner
IMS Indian Medical Service
JAR Junior Assistant Resident
JHMO Junior Hospital Medical Officer
JMS Junior Medical Student
LAc Licensed Acupuncturist
LAT Licensed Athletic Trainer
LATC Licensed Athletic Trainer, Certified
LCSW Licensed Clinical Social Worker
LD Licensed Dietitian
LDS Licentiate in Dental Surgery
LISW Licensed Independent Social Worker
LM Licentiate in Midwifery
LMFCC Licensed Marriage, Family and Child Counselor
LMFT Licensed Marriage and Family Therapist
LMT Licensed Massage Therapist
LOT Licensed Occupational Therapist
LPC Licensed Professional Counselor
LPCC Licensed Professional Certified Counselor
LPN Licensed Practical Nurse
LPT Licensed Physical Therapist
Licensed Psychiatric Technician
LPTN Licensed Psychiatric Technical Nurse
LRCP Licentiate of the Royal College of Physicians of England
LRCP (Edin) Licentiate of the Royal College of Physicians (Edinburgh)
LRCP (Ireland) Licentiate of the Royal College of Physicians (Ireland)
LRCS Licentiate of the Royal College of Surgeons

LRFPS Licentiate of the Royal Faculty of Physicians and Surgeons
LSW Licensed Social Worker
LT Laboratory Technician
LVN Licensed Visiting Nurse
Licensed Vocational Nurse
MA Master of Arts
Medical Assistant
MACCC Master Arts, Certified Clinical Competence
MASc Master of Ayurvedic Science
MBA Master of Business Administration
MBBS Bachelor of Medicine and Bachelor of Surgery
MC Master of Chirurgiae
MCE Medicare Code Editor
MChD Master of Dental Surgery
MChOrth Master of Orthopaedic Surgery
MChOtol Master of Otology
MCISci Master of Clinical Science
MCommH Master of Community Health
MD Doctor of Medicine
MDD Doctor of Dental Medicine
MDentSc Master of Dental Science
MDS Master of Dental Surgery
MDT Mechanical Diagnostic Therapist
ME Medical Examiner
MEDEX Extension of physician (physician assistant program using former medical corpsman; medicus)
MEDIHC Military Experience Directed into Health Careers
MEDScD Doctor of Medical Science
MT Med Tech
Medical Technician
Medical Technologist
MFCC Marriage, Family, and Child Counselor
MFST Medical Field Service Technician
MHT Mental Health Technician
ML Licentiate in Midwifery
MLDT Manual Lymph Drainage Therapist
MLPN Medical Licensed Practical Nurse
MLT(ASCP) Medical Laboratory Technician (American Society of Clinical Pathologists)
MLT(AMT) Medical Laboratory Technician (American Medical Technologists)
MMed Master of Medicine

MMS, MMSc Master of Medical Science
MMSA Master of Midwifery, Society of Apothecaries
MMSc Master of Medical Science
MNSc Master of Nursing Science
MO Master of Obstetrics
Master of Osteopathy
MOC Medical Officer on Call
MOD Medical Officer of the Day
MOH Medical Officer of Health
MOOW Medical Officer of the Watch
MPM Master of Psychological Medicine
MPH Master of Public Health
MPharm Master in Pharmacy
MRad Master of Radiology
MRC Master of Rehabilitation Counseling
MRCP Member of the Royal College of Physicians
MRCP (Edin) Member of the Royal College of Physicians (Edinburgh)
MRCP (Ireland) Member of the Royal College of Physicians (Ireland)
MRCS Member of the Royal College of Surgeons
MRL Medical Records Librarian
MRT Medical Records Technician
MS Master of Science
Master of Surgery
MS I, II, III, IV Medical Student: first, second, third, and fourth year
MSCCC Master Sciences, Certified Clinical Competence
MScD Doctor of Medical Science
Master of Dental Science
MScMed Master of Science in Medicine
MScN Master of Science in Nursing
MSD Master of Science in Dentistry
MSHyg Master of Science in Hygiene
MSM Master of Medical Science
MSN Master of Science in Nursing
MSPH Master of Science in Public Health
MSPhar Master of Science in Pharmacy
MS Rad Master of Science in Radiology
MSSc Master of Sanitary Science
MSSE Master of Science in Sanitary Engineering
MSurg Master of Surgery
MSW Master of Social Welfare
Master of Social Work

Medical Social Worker
MT Medical Technologist
Medical Transcriptionist
Monitor Technician
MTA Medical Technical Assistant
MT(AMT) Medical Technologist (American Medical Technologists)
MT(ASCP) Medical Technologist (American Society of Clinical Pathologists)
MT(ASCP)SBB Medical Technologist (American Society of Clinical Pathologists), Specialist Blood Bank
MTBC Music Therapist-Board Certified
MTO Medical Transport Officer
MTR Music Therapist, Registered
MTRS Licensed Master Therapeutic Recreation Specialist
MV Veterinary Physician; Medicus Veterinarius
MVD Doctor of Veterinary Medicine
NA Network Administrator
Nurse Anesthetist
NCT Nursing Care Technician
NCTMB Nationally Certified Therapeutic Massage and Bodywork
ND Doctor of Naturopathy
Naturopathic Doctor
Nursing Doctorate
NDP Nurse Discharge Planner
NIRMP National Intern and Resident Matching Program
NM(ASCP) Technologist in Nuclear Medicine (American Society of Clinical Pathologists)
NMD Doctor of Naturopathic Medicine
NMT(R) Nuclear Medicine Technologist Registered
NOA Nurse Obstetric Assistant
NOSTA Naval Ophthalmic Support and Training Activity
NNP Neonatal Nurse Practitioner
NP Nurse Practitioner
NPOD Neuropsychiatric Officer of the Day
OA Orthopedic Assistant
OccTh Occupational Therapist
OCN Oncology Certified Nurse
OD Doctor of Optometry
Officer-of-the-Day

OHN Occupational Health Nurse
OHT Occupational Health Technician
ON Office Nurse
Orthopedic Nurse
ONC Orthopedic Nursing Certificate
OphD Doctor of Ophthalmology
ORN Orthopedic Nurse
ORT Operating Room Technician
Registered Occupational Therapist
Osteo Osteopathologist
OT Occupational Therapist
OTC Orthopedic Technician, Certified
OTL Orthopedic Technician, Licensed
OTR Occupational Therapist, Registered
OTRL Occupational Therapist, Registered Licensed
PA Physician Assistant
PAC, PA-C Physician Assistant, Certified
PA-S Physician Assistant, Student
PBM Pharmacy Benefit Manager
PC Psychiatric Counselor
PCLN Psychiatric Consultation Liaison Nurse
PCMO Principal Clinical Medical Officer
PD Doctor of Pharmacy
Phar G Graduate in Pharmacy
PharmD Doctor of Pharmacy; Pharmaciae Doctor
PhC Pharmaceutical Chemist
PhD Doctor of Pharmacy; Pharmaciae Doctor
Doctor of Philosophy; Philosophiae Doctor
PhG Graduate in Pharmacy
PHN Public Health Nurse
PHNC Public Health Nurse Coordinator
PhTD Doctor of Physical Therapy
PMO Principal Medical Officer
PN Practical Nurse
PNA Pediatric Nurse Associate
PNC Psychiatric Nurse Clinician
PNNP Perinatal Nurse Practitioner
PNO Principal Nursing Officer
PNP Pediatric Nurse Practitioner
PNS Practical Nursing Student
Pod D Doctor of Podiatry
PSMT Psychiatric Services Management Team
PST Patient Service Technician

QMRP Qualified Mental Retardation Professional
RACP Royal Australasian College of Physicians
RCGP Royal College of General Practitioners
RCP Respiratory Care Practitioner
RCPT Royal College of Physicians of Thailand
RCT Registered Care Technologist
RD Registered Dietitian
RDA Registered Dental Assistant
RDCS Registered Diagnostic Cardiac Sonographer
RDH Registered Dental Hygienist
RDMS Registered Diagnostic Medical Sonographer
R. EEG T Registered Electroencephalographic Technician
R. EP T Registered Evoked Potential Technologist
RGN Registered General Nurse
RHIA Registered Health Information Administrator
RHIT Registered Health Information Technologist
RHU Registered Health Underwriter
RKT Registered Kinesiotherapist
RMA Registered Medical Assistant
RMO Resident Medical Officer
Responsible Medical Officer
RMT Registered Music Therapist
RN Registered Nurse
RNA Registered Nurse Anesthetist
RNC Registered Nurse, Certified
RNCD Registered Nurse, Chemical Dependency
RNCNA Registered Nurse, Certified in Nursing Administration
RNCNAA Registered Nurse, Certified in Nursing Administration Advanced
RNCS Registered Nurse, Certified Specialist
RNLP Registered Nurse, license pending
RNMT Registered Nuclear Medicine Technologist
RNP Registered Nurse Practitioner
RP Registered Pharmacist
RPAC Registered Physician's Assistant Certified

RPFT Registered Pulmonary Function Therapist

RPh Registered Pharmacist

RPT Registered Physical Therapist

RPTA Registered Physical Therapist Assistant

RRA Registered Record Administrator

RRNA Resident Registered Nurse Anesthetist

RRT Registered Respiratory Therapist

RSCN Registered Sick Children's Nurse

RSO Resident Surgical Officer

RT Radiologic Technologist
Registered Technologist
Respiratory Therapist

RT(ARRT) Registered Technologist (American Registry of Radiologic Technologists)

RT(N) Registered Technologist in Nuclear Medicine

RT(N)(AART) Registered Technologist in Nuclear Medicine (American Registry of Radiologic Technologists)

RTR Recreational Therapist, Registered

RT(R)(ARRT) Registered Technologist in Radiography (American Registry of Radiologic Technologists)

RT(T)(AART) Radiologic Technologist in Radiation Therapy (American Registry of Radiologic Technologists)

RVT Registered Vascular Technologist

SA Surgeon's Assistant
Surgical Assistant

SAC Substance Abuse Counselor

SAMO Senior Administrative Medical Officer

SAR Senior Assistant Resident

ScD Doctor of Science

SCM State Certified Midwife

SCMO Senior Clerical Medical Officer

SCT Specialist in Cytotechnology

SED Surgeon, Emergency Department

SEN State Enrolled Nurse

SEO Surgical Emergency Officer

SG Surgeon General

SGO Society of Gynecologic Oncologists
Society of Gynecologic Oncology

SHMO Senior Hospital Medical Officer

SHO Senior House Officer

SM Master of Science

SMI Senior Medical Investigator

SMO Senior Medical Officer

SMOH Senior Medical Officer of Health

SN Student Nurse

SNA Student Nursing Assistant

SNM Student Nurse Midwife

SNP School Nurse Practitioner

SP Speech Pathologist

SPA Student Physician's Assistant

SPN Student Practical Nurse

SR Senior Resident

SRP State Registered Physiotherapist

SRT Stroke Rehabilitation Technician

TAS Therapeutic Activities Specialist

TMA Trained Medication Aide

UC Unit Coordinator

UL Unit Leader

USFMG United States foreign medical graduate

USMG United States medical graduate

Vet Med Veterinary Medicine

Vet Sci Veterinary Science

VMC Village Malaria Communicator

VMD Doctor of Veterinary Medicine;
Veterinariae Medicinae Doctor

VN Visiting Nurse
Vocational Nurse

VRTA Vocational Rehabilitation Therapy Assistant

WC Ward Clerk

WOC(ET) Wound Ostomy Care, Enterostomal Therapy (nurse)

WS Ward Secretary

XDFHom Diploma of the Faculty of Homeopathy

XRT X-Ray Technician

Appendix 5
Common Medical Abbreviations and Acronyms

α alpha: Bunsen's solubility coefficient; first in a series; specific rotation term; heavy chain class corresponding to IgA

a (specific) absorption (coefficient) (USUALLY ITALIC); (total) acidity; area; (systemic) arterial (blood) (SUBSCRIPT); asymmetric; atto-

A absorbance; adenosine (or adenylic acid); alveolar gas (SUBSCRIPT); ampere

Å angstrom; Ångström unit

AA amino acid; aminoacyl

AB abortion

Ab antibody

ABG arterial blood gas

abl Abelson murine leukemia (virus)

ABLB alternate binaural loudness balance (test)

ABO blood group system

ABR abortus-Bang-ring (test); auditory brainstem response (audiometry)

γ-Abu γ-aminobutyric acid

ABVD adriamycin (doxorubicin), bleomycin, vinblastine, and dacarbazine

AC acetate; acromioclavicular; atriocarotid

Ac acetyl; actinium

aC arabinosylcytosine

a.c. [L.] *ante cibum,* before a meal

AC/A accommodation convergence-accommodation (ratio)

ACE angiotensin-converting enzyme

ACEI angiotensin-converting enzyme inhibitor

AcG accelerator globulin

ac-g accelerator globulin

Ach acetylcholine

aCL anticardiolipin (antibody)

ACP acyl carrier protein

ACTH adrenocorticotropic hormone (corticotropin)

AD [L.] *auris dextra,* right ear; Alzheimer disease

ADA Americans with Disabilities Act

Ade adenine

ADH antidiuretic hormone

ADLs activities of daily living

ad lib. [L.] *ad libitum,* freely, as desired

Ado adenosine

ADP adenosine 5′-diphosphate

A-E above elbow (amputation)

AFB acid-fast bacillus

AFORMED alternating failure of response, mechanical, to electrical depolarization

AFP α-fetoprotein

Ag antigen; [L.] *argentum,* silver

AHF antihemophilic factor

AHG antihemophilic globulin

AID artificial insemination donor

AIDS acquired immunodeficiency syndrome

AIH artificial insemination by husband; artificial insemination, homologous

A-K above knee (amputation)

Al aluminum

Ala alanine (or its mono- or diradical)

ALA δ-aminolevulinic acid

ALD adrenoleukodystrophy

ALL acute lymphocytic leukemia

ALS advanced life support; antilymphocyte serum

ALT alanine aminotransferase

Am americium

AML acute myelogenous leukemia

AMP adenosine monophosphate (adenylic acid)

amu atomic mass unit

ANA antinuclear antibody

ANF antinuclear factor

ANOVA analysis of variance

ANS autonomic nervous system

ANUG acute necrotizing ulcerative gingivitis

APA antipernicious anemia (factor)

APC antigen-presenting cell

A-P-C adenoidal-pharyngeal-conjunctival (virus)

APS antiphospholipid syndrome

APTT activated partial thromboplastin time

Ar argon

araC arabinosylcytosine (cytarabine)

ARDS adult respiratory distress syndrome

ARF acute renal failure; acute rheumatic fever

Arg arginine (or its mono- or diradical)

AS [L.] *auris sinistra,* left ear

As arsenic

ASA acetylsalicylic acid (aspirin)

ASCUS atypical squamous cells of undetermined significance

ASHD arteriosclerotic heart disease

Asn asparagine (or its mono- or diradical)

ASO antistreptolysin O

Asp aspartic acid (or its radical forms)

AST aspartate aminotransferase

At astatine

ATFL anterior talofibular ligament

ATL adult T-cell leukemia; adult T-cell lymphoma

atm (standard) atmosphere

ATP adenosine 5'-triphosphate

ATPase adenosine triphosphatase

ATPD ambient temperature and pressure, dry

ATPS ambient temperature and pressure, saturated (with water vapor)

at. wt. atomic weight

AU [L.] *auris utraque,* each ear, both ears

Au [L.] *aurum,* gold

AV, A-V arteriovenous; atrioventricular

AVN atrioventricular node

AVP antiviral protein

AW atomic weight

ax. axis

AZT azidothymidine (zidovudine)

B barometric (pressure) (SUBSCRIPT); boron

b blood (SUBSCRIPT)

Ba barium

BADL basic activities of daily living

BAER brainstem auditory evoked response

BAL British anti-lewisite (dimercaprol); bronchoalveolar lavage

BALB binaural alternate loudness balance (test)

BBB blood-brain barrier

BCG bacille Calmette-Guérin (vaccine)

BE barium enema

Be beryllium

B-E below elbow (amputation)

Bi bismuth

b.i.d. [L.] *bis in die,* twice a day

BIDS brittle hair, impaired intelligence, decreased fertility, short stature (syndrome)

BiPAP bilevel positive airway pressure

Bk berkelium

BM bowel movement

BMI body mass index

bp base pair

BP blood pressure; boiling point; *British Pharmacopoeia*

BPF bronchopleural fistula

BPH benign prostatic hyperplasia

Bq becquerel (SI unit of radionuclide activity)

Br bromine

BRAT banana, rice cereal, applesauce, toast (diet)

BSA body surface area

BSER brainstem evoked response (audiometry)

BT bleeding time

BTPS body temperature, ambient pressure, saturated (with water vapor)

BTU British thermal unit

BUN blood urea nitrogen

BUS Bartholin glands, urethra, Skene (glands)

C calorie (large); carbon; Celsius; centigrade; clearance (rate, renal) (FOLLOWED BY A SUBSCRIPT); compliance; concentration; cylindrical (lens); cytidine

c calorie (small); capillary (blood) (SUBSCRIPT); centi-

CA cancer; carcinoma; cardiac arrest; chronologic age; croup-associated (virus); cytosine arabinoside

Ca calcium; cathodal; cathode

ca [L.] *circa,* about, approximately

c-a cardioarterial

CABG coronary artery bypass graft

Cal calorie (large)

cal calorie (small)

cAMP cyclic adenosine monophosphate

CAP catabolite (gene) activator protein

CAPD continuous ambulatory peritoneal dialysis

CAT computerized axial tomography

CBC complete blood (cell) count

CBG corticosteroid-binding globulin
Cbz carbobenzoxy (chloride)
CC chief complaint
cc, c.c. cubic centimeter
CCK cholecystokinin
CCNU chloroethylcyclohexylnitrosourea (lomustine)
CCU coronary care unit; critical care unit
Cd cadmium
cd candela
CDC Centers for Disease Control and Prevention
cDNA complementary DNA
CDP cytidine 5′-diphosphate
Ce cerium
CEA carcinoembryonic antigen
CELO chicken embryo lethal orphan (virus)
CEP congenital erythropoietic porphyria
CF complement fixation; coupling factor; cystic fibrosis
Cf californium
CG chorionic gonadotropin
CGA catabolite gene activator
cGMP cyclic guanosine monophosphate
CGS, cgs centimeter-gram-second (system, unit)
Ch¹ Christchurch (chromosome)
CHF congestive heart failure
CHO carbohydrate
CI color index; *Colour Index*
Ci curie
CJD Creutzfeldt-Jakob disease
CK creatine kinase
Cl chlorine
CL cardiolipin
CLL chronic lymphocytic leukemia
CLQ cognitive laterality quotient
Cm curium
cM centimorgan
cm centimeter
CMC carpometacarpal
CMI cell-mediated immunity
CML chronic myelogenous leukemia
CMP cytidine monophosphate
CMV controlled mechanical ventilation; cytomegalovirus
CNS central nervous system
Co cobalt
c/o complains of

CoA coenzyme A
COG center of gravity
conA concanavalin A
COPD chronic obstructive pulmonary disease
CP cerebral palsy
CPAP continuous (or constant) positive airway pressure
CPD cephalopelvic disproportion
CPM continuous passive motion
CPPB continuous positive-pressure breathing
CPPV continuous positive-pressure ventilation
CPR cardiopulmonary resuscitation
cps cycles per second
Cr chromium; creatinine
CR conditioned reflex; crown-rump (length)
CRD chronic respiratory disease
CRH corticotropin-releasing hormone
CRL crown-rump length
CRP cross-reactive protein
CRST calcinosis cutis, Raynaud phenomenon, sclerodactyly, telangiectasia (syndrome)
Cs cesium
C&S culture and sensitivity
CSD catscratch disease
CSF cerebrospinal fluid
CT computed tomography
CTP cytidine 5′-triphosphate
CTR cardiothoracic ratio
Cu [L.] *cuprum,* copper
CV cardiovascular
CVA cerebrovascular accident
CVP central venous pressure
CXR chest x-ray
Cyd cytidine
CYP cytochrome P-450 (enzyme)
Cys cysteine
Cyt cytosine
δ delta; heavy chain class corresponding to IgD
Δ delta; change; heat
D dead (space gas) (SUBSCRIPT); deciduous; deuterium; dihydrouridine (in nucleic acids); diopter; [L.] *dexter,* right (opposite of left); vitamin D potency of cod liver oil

d deci-

d- dextrorotatory

D- prefix indicating that a molecule is sterically analogous to D-glyceraldehyde

dA deoxyadenosine

da deca-

DA developmental age

dAdo deoxyadenosine

dAMP deoxyadenylic acid

DANS 1-dimethylaminonaphthalene-5-sulfonic acid

dB decibel

db diabetes

D&C dilation and curettage

DCG dacryocystography

DCI dichloroisoproterenol

dCMP deoxycytidylic acid

DDT dichlorodiphenyltrichloroethane (chlorophenothane)

D&E dilation and evacuation

DEF decayed, extracted, or filled (permanent teeth)

def decayed, extracted, or filled (deciduous teeth)

DES diethylstilbestrol

DET diethyltryptamine

DEV duck embryo vaccine; duck embryo virus

DEXA dual-energy x-ray absorptiometry

DF decayed and filled (permanent teeth)

df decayed and filled (deciduous teeth)

dGMP deoxyguanosine monophosphate; deoxyguanylic acid

DHEA dehydro-3-epiandrosterone

Dia diabetes

DIC disseminated intravascular coagulation

DIP desquamative interstitial pneumonia; distal interphalangeal (joint)

DJD degenerative joint disease

dM decimorgan

DMD Duchenne muscular dystrophy

DMF decayed, missing, or filled (permanent teeth)

dmf decayed, missing, or filled (deciduous teeth)

DMSO dimethyl sulfoxide

DMT *N,N*-dimethyltryptamine

DN dibucaine number

DNA deoxyribonucleic acid

DNase, DNAse deoxyribonuclease

DNP deoxyribonucleoprotein; 2,4-dinitrophenol

DNR do not resuscitate

DOA dead on arrival

DOC deoxycorticosterone

DOM 2,5-dimethoxy-4-methylamphetamine

DPN diphosphopyridine nucleotide

DPT dipropyltryptamine; diphtheria, pertussis, and tetanus (vaccine)

DR degeneration reaction, reaction of degeneration

dr dram

DRG diagnosis-related group

DRVVT dilute Russell viper venom test

D-S Doerfler-Stewart (test)

DSA digital subtraction angiography

dsDNA double-stranded DNA

DT delirium tremens; duration of tetany

dT deoxythymidine

dTDP deoxythymidine 5′-diphosphate

dThd thymidine

DTIC dimethyltrizenoimidazole carboxamide (dacarbazine)

dTMP deoxythymidylic acid

DTP diphtheria and tetanus toxoids and pertussis vaccine; distal tingling on percussion (Tinel sign)

DTPA diethylenetriamine pentaacetic acid

DTR deep tendon reflex

dTTP deoxythymidine 5′-triphosphate

Dx diagnosis

Dy dysprosium

ϵ epsilon; molar absorption coefficient; heavy chain class corresponding to IgE

E exa-; extraction (ratio)

EB Epstein-Barr (virus)

EBV Epstein-Barr virus

ECF extracellular fluid

ECF-A eosinophilic chemotactic factor of anaphylaxis

ECG electrocardiogram

ECHO enterocytopathogenic human orphan (virus)

ECM erythema chronicum migrans

ECMO extracorporeal membrane oxygenation

ECS electrocerebral silence

ECT electroconvulsive therapy

ED effective dose

EDTA ethylenediaminetetraacetic acid (edathamil, edetic acid)

EEG electroencephalogram

EENT eye, ear, nose, and throat

EIA enzyme immunoassay

EKG electrocardiogram

EKY electrokymogram

ELISA enzyme-linked immunosorbent assay

EMF electromotive force

EMG electromyogram; exomphalos, macroglossia, and gigantism (syndrome)

EMS emergency medical services

ENG electronystagmography

ENT ear, nose, and throat

EOG electrooculography

EPAP expiratory positive airway pressure

ER emergency room; endoplasmic reticulum

Er erbium

ERBF effective renal blood flow

ERCP endoscopic retrograde cholangiopancreatography

ERG electroretinogram

ERPF effective renal plasma flow

ERV expiratory reserve volume

Es einsteinium

ESEP extreme somatosensory evoked potential

ESP extrasensory perception

ESR electron spin resonance; erythrocyte sedimentation rate

ESRD end-stage renal disease

EtOH ethyl alcohol

Eu europium

ev, eV electron-volt

F Fahrenheit; Faraday (constant); fertility (factor); field (of vision); fluorine; force; fractional (concentration); free (energy)

f femto-; (respiratory) frequency

F₁ first filial generation

Fab fragment of antibody molecule involved in antigen binding

FAD familial Alzheimer disease; flavin(e) adenine dinucleotide

FANA fluorescent antinuclear antibody (test)

FB foreign body

FBS fasting blood sugar

Fc constant fragment of an antibody molecule

FDA Food and Drug Administration

Fe [L.] *ferrum,* iron

FEF forced expiratory flow

FET forced expiratory time

FEV forced expiratory volume

FF filtration fraction

FFD focusfilm distance

FHR fetal heart rate

FHT fetal heart tone

FIA fluorescent immunoassay

FIGLU formiminoglutamic (acid)

FISH fluorescent in situ hybridization

Fm fermium

FMN flavin(e) mononucleotide

fps, FPS foot-pound-second (system, unit)

Fr francium; French (gauge, scale)

FRC functional residual capacity (of lungs)

FRF follicle-stimulating hormone-releasing factor

FRS firstrank symptom

Fru fructose

FSH follicle-stimulating hormone

FSH-RF follicle-stimulating hormone-releasing factor

FSH-RH follicle-stimulating hormone-releasing hormone

FTA-ABS fluorescent treponemal antibody-absorption (test)

FU fluorouracil

FUO fever of unknown origin

FVC forced vital capacity

Fw F wave (fibrillatory wave, flutter wave)

Fx fracture

γ gamma; Ostwald solubility coefficient; the third in a series; heavy chain class corresponding to IgG

μg microgram

G giga-; glucose; gravitation (newtonian constant of); gravida (obstetric history); guanosine (or guanylic acid)

g gram

Ga gallium

GABA γ-aminobutyric acid

GABHS group-A β-hemolytic streptococcus

Gal galactose

GC gonococcus, gonorrhea

Gd gadolinium
GDP guanosine 5′-diphosphate
Ge germanium
GERD gastroesophageal reflux disease
GFR glomerular filtration rate
GGT γ-glutamyltransferase
GH glenohumeral; growth hormone
GHB γ-hydroxybutyrate
GHRF, GH-RF growth hormone-releasing factor
GHRH, GH-RH growth hormone-releasing hormone
GI gastrointestinal; gingival index
GIP gastric inhibitory polypeptide
GLC gas-liquid chromatography
Gln glutamine; glutaminyl
Glu glutamic acid; glutamyl
Gly glycine; glycyl
GMP guanosine monophosphate (guanylic acid)
GMS Gomori (or Grocott) methenamine silver (stain)
GnRH gonadotropin-releasing hormone
GOT glutamic-oxaloacetic transaminase (aspartate aminotransferase)
GPI Gingival-Periodontal Index
GPT glutamic-pyruvic transaminase (alanine aminotransferase)
gr grain
GSH growth-stimulating hormone
GSR galvanic skin response
GSSG oxidized glutathione
gt. [L.] *gutta*, a drop
GTP guanosine 5′-triphosphate
gtt. [L.] *guttae*, drops
GTT glucose tolerance test
GU genitourinary
Guo guanosine
GVHD graft-versus-host disease
Gy gray (unit of absorbed dose of ionizing radiation)
GYN gynecology
H henry; hydrogen; hyperopia; hyperopic
h hecto-
h Planck constant
α-h the right-handed helical form assumed by many proteins
^{1}H hydrogen-1 (protium, light hydrogen)
^{2}H hydrogen-2 (deuterium, heavy hydrogen)

^{3}H hydrogen-3 (tritium, radioactive hydrogen)
H$^+$ hydrogen ion
HA hyaluronic acid
Ha hahnium
HAV hepatitis A virus
Hb hemoglobin
HbA adult hemoglobin
HbA$_1$ major component of adult hemoglobin
HbA$_2$ minor fraction of adult hemoglobin
HbAS heterozygosity for hemoglobin A and hemoglobin S (sickle cell trait)
HB$_c$Ag hepatitis B core antigen
HbCO carboxyhemoglobin
HB$_e$ hepatitis B early antigen
HB$_e$Ab hepatitis B early antibody
Hb$_e$Ag hepatitis B early antigen
HbF fetal hemoglobin
HBIG hepatitis B immune globulin
HbO$_2$ oxygenated hemoglobin, oxyhemoglobin
HbS sickle cell hemoglobin
HB$_s$Ab hepatitis B surface antibody
HB$_s$Ag hepatitis B surface antigen
HBV hepatitis B virus
HCFA Health Care Financing Administration
HCG human chorionic gonadotropin
HCS human chorionic somatomammotropin (human placental lactogen)
Hct hematocrit
HDL high-density lipoprotein
HDRV human diploid (cell strain) rabies vaccine
He helium
H&E hematoxylin and eosin (stain)
HEMPAS hereditary erythroblastic multinuclearity associated with positive acidified serum
Hf hafnium
HFJV high-frequency jet ventilation
HFOV high-frequency oscillatory ventilation
HFPPV high-frequency positive-pressure ventilation
HFV high-frequency ventilation
Hg [L.] *hydrargyrum,* mercury
HGE human granulocytic ehrlichiosis

HGH human (pituitary) growth hormone
HGSIL high-grade squamous intraepithelial lesion
HI hemagglutination inhibition (test, titer)
His histidine
His- histidyl
-His histidino
HIV human immunodeficiency virus
HI hyperopia, latent
HLA human lymphocyte antigen
Hm hyperopia, manifest (hypermetropia)
HME human monocytic ehrlichiosis
HMG human menopausal gonadotropin
HMO health maintenance organization
HMWK high molecular weight kininogen
Ho holmium
HPF high-power field
HPI history of present illness
HPL human placental lactogen
HPLC high-performance liquid chromatography
HPV human papillomavirus
HS, h.s. [L.] *hora somni,* at bedtime
HSV herpes simplex virus
Ht hyperopia, total
5-HT 5-hydroxytryptamine (serotonin)
HTLV human T-cell lymphocytotrophic virus
HVL half-value layer
Hx (medical) history
Hyp hydroxyproline
Hz hertz
I inspired (gas) (SUBSCRIPT); iodine
123I iodine-123 (radioisotope)
125I iodine-125
131I iodine-131
IADL instrumental activities of daily living
IAP intermittent acute porphyria
ICD *International Classification of Diseases (of the World Health Organization)*
ICDA *International Classification of Diseases, Adapted (for Use in the United States)*
ICF intracellular fluid
ICP intracranial pressure
ICSH interstitial cell-stimulating hormone
ICU intensive care unit
ID infective dose
I&D incision and drainage

IDU idoxuridine
IF initiation factor; intrinsic factor
IFN interferon
Ig immunoglobulin
IGF insulin-like growth factor
IH infectious hepatitis
IL interleukin
ILA insulin-like activity
Ile isoleucine
IM infectious mononucleosis; internal medicine; intramuscular(ly)
IMP inosine monophosphate (inosinic acid)
IMV intermittent mandatory ventilation
In indium
Ino inosine
INR international normalized ratio
I&O (fluid) intake and output
IOML infraorbitomeatal line
IP interphalangeal; intraperitoneal(ly)
IPAP inspiratory positive airway pressure
IPPB intermittent positive-pressure breathing
IPPV intermittent positive-pressure ventilation
IPV inactivated poliovirus vaccine
IQ intelligence quotient
Ir iridium
IRV inspiratory reserve volume
ISI International Sensitivity Index
ITP idiopathic thrombocytopenic purpura; inosine 5'-triphosphate
IU International Unit
IUCD intrauterine contraceptive device
IUD intrauterine device
I.V. intravenous, intravenously; intraventricular
J joule
J flux (density)
K [Modern L.] *kalium,* potassium; kelvin
k kilo-
K_M Michaelis constant
kat katal
kb kilobase
kc kilocycle
kcal kilocalorie
KCT kaolin clotting time
kg kilogram
KJ knee jerk
Kr krypton
KS Kaposi sarcoma
17-KS 17-ketosteroid

kV kilovolt

kVp kilovolt peak

KW Keith-Wagener (retinal changes); Kimmelstiel-Wilson (disease)

μl, μL microliter

L inductance; left; [L.] *limes,* boundary, limit; liter

l liter

L- prefix indicating that a molecule is sterically analogous to L-glyceraldehyde

La lanthanum

LA lupus anticoagulant

LAP leucine aminopeptidase

LATS long-acting thyroid stimulator

LBT lupus band test

LC lethal concentration

LCAT lecithin-cholesterol acyltransferase

LCM lymphocytic choriomeningitis (virus)

LD lethal dose

LDH lactate dehydrogenase

LDL low-density lipoprotein

LE left eye; lupus erythematosus

LEEP loop electrosurgical excision procedure

LES lower esophageal sphincter

LETS large external transformation-sensitive (fibronectin)

Leu leucine

LFA left frontoanterior (fetal position)

LFP left frontoposterior (fetal position)

LFT left frontotransverse (fetal position)

LGSIL low-grade squamous intraepithelial lesion

LGV lymphogranuloma venereum

LH luteinizing hormone

LH/FSH-RF luteinizing hormone/follicle-stimulating hormone-releasing factor

LH-RF luteinizing hormone-releasing factor

LH-RH luteinizing hormone-releasing hormone

Li lithium

LLQ left lower quadrant

LMA left mentoanterior (fetal position)

LMP left mentoposterior (fetal position)

LMT left mentotransverse (fetal position)

LNPF lymph node permeability factor

LOA left occipitoanterior (fetal position)

LOP left occipitoposterior (fetal position)

LOT left occipitotransverse (fetal position)

LPF low-power field

LPH lipotropic pituitary hormone (lipotropin)

Lr lawrencium

LRH luteinizing hormone-releasing hormone

LSA left sacroanterior (fetal position)

LSD lysergic acid diethylamide

LSP left sacroposterior (fetal position)

LST left sacrotransverse (fetal position)

LTH luteotropic hormone

LTM long-term memory

LTR long terminal repeat

Lu lutetium

LUQ left upper quadrant

LVET left ventricular ejection time

LVH left ventricular hypertrophy

Lw (FORMER SYMBOL FOR) lawrencium (now Lr)

Lys lysine (or its radicals in peptides)

μ mu; micro-; heavy chain class corresponding to IgM

M mega-; molar; moles (per liter); morgan; myopia; myopic

m mass; meter; molar

μμ micromicro-

μm micrometer

mμ millimicron

MA mental age

mA milliampere

MAA macroaggregated albumin

M-Am compound myopic astigmatism

MAC *Mycobacterium avium* complex

MAI *Mycobacterium avium-intracellulare*

MAO monoamine oxidase

MAOI monoamine oxidase inhibitor

MAP mean aortic pressure

mA-S milliampere-second

Mb myoglobin

MBC maximum breathing capacity

MbCO carbon monoxide myoglobin

MbO$_2$ oxymyoglobin

MCH mean corpuscular hemoglobin

MCHC mean corpuscular hemoglobin concentration

mCi millicurie

MCP metacarpophalangeal

MCV mean corpuscular volume

Md mendelevium

MDF myocardial depressant factor
MDI metered-dose inhaler
Me methyl
MEDLARS Medical Literature Analysis and Retrieval System
MEP maximal expiratory pressure
mEq, meq milliequivalent
MET metabolic equivalent of task
Met methionine
met-Hb methemoglobin
met-Mb metmyoglobin
MEV million electron-volts (10^6 ev)
Mg magnesium
mg milligram
MHC major histocompatibility complex
mho siemens unit
MHz megahertz
MI myocardial infarction
MID minimal infecting dose
MIP maximum inspiratory pressure
MK menaquinone (vitamin K_2)
MKS, mks meter-kilogram-second (system, unit)
mL, ml milliliter
MLC mixed lymphocyte culture (test)
MLD minimal lethal dose
mm millimeter
mmol millimole
MMPI Minnesota Multiphasic Personality Inventory
MMR measles-mumps-rubella (vaccine)
Mn manganese
MO medical officer; mineral oil
Mo molybdenum
mol mole
mol wt molecular weight
MOM milk of magnesia
MOPP Mustargen (mechlorethamine), Oncovin (vincristine), procarbazine, and prednisone
mor. sol. [L.] *more solito,* as usual, as customary
MPD maximal permissible dose
MPS mononuclear phagocyte system
MR milk-ring (test)
M_r molecular (weight) ratio
MRD, mrd minimal reacting dose
MRI magnetic resonance imaging
mRNA messenger ribonucleic acid

MS multiple sclerosis; morphine sulfate
ms millisecond
msec millisecond
MSG monosodium glutamate
MSH melanocyte-stimulating hormone
mtDNA mitochondrial deoxyribonucleic acid
MTP metatarsophalangeal (joint)
Mu Mache unit
MUGA multiple-gated acquisition (imaging)
Mv mendelevium
mV millivolt
MVE Murray Valley encephalitis (virus)
MVV maximal voluntary ventilation
MW molecular weight
My myopia
ν nu; kinematic viscosity
N newton; nitrogen; normal (concentration)
n index of refraction; nano-
NA *Nomina Anatomica*
Na [Modern L.] *natrium,* sodium
NAD nicotinamide adenine dinucleotide; no acute distress
NAD$^+$ nicotinamide adenine dinucleotide (oxidized form)
NADH nicotinamide adenine dinucleotide (reduced form)
NADP nicotinamide adenine dinucleotide phosphate
NADP$^+$ nicotinamide adenine dinucleotide phosphate (oxidized form)
NADPH nicotinamide adenine dinucleotide phosphate (reduced form)
NAME nevi, atrial myxoma, myxoid neurofibromas, and ephelides (syndrome)
Nb niobium
NCV nerve conduction velocity
Nd neodymium
NE norepinephrine; not examined
Ne neon
NEEP negative end-expiratory pressure
NF National Formulary
ng nanogram
NGF nerve growth factor (antigen)
Ni nickel
NIH National Institutes of Health
NK natural killer (cell)
NKA no known allergies
NLM National Library of Medicine

nm nanometer
NMN nicotinamide mononucleotide
No nobelium
Np neptunium
NREM nonrapid eye movement (sleep)
nRNA nuclear ribonucleic acid
NS normal saline
NSAID nonsteroidal antiinflammatory drug
NSR normal sinus rhythm
NUG necrotizing ulcerative gingivitis
Ω omega; ohm
O [L.] *oculus,* eye; opening (in formulas for electrical reactions); oxygen
o- ortho-
OAV oculoauriculovertebral (dysplasia, syndrome)
OB obstetrics
OB/GYN obstetrics (and) gynecology
OBS organic brain syndrome
OC oral contraceptive
OCD obsessive-compulsive disorder
OD [L.] *oculus dexter,* right eye; overdose
ODD oculodentodigital (dysplasia, syndrome)
Oe oersted (centimeter-gram-second unit of magnetic field strength)
OFD orofaciodigital (dysostosis, syndrome)
OKT Ortho-Kung T (cell)
OML orbitomeatal line
OMM ophthalmomandibulomelic (dysplasia, syndrome)
OMS organic mental syndrome
OP osmotic pressure; outpatient
O&P ova and parasites
OPV oral poliovirus vaccine
OR operating room
ORD optical rotatory dispersion
Orn ornithine (or its radical)
Oro orotate; orotic acid
OS [L.] *oculus sinister,* left eye
Os osmium
OSHA Occupational Safety and Health Administration
OT occupational therapy; (Koch) old tuberculin
OTC over the counter (nonprescription drug)
OU [L.] *oculus uterque,* each eye (both eyes)

OXT oxytocin
oz ounce
P para (obstetric history); partial (pressure); peta-; phosphorus, phosphoric (residue); plasma (concentration); pressure
p pico-; pupil
p- *para-*
³²P phosphorus-32
P₁ first parental generation
Pa pascal; protactinium
PABA paraaminobenzoic acid
PAF platelet-aggregating (or -activating) factor
PAH paraaminohippuric (acid)
PAO₂ partial pressure of arterial oxygen
PAS paraaminosalicylic (acid), periodic acid-Schiff (reagent)
PASA paraaminosalicylic acid
PAT paroxysmal atrial tachycardia
Pb [L.] *plumbum,* lead
PBG porphobilinogen
p.c. [L.] *post cibum,* after a meal
PCB polychlorinated biphenyl
Pco₂ partial pressure of carbon dioxide
PCP phencyclidine
PD prism diopter
Pd palladium
PDGF platelet-derived growth factor
PDLL poorly differentiated lymphocytic lymphoma
PEEP positive end-expiratory pressure
PEG percutaneous endoscopic gastrostomy
PET positron emission tomography
PFT pulmonary function test
PG prostaglandin
pg picogram
PGA prostaglandin A
PGB prostaglandin B
PGE prostaglandin E
PGF prostaglandin F
Ph phenyl
pH hydrogen ion concentration
Ph¹ Philadelphia (chromosome)
PHA phytohemagglutinin (antigen)
Phe phenylalanine (or its radical)
PhG [L.] *Pharmacopoeia Germanica,* German Pharmacopeia
PICC peripherally inserted central catheter
PID pelvic inflammatory disease

PIF prolactin-inhibiting factor

PIP proximal interphalangeal (joint)

PK pyruvate kinase

pK negative logarithm of the ionization constant (K_a) of an acid

PKU phenylketonuria

PM post mortem

Pm promethium

pm picometer

PMN polymorphonuclear (leukocyte)

PMS premenstrual syndrome

PND paroxysmal nocturnal dyspnea; post-nasal drip

PNP platelet neutralization procedure

PNPB positive-negative pressure breathing

PO [L.] *per os,* by mouth

Po polonium

PO$_2$, Po$_2$ partial pressure of oxygen

POEMS polyneuropathy, organomegaly, endocrinopathy, monoclonal gammopathy, and skin changes (syndrome)

POMP prednisone, Oncovin (vincristine sulfate), methotrexate, and Purinethol (6-mercaptopurine)

POR problem-oriented (medical) record

PP pyrophosphate

PPCA proserum prothrombin conversion accelerator

PPD purified protein derivative (of tuberculin)

PPLO pleuropneumonia-like organism

ppm parts per million

PPO 2,5-diphenyloxazole

PPPPP pain, pallor, pulselessness, paresthesia, paralysis

PPPPPP pain, pallor, pulselessness, paresthesia, paralysis, prostration

PPV positive pressure ventilation

Pr praseodymium; presbyopia

PRA plasma renin activity

PRF prolactin-releasing factor

PRL prolactin

p.r.n. [L.] *pro re nata,* as needed

Pro proline (or its radicals)

psi pounds per square inch

PSV pressure-supported ventilation

PT physical therapy; prothrombin time

Pt platinum

PTA phosphotungstic acid; plasma thromboplastin antecedent; prior to admission

PTAH phosphotungstic acid hematoxylin

PTCA percutaneous transluminal coronary angioplasty

PTH parathyroid hormone

PTU propylthiouracil

Pu plutonium

PUO pyrexia of unknown origin

PUPPP pruritic urticarial papules and plaques of pregnancy

PUVA (oral administration of) psoralen (and subsequent exposure to) ultraviolet light of A wavelength (UV-A)

PVC polyvinyl chloride; premature ventricular contraction

PVP polyvinylpyrrolidone (povidone)

Q coulomb

Q̇ volume of blood flow

Qco$_2$ microliters CO_2 given off per milligram of dry weight of tissue per hour

q.d. [L.] *quaque die,* every day

q.i.d. [L.] *quater in die,* 4 times a day

QNS quantity not sufficient

Qo oxygen consumption

Qo$_2$ oxygen consumption

q.s. [L.] *quantum satis,* as much as is enough; [L.] *quantum sufficiat,* as much as may suffice; quantity sufficient

R gas constant (8.315 joules); (organic) radical; [L.] *recipe,* take; resistance determinant (plasmid); resistance (electrical); resistance (unit) (in the cardiovascular system); respiration; respiratory (exchange ratio); roentgen

r racemic; roentgen

RA rheumatoid arthritis

Ra radium

rad radian

RAS reticular activating system

RAST radioallergosorbent test

RAV Rous-associated virus

RAW resistance, airway

Rb rubidium

RBC, rbc red blood cell; red blood (cell) count

RBF renal blood flow

RD reaction of degeneration; reaction of denervation

RDA recommended daily allowance

rDNA ribosomal deoxyribonucleic acid
RDS respiratory distress syndrome
RDW red (cell) diameter (or distribution) width
RE right ear; right eye
Re rhenium
REM rapid eye movement (sleep); reticular erythematous mucinosis
rem roentgen-equivalent-man
rep roentgen equivalent-physical
RF release factor; rheumatoid factor
RFA right frontoanterior (fetal position)
RFLP restriction fragment length polymorphism
RFP right frontoposterior (fetal position)
RFT right frontotransverse (fetal position)
RH releasing hormone
Rh Rhesus (Rh blood group); rhodium
RIA radioimmunoassay
Rib ribose
RLL right lower lobe
RLQ right lower quadrant
RMA right mentoanterior (fetal position)
RML right middle lobe
RMP right mentoposterior (fetal position)
RMT right mentotransverse (fetal position)
Rn radon
RNA ribonucleic acid
RNase ribonuclease
RNP ribonucleoprotein
ROA right occipitoanterior (fetal position)
ROM range of motion
ROP right occipitoposterior (fetal position)
ROT right occipitotransverse (fetal position)
RP retinitis pigmentosa
RPF renal plasma flow
rpm revolutions per minute
RPR rapid plasma reagin (test)
RQ respiratory quotient
rRNA ribosomal ribonucleic acid
RS respiratory syncytial (virus)
Rs response
RSA right sacroanterior (fetal position)
RSP right sacroposterior (fetal position)
RST right sacrotransverse (fetal position)
RSV respiratory syncytial virus; Rous sarcoma virus
rTMP ribothymidylic acid
Ru ruthenium

RUL right upper lobe
RUQ right upper quadrant
RV residual volume
RVH right ventricular hypertrophy
℞ [L.] *recipe,* (the first word on a prescription), take; prescription; treatment
σ sigma; reflection coefficient; standard deviation; 1 millisecond (0.001 sec)
S [L.] *sinister,* left; saturation (of hemoglobin) (FOLLOWED BY SUBSCRIPT O_2 or CO_2); siemens; spherical (lens); sulfur; Svedberg (unit)
S-A sinoatrial
SaO$_2$ oxygen saturation (of) arterial (oxyhemoglobin)
sat. saturated
sat. sol. saturated solution
Sb [L.] *stibium,* antimony
SBE subacute bacterial endocarditis
SC sternoclavicular; subcutaneous(ly)
Sc scandium
sc subcutaneous(ly)
SCID severe combined immunodeficiency
SD standard deviation; streptodornase
SDA specific dynamic action
Se selenium
Ser serine
Sf Svedberg flotation (constant, unit)
SGOT serum glutamic-oxaloacetic transaminase (aspartate aminotransferase)
SGPT serum glutamic-pyruvic transaminase (alanine aminotransferase)
SH serum hepatitis
SI [French] Système International d'Unités; International System of Units
Si silicon
SID source-to-image (-receptor) distance
SIDS sudden infant death syndrome
sig. [L.] *signa,* affix a label, inscribe
SIMV spontaneous intermittent mandatory ventilation; synchronized intermittent mandatory ventilation
SISI small-increment (or short-increment) sensitivity index (test)
SK streptokinase
SLE systemic lupus erythematosus
SLR straight leg raising
Sm samarium
Sn [L.] *stannum,* tin

SOAP subjective (data), objective (data), assessment, and plan (problem-oriented medical record)

SOB short(ness) of breath

sol., soln solution

sp species

SPCA serum prothrombin conversion accelerator (factor VII)

SPECT single photon emission computed tomography

SPF sun protection (or protective) factor

sp. gr. specific gravity

sph spherical (lens)

spm suppression and mutation

spp species (plural)

SQ subcutaneous

Sr strontium

SRF somatotropin-releasing factor

SRF-A slow-reacting factor of anaphylaxis

SRIF somatotropin-release-inhibiting factor

sRNA soluble ribonucleic acid

SRS slow-reacting substance

SRS-A slow-reacting substance of anaphylaxis

ssDNA single-stranded deoxyribonucleic acid

ssp subspecies

SSRI selective serotonin reuptake inhibitor

stat. [L.] *statim,* immediately, at once

STD sexually transmitted disease

STEL short-term exposure limit

STH somatotropic hormone

STM short-term memory

STPD standard temperature ($0°$ C) and pressure (760 mm Hg absolute), dry

Sv sievert (unit)

SVT supraventricular tachycardia

T temperature, absolute (Kelvin); tension (intraocular); tera-; tesla; tetanus (toxoid); tidal (volume) (SUBSCRIPT); tocopherol; transverse (tubule); tritium; tumor (antigen)

T absolute temperature (Kelvin)

t (metric) ton; temperature (Celsius); tritium

T$_3$ 3,5,5'-triiodothyronine

T$_4$ tetraiodothyronine (thyroxine)

T− (FOLLOWED BY NUMBER) decreased tension (intraocular)

T+ (FOLLOWED BY NUMBER) increased tension (intraocular)

α-T α-tocopherol

TA *Terminologia Anatomica*

Ta tantalum

TAD transient acantholytic dermatosis

TAF tumor angiogenesis factor

TAR thrombocytopenia with absent radius (syndrome)

TAT thematic apperception test

TB tuberculosis

Tb terbium

TBP thyroxine-binding protein

TBV total blood volume

Tc technetium

^{99m}Tc technetium-99m

T&C type and crossmatch

TCA tricarboxylic acid; trichloracetic acid

TCN talocalcaneonavicular (joint)

Td tetanus-diphtheria (toxoids, adult type)

TDP ribothymidine 5'-diphosphate

Te tellurium

TEDD total end-diastolic diameter

TEN toxic epidermal necrolysis

TESD total end-systolic diameter

Th thorium

THC tetrahydrocannabinol

Thr threonine (or its radicals)

Ti titanium

TIA transient ischemic attack

t.i.d. [L.] *ter in die,* 3 times a day

tinct tincture

TITh 3,5,3'-triiodothyronine

TKO to keep (venous infusion line) open

Tl thallium

TLC tender, loving care; thin-layer chromatography; total lung capacity

TLV threshold limit value

TM transport maximum

Tm thulium; tubular maximal (excretory capacity of kidneys)

T$_m$ temperature midpoint (Kelvin)

t$_m$ temperature midpoint (Celsius)

TMJ temporomandibular joint

TMT tarsometatarsal

TMV tobacco mosaic virus

Tn (normal intraocular) tension

TNF tumor necrosis factor

TNM tumor, node, metastasis (tumor staging)

TORCH toxoplasmosis, other, rubella, cytomegalovirus, and herpes simplex (maternal infections)

TPA, t-PA tissue plasminogen activator
TPHA *Treponema pallidum* hemagglutination (test)
TPI *Treponema pallidum* immobilization (test)
TPN total parenteral nutrition
TPR temperature, pulse, and respirations
tr tincture
TRH thyrotropin-releasing hormone (stimulation test)
TRIC trachoma inclusion conjunctivitis (organism)
tRNA transfer ribonucleic acid
Trp tryptophan (and its radicals)
TSH thyroid-stimulating hormone
TSS toxic shock syndrome
TSTA tumor-specific transplantation antigen
TTP thrombotic thrombocytopenic purpura
TU toxic unit, toxin unit
Tyr tyrosine (and its radicals)
U unit; uranium; uridine (in polymers); urinary (concentration)
UA urinalysis
UDP uridine diphosphate
UDPG uridine diphosphoglucose
UGIS upper gastrointestinal series
UMP uridine monophosphate (uridylic acid)
ung. [L.] *unguentum,* ointment
u-PA urokinase
Urd uridine
URI upper respiratory infection
UTI urinary tract infection
UTP uridine triphosphate
UV ultraviolet
V vanadium; vision; visual (acuity); volt; volume (frequently with subscripts denoting location, chemical species, and conditions)
V̇ ventilation; gas flow (frequently with subscripts indicating location and chemical species); ventilation
v venous (blood); volt
V$_1$-V$_6$ unipolar precordial electrocardiogram chest leads
VA viral antigen
V̇$_A$ alveolar ventilation

V-A ventriculoatrial
Val valine (and its radicals)
VATER vertebral (defects), (imperforate) anus, tracheoesophageal (fistula) with esophageal atresia, and radial and renal dysplasia (complex)
VC vision, color; vital capacity
VCE vagina, (ecto)cervix, endocervical (canal)
V$_D$ (physiologic) dead space
VDRL Venereal Disease Research Laboratory (test)
VHDL very-high-density lipoprotein
VIP vasoactive intestinal polypeptide
VLDL very-low-density lipoprotein
VMA vanillylmandelic acid (test)
V$_{max}$ maximal velocity
VP vasopressin
V/Q ventilation/perfusion ratio
VR vocal resonance
VS volumetric solution
V$_T$ tidal volume
W watt; [German] *Wolfram,* tungsten
Wb weber
WBC white blood cell; white blood (cell) count
WD well-developed
WDLL well-differentiated lymphocytic (or lymphatic) lymphoma
WHO World Health Organization
WN well-nourished
X xanthosine
Xao xanthosine
Xe xenon
^{133}Xe xenon-133
XU excretory urogram
Y yttrium
YAG yttrium-aluminum-garnet (laser)
Yb ytterbium
Z carbobenzoxy (chloride)
ZEEP zero end-expiratory pressure
ZES Zollinger-Ellison syndrome
Zn zinc
^{65}Zn zinc-65
Zr zirconium
ZSR zeta sedimentation ratio